THE *PAST & PRESENT* BOOK SERIES

General Editor
PETER COSS

Malleable Anatomies

Malleable Anatomies

Models, Makers, and Material Culture in Eighteenth-Century Italy

LUCIA DACOME

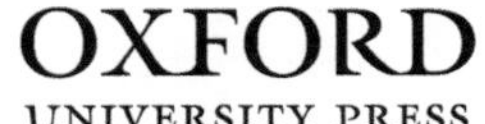

OXFORD
UNIVERSITY PRESS

Great Clarendon Street, Oxford, OX2 6DP,
United Kingdom

Oxford University Press is a department of the University of Oxford. It furthers the University's objective of excellence in research, scholarship, and education by publishing worldwide. Oxford is a registered trade mark of Oxford University Press in the UK and in certain other countries

First Edition published in 2017

Impression: 1

Published in the United States of America by Oxford University Press
198 Madison Avenue, New York, NY 10016, United States of America

British Library Cataloguing in Publication Data
Data available

Library of Congress Control Number: 2016957137

ISBN 978–0–19–873618–9

Printed and bound by
CPI Group (UK) Ltd, Croydon, CR0 4YY

To Joseph, Almea, and Alberto

Acknowledgements

When I set off to investigate the history of mid-eighteenth-century anatomical displays, I did not expect to encounter a world that is still today so profoundly enmeshed in networks of social relations. In a sense, this very study may be regarded as a reflection of how the history of anatomical specimens is a story of long-term social entanglements involving both humans and non-humans. The book was written over a long period of time and in many different locations, and I am delighted to have the opportunity to express my gratitude to all of those who have supported its development along the way. I was fortunate to receive the kindness and generosity of so many friends and colleagues that I wish to apologize in advance if I miss anyone.

This book started out as a post-doctoral project at the Wellcome Trust Centre for the History of Medicine at UCL. I have fond memories of the time I spent at the Centre, where I learnt a great deal from its lively scholarly community. I wish to thank Hal Cook, my sponsor at the time, who followed the early stages of the project with encouragement, support, and intellectual openness. I owe a long-term debt of gratitude to Simon Schaffer, whose unique capacity to blend creativity, vision, scholarship, and intellectual generosity has provided me with a vital and enduring source of inspiration. I am also especially indebted to Sandra Cavallo, Mary Fissell, Ludmilla Jordanova, Jeanne Peiffer, and Mary Terrall, who during the development of this project have become invaluable intellectual interlocutors and have offered friendship, support, and insights.

For reading and offering helpful comments on parts of this work, in addition to those just mentioned, I am grateful to Paola Bertucci, James Delbourgo, Simon Ditchfield, Maria Pia Donato, Maria Teresa Fattori, Anita Guerrini, Nick Hopwood, and Pamela Long. In addition, I have had the privilege of receiving stimulating suggestions and insights from anonymous referees and tenure reviewers. I have also greatly benefited from conversations, exchanges, and consultations with numerous colleagues and friends including Katey Anderson, Cesarina Casanova, Marta Cavazza, Silvia Contarini, Roger Cooter, Silvia De Renzi, Giovanna Fiume, David Gentilcore, Giacomo Giacobini, Colin Jones, Anna Maerker, Michelle Murphy, Ottavia Niccoli, Claudia Pancino, Katy Park, Alessandro Pastore, Renata Peters, Gianna Pomata, Alessandro Ruggeri, Franco Ruggeri, Raffaella Sarti, Pamela Smith, Emma Spary, Leen Spruit, Joan Steigerwald, Claudia Stein, and Claudia Swan.

While working on this project, I have had the privilege of meeting friends and colleagues who have provided models of intellectual and scholarly vision. I am very thankful to Pauline M.H. Mazumdar for her extraordinary commitment to the history of medicine and for her intellectual openness and curiosity, as well as her support. It is an honour to hold the Pauline M.H. Mazumdar Chair in the History of Medicine that was endowed by her and her husband Dipak Mazumdar. Since my arrival in Toronto, Natalie Zemon Davis has provided an invaluable and incessant source of inspiration and a vibrant sense of community and purpose.

The research for this book has taken me to many different archives and libraries, including the Archives du Palais Princier in Monaco, the Archivio dell'Accademia di Belle Arti di Bologna, the Archivio di Stato di Bologna, the Archivio di Stato di Milano, the Archivio di Stato di Napoli, the Archivio di Stato di Palermo, the Archivio di Stato di Torino, the Archivio Storico del Comune di Palermo, the Archivio storico dell'Accademia della Crusca, The Beinecke Rare Book & Manuscript Library, the Biblioteca Centrale della Regione Siciliana, the Biblioteca Comunale dell'Archiginnasio di Bologna, the Biblioteca Comunale di Palermo, the Biblioteca della Società Napoletana di Storia Patria di Napoli, the Biblioteca Universitaria di Bologna, the Wellcome Library, and many more. I wish to thank the staff of all of these institutions that have made my work possible. For reasons of space, not everybody can be mentioned individually here. However, a special acknowledgement is due to the staff of the Archivio di Stato di Bologna, where I spent many happy hours studying manuscript documents in a friendly, helpful, and supportive atmosphere, and to Diana Tura for allowing me to access documents even in the most adverse of circumstances. I wish to thank the Malvasia family for their hospitality and for allowing me to peruse their family papers, and the Isolani family for giving me access to their private archives. I am also grateful to the Archivio Arcivescovile di Bologna and the archives of the parishes of Santa Maria Maddalena, San Martino Maggiore, and San Martino di Bertalia for allowing me to carry out research in their archives, to Massimo Zini for granting me access to the documents at the Accademia delle Scienze in Bologna, and to Isidoro Turdo who offered valuable assistance at the Biblioteca Centrale della Regione Siciliana in Palermo. Special thanks are due to Armando Antonelli, who graciously allowed me to study the documents of the Archivio Storico del Monte del Matrimonio in Bologna while the archive was being refurbished. I am also thankful to the staff at The William Andrews Clark Memorial Library at UCLA, and especially to Scott Jacobs, for creating a supportive and friendly working environment at the time I was an Ahmanson-Getty postdoctoral fellow there and, more recently, for swiftly providing me with a reproduction of the map of eighteenth-century Italy's postal routes.

None of the work I have undertaken would have been possible without the financial support and generosity that I have received over the years. The Wellcome Trust supported a Postdoctoral Research Fellowship at the Wellcome Trust Centre for the History of Medicine at UCL (Grant Number 66517/Z/01/Z), which allowed me to begin the project. I was then fortunate enough to receive an Ahmanson-Getty Postdoctoral Fellowship at the Centre for Seventeenth- and Eighteenth-Century Studies and the Clark Library at UCLA, for the project 'Vital Matters' under the lead of Helen Deutsch and Mary Terrall. A Marie Curie fellowship from the European Commission, which was based at the Centre Alexandre Koyré/CNRS in Paris, allowed me to expand my investigation of the history of eighteenth-century anatomical modelling and its practitioners under the sponsorship of Jeanne Peiffer. The later stages of this project were supported by a Connaught start-up grant from the University of Toronto, an SSHRC Standard Research Grant, SSHRC-SIG funding, a Victoria College Senate Research Grant and a Victoria College Publication Grant. In 2013, a three-month Visiting Scholar Residential Fellowship in the Research Group 'Art and Knowledge in Pre-Modern Europe' directed by Sven Dupré at the Max Planck Institute for the History of Science, in Berlin, offered a congenial environment to finalize the manuscript for submission. It was a pleasure to return to an institution where I had enjoyed many opportunities for intellectual exchange as postdoctoral fellow in Department II under the leadership of Lorraine Daston. I wish to express my deep gratitude to all of these institutions for their generosity and support. I am also grateful to Giuliano Pancaldi at the CIS-International Centre for the History of Science at the University of Bologna, to Mary Fissell, Randall Packard, Christine Ruggere, and the late Harry Marks at the Department of the History of Medicine at Johns Hopkins University, and to Ofer Gal and Hans Pols at the Unit for History and Philosophy of Science at the University of Sydney, for hosting me as a visiting scholar at their institutions while I was working on this project.

Early versions of this material were presented as papers at conferences and colloquia. Although I cannot mention all of them here, I would like to thank participants at various meetings of the AAHM, CSHM, CSHPS, HSS, ICHSTM, RSA and the Three Societies' Meetings, for their questions and comments. I am also grateful to numerous colleagues, including Patrice Bret, Sandra Cavallo, Hal Cook, Adriana Craciun, Helen Deutsch, Nick Dew, Maria Pia Donato, Sven Dupré, Maria Teresa Fattori, Valeria Finucci, Mary Fissell, Adeline Gargam, David Gentilcore, Deborah Harkness, Sonia Horn, Colin Jones, Peter Murray Jones, Ludmilla Jordanova, Lauren Kassell, Graham Mooney, Michelle Murphy, Jeanne Peiffer, Eileen Reeves, Pamela Smith, and Mary Terrall, who kindly invited me to present parts of this work at their institutions or at conferences, meetings, and panels organized by them. I wish to thank the audiences of all these venues for their valuable and helpful feedback.

A number of friends and colleagues have facilitated this project in many different ways. Besides helping me navigate the archival and library system in Palermo, Giovanna Fiume made my stay in the city delightful and introduced me to some of the city's impressive treasures and communities. I am grateful to Muna Salloum for her translation of Mohammed Ibn Uthmân Al-Meknassî's text. I thank Maria Teresa Fattori and Paolo Prodi for letting me see their edition of Benedict XIV's letters to Paolo Magnani before it was published, Elio Vassena for giving me access to his unpublished dissertation (Tesi di Laurea), Domenico Medori for sharing his thorough knowledge of the Bolognese archives, and Maricetta Parlatore for kindly communicating some details related to her restoration of Anna Morandi's self-portrait.

Entering the digital age does not seem to have made the process of publishing pictures much easier, and I am thankful to all those individuals and institutions that made the task of gathering a large number of images more manageable. I thank the Museo di Palazzo Poggi in Bologna and, in particular, Cristina Nisi and Fulvio Simoni, for providing a large number of pictures for this book. I am very grateful to the Museo Cappella di Sansevero in Naples and, especially, Bruno Crimaldi for allowing me to take a close look at Giuseppe Salerno's anatomical machines and for providing several pictures, and to Vincenzo Martorana for kindly letting me use his photograph of ex-votos in Sicily. I owe a special debt of gratitude to Noa Uri for her artistic advice on the cover of the book.

I am very grateful to the Past and Present Society, and in particular to Alex Walsham, who first expressed interest in the project as the editor of the Past and Present Book Series, and to subsequent editors, Matthew Hilton and Peter Cross, for their continued interest and patience. It is an honour to complete this project under the umbrella of such an inspiring scholarly genealogy. At Oxford University Press I was very fortunate to be able to rely on the unstinting support of Stephanie Ireland and Cathryn Steele, who have graciously accompanied the completion of the book with encouragement and patience. It was a pleasure to work with them. Cathryn closely followed the later stages of the book and helped me to acquire the rights and permissions to publish the pictures, and I am very thankful for her help. I am also indebted to Brian North for copy editing this work with admirable care and patience, to Lydia Shinoj for managing the production process with great efficiency, to Hayley Buckley for careful proofreading, and to Rio Ruskin-Tompkins for skillfully producing the cover.

In the later stages of the book's development I have had the privilege of being surrounded by talented graduate students and young scholars. Some of them have also helped me finalize this book. I am particularly grateful to Delia Gavrus and Daniel Carens-Nedelsky, who proofread earlier drafts of some of the chapters, to Jennifer Fraser and Sarah Rolfe Prodan, who carefully and patiently read the penultimate versions and made many helpful suggestions that have improved the text, and to Esther Atkinson, Daisy Dowdall, and Vanessa McCarthy for editorial assistance. Esther also skilfully compiled the index and was a great help in the final proofreading. Adam Barker offered assistance with the translation of some of the Latin texts.

An earlier version of Chapter 1 was published in Maria Pia Donato and Jill Kraye (eds.), *Conflicting Duties: Science, Medicine and Religion in Rome, 1550–1750* (London, the Warburg Institute, 2009), 353–74. I wish to thank the publisher and the editors for their permission to publish an expanded version. Parts of the materials presented in some of the other chapters appeared in different forms in the following essays: '"Un certo e quasi incredibile piacere": cera e anatomia nel Settecento', *Intersezioni*, 25:3 (2005), 415–36; 'Waxworks and the Performance of Anatomy in Mid-Eighteenth-Century Italy', *Endeavour*, 30:1 (2006), 29–35; 'Women, Wax and Anatomy in the "Century of Things"', *Renaissance Studies*, 21:4 (2007), 522–50; 'Ai confini del mondo naturale: anatomia e santità nell'opera di Prospero Lambertini', in Maria Teresa Fattori (ed.), *Storia, medicina e diritto nei trattati di Prospero Lambertini—Benedetto XIV* (Rome, Edizioni di Storia e Letteratura, 2013), 318–38; '"Une dentelle très bien agencée et très precise": les femmes et l'anatomie dans l'Europe du dix-huitième siècle', in Adeline Gargam (ed.), *Sur les traces d'Hypatie. Réalités et représentations des femmes de sciences avant Marie Curie* (Dijon: Editions universitaires de Dijon, 2014), 157–75; and 'A Crystal Womb', in Nick Hopwood, Rebecca Flemming and Lauren Kassell (eds.), *Reproduction: From Antiquity to the Present Day* (Cambridge: Cambridge University Press, forthcoming).

My family and friends have offered me love and encouragement throughout the duration of this project. I wish to give special thanks my parents, Almea Bertozzi and Alberto Dacome, for providing me with a model of intellectual curiosity and integrity as well as for their continued support and generosity. My greatest debt is to Joseph Berkovitz who has read many drafts of this work, heard all about it, and patiently provided insights at all levels, from methodological frameworks and broader philosophical implications all the way down to the minutiae of editing. He has also forbearingly followed me to numerous archival expeditions in many different locations. Still, he has faced all the ups and downs of this long project with unfailing cheerfulness and good spirits, and has infused the years of this book's realization with warmth, wit, humour, and love. I wish to dedicate this book to him as well as to my parents.

Table of Contents

List of Plates xv
List of Figures xix
List of Abbreviations xxi

Introduction 1

1. Prospero's Tools 24
2. Artificer and Connoisseur 56
3. Anatomy, Embroidery, and the Fabric of Celebrity 93
4. Women, Wax, and Anatomy 130
5. Blindfolding the Midwives 163
6. Transferring Value 192
7. Injecting Knowledge 215

Epilogue: Becoming Obsolete 254

Select Bibliography 261
Index 295

List of Plates

1. Wax models of the kidneys by Ercole Lelli (courtesy of Museo di Palazzo Poggi—Università di Bologna)
2. Map of the postal routes of the Italian peninsula (1774) (courtesy of the William Andrews Clark Memorial Library, University of California, Los Angeles)
3. Portrait of Prospero Lambertini (1739/40) (courtesy of Istituzione Bologna Musei, Collezioni Comunali d'Arte, Bologna)
4. Anatomy room, Institute of the Sciences (courtesy of Museo di Palazzo Poggi—Università di Bologna)
5. *Insignia degli Anziani* depicting Laura Bassi's dramatic appearance in Bologna's anatomical theatre (1734) (courtesy of Archivio di Stato di Bologna—Ministero dei beni e delle attività culturali e del turismo)
6. *Insignia degli Anziani* commemorating the visit of the Polish Prince Frederick Christian to the Institute of the Sciences (1739) (courtesy of Archivio di Stato di Bologna—Ministero dei beni e delle attività culturali e del turismo)
7. Two wooden écorchés in Bologna's anatomical theatre by Silvestro Giannotti and Ercole Lelli (courtesy of the Biblioteca Comunale dell'Archiginnasio di Bologna)

8 & 9. Wax figures of a woman and a man by Ercole Lelli (courtesy of Museo di Palazzo Poggi—Università di Bologna)

10–13. Series of four écorché figures by Ercole Lelli (courtesy of Museo di Palazzo Poggi—Università di Bologna)

14 & 15. Female and male skeletons by Ercole Lelli (courtesy of Museo di Palazzo Poggi—Università di Bologna)

16. Bologna's anatomical theatre (courtesy of the Biblioteca Comunale dell'Archiginnasio di Bologna)
17. Expulsion of Adam and Eve from the Garden of Eden by Jacopo della Quercia (courtesy of Archivio Fotografico Soprintendenza Belle Arti—Bologna)
18. Ercole Lelli, 'Self-Portrait' (courtesy of Museo di Palazzo Poggi—Università di Bologna)
19. Model of the human arm (courtesy of Museo Galileo, Florence—photo by Franca Principe)
20. Model of unborn twins by Angélique-Marguerite Le Boursier du Coudray (courtesy of the Musée Flaubert et d'histoire de la médecine, CHU-Hôpitaux de Rouen, France)
21. *Insignia degli Anziani* depicting women working in a silk factory (1750) (courtesy of Archivio di Stato di Bologna—Ministero dei beni e delle attività culturali e del turismo)

22. Anna Morandi, self-portrait (courtesy of Museo di Palazzo Poggi—Università di Bologna)
23. Anna Morandi, self-portrait: detail (courtesy of Museo di Palazzo Poggi—Università di Bologna)
24. Anna Morandi, self-portrait: detail (courtesy of Museo di Palazzo Poggi—Università di Bologna)
25. Table of the eye by Anna Morandi (courtesy of Museo di Palazzo Poggi—Università di Bologna)
26. Table of the eye by Anna Morandi (courtesy of Museo di Palazzo Poggi—Università di Bologna)
27. Table of the larynx by Anna Morandi (courtesy of Museo di Palazzo Poggi—Università di Bologna)
28. Model of the hands by Anna Morandi (courtesy of Museo di Palazzo Poggi—Università di Bologna)
29. Table of the tongue by Anna Morandi (courtesy of Museo di Palazzo Poggi—Università di Bologna)
30. Self-portrait of Anna Morandi and portrait of her husband Giovanni Manzolini (courtesy of Museo di Palazzo Poggi—Università di Bologna)
31. Portrait of Giovanni Manzolini by Anna Morandi: detail (courtesy of Museo di Palazzo Poggi—Università di Bologna)
32. Model of the foot by Giovanni Manzolini and Anna Morandi (courtesy of Museo di Palazzo Poggi—Università di Bologna)
33. Ex-votos in wax (courtesy of Vincenzo Martorana)
34. Sacra Famiglia (Holy Family) by Angelo Piò (courtesy of Archivio Fotografico Soprintendenza Belle Arti—Bologna—photo by Marco degli Degli Esposti—Equipe Fotostudio)
35. Sacra Famiglia (Holy Family) by Angelo Piò: detail (courtesy of Archivio Fotografico Soprintendenza Belle Arti—Bologna—photo by Marco degli Degli Esposti—Equipe Fotostudio)
36. Model of the pelvis by Giovanni Manzolini and Anna Morandi (courtesy of Museo di Palazzo Poggi—Università di Bologna)
37. Table displaying two wax models of the womb by Giovanni Manzolini and Anna Morandi (courtesy of Museo di Palazzo Poggi—Università di Bologna)
38. Clay models of the gravid uterus (courtesy of Museo di Palazzo Poggi—Università di Bologna)
39. Midwifery machine by Antonio Cartolari (courtesy of Museo di Palazzo Poggi—Università di Bologna)
40. Series of clay wombs presenting unborn children in anomalous situations (courtesy of Museo di Palazzo Poggi—Università di Bologna)
41. Model of the gravid uterus with nine-month-old unborn twins (courtesy of Museo di Palazzo Poggi—Università di Bologna)
42. Model of the gravid uterus with unborn child (courtesy of Museo di Palazzo Poggi—Università di Bologna)

43. Portrait of Giovanni Antonio Galli (1775) (courtesy of Museo di Palazzo Poggi—Università di Bologna)
44. Wax model of a malformed newborn child (courtesy of Museo di Palazzo Poggi—Università di Bologna)
45. Model of the gravid uterus with unborn child in unordinary situation (courtesy of Museo di Palazzo Poggi—Università di Bologna)
46. Model of the gravid uterus with unborn child in unordinary situation (courtesy of Museo di Palazzo Poggi—Università di Bologna)
47. Night eruption of Mount Vesuvius on 20 October 1767 (courtesy of Division of Rare and Manuscript Collections, Cornell University Library)
48. Portrait of Raimondo di Sangro, *c.*1759 (?) (courtesy of Alòs edizioni—Naples, photo by Massimo Velo)
49. William Hamilton escorting the Neapolitan sovereigns to see the current of lava from Mount Vesuvius on the night of 11 May 1771 (courtesy of Division of Rare and Manuscript Collections, Cornell University Library)
50. 'Anatomical machine' (female) by Giuseppe Salerno (courtesy of Alòs edizioni—Naples, photo by Massimo Velo)
51. 'Anatomical machine' (male) by Giuseppe Salerno (courtesy of Alòs edizioni—Naples, photo by Massimo Velo)
52. 'Anatomical machine' (male) by Giuseppe Salerno: detail (courtesy of Renata Peters)
53. 'Anatomical machine' (female) by Giuseppe Salerno: detail (courtesy of Renata Peters)
54. Seating plan for Giuseppe Salerno's anatomical demonstration of 1789 at the Palermitan Senate (courtesy of the Archivio Storico del Comune di Palermo)

List of Figures

0.1 Title page of *De Bononiensi Scientiarum et Artium Instituto atque Academia Commentarii*, where the picture depicts the façade of Palazzo Poggi in Bologna, the site of the Institute of the Sciences (courtesy of Division of Rare and Manuscript Collections, Cornell University Library) 2

1.1 Prospero Lambertini (Pope Benedict XIV) portrayed in the act of writing (courtesy of the Biblioteca Diocesana Vigilianum, Trento, Italy) 25

1.2 Prospero Lambertini (Pope Benedict XIV) portrayed in the act of writing his way to St Peter (courtesy of the Biblioteca Diocesana Vigilianum, Trento, Italy) 26

1.3 Portrait of Prospero Lambertini (Pope Benedict XIV) depicted as wielding a pen in the frontispiece of Louis-Antoine Caraccioli's *Vita del papa Benedetto XIV* (courtesy of the Thomas Fisher Rare Book Library, University of Toronto) 27

1.4 Decorations in St Peter's Basilica for the ceremony of beatification and canonization celebrated by Pope Benedict XIV (courtesy of John M. Kelly Library, University of St Michael's College) 54

2.1 Drawing of the anatomy room (photo of original document held in Archivio di Stato di Bologna and provided by Museo di Palazzo Poggi; courtesy of Museo di Palazzo Poggi—Università di Bologna) 72

2.2 William Pether, 'Three Persons Viewing the Gladiator by Candlelight' (courtesy of Photography © The Art Institute of Chicago) 89

3.1 Three women reading, sewing, and knitting in a domestic setting (courtesy of Ottavia Niccoli) 109

3.2 Portrait of Anna Morandi Manzolini (courtesy of the University of Wisconsin—Madison Libraries) 110

3.3 'Anatomia': Allegory of anatomy (courtesy of Rare Books and Special Collections, McGill University Library) 115

4.1 Giuseppe Maria Mitelli, 'Vedere' ('Seeing') (courtesy of Civica Raccolta delle Stampe 'Achille Bertarelli', Castello Sforzesco, Milan) 148

4.2 Anna Morandi's membership invoice, issued by the *Unione di Sant'Anna* (courtesy of Museo di Palazzo Poggi—Università di Bologna) 157

7.1 Limewood models of the ear (courtesy of Wellcome Library, London) 219

7.2 Francesco Celebrano, 'Maritime Carriage invented by the Prince of Sansevero' (courtesy of The Metropolitan Museum of Art, New York, Thomas J. Watson Library) 230

List of Abbreviations

AAB	Archivio Arcivescovile di Bologna
AABAB	Archivio dell'Accademia di Belle Arti di Bologna
AOM	Archives of the Order of Malta
ASB	Archivio di Stato di Bologna
ASM	Archivio di Stato di Milano
ASN	Archivio di Stato di Napoli
ASTo	Archivio di Stato di Torino
ASV	Archivio Segreto Vaticano
BAV	Biblioteca Apostolica Vaticana
BCABo	Biblioteca Comunale dell'Archiginnasio di Bologna
BCP	Biblioteca Comunale di Palermo
BNF	Bibliothèque nationale de France
BUB	Biblioteca Universitaria di Bologna
cart.	cartone/folder
fasc.	fascicolo/fascicle
fol./fols.	folio/s
Lib.	Liber
NLM	The National Library of Malta (Valletta).
SAAS-SIPA	Soprintendenza Archivistica della Sicilia-Archivio di Stato, Palermo

Introduction

BEGINNINGS

The story that marks the creation of anatomical collections in mid-eighteenth-century Italy has the aura of a mythical beginning. It takes place in Bologna, the second largest urban centre in the Papal States. Imagine entering an imposing Renaissance palace, a beautiful senatorial residence turned into an academy, and catching a glimpse of a man visiting the site. The individual in question is Prospero Lambertini (1675–1758), a Bolognese clergyman recently returned to his native city as the newly appointed archbishop and cardinal. The building is the Institute of the Sciences, the academy founded by the savant and soldier Luigi Ferdinando Marsigli (1658–1730) in 1711 (and inaugurated in 1714) with the purpose of creating a 'Solomon's house', gathering all knowledge under the same roof (Figure 0.1).[1] One can almost visualize Lambertini, sporting a characteristically red cardinal's gown, walking along the building's grand halls and corridors and perusing its displays. As the story has it, he is actually heading towards a specific corner: the tables of two wax models of the kidney, one normal and one anomalous (Plate 1). As he reaches them, he admires them, inquires about their author, and asks: why should the senators not provide the Institute with an anatomical museum?[2]

This study begins with this episode to explore how, in the years and decades following Lambertini's visit to the Institute, anatomical models were propelled to the forefront of the anatomical world. It investigates the 'mania' for anatomical displays

[1] On the Institute of the Sciences, see *I materiali dell'Istituto delle Scienze: Catalogo della mostra, Bologna, settembre–novembre 1979* (Bologna: CLUEB, 1979); Annarita Angelini (ed.), *Anatomie Accademiche*, vol. 3: *L'Istituto delle Scienze e l'Accademia* (Bologna: Il Mulino, 1993); Annarita Angelini, 'L'Institut des Sciences de Bologne entre les "théâtres du monde" et les laboratoires de science expérimentale', in Daniel-Odon Hurel and Gérard Laudin (eds.), *Académies et sociétés savantes en Europe (1650–1800)* (Paris: Honoré Champion, 2000), 177–97; Marta Cavazza, 'La "Casa di Salomone" realizzata?', in *I materiali dell'Istituto delle Scienze*, 42–54; Marta Cavazza, *Settecento inquieto: Alle origini dell'Istituto delle Scienze di Bologna* (Bologna: Il Mulino, 1990); Marta Cavazza, 'Innovazione e compromesso. L'Istituto delle Scienze e il sistema accademico bolognese del Settecento', in Adriano Prosperi (ed.), *Storia di Bologna*, vol. 3: *Bologna nell'età moderna (secoli XVI–XVIII)*, part II: *Cultura, istituzioni culturali, Chiesa e vita religiosa* (Bologna: Bononia University Press, 2008), 317–74.

[2] Francesco Maria Zanotti, 'De anatome in Institutum introducenda', in *De Bononiensi Scientiarum et Artium Instituto atque Academia Commentarii*, vol. 2/I (Bologna: Lelio dalla Volpe, 1745), 44–6. At the time of its foundation the Institute did not include the study of anatomy; see ibid. On anatomical teaching in seventeenth- and eighteenth-century Bologna, see Marta Cavazza, 'Aspetti dell'insegnamento dell'anatomia a Bologna nel Seicento e Settecento', in Giuseppe Olmi and Claudia Pancino (eds.), *Anatome: Sezione, scomposizione, raffigurazione del corpo nell'età moderna* (Bologna: Bononia University Press, 2012), 59–77.

DE BONONIENSI
SCIENTIARUM
ET
ARTIUM
INSTITUTO ATQUE ACADEMIA
COMMENTARII.
TOMUS QUARTUS.

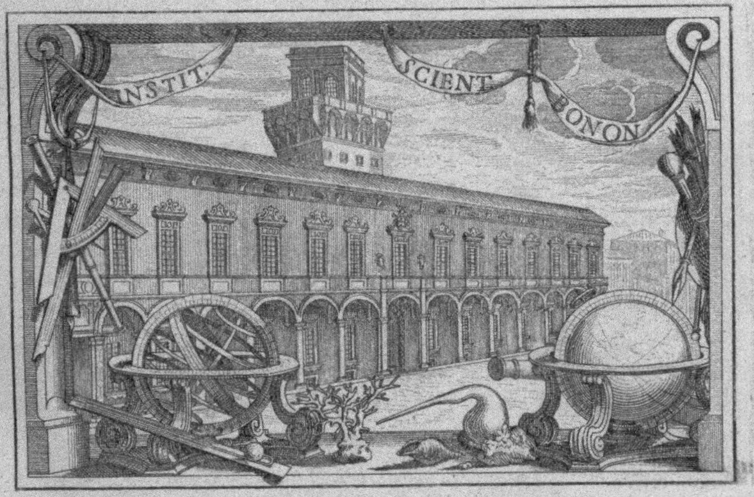

BONONIAE

Typis Lælii a Vulpe Inſtituti Scientiarum Typographi . MDCCLVII.
SUPERIORUM PERMISSU.

Figure 0.1 Title page of *De Bononiensi Scientiarum et Artium Instituto atque Academia Commentarii*, where the picture depicts the façade of Palazzo Poggi in Bologna, the site of the Institute of the Sciences.

that swept the Italian peninsula in the mid-eighteenth century, and traces the fashioning of anatomical models as important social, cultural, and political as well as medical tools. How did anatomical models inscribe and mediate bodily knowledge? How did they change the way in which anatomical knowledge was created and communicated? And how did they affect the lives of those involved in their production and viewing? In a way, the story of Lambertini's visit to the Institute of the Sciences introduces us to some of the features that ended up characterizing the domain of anatomical modelling. It calls attention to the presence in Bologna of the kind of knowledge and expertise that was required to make anatomical models. It also points to the transformation of the proverbially gruesome practice of anatomy into an enthralling experience that engaged audiences' senses and affects. Indeed, anatomical models provided an impressive means to overcome the shortcomings of bodily fluids, bad smells, and fears of contamination that characterized the messy setting of anatomical dissection. Offering a worthy complement to the famous ritual of the public anatomy lesson, modelling defined a more controllable, detailed, and pleasurable medium of anatomical knowledge.[3] Different audiences alternated in front of anatomical displays, and increasing numbers of viewers marvelled at the models' visual and material rendering of the complex language of anatomy. Although, given the models' rarity and cost, only a few could possess them, many shared the experience of delight and amazement that was prompted by their viewing. We could think of Lambertini as one of the many lay viewers who enjoyed such an experience, an early witness of anatomical models' lure and promise. Lambertini, however, turned out to be no ordinary spectator. At the time in which he visited the Institute and launched the idea of an anatomical museum, nobody could imagine that in less than a decade he would become pope. Nor could anyone have anticipated that in this capacity he would be instrumental in the development of anatomical modelling in Bologna and, indirectly, in the Italian peninsula as a whole.

Studies of eighteenth-century anatomical displays in the Italian peninsula have largely focused on the collection of the Royal Museum of Physics and Natural History ('La Specola'), which opened in Florence in 1775, and defined new parameters of anatomical wax modelling that ended up being shared, and sometimes challenged, by others.[4] This literature has paved the way for an analysis of the

[3] On the public anatomy lesson in Bologna, see the classic article by Giovanna Ferrari, 'Public Anatomy Lessons and the Carnival: The Anatomy Theatre of Bologna', *Past & Present*, 117 (1987), 50–106.

[4] See Ludmilla Jordanova, *Sexual Visions: Images of Gender in Science and Medicine between the Eighteenth and Twentieth Centuries* (Madison: University of Wisconsin Press, 1989), chapter 3; Renato G. Mazzolini, 'Plastic Anatomies and Artificial Dissections', in Soraya de Chadarevian and Nick Hopwood (eds.), *Models: The Third Dimension of Science* (Stanford: Stanford University Press, 2004), 43–70; Monika von Düring, Georges Didi-Huberman, and Marta Poggesi, *Encyclopaedia Anatomica: A Complete Collection of Anatomical Waxes* (Cologne: Taschen, 1999); Francesco Paolo De Ceglia, 'Rotten Corpses, a Disembowelled Woman, a Flayed Man: Images of the Body from the End of the 17th to the Beginning of the 19th Century: Florentine Wax Models in the First-Hand Accounts of Visitors', *Perspectives on Science*, 14:4 (2006), 417–56; Francesco Paolo De Ceglia, 'The Importance of Being Florentine: A Journey around the World for Wax Anatomical Venuses', *Nuncius*, 26:1 (2011), 83–108; Anna Maerker, '"Turpentine Hides Everything": Autonomy and Organization

variety of social, cultural, and political factors that lay behind the development of anatomical modelling in the late eighteenth century. Considering the anatomical collections of Florence and Vienna, Anna Maerker's rich and insightful *Model Experts* sheds light on how the politics that underpinned changing notions of expertise in state service affected views of public education and the rise of public museums. As Maerker herself notes, however, the anatomical collection of La Specola did not develop in a vacuum.[5] In the decades preceding its creation, a series of anatomical displays scattered around the Italian peninsula had introduced different audiences to the anatomy of the inner body. With few exceptions, little is known about these collections. However, they marked the emergence of new practices and spaces of production and consumption of anatomy and bodily knowledge as a whole. Focusing on these early stages of the practice of anatomical modelling, this study investigates the social lives of some of these displays.[6] Reconstructing the fashioning of anatomical models as special media that inscribed bodily knowledge, it follows the transformation of Bologna into a capital of anatomical display.[7] Moreover, it explores how anatomical modelling developed in the

in Anatomical Model Production for the State in Late Eighteenth-Century Florence', *History of Science*, 45:3 (2007), 257–86; Anna Maerker, *Model Experts: Wax Anatomies and Enlightenment in Florence and Vienna, 1775–1815* (Manchester: Manchester University Press, 2011); Anna Maerker, 'Florentine Anatomical Models and the Challenge of Medical Authority in Late Eighteenth-Century Vienna', *Studies in History and Philosophy of Science, Part C: Studies in History and Philosophy of Biological and Biomedical Sciences*, 43:3 (2012), 730–40; Rebecca Messbarger, 'The Re-Birth of Venus in Florence's Royal Museum of Physics and Natural History', *Journal of the History of Collections*, 25:2 (2013), 195–215; Joanna Ebenstein, 'Ode to an Anatomical Venus', *Women's Studies Quarterly*, 40:3/4 (2012), 346–52. See also *La ceroplastica nella scienza e nell'arte: Atti del I Congresso Internazionale, Firenze, 3–7 giugno 1975*, vols. 1 and 2 (Florence: Leo S. Olschki, 1977); Thomas N. Haviland and Lawrence Charles Parish, 'A Brief Account of the Use of Wax Models in the Study of Medicine', *Journal of the History of Medicine and Allied Sciences*, 25:1 (1970), 52–75; Michel Lemire, *Artistes et mortels* (Paris: Chabaud, 1990).

5 Maerker, *Model Experts*, 65–7.

6 On the social lives of things, see the classic Arjun Appadurai (ed.), *The Social Life of Things: Commodities in Cultural Perspective* (Cambridge: Cambridge University Press, 1986); Igor Kopytoff, 'The Cultural Biography of Things: Commoditization as Process', in ibid., 64–91. See also Chris Gosden and Yvonne Marshall (eds.), *The Cultural Biography of Objects*, special issue of *World Archaeology*, 31:2 (1999), 169–78; Jody Joy, 'Reinvigorating Object Biography: Reproducing the Drama of Object Lives', *World Archaeology*, 41:4 (2009), 540–56; David Pantalony, 'Biography of an Artifact: The Theratron Junior and Canada's Atomic Age', *Scientia Canadensis: Canadian Journal of the History of Science, Technology and Medicine*, 34: 1 (2011), 51–63.

7 On anatomical collections in mid-eighteenth-century Bologna, see Vincenzo Busacchi, 'Le cere anatomiche dell'Istituto delle Scienze', in *I materiali dell'Istituto delle Scienze*, 230–8; Maurizio Armaroli (ed.), *Le cere anatomiche bolognesi del Settecento: Catalogo della mostra organizzata dall'Università degli Studi di Bologna nell'Accademia delle Scienze* (Bologna: CLUEB, 1981); Elio Vassena, *La fortuna dei ceroplasti bolognesi del Settecento* (Tesi di Laurea, Storia della Critica d'Arte, Università di Bologna, 1996–7); Agostino Tripaldi, *Le cere anatomiche bolognesi del Settecento tra arte e scienza* (Tesi di Laurea, Storia della Scienza, Università di Bologna, 1997–8); Rebecca Messbarger, 'Waxing Poetic: Anna Morandi Manzolini's Anatomical Sculptures', *Configurations*, 9:1 (2001), 65–97; Rebecca Messbarger, 'Re-Membering a Body of Work: Anatomist and Anatomical Designer Anna Morandi Manzolini', *Studies in Eighteenth Century Culture*, 32:1 (2003), 123–54; Rebecca Messbarger, *The Lady Anatomist: The Life and Work of Anna Morandi Manzolini* (Chicago: University of Chicago Press, 2010); Claudia Pancino, 'Questioni di genere nell'anatomia plastica del Settecento bolognese', *Studi tanatologici*, 2 (2007), 317–32; Lucia Dacome, '"Un certo e quasi incredibile piacere": cera e anatomia nel Settecento', *Intersezioni*, 25:3 (2005), 415–36; Lucia Dacome, 'Waxworks and the Performance of Anatomy in

same period in other venues such as Palermo and Naples. Anatomical displays ended up being among these cities' notable monuments and became an integral part of the culture of the Grand Tour, the European journey undertaken by members of the elite for pleasure, culture, health, and education (see Plate 2 for a map of the Italian peninsula prepared for Grand Tour travellers).[8] This book investigates how in the Italian peninsula anatomical modelling developed at the crossroads of medical teaching, religious ritual, antiquarian, artisanal and artistic cultures, and Grand Tour display. I argue that the meanings of mid-eighteenth-century anatomical models were neither fixed nor unambiguous. Rather, they varied according to their spaces and sites of production and viewing, as well as to their different employments as pedagogical tools in medical and artistic settings, and as curiosities, artworks, Grand Tour collectibles, luxury goods, cultural currencies, or home decorations. Furthermore, I consider the significance of materials in substantiating models' capacity to inscribe and mediate anatomical knowledge.[9]

LIFELIKE MATTERS

Wax featured as a core material used in the making of anatomical models. Other materials—usually also malleable ones, like clay—were also used. Still, the majority of the anatomical models considered in this work were made in wax. The reasons underpinning the widespread use of wax in anatomical modelling were manifold. Throughout the early modern period, wax was regarded as a particularly versatile

Mid-18th-Century Italy', *Endeavour*, 30:1 (2006), 29–35; Lucia Dacome, 'Women, Wax and Anatomy in the "Century of Things"', *Renaissance Studies*, 21:4 (2007), 522–50; Lucia Dacome, 'The Anatomy of the Pope', in Maria Pia Donato and Jill Kraye (eds.), *Conflicting Duties: Science, Medicine and Religion in Rome, 1550–1750* (London: Warburg Institute, 2009), 353–74; Lucia Dacome, 'Ai confini del mondo naturale: anatomia e santità nell'opera di Prospero Lambertini', in Maria Teresa Fattori (ed.), *Storia, medicina e diritto nei trattati di Prospero Lambertini—Benedetto XIV* (Rome: Edizioni di Storia e Letteratura, 2013), 319–38.

[8] Among the many studies on the Grand Tour, see Andrew Wilton and Ilaria Bignamini (eds.), *Grand Tour: The Lure of Italy in the Eighteenth Century* (London: Tate Gallery Publishing, 1996); Chloe Chard and Helen Langdon (eds.) *Transports: Travel, Pleasure and Imaginative Geography, 1600–1830* (New Haven: Yale University Press, 1996); Edward Chaney, *The Evolution of the Grand Tour: Anglo-Italian Cultural Relations since the Renaissance* (London: Frank Cass, 1998); Chloe Chard, *Pleasure and Guilt on the Grand Tour: Travel Writing and Imaginative Geography: 1600–1830* (Manchester: Manchester University Press, 1999); Melissa Calaresu, 'Looking for Virgil's Tomb: The End of the Grand Tour and the Cosmopolitan Ideal in Europe', in Jaś Elsner and Joan Pau Rubiés (eds.), *Voyages and Visions: Towards a Cultural History of Travel* (London: Reaktion Books, 1999), 138–61; Jeremy Black, *The British Abroad: The Grand Tour in the Eighteenth Century* (Stroud: The History Press, 2003); Jeremy Black, *Italy and the Grand Tour* (New Haven: Yale University Press, 2003); Barbara Ann Naddeo, 'Cultural Capitals and Cosmopolitanism in Eighteenth-Century Italy: The Historiography and Italy on the Grand Tour', *Journal of Modern Italian Studies*, 10:2 (2005), 183–99; Paula Findlen, Wendy Wassyng Roworth, and Catherine M. Sama (eds.), *Italy's Eighteenth Century: Gender and Culture in the Age of the Grand Tour* (Stanford: Stanford University Press, 2009); Rosemary Sweet, *Cities and the Grand Tour: The British in Italy, c.1690–1820* (Cambridge: Cambridge University Press, 2012).

[9] On the role of materials in early modern natural inquiries, see Ursula Klein and Emma C. Spary (eds.), *Materials and Expertise in Early Modern Europe: Between Market and Laboratory* (Chicago: University of Chicago Press, 2010).

material: not only the object of mundane consumption and a core commodity sold in apothecary shops, but also a substance that mediated magic rituals and informed devotional practices.[10] Moreover, it acted as a landmark of public ceremonies, funerals, and liturgies.[11] The amount of wax employed for illumination and decoration in such ceremonies underscored the significance and grandiosity of the event and, in the case of funerary rituals, the social standing of the deceased.[12] What follows examines how using wax to chart the human body offered the opportunity to reclaim and control some of its cultural and physical plasticity. In particular, it explores how anatomical waxworks transformed wax's material features into privileged markers of the natural world. Indeed, being soft, malleable, palpable, and moist looking, wax was taken to be particularly well suited to 'imitate the state of life'.[13] Features such as malleability and palpability were considered characteristic of the living body, and could therefore appropriately express lifelikeness.[14] Yet, making sure that a material like wax could portray the body effectively was no straightforward matter. Rather, it entailed a laborious process and sometimes a long journey.

Often produced in the Ottoman territories, the wax of the Levant was frequently employed to make anatomical models. Considered the finest type of wax because it could be easily and rapidly whitened, it was sometimes preserved in soil before being shipped across the Mediterranean.[15] Being a porous material, wax was considered prone to absorbing bad air and was therefore regarded as a potential carrier of disease.[16] As a consequence, it was often quarantined in the ports of

[10] See Dacome, 'Women, Wax and Anatomy'; Guido Antonio Guerzoni, 'Uses and Abuses of Beeswax in the Early Modern Age: Two Apologues and a Taste', in Andrea Daninos (ed.), *Waxing Eloquent: Italian Portraits in Wax* (Milan: Officina Libraria, 2012), 43–59.

[11] See James Shaw and Evelyn S. Welch, *Making and Marketing Medicine in Renaissance Florence* (Amsterdam: Rodopi, 2011), chapter 6.

[12] See Sharon T. Strocchia, *Death and Ritual in Renaissance Florence* (Baltimore: Johns Hopkins University Press, 1992), esp. 128–9.

[13] In 1793, the French military surgeon René-Nicolas Desgenettes, remarked that after many attempts carried out with different materials, wax appeared to be preferable to all the other substances used in making artificial anatomies because of 'its transparency, ability to melt' and absorb all possible colours and degrees of thickness. Moreover, it was unassailable by insects and could be coated with a transparent, 'spirituous' varnish that made it possible to wash it, preserve its properties and freshness, and impart to it 'that greasy and moist appearance that perfectly imitates the state of life'; see René-Nicolas Desgenettes, 'Réflexions générales sur l'utilité de l'anatomie artificielle; et en particulier sur la collection de Florence, et la necessité d'en former de semblables en France', *Journal de médecine, chirurgie et pharmacie*, 94 (1793), 162–76 and 233–52 (citation pp. 170–1). At the turn of the nineteenth century, Giovanni Tumiati, professor of anatomy and obstetrics in Ferrara, similarly characterized wax as a material that was particularly apt to express lifelikeness due to its softness; see Giovanni Tumiati, *Elementi d'anatomia*, vol. 2 (Ferrara: Pomatelli, 1800), 192ff. On the significance of wax's material properties for anatomical modelling, see also Dacome, 'Women, Wax and Anatomy'.

[14] For instance, Bernard le Bovier de Fontenelle linked the palpable character of Ruysch's preparation with their lifelikeness, see Bernard le Bovier de Fontenelle, 'Éloge de M. Ruysch', in *Histoire de l'Académie Royale des Sciences, Année 1731* (Paris: Imprimerie Royale, 1733), 100–9.

[15] [Louis-Benjamin Francœur, François Étienne Molard, Louis Sébastien Lenormand, et al.], *Dictionnaire technologique, ou Nouveau dictionnaire universel des arts et métiers, et de l'économie industrielle et commerciale, par une société de savans et d'artistes*, vol. 5 (Paris: Thomine et Fortic, 1824), 305–6.

[16] On early modern preoccupations with bad air, see Sandra Cavallo and Tessa Storey, *Healthy Living in Late Renaissance Italy* (Oxford: Oxford University Press, 2013), esp. chapter 3.

destination. Once in Bologna, 'both local and foreign wax' had to be further inspected by apothecaries and *pro tempore* officials before it could leave the customs office.[17] As it finally reached the skilled hands of artificers, wax would first have to be whitened and then coloured through the mixing of pigments before it could be modelled into anatomical sculptures.[18] The result was striking. As Roberta Panzanelli has put it, coloured waxworks were regarded as having the capacity to generate a sense of 'compelling presence' and were taken to act as substitutes rather than representations. Bridging the distance with 'a segment of reality removed by time or space', they heightened 'the experience of the encounter' and transformed the viewer 'from the beholder of an image to an eyewitness'.[19] Likewise, anatomical waxworks were considered actual embodiments rather than depictions, and were viewed and studied as artefacts that conveyed knowledge in their own right.[20]

As is well known, even before being systematically employed in the realm of anatomy, wax had long been used to portray the human body in religious and artistic settings. For instance, wax votives contributed to long-standing devotional traditions in which two- and three-dimensional representations of bodily parts affected by accidents and illnesses were meant to invoke or acknowledge divine intervention.[21] Wax figures and écorchés (models of flayed anatomical statues) could furthermore be found in the workshops of artists and in cabinets of curiosities as well as on the desks of physicians and surgeons.[22] Yet, as artificers,

[17] Archivio di Stato di Bologna (henceforth ASB), Miscellanea delle Arti, B XII, n. 59, 26 January 1748.

[18] On the whitening of wax see, for instance, the entry for 'Blanchir la cire' in Denis Diderot and Jean Le Rond d'Alembert (eds.), *Encyclopédie, ou dictionnaire raisonné des sciences, des arts et des métiers*, vol. 2 (Paris: Briasson et al., 1751), 273–4.

[19] Uta Kornmeier, 'Almost Alive: The Spectacle of Verisimilitude in Madame Tussaud's Waxworks', in Roberta Panzanelli (ed.), *Ephemeral Bodies: Wax Sculpture and the Human Figure* (Los Angeles: Getty Research Institute, 2008), 67–81 (citation p. 74); Roberta Panzanelli, 'Compelling Presence: Wax Effigies in Renaissance Florence', in ibid., 13–39, esp. 17. See also Roberta Panzanelli, 'Introduction: The Body in Wax, the Body of Wax', in ibid., 1–12; Georges Didi-Huberman, 'Viscosities and Survivals: Art History Put to the Test by the Material', in ibid., 154–69.

[20] The understanding of anatomical wax models and preparations as 'material embodiments of scientific knowledge' continued into the nineteenth century; see Carin Berkowitz, 'Systems of Display: The Making of Anatomical Knowledge in Enlightenment Britain', *The British Journal for the History of Science*, 46:3 (2013), 359–87.

[21] See Fabio Bisogni, 'Ex voto e la scultura in cera nel tardo Medioevo', in Andrew Ladis and Shelley E. Zuraw (eds.), *Visions of Holiness: Art and Devotion in Renaissance Italy* (Athens: Georgia Museum of Art, 2001), 67–91; Megan Holmes, 'Ex-votos: Materiality, Memory and Cult', in Michael W. Cole and Rebecca E. Zorach (eds.), *The Idol in the Age of Art: Objects, Devotions and the Early Modern World* (Farnham: Ashgate, 2009), 159–82; Panzanelli, 'Compelling Presence'.

[22] For an account of the 'lost wax' ('*cera persa*') technique, namely, the creation of wax models of sculptures that were then re-cast in a different material such as bronze, see Giorgio Vasari, *Le vite de' più eccellenti pittori scultori e architettori*, 2nd edn., vol. 1 (parts I and II) (Florence: Giunti, 1568), chapter 9. Well into the eighteenth century, this technique continued to be used in the making of precious objects. For instance, in 1761 the Orsini family wanted to acquire a set of rubies and diamonds and asked an artificer to create wax models of the jewels; see UCLA, Charles E. Young Research Library, Orsini Archive, Collection 902, Box 389, Letters of 14, 18, and 21 April 1761 from Carlo Ungano in Napoli. For a famous reference to the presence of anatomical models in physicians' cabinets, see the portrait of Volcher Coiter (1534–1576), which depicts the physician standing next to a small écorché figure with a hand resting on the life-size model of a flayed arm. On Coiter's portrait and his interest in anatomical models, see Nancy G. Siraisi, *The Clock and the Mirror: Girolamo Cardano*

anatomists, and collectors started to assemble anatomical models and place specimens into displays that catered to lay audiences as well as to artists and medical practitioners, anatomical modelling was off to a new start and informed a new space of anatomical encounter. Reconstructing the social settings, cultural environments, gender relations, institutional demands, and visual and material domains that substantiated the status of anatomical models as impressive tools of bodily knowledge, this work sets off to write a microhistory of things.

THE CENTURY OF THINGS

The eighteenth century was the century of things. Ever more things were created, collected, used, consumed, and moved around. Things also promised to trigger a new era of knowledge. In 1737, the savant and traveller Francesco Algarotti (1712–1764) famously singled out 'things' as the characteristic feature of a new function of knowledge in society: 'Let the century of things arise again for us', he wrote in the dedicatory letter opening his *Newtonianism for the Ladies*, and 'let knowledge' serve to improve and 'adorn society' rather than 'harden the soul and make it quarrel over an old and obsolete phrase'.[23] As a distinguishing mark of this new era, 'things', the objects of natural knowledge, promised to free new audiences, including women, from the tyranny of baroque pedantry and instead bring about beneficial and pleasurable knowledge. Anatomical models promised to do just that. Coloured, soft, malleable, and often life-size, they afforded a more intimate and polite ambiance to the encounter with details of the inner body. Praised for their beauty, they promised to foster anatomical knowledge and mediate it in a delightful way. Staging an impressive and potentially portable archive of the body, they shed light on the human body's proverbial mysteries and uncertainties. By the mid-eighteenth century, the view that the workings of the human body relied on solid anatomical parts was widely adopted in the medical world. Yet, many continued to experience their bodies as fluid and porous entities that worked in unpredictable and ambiguous ways.[24] Anatomical models offered to tackle this persistent sense of opacity by presenting viewers with solid (however soft and malleable) bodily parts that were lodged inside them. Inaugurating a new era of purported corporeal transparency, they left audiences amazed, instructed, delighted, and occasionally perplexed. Upon turning their eyes away from the models, some could

and Renaissance Medicine (Princeton: Princeton University Press, 1997), 111–13. The physician Theodore Turquet de Mayerne (1573–1655) similarly kept on his table the 'proportion of a man in wax, to set forth ye ordure & composure of every part'; quoted in Brian Nance, *Turquet de Mayerne as Baroque Physician: The Art of Medical Portraiture* (Amsterdam: Rodopoi, 2001), 24. On the history of écorché figures, see Boris Röhrl, *History and Bibliography of Artistic Anatomy: Didactics for Depicting the Human Figure* (Hildesheim: G. Olms, 2000).

[23] Francesco Algarotti, *Il newtonianismo per le dame, ovvero, Dialoghi sopra la luce e i colori* (Naples [Milan]: n.p., 1737), xii. Unless otherwise stated, translations are my own.

[24] See, for instance, Barbara Duden, *The Woman Beneath the Skin: A Doctor's Patients in Eighteenth-Century Germany*, trans. Thomas Dunlap (Cambridge, MA: Harvard University Press, 1991).

not stop thinking about, or even visualizing, what they had seen.[25] Yet, following a period in which the utility of anatomy had been called into question, anatomical models ended up being fashioned as sites of authenticity, tokens of trustworthy bodily knowledge that provided visually powerful celebrations of anatomy's claims and promises.

Looking back at the anatomical collections that had been on display in the previous decades in Bologna, in 1777 the famous anatomist and natural philosopher Luigi Galvani (1737–1798) pointed to the advantages of models' material features, especially their solidity, for the study of anatomy.[26] He remarked that when bodily parts were taken out of a cadaver, they lost what was 'natural and true': once exposed to the air, they dried out and wrinkled, and when placed on a table they flattened and lost shape. By contrast, thanks to their malleability, reliable colouring, imperishable character, and capacity to capture detail and attain proper bulk and shape, anatomical waxworks could express natural features with absolute precision and convey fundamental anatomical characteristics such as form, position, direction, and development of bodily parts.[27] As a consequence, they were to be considered particularly accurate and truthful—even truer, in fact, than the natural body itself.

Authoritative as they may appear, Galvani's words are deceptively simple. They seem to point to a purportedly self-evident process of knowledge production. In fact, transforming an object like an anatomical model into an effective tool of knowledge—one that could be even more fitting than the natural body—was no straightforward matter. Rather, it entailed a complex, polyphonic process that involved the models' makers, viewers, patrons, and collectors as well as materials, techniques, skills, spaces and modes of display, social and visual conventions, and much more. This study examines how models set the stage for a complex encounter between the gaze of viewers and the authority of makers, between shifting approaches to the unveiling of the human body and codified forms of visual and material representation. In order to reconstruct the genealogy of claims about the models' capacity to chart the human body in an accurate and truthful way, it investigates the different constituencies and the contingencies that were involved in the making and employment of anatomical models. I argue that the stratification of meanings and values that came to characterize mid-eighteenth-century anatomical displays was shaped within networks that were socially and culturally embedded,

[25] See Giovanni Lodovico Bianconi, *Lettere del consigliere Gian Lodovico Bianconi [...] sopra il libro del Canonico Luigi Crespi, Bolognese, intitolato Felsina pittrice* (Milan: Tipografia de' Classici italiani, 1802), 11–12; Louise-Élisabeth Vigée-Lebrun, *Souvenirs de Madame Vigée Le Brun*, vol. 1 (Paris: Charpentier et Cie, 1869), 237–8.

[26] Luigi Galvani, *De Manzoliniana supellectili, oratio, habita in Scientiarum et Artium Instituto cum ad anatomen in tabulis ab Anna Manzolina perfectis pubblice tradendam aggrederetur anno MDCCLXXVII*, in *Opere edite ed inedite del professore Luigi Galvani, raccolte e pubblicate per cura dell'Accademia delle Scienze dell'Istituto di Bologna* (Bologna: Emidio Dall'Olmo, 1841), 41–58, esp. 45–58.

[27] Ibid., esp. 47–51.

and extended well beyond the medical world.[28] Moreover, I consider how, upon entering consumer, travel, and celebrity cultures and patronage networks, a local artisanal practice like wax modelling was transformed into a medium that could substantiate normative accounts of the body and, accordingly, promised privileged access to the understanding of human nature.[29] Situating anatomical modelling in the context of rituals and practices that endowed objects with special power—such as the worlds of devotion and antiquarian culture—I further investigate the significance of proximity in knowledge-making processes based on the direct experience of things. In a related manner, I explore how models owed some of their capacity to generate approval to their ability to forge affective bonds that reworked and restaged rituals of adoration into practices of knowledge.[30]

BETWEEN PATRONAGE AND COMMERCE

As in the case of many early modern collections, it all started with the munificence of a mighty patron. The story opens in Bologna in the early 1730s, where Prospero Lambertini engaged in promoting anatomy in his capacity as the local archbishop. After becoming Pope Benedict XIV, Lambertini became a major patron of the anatomical collections of Bologna and a key player in the fashioning of the Italian peninsula as a centre of anatomical modelling. While much of the literature on Lambertini views his support for natural and anatomical knowledge as related to his characterization as 'the Enlightenment pope', I situate Lambertini's patronage of anatomical displays in the context of his engagement as an assessor of sanctity who appealed to anatomical knowledge as a means of tracing and verifying the signs of holy embodiment.[31] In a related manner, I suggest that the significance that the pope attributed to anatomical models as markers of the natural body played a part in the fashioning of anatomical collections as sites of knowledge about human nature.

Of course, the Italian peninsula was not the only setting in which the creation of anatomical displays generated much interest and widespread approval.[32] Still, in

[28] On anatomical practices conducted outside the world of learned medicine in the pre-modern period, see Katharine Park, *Secrets of Women: Gender, Generation and the Origins of Human Dissection* (New York: Zone Books, 2006).

[29] On eighteenth-century views of human nature see, for instance, Christopher Fox, Roy Porter, and Robert Wokler (eds.), *Inventing Human Science: Eighteenth-Century Domains* (Berkeley: University of California Press, 1995).

[30] On anatomical displays' affective power, see Samuel J.M.M. Alberti, 'The Museum Affect: Visiting Collections of Anatomy and Natural History', in Aileen Fyfe and Bernard Lightman (eds.), *Science in the Marketplace: Nineteenth-Century Sites and Experiences* (Chicago: University of Chicago Press, 2007), 371–403; Rina Knoeff, 'Touching Anatomy: On the Handling of Anatomical Preparations in the Anatomical Cabinets of Frederik Ruysch (1638–1731)', *Studies in History and Philosophy of Science, Part C: Studies in History and Philosophy of Biological and Biomedical Sciences*, 49 (2015), 32–44.

[31] See Dacome, 'The Anatomy of the Pope'; Dacome, 'Ai confini del mondo naturale'.

[32] See Jonathan Simon, 'The Theatre of Anatomy: The Anatomical Preparations of Honoré Fragonard', *Eighteenth-Century Studies*, 36:1 (2002), 63–79; Simon Chaplin, 'Nature Dissected, or Dissection Naturalized? The Case of John Hunter's Museum', *Museum and Society*, 6:2 (2008), 135–51; Simon Chaplin, 'John Hunter and the "Museum Oeconomy", 1750–1800' (PhD Thesis, King's College London, 2009);

the mid-eighteenth century the convergence of Grand Tour culture, artistic and artisanal practices, antiquarian pursuits, and consolidated practices of worship of holy bodies and sacred objects transformed cities like Bologna, Palermo, and Naples into particularly propitious sites for the development of new collective rituals related to the display and viewing of bodily parts. Notably, some of the enthusiasm for anatomical displays was lodged in the long-standing interest in curiosities, which throughout the early modern period had informed the creation of displays that defined and showcased the natural world. Likewise, the value of anatomical models increased with the surge in the prestige of cabinets and collecting practices that received courtly patronage.[33] Although over time the court had changed its role as a focal point in the production of natural knowledge, in the eighteenth century it continued to act as an important source of patronage, often through the sponsorship of academies, libraries and museums, and increased ties with universities. Making anatomical models was expensive and time-consuming, and few could afford them. Anatomical models were thus well suited to the resources, collecting habits, and patronage strategies of courts and patrician households, and offered desirable additions to their cabinets. By articulating orderly arrangements of anatomical parts, models furthermore presented the audiences that they pledged to educate with remarkable instances of bodily control, and accordingly staged an impressive promise of corporeal governance and hegemony over the body politic. Not surprisingly, a number of European courts entered a race to acquire anatomical models, and those who could afford them delighted in adding them to their collections. It was not only Pope Benedict XIV who supported the creation of anatomical collections. Many other eighteenth-century European sovereigns also commissioned, acquired, and displayed anatomical models, including

Simon Chaplin, 'The Divine Touch, or Touching Divines: John Hunter, David Hume and the Bishop of Durham's Rectum', in Helen Deutsch and Mary Terrall (eds.), *Vital Matters: Eighteenth-Century Views of Conception, Life, and Death* (Toronto: University of Toronto Press, 2012), chapter 10; Joan B. Landes, 'Wax Fibers, Wax Bodies and Moving Figures: Artifice and Nature in Eighteenth-Century Anatomy', in Panzanelli (ed.), *Ephemeral Bodies*, 41–65; Lyle Massey, 'On Waxes and Wombs: Eighteenth-Century Representations of the Gravid Uterus', in ibid., 83–105; Berkowitz, 'Systems of Display'. On the longer history of anatomical modelling, see Thomas Schnalke, *Diseases in Wax: The History of the Medical Moulage*, trans. Kathy Spatschek (Carol Stream, IL: Quintessence Books, 1995); Martin Kemp and Marina Wallace, *Spectacular Bodies: The Art and Science of the Human Body from Leonardo to Now* (Berkeley: University of California Press, 2000); Nick Hopwood, *Embryos in Wax: Models from the Ziegler Studio* (Cambridge: Whipple Museum for the History of Science, University of Cambridge; Bern: Institute of the History of Medicine, University of Bern, 2002); Samuel J.M.M. Alberti, 'Wax Bodies: Art and Anatomy in Victorian Medical Museums', *Museum History Journal*, 2:1 (2009), 7–36; Samuel J.M.M. Alberti, *Morbid Curiosities: Medical Museums in Nineteenth-Century Britain* (Oxford: Oxford University Press, 2011); Elizabeth Stephens, *Anatomy as Spectacle: Public Exhibitions of the Body from 1700 to the Present* (Liverpool: Liverpool University Press, 2011); Carin Berkowitz, 'The Beauty of Anatomy: Visual Displays and Surgical Education in Early Nineteenth-Century London', *Bulletin of the History of Medicine*, 85:2 (2011), 248–78; Anna Maerker, 'Anatomizing the Trade: Designing and Marketing Anatomical Models as Medical Technologies, c.1700–1900', *Technology and Culture*, 54:3 (2013), 531–62.

[33] On collecting practices in early modern Italy see, for instance, Giuseppe Olmi, *L'inventario del mondo: Catalogazione della natura e luoghi del sapere nella prima età moderna* (Bologna: Il Mulino, 1992); Paula Findlen, *Possessing Nature: Museums, Collecting, and Scientific Culture in Early Modern Italy* (Berkeley: University of California Press, 1994).

Peter the Great, his daughter Elizabeth, and Catherine II of Russia; Leopold II of Tuscany and his brother, the Holy Roman Emperor Joseph II; Charles Emmanuel III of Savoy; Christian VII of Denmark; and Charles de Bourbon of Naples.

Yet, just as elsewhere, in the Italian peninsula anatomical displays were not merely an expression of the continuing significance of patronage culture. Commerce and consumption were as much a part of the landscape of anatomical modelling as was patronage, and anatomical displays developed within networks that involved trading and advertising.[34] In turn, models acted as cultural assets and could serve as currencies that had the capacity to transfer value.[35] Their prohibitive costs and relative rarity further conferred upon them double status as tools of knowledge and luxury goods.[36] At a time of intense debate over the consequences of lavish consumption, their educational value offered their collectors the opportunity to acquire expensive objects without incurring the pitfalls traditionally associated with luxury, such as the risk of bringing about both physical and moral ruin.

TOURING AND VIEWING

Grand Tour travellers featured as particularly avid consumers of anatomical displays. In April 1776, Samuel Johnson famously stated that 'a man who has not been in Italy, is always conscious of an inferiority, from his not having seen what it

[34] On the trade and consumption of early modern curiosities, natural specimens, and artefacts, see Pamela H. Smith and Paula Findlen (eds.), *Merchants and Marvels: Commerce, Science, and Art in Early Modern Europe* (New York: Routledge, 2002); Harold J. Cook, *Matters of Exchange: Commerce, Medicine, and Science in the Dutch Golden Age* (New Haven: Yale University Press, 2007). While much attention has been devoted to the thriving consumer cultures of eighteenth-century Britain and France, interest in the patterns of consumption that developed in the Italian peninsula has primarily focused on the Renaissance period. On consumer culture in Renaissance Italy, see Evelyn S. Welch, *Shopping in the Renaissance: Consumer Cultures in Italy, 1400–1600* (New Haven: Yale University Press, 2005); Michelle O'Malley and Evelyn Welch (eds.), *The Material Renaissance* (Manchester: Manchester University Press, 2007). On consumption in eighteenth-century Britain and France, see Neil McKendrick, John Brewer, and John H. Plumb (eds.), *The Birth of a Consumer Society: The Commercialization of Eighteenth-Century England* (London: Europa, 1982); John Brewer and Roy Porter (eds.), *Consumption and the World of Goods* (London: Routledge, 1993); Daniel Roche, *Histoire des choses banales. Naissance de la consommation dans les sociétés traditionnelles (XVIIe–XIXe siècle)* (Paris: Fayard, 1997); Maxine Berg and Helen Clifford (eds.), *Consumers and Luxury: Consumer Culture in Europe, 1650–1850* (Manchester: Manchester University Press, 1999); Maxine Berg and Elizabeth Eger (eds.), *Luxury in the Eighteenth Century: Debates, Desires and Delectable Goods* (Basingstoke: Palgrave, 2003).

[35] This aspect of anatomical modelling is discussed in Chapters 6 and 7.

[36] On the commercialization of anatomical preparations and their fashioning as luxury goods in seventeenth-century Netherlands, see Cook, *Matters of Exchange*; Harold J. Cook, 'Time's Bodies: Crafting the Preparation and Preservation of Naturalia', in Smith and Findlen (eds.), *Merchants and Marvels*, 223–47; Dániel Margócsy, 'Advertising Cadavers in the Republic of Letters: Anatomical Publications in the Early Modern Netherlands', *The British Journal for the History of Science*, 42:2 (2009), 187–210; Dániel Margócsy, 'A Museum of Wonders or a Cemetery of Corpses? The Commercial Exchange of Anatomical Collections in Early Modern Netherlands', in Sven Dupré and Christoph Herbert Lüthy (eds.), *Silent Messengers: The Circulation of Material Objects of Knowledge in the Early Modern Low Countries* (Berlin: LIT Verlag, 2011), 185–215; Dániel Margócsy, *Commercial Visions: Science, Trade, and Visual Culture in the Dutch Golden Age* (Chicago: University of Chicago Press, 2014).

is expected a man should see'.[37] By then, anatomical displays such as the ones housed in Bologna and Naples had been included among the sights that one was expected to visit along Grand Tour routes. This study situates anatomical displays in the context of the conspicuous movement of people, artefacts, specimens, books, letters, stories, and gossip, which characterized the culture of the Grand Tour.[38] It suggests that if anatomical models became so popular among travellers, it was also because they played a part in the development of the observational practices that were incidental to Grand Tour culture. To some, visiting anatomical collections became something of a rite of passage. In 1761, the self-proclaimed 'Chevalier' and 'Opthalmiater Royal' John Taylor (1703–1772) boasted of having seen 'all the most noted cabinets of anatomical preparations in Europe', both 'those belonging to particular states, academies, universities, and societies of the learned' and to 'particular persons', indicating that he 'could write volumes' on what he had seen there.[39] As part of his 'travels and adventures', Taylor toured the Italian peninsula. While in Naples, he had in his care the son of Raimondo di Sangro (1710–1771), the seventh Prince of San Severo. As we shall see in Chapter 7, di Sangro, who was described by Taylor as 'a most extraordinary genius', housed in his palace a remarkable anatomical display.[40] Like Taylor, many other travellers engaged in anatomical pilgrimages and wandered around the workshops, cabinets, homes, and academies where anatomical models and preparations were made and displayed. The Grand Tour equally set models in motion: it fashioned them as worthy matter for travel literature and created the occasion for purchase, transport, and theatrical demonstrations. This study explores how mobility had a transformative power and subjected models to processes of change and reconfiguration, which cross-pollinated with—and were sometimes short-circuited by—local practices. In a related manner, it considers how the very information networks, which crucially contributed

[37] James Boswell, *The Life of Samuel Johnson, LL.D., Comprehending an Account of His Studies and Numerous Works*, vol. 2 (London: Henry Baldwin for Charles Dilly, 1791), 61.

[38] On anatomical tourism in early modern Netherlands, see Rina Knoeff, 'The Visitor's View: Early Modern Tourism and the Polyvalence of Anatomical Exhibits', in Lissa Roberts (ed.), *Centres and Cycles of Accumulation in and around the Netherlands during the Early Modern Period* (Berlin: LIT Verlag, 2011), 155–75. On travel, movement, and the making of natural knowledge, see Mary Terrall, *The Man Who Flattened the Earth: Maupertuis and the Sciences in the Enlightenment* (Chicago: University of Chicago Press, 2002); Marie Noëlle Bourguet, Christian Licoppe, and H. Otto Sibum (eds.), *Instruments, Travel and Science: Itineraries of Precision from the Seventeenth to the Twentieth Century* (London: Routledge, 2002); Simon Schaffer et al. (eds.), *The Brokered World: Go-Betweens and Global Intelligence, 1770–1820* (Sagamore Beach, MA: Watson Publishing International, 2009); Kapil Raj and Mary Terrall (eds.), 'Circulation and Locality in Early Modern Science', special issue, *The British Journal for the History of Science*, 43:4 (2010); Dupré and Lüthy (eds.), *Silent Messengers*; Paola Bertucci, 'Enlightened Secrets: Silk, Intelligent Travel, and Industrial Espionage in Eighteenth-Century France', *Technology and Culture*, 54:4 (2013), 820–52; Pedro M.P. Raposo et al., 'Moving Localities and Creative Circulation: Travels as Knowledge Production in 18th-Century Europe', *Centaurus*, 56:33 (2014), 167–88.

[39] John Taylor, 'The Life &c.', in *The History of the Travels and Adventures of the Chevalier John Taylor, Ophthalmiater*, vol. 1 (London: J. Williams, 1761), 66.

[40] Ibid., 8. The name of the Prince of San Severo has been spelled differently, including 'Sansevero', 'S. Severo', and 'San Severo'. In order to use it consistently, and reflect the way di Sangro's contemporaries and, especially, Grand Tour travellers, often referred to him, his palace, and chapel, in what follows I will use the spelling 'San Severo'.

to the fortune of anatomical displays, underwent failures and friction, and how even the stories that circulated about anatomical models and their modellers did not necessarily match each other. In the complex process of translating local knowledge into Grand Tour narratives that fed a transnational readership, things could get mixed up.

The reasons underscoring Grand Tourists' interest in anatomical models were, of course, various. Alongside the search for warmer climates and the pursuit of better health, the longing for fresh contact with antiquities and curiosities scattered around the Italian peninsula scored high among the motivations that led many to undertake the expensive, uncomfortable, and often dangerous journey.[41] Indeed, part of the lure of the Grand Tour lay in the characterization of Italy as a land that was remarkable for 'its profusion of objects of exceptional singularity'.[42] Anatomical models promised to cater to this diverse range of expectations. While they were remarkable objects that mediated knowledge of human nature, they also helped to hone the skills required in the contemplation of classical statues, one of Grand Tourists' favourite engagements. By the eighteenth century, classical statues had gained a significant place in the history of anatomy. Notably, the famous statue of Polykleitos (or Polycleitus) had informed the notion of a bodily canon, linking the idea of a physical norm with views of a healthy body.[43] As Valerie Traub has observed, at a time of global expansion the adoption of classical sculpture to define the normative body of anatomy offered an important positioning tool: by singling out classical proportions as a universalizing ideal, anatomy defined a corporeal norm against which other bodies could be gauged. While doing so, it promised to grant European bodies a place of centrality on the global map.[44] Anatomical models participated in this act of positioning. Many among the anatomical models that were on display along Grand Tour routes variously evoked the corporeal norm that was rooted in classical sculpture and was echoed in early modern anatomical literature. In doing so, they mediated this norm to wide audiences, including those tourists, such as the French naturalist and mathematician Charles-Marie de La Condamine (1701–1774), who travelled to southern Europe as well as across the Atlantic.[45] Notably, the southern European locations of a number of anatomical displays, such as Naples and Palermo, signposted both geographical and corporeal

[41] On travelling to Italy for health purposes, see Black, *Italy and the Grand Tour*, 116.

[42] Chard, *Pleasure and Guilt*, 19, quoted in Naddeo, 'Cultural Capitals', 186.

[43] Galen mentioned the statue of Polykleitos as an example of a body where all the 'parts are in perfect proportions with each other' and is 'well balanced in every way'; see Claudius Galen, 'On Mixtures, Book 1', in *Selected Works*, ed. and trans. P.N. Singer (Oxford: Oxford University Press, 1997), 229. In the early modern period, Andreas Vesalius singled out the canon of Polykleitos as a cogent example of the average body, which ideally had to be used in public anatomies lessons; see Sachiko Kusukawa, *Picturing the Book of Nature: Image, Text and Argument in Sixteenth-Century Human Anatomy and Medical Botany* (Chicago: Chicago University Press, 2012), 213–15.

[44] Valerie Traub, 'The Nature of Norms in Early Modern England: Anatomy, Cartography, *King Lear*', *South Central Review*, 26:1/2 (2009), 42–81.

[45] On La Condamine's transatlantic travels, see Mary Louise Pratt's classic *Imperial Eyes: Travel Writing and Transculturation*, 2nd edn. (London: Routledge, 2008), chapter 2; Neil Safier, *Measuring the New World: Enlightenment Science and South America* (Chicago: University of Chicago Press, 2008).

borderlands. When in 1766 the surgeon and anatomical modeller Anthonius Mayer (or Majer), who displayed his anatomical cabinet in Naples, donated a number of models to the Grand Master of Malta, he participated in delineating the boundaries of the canonic anatomical body along the edges of the Grand Tour.[46]

In addition to generating audiences for anatomical displays, Grand Tour culture also produced knowledge about models and their makers. This study draws attention to the variety of media—books, periodicals, images, artefacts, etc.—that variously shaped this knowledge. Over the course of the eighteenth century, Grand Tourists' reports about their dazzling encounters with models became major agents of publicity for anatomical displays. In fact, not all anatomical cabinets reached the same level of popularity, and those that did were usually included among the attractions of the Grand Tour. In Bologna, for instance, the hospital of Santa Maria della Morte, which supplied cadavers for the making of anatomical models, housed an anatomy room. Yet, its models and preparations were locked up behind closed doors, and remained largely unknown. When, in 1764, a former assistant offered a 'skeleton' and four anatomical preparations to the hospital's governors (*Assunti*), the hospital gladly accepted the donation. However, the specimens ended up being used only by the restricted few who could access its anatomy room.[47] By contrast, the anatomical collections that joined the Grand Tour spectacle of artistic, antiquarian, religious, and natural specimens, obtained a high degree of visibility. As tourists recorded what they saw in travel diaries, they fed readers' curiosity and expectations. As their travel reports ended up serving as guides for other travellers, they also shaped Grand Tour itineraries and informed the experience of many viewers.[48] Gazettes and periodicals equally spread the news about the impressive anatomical cabinets that were mushrooming across Europe. As the gaze of foreigners conferred special value on anatomical models, it turned them into a part of the local heritage: it stimulated a sense of belonging and kindled hope that they could provide a sustained source of pride and prosperity.[49] This study sets out to investigate the history of mid-eighteenth-century anatomical displays at the point of encounter between locals and travellers. While much of the literature on the Grand Tour has focused on tourists, less attention has been drawn to the point of view of the local communities that were visited by travellers. In fact, locals were just as

[46] See The National Library of Malta (henceforth NLM), Archives of the Order of Malta (henceforth AOM) 637 (Deliberazioni della Camera del Tesoro, 1763–1769), fols. 109r–v. Mayer is generally mentioned in the primary sources by his surname as Mayer or Majer. His first name in Latin and Italian sources is, respectively, 'Anthonius' or 'Antonio'. On Grand Tourists' fashioning of Southern Italy as a European borderland, see Nelson Moe, *The View from Vesuvius: Italian Culture and the Southern Question* (Berkeley: University of California Press, 2002); Naddeo, 'Cultural Capitals', 186–8.

[47] ASB, Ospedale di Santa Maria della Morte, Atti di Congregazione, Serie VIII, Busta 42, Lib. 9, 22 January 1764.

[48] On travellers as mediators of knowledge, see Schaffer et al. (eds.), *The Brokered World.*

[49] Notably, while the anatomical models and preparations that were located in the hospital of Santa Maria della Morte were relegated to historical oblivion and, apparently, did not survive to this day, the anatomical displays that were on view along Grand Tour routes have often enjoyed long histories (though, admittedly, with mixed fortunes in terms of care and conservation).

much part of the Grand Tour culture as travellers were. In the case of anatomical models, the Grand Tour offered local artificers, patrons, and collectors a special opportunity to impart value and visibility to their own pursuits. Propelling their makers to the forefront of the anatomical world, it bolstered their status as anatomical celebrities.

ANATOMICAL CELEBRITIES

Scholars have identified the emergence of a celebrity culture that developed in the eighteenth century side by side with a long-lasting culture of fame, sometimes intersecting and overlapping with it.[50] They have suggested that the emerging phenomenon of eighteenth-century celebrity went beyond the traditional engines of fame such as 'royal recognition, state honours, religious canonization', and 'the laurels of artistic achievement'.[51] Rather, its origins could be linked with the rise of eighteenth-century consumer societies and the development and dissemination of media such as periodicals, the popular press, printed images, and the theatre, all of which allowed 'widespread recognition for the celebrities of the day' and their capacity to engage new and potentially adoring audiences.[52] While all these factors came to a particularly favourable convergence in London and Paris, they characterized much of eighteenth-century European urban culture as a whole.

This book explores how this culture of renown extended to the world of anatomical modelling and affected the lives of a number of artificers, including a woman like Anna Morandi Manzolini (1714–1774), who became an anatomical celebrity.[53] Historians have highlighted artisans' position of centrality in the theatrical

[50] On fame and celebrity in the eighteenth century, see Stella Tillyard, 'Celebrity in 18th-Century London', *History Today*, 55:6 (June 2005), 20–7; Claire Brock, *The Feminization of Fame, 1750–1830* (Basingstoke: Palgrave Macmillan, 2006); Elizabeth Barry, 'From Epitaph to Obituary: Death and Celebrity in Eighteenth-Century British Culture', *International Journal of Cultural Studies*, 11:3 (2008), 259–75; Uta Kornmeier, 'The Famous and the Infamous Waxworks as Retailers of Renown', ibid., 276–88; Tom Mole, 'Lord Byron and the End of Fame', ibid., 343–61; Fred Inglis, *A Short History of Celebrity* (Princeton: Princeton University Press, 2010), chapters 3 and 4; Felicity Nussbaum, *Rival Queens: Actresses, Performance, and the Eighteenth-Century British Theater* (Philadelphia: University of Pennsylvania Press, 2010); Laura Engel, *Fashioning Celebrity: Eighteenth-Century British Actresses and Strategies for Image Making* (Columbus: Ohio State University Press, 2011); Bärbel Czennia (ed.), *Celebrity: The Idiom of a Modern Era* (New York: AMS Press, 2013); Antoine Lilti, *Figures publiques: l'invention de la célébrité, 1750–1850* (Paris: Fayard, 2014). On the role of the visual in celebrity culture, see Joshua Gamson, *Claims to Fame: Celebrity in Contemporary America* (Berkeley: University of California Press, 1994), 17.

[51] Elizabeth Barry, 'Celebrity, Cultural Production and Public Life', *International Journal of Cultural Studies*, 11:3 (2008), 251–8 (citation p. 252).

[52] Ibid., 253.

[53] On Anna Morandi Manzolini, see Vittoria Ottani and Gabriella Giuliani-Piccari, 'L'opera di Anna Morandi Manzolini nella ceroplastica anatomica bolognese', in *Alma Mater Studiorum: La presenza femminile dal XVIII al XX secolo; Ricerche sul rapporto Donna/Cultura universitaria nell'Ateneo bolognese* (Bologna: CLUEB, 1988), 81–103; Messbarger, 'Waxing Poetic'; Messbarger, 'Re-Membering a Body of Work'; Messbarger, *The Lady Anatomist*; Jeanne Peiffer, 'L'âme, le cerveau et les mains: l'autoportrait d'Anna Morandi', in Thérèse Chotteau et al., *Rencontres entre artistes et mathématiciennes: Toutes un peu les autres* (Paris: Harmattan, 2001), 72–7; Ilaria Bianchi, 'Femminea natura degli studi sopra i cadaveri: L'arte della scienza di Anna Morandi Manzolini', *Annuario della scuola di specializzazione in storia dell'arte dell'Università di Bologna*, 3 (2002), 21–41; Dacome, 'Waxworks'; Dacome,

culture of demonstration that characterized eighteenth-century presentations of natural and anatomical knowledge to different audiences.[54] Less attention, however, has been drawn to how artisans' involvement in these spectacular performances turned some of them into cherished celebrities. The case of mid-eighteenth-century anatomical modellers is, in this sense, significant. This study considers how modellers were driven to the forefront of the anatomical world and became anatomical celebrities.[55] In a related manner, it examines how they navigated across anatomical, artistic, artisanal, religious, and antiquarian domains—and produced artistic and devotional objects as well as anatomical models—but became renowned thanks to their involvement in anatomical practice.

By the early eighteenth century, artists and anatomists had consolidated a common history of anatomical visualizations. As anatomical representation became an important means to support claims about anatomy's capacity to chart the human body, the training of the anatomist's eye required the proficiency of the artist's hand. For their part, artists needed anatomists too. Although the role of anatomy in art continued to stir controversy, many early modern artists espoused the principle that knowledge of the inner body allowed for an accurate representation of its surface. In fact, for all their reciprocation, artists and anatomists could find

'Women, Wax and Anatomy'; Lucia Dacome, '"Une dentelle très bien agencée et très precise": les femmes et l'anatomie dans l'Europe du dix-huitième siècle', in Adeline Gargam (ed.), *Femmes de science de l'Antiquité au XIXe siècle: Réalités et représentations* (Dijon: Editions Universitaires de Dijon, 2014), 157–75; Miriam Focaccia (ed.), *Anna Morandi Manzolini: Una donna fra arte e scienza; immagini, documenti, repertorio anatomico* (Florence: Leo S. Olschki, 2008); Rose Marie San Juan, 'The Horror of Touch: Anna Morandi's Wax Models of Hands', *Oxford Art Journal*, 34:3 (2011), 433–47; Rose Marie San Juan, 'Dying Not to See: Anna Morandi's Wax Model of the Sense of Sight', *Oxford Art Journal*, 36:1 (2013), 39–54. See also Marta Cavazza, 'Dottrici e lettrici dell'Università di Bologna nel Settecento', *Annali di Storia delle università italiane*, 1 (1997), esp. 120–2; Gabriella Berti Logan, 'Women and the Practice and Teaching of Medicine in Bologna in the Eighteenth and Early Nineteenth Centuries', *Bulletin of the History of Medicine*, 77:3 (2003), esp. 512–16; Jeanne Peiffer and Véronique Roca, 'Corps moulés, corps façonnés: Autoportraits de femmes', in Chotteau et al., *Rencontres*, 56–91; Jeanne Peiffer, 'La recherche dans et hors ses murs', *Cahiers art et science*, 7 (2002), 47–63. Contemporaries of Anna Morandi Manzolini used both her maiden name, Morandi, and her husband's surname, Manzolini, to refer to her. In what follows, I will use Morandi's own family name.

54 On the eighteenth-century culture of theatrical scientific demonstration, see, for instance, Simon Schaffer, 'Natural Philosophy and Public Spectacle in the Eighteenth Century', *History of Science*, 21:1 (1983), 1–43; Jan Golinski, 'A Noble Spectacle: Phosphorus and the Public Cultures of Science in the Early Royal Society', *Isis*, 80:1 (1989), 11–39; Jan Golinski, *Science as Public Culture: Chemistry and Enlightenment in Britain, 1760–1820* (Cambridge: Cambridge University Press, 1992); Larry Stewart, *The Rise of Public Science: Rhetoric, Technology, and Natural Philosophy in Newtonian Britain, 1600–1750* (Cambridge: Cambridge University Press, 1992); Geoffrey V. Sutton, *Science for a Polite Society: Gender, Culture, and the Demonstration of Enlightenment* (Boulder: Westview Press, 1995); Bernadette Bensaude-Vincent and Christine Blondel (eds.), *Science and Spectacle in the European Enlightenment* (Aldershot: Ashgate: 2008), Simon Werrett, *Fireworks: Pyrotechnic Arts and Sciences in European History* (Chicago: University of Chicago Press, 2010).

55 While I follow scholars' suggestion to distinguish between fame and celebrity, I depart slightly from Antoine Lilti's characterization of fame as posthumous and related to posterity. Rather, I maintain that in the case of mid-eighteenth-century anatomical modellers, their access to renown could be characterized in terms of both fame and celebrity: not only did modellers acquire fame thanks to their accomplishments, they became celebrities as they enjoyed special public exposure and were revered by adoring audiences. Accordingly, in this work I will use either term when referring to them, depending on the emphasis placed on one or the other aspect of renown enjoyed by the modellers. On Lilti's emphasis on the posthumous character of fame, see Lilti, *Figures publiques*, 12–14.

themselves sitting next to each other in front of the same anatomical specimen without necessarily agreeing on what they saw. As a consequence, anatomists who recruited artists to illustrate anatomy books frequently stressed the necessity of scrutinizing the artists' work.[56] The artists were not impressed. When, in the 1710s, the Bolognese artist Angelo Michele Cavazzoni (1672–1743) engaged in illustrating Giambattista Morgagni's *Adversaria anatomica*, he complained that the anatomist interfered over and over again with his work in order to modify or even erase his sketches. Although Cavazzoni drew truthfully what he saw, and depicted the parts of the cadavers that lay in front of him 'with the greatest exactitude', Morgagni seemed endlessly dissatisfied.[57] In the case of Cavazzoni, the hand of the artist was subordinated to the eye of the anatomist. Yet, when, in the mid-eighteenth century, the Bolognese artists Ercole Lelli (1702–1766), Giovanni Manzolini (1700–1755), and Anna Morandi joined the world of anatomy by making anatomical specimens, they not only enjoyed complete control over their creations but also rapidly leapt to fame. Being in charge of all the phases of production and display of anatomical models (i.e. anatomical dissection, modelling, display, and demonstration), they engaged in dramatic performances in which they showcased their anatomical knowledge and became protagonists of the grand spectacle of the body that lured and instructed both local and itinerant viewers.[58]

This study investigates this diversified world of anatomy. Highlighting the place of centrality occupied by artificers in anatomical modelling, it shifts attention from a traditional image of anatomy as an elite pursuit largely carried out by university-trained men to the artisanal dimension of anatomical practice. Moreover, it considers the forms of labour, occupational roles, practices, and skills of the practitioners who were involved in the production and use of the models. Literature on the place of artisans in the world of natural knowledge has identified in the eighteenth century a break in the tradition that viewed artisanal skill as integral to knowledge-making processes.[59] However, the history of mid-eighteenth-century anatomical modelling presents a situation in which artisans continued to be at the centre of the relationship between making and knowing. In order to explore this setting, I investigate the relationship between the place of anatomical modellers in the worlds of artificers and natural inquirers and the power and value of the models.

[56] On the relationship between early modern artists and anatomists, see, for instance, Kusukawa, *Picturing the Book of Nature*.

[57] See Biblioteca Comunale 'Aurelio Saffi' (Forlì), Fondo Morgagni, vol. 36, fols. 78r–v. See also Roberto Ciardi, 'L'anatomista e il pittore', in *Morgagni e l'iconografia anatomica tra '600 e '800* (Forlì: Comune di Forlì, 1982), 23. Cavazzoni's text was not published but became known in the anatomical world.

[58] See Dacome, 'Waxworks'.

[59] See, for instance, Pamela H. Smith, *The Body of the Artisan: Art and Experience in the Scientific Revolution* (Chicago: University of Chicago Press, 2004); Bert De Munck, 'Artisans, Products and Gifts: Rethinking the History of Material Culture in Early Modern Europe', *Past & Present*, 224:1 (2014), 39–74. On making and knowing in the pre-modern period, see also Pamela H. Smith and Benjamin Schmidt (eds.), *Making Knowledge in Early Modern Europe: Practices, Objects, and Texts, 1400–1800* (Chicago: University of Chicago Press, 2007); Pamela H. Smith, Amy R.W. Meyers, and Harold J. Cook (eds.), *Ways of Making and Knowing: The Material Culture of Empirical Knowledge* (Ann Arbor: University of Michigan Press, 2014).

Likewise, I examine how a female artificer like Anna Morandi became a protagonist of the early stages of anatomical modelling and a celebrity in her own right.

In recent years, Morandi's life and work have started to draw scholarly attention, and Rebecca Messbarger has completed a noteworthy biography of the famous modeller and anatomist.[60] While Messbarger's *The Lady Anatomist* highlights Morandi's place within the neglected heritage of the great women of science, in what follows I situate Morandi's activities in the tradition of early modern women who participated in practices of knowledge production through hands-on activities.[61] More specifically, I examine how Morandi addressed contemporary calls for women's participation in the anatomical world by reinterpreting the forms of know-how developed within an established tradition of female wax modellers. I approach Morandi's life in the context of a composite historical stage where the interplay of practices and spaces of knowledge, gender conventions, Grand Tour culture, and the emerging culture of celebrity, made it possible for a woman to gain renown and become a famous anatomical practitioner while complying with the codes of female conduct. In order to reconstruct how anatomy came to be fashioned as a realm of practice and knowledge that could not only accommodate women but also give them prominence and celebrity, I also analyse some of the features that enabled thinking about anatomical practice as a pursuit whose spaces, materials, and techniques could be characterized in gendered terms. For instance, I explore the relationship between claims to knowledge associated with anatomical modelling and situated practices that were largely associated with the realms of domesticity and maternity. I also consider how the culture of celebrity linked the making of public figures with the rise of curiosity about their personal lives and, in so doing, created forms of imagined intimacy between celebrities and their audiences.[62] Since women's personal lives were traditionally under public scrutiny, they occupied a special place within celebrity culture.[63] This study investigates how the making of Morandi's anatomical celebrity was articulated in a way that linked her public figure as an anatomical practitioner with her family life and even with her mothering body.

ENTANGLED LIVES

A significant number of the models considered in this work have survived to this day and continue to enjoy an impressive visual lure. In fact, their visual power is so

[60] Messbarger, *The Lady Anatomist.*

[61] See Elaine Leong, 'Making Medicines in the Early Modern Household', *Bulletin of the History of Medicine*, 82:1 (2008), 145–68; Alisha Rankin, *Panaceia's Daughters: Noblewomen as Healers in Early Modern Germany* (Chicago: University of Chicago Press, 2013); Sharon T. Strocchia (ed.), 'Women and Healthcare in Early Modern Europe', special issue, *Renaissance Studies*, 28:4 (2014); Meredith K. Ray, *Daughters of Alchemy: Women and Scientific Culture in Early Modern Italy* (Cambridge, MA: Harvard University Press, 2015).

[62] See Lilti, *Figures publiques*, 14–15.

[63] On women's participation in eighteenth-century celebrity culture, see Brock, *The Feminization of Fame*; Nussbaum, *Rival Queens*; Engel, *Fashioning Celebrity*; Czennia (ed.), *Celebrity*, part 2.

striking that it runs the risk of becoming historically blinding. As Nick Hopwood has observed in his discussion of the wax models of embryos from the Ziegler studio, 'the historical challenge' in the study of such objects 'is to get behind the finished products'.[64] Focusing on the making and early viewing of anatomical displays, this study addresses this challenge by investigating the networks of social interactions that shaped the models and their biographies, and that involved materials, spaces, techniques, skills, and visual vocabularies as well as makers, viewers, users, patrons, and collectors. Highlighting the inherent fluidity and mutability that characterized anatomical modelling, it explores the circumstances and contingencies that, in these early stages, contributed to transforming wax models of the body into proficient tools of corporeal knowledge. In order to do so, this work adopts a biographical approach that considers the entangled lives of the models and the people who were involved in their production and early use. Anatomical models often included actual bodily parts. As such, they complicate our understanding of projected boundaries between humans and non-humans. This is all the more the case if we consider that some of the anatomical specimens studied in this work were taken to stage revivified human bodies.

While considering the entangled lives of models, this work builds on the suggestion that things are enmeshed in networks of agency, and should be regarded as modes of world-making (rather than mere world-mirroring), which generate both effects and affects and ask viewers and users to engage with their demands.[65] The task of tracing the agency of things is notoriously daunting. Such an agency is difficult to locate and is ontologically slippery. Even Arjun Appadurai's and Igor Kopytoff's seminal insights into the 'social lives' of things have themselves become the object of scrutiny.[66] Yet, the study of the entangled lives of models and people, and the reconstruction of how they mutually constituted, affected, and transformed their biographical trajectories, can offer a felicitous point of entry into the

[64] Hopwood, *Embryos in Wax*, 2. On the study of past visual and material cultures, see Ludmilla Jordanova, *The Look of the Past: Visual and Material Evidence in Historical Practice* (Cambridge: Cambridge University Press, 2012).

[65] See Alfred Gell's classic *Art and Agency: An Anthropological Theory* (Oxford: Clarendon Press, 1998); Bruno Latour, *Reassembling the Social: An Introduction to Actor-Network-Theory* (Oxford: Oxford University Press, 2005); William J.T. Mitchell, *What Do Pictures Want? The Lives and Loves of Images* (Chicago: University of Chicago Press, 2005).

[66] See, for instance, Frank Trentmann, 'Materiality in the Future of History: Things, Practices, and Politics', special issue on Material Culture, *Journal of British Studies*, 48:2 (2009), 283–307. In 2002, Carl Knappett noticed that emphasis on social lives of things had become 'something of a mantra in material culture studies', and called for further inquiry into the processes whereby objects come to be socially alive; see Carl Knappett, 'Photographs, Skeuomorphs and Marionettes: Some Thoughts on Mind, Agency and Object', *Journal of Material Culture*, 7:1 (2002), 97–117 (citation p. 97). Later on, Jonathan Gil Harris pointed out that the view that things have social lives may be at risk of generating a 'linear understanding of the temporality of objects' that does not take into account that things inscribe multiple temporalities and bear the traces of different moments embedded in them; see Jonathan Gil Harris, *Untimely Matter in the Time of Shakespeare* (Philadelphia: University of Pennsylvania Press, 2009), esp. 8–9. However, as Jody Joy has observed, objects' biographies 'do not necessarily follow a linear pattern'. Rather, objects can have simultaneous lives and join and leave different webs of social relations. Likewise, the lives of things could extend 'over a series of human lifetimes' and are affected by shifting 'attitudes and perceptions of the past'; see Joy, 'Reinvigorating Object Biography', esp. 543–4.

complexity of anatomical models' own stories.[67] Whilst the meanings of the objects considered in this work have shifted at different points of their biographies, this study focuses on their historical entanglements at the time of their creation and early existence. It considers how the first communities of users and viewers who entered into contact with them participated in fashioning them as powerful tools of knowledge.[68] It concludes by drawing some attention to the circumstances that marked the close of this particular phase of their lives.[69]

In order to reconstruct the various aspects and specificities of the entangled lives of anatomical models, this study adopts a microhistorical approach that closely follows the threads of their intricate historical fabric. Accordingly, it embraces a reduced scale of historical observation, and privileges an in-depth investigation of smaller units of analysis to retrieve the voices, domains of experience, and social relations that accompanied the creation and early use of mid-eighteenth-century anatomical displays. The adoption of a biographical lens has characterized much microhistorical work, making it possible to retrieve the silenced voices of forgotten historical actors.[70] Extending this focus to things can sustain the effort to repopulate our histories with their entangled lives. Objects moulded lives as much as people modelled objects. As such, their stories allow us to reach out to historical actors who had limited access to other forms of expression, recording, and communication. In the case of the anatomical models considered in this work, the adoption of a biographical focus also provides a special point of entry into the specific conditions that determined these objects' capacity to create and convey

[67] On the entanglements of humans and non-humans see, for instance, Nicholas Thomas' classic *Entangled Objects: Exchange, Material Culture, and Colonialism in the Pacific* (Cambridge, MA: Harvard University Press, 1991); Ian Hodder, *Entangled: An Archaeology of the Relationships Between Humans and Things* (Oxford: Wiley Blackwell, 2012). On the notion of entanglement, see also, among others, Karen Barad, *Meeting the Universe Halfway: Quantum Physics and the Entanglement of Matter* (Durham: Duke University Press, 2007); Joan Steigerwald, 'The Subject as Instrument: Galvanic Experiments, Organic Apparatus and Problems of Calibration', in Erika Dyck and Larry Stewart (eds.), *The Uses of Humans in Experiment: Perspectives from the 17th to the 20th Century* (Leiden: Brill, forthcoming).

[68] While doing so, I draw on historians' emphasis on the significance of communities of readers as 'interpretive communities'; see, for instance, Roger Chartier, *The Order of Books: Readers, Authors and Libraries in Europe between the Fourteenth and the Eighteenth Centuries*, trans. Lydia C. Cochrane (Stanford: Stanford University Press, 1994), chapter 1.

[69] While historians of science have largely focused on the historical analysis of the production and use of scientific and medical objects, less attention has been devoted to understanding the different phases of objects' lives. Among the exceptions, see Simon Schaffer, 'Easily Cracked: Scientific Instruments in States of Disrepair', *Isis*, 102:4 (2011), 706–17; Simon Werrett, 'Recycling in Early Modern Science', *The British Journal for the History of Science*, 46:4 (2013), 627–46; Rina Knoeff and Robert Zwijnenberg (eds.), *The Fate of Anatomical Collections* (Farnham: Ashgate, 2015).

[70] The literature on microhistory is vast; see, for instance, Giovanni Levi, 'On Microhistory', in Peter Burke (ed.), *New Perspectives on Historical Writing*, 2nd edn. (Cambridge: Polity Press, 2001), 97–119; Edward Muir and Guido Ruggiero (eds.), *Microhistory and the Lost Peoples of Europe: Selections from Quaderni Storici* (Baltimore: Johns Hopkins University Press, 1991); Carlo Ginzburg, 'Microhistory: Two or Three Things That I Know About It', trans. John Tedeschi and Anne C. Tedeschi, *Critical Inquiry*, 20:1 (1993), 10–35; Francesca Trivellato, 'Is There a Future for Italian Microhistory in the Age of Global History?', *California Italian Studies*, 2:1 (2011), 1–26. For a discussion of microhistory in the history of the sciences, see Soraya de Chadarevian, 'Microstudies Versus Big Picture Accounts?', *Studies in History and Philosophy of Science, Part C: Studies in History and Philosophy of Biological and Biomedical Sciences*, 40:1 (2009), 13–19.

knowledge and the circumstances that made them subsequently slip into obsolescence. The result is an investigation of the role of artefacts in the production and communication of bodily knowledge, the relationship between local practices and anatomy's normative claims about human nature, the creation of distinctive relations between making and knowing, and the shaping of new audiences that, also thanks to the models, became responsive to the claims and promises of anatomical knowledge. Other stories may be told. The main protagonists of this story, the models, call for further narratives about other segments of their longer, entangled existences along with, and beyond, their visually luring and blinding power.

THE OUTLINE

This book largely unfolds chronologically. It takes its start from the project of an anatomy room at the Bolognese Institute of the Sciences, and charts the early development of anatomical modelling in Bologna, Naples, and Palermo. Each chapter has a specific analytical focus. Chapters 1 to 6 explore the different perspectives of commissioners, makers, viewers, and users in the context of Bolognese anatomical modelling, whereas Chapter 7 follows the echoes of Bolognese anatomical modelling to the southern Italian cities of Naples and Palermo. More specifically, Chapter 1 considers Prospero Lambertini's patronage of anatomy and anatomical modelling in Bologna and antiquarian displays in Rome. In particular, it situates Lambertini's support for anatomical displays in the context of his pursuits as an assessor of sanctity who saw in anatomy a powerful tool to discern the signs of holy embodiment. Shifting perspective from patrons to makers, Chapter 2 follows the circumstances underpinning the creation of an anatomy room at the Bolognese Institute of the Sciences and examines the occupational trajectory of Ercole Lelli, the artificer in charge of realizing its models. Reconstructing Lelli's multifaceted skills as an artisan, an artist, and a broker, it draws attention to how Lelli relied on his manual and artisanal skills to act as a go-between across artisanal, anatomical, artistic, and antiquarian domains, ultimately fashioning himself as a connoisseur. In a related manner, it considers the fashioning of the anatomy room as a site for the training of the eyes of surgeons, artists, and connoisseurs. Chapter 3 furthers the analysis of the place of modellers as protagonists of the mid-eighteenth-century world of anatomical modelling. In particular, it focuses on the anatomical practice of Anna Morandi and her husband Giovanni Manzolini, who together created a collection of anatomical waxworks in their home, and investigates the role of the domestic setting as a complex, multi-functional venue of anatomical pursuit, which was characterized by shifting boundaries between shared and secluded spaces of knowledge. Chapter 4 follows Anna Morandi's activities after the death of her husband, and reconstructs the setting in which she sought and obtained the patronage of Pope Benedict XIV. It situates Morandi's waxworks in the context of a diversified world of wax modelling that was characterized by patterns of continuity and discontinuity between devotional, artistic, and anatomical displays. Chapter 5 turns to the collection of midwifery models, which was gathered by the Bolognese surgeon and man-midwife Giovanni Antonio Galli (1708–1782), and was subsequently acquired by Pope Benedict XIV who donated it to the Institute of the Sciences. Shifting attention away from makers and viewers of anatomical models to hands-on users, this chapter reconstructs how the models' translations of embodied skill and tacit knowledge into the visual and material language of anatomy contributed to redefining midwives' realm of competence and expertise. While seeking to extract historical meaning out of the analysis of how models inscribed knowledge, it explores how midwifery models redefined the relationship between skill, knowledge, and expertise. Chapters 6 and 7 turn to collectors to investigate how anatomical models were subject to processes of valorization. More specifically, Chapter 6 considers the acquisition of Morandi's collection by the nobleman and senator Girolamo Ranuzzi and examines how her models served as testimonials that added value to Ranuzzi's undertakings. Chapter 7 similarly examines the role of anatomical models as cultural currencies capable of transferring value. It does so by adopting a comparative perspective that opens with the story of an anatomical skeleton that was supposed to travel from Palermo to Bologna but did not arrive at its destination, ending up in Raimondo di Sangro's Palace in Naples. By extending the study of the early stages of anatomical modelling to a new setting, this chapter complements previous chapters by highlighting how geography and locality played an important part in shaping mid-eighteenth-century anatomical modelling. Moreover, it draws attention to aspects of anatomical modelling that were common to the various collections and yet locally defined, such as the role of diverse audiences and Grand Tour spectacle in shaping the culture of anatomical displays, the link between claims to knowledge and techniques of visualization, shifting views of the natural and the artificial, and the processes of valorization that were incidental to the fashioning anatomical displays as privileged sites of bodily knowledge.

1

Prospero's Tools

'MAGNUS IN FOLIO, PARVUS IN SOLIO'

Prospero Lambertini's key role in the development of anatomical modelling has often been read in the context of the fashioning of his persona as a savant. Lambertini—Pope Benedict XIV—was remembered by his contemporaries as a learned man who had little patience with government.[1] In both visual and verbal settings, Lambertini's historical memory has accordingly been associated with his scholarly activities. On the dilapidated statue *Il Pasquino*, which since the sixteenth century had become a popular site in Rome for displaying notes that lampooned the Church and the aristocracy, the people of Rome mocked his pontificate as 'magnus in folio, parvus in solio' ('big on paper, small on the throne').[2] Lambertini himself was frequently portrayed with a pen in his hand. Notably, in 1740, just before becoming pope, he was depicted by the Bolognese artist Giuseppe Maria Crespi holding a pen in one hand, while seemingly tearing a page with the other, perhaps from the manuscript of his work on beatification and canonization, his *De servorum Dei beatificatione et canonizatione beatorum* (1734–8) (Plate 3). The work had been published a few years earlier, and marked his career as an author and a clergyman. A number of illustrations similarly represented Lambertini in the act of writing. In one illustration, he is portrayed as busily writing while the symbols of the pontificate stand right behind him as if waiting for him to finish (Figure 1.1). In another picture, Lambertini is caught in the act of writing his way to St Peter's Basilica while seemingly receiving divine approval (Figure 1.2). Finally, he is depicted as wielding a pen in the image that was also to appear in the frontispiece of the Italian translation of his biography by Louis-Antoine Caraccioli (Figure 1.3).

Such portraits of the writing pope fit well with Lambertini's historical representation as a *pape savant* and a patron of knowledge, a portrayal that has also been established through a whole repertoire of quotations that included words of praise from savants such as Voltaire (who dedicated his play *Mahomet* to him), Montesquieu (who called him 'a learned man who befriended the learned'), and

[1] Louis-Antoine Caraccioli, *The Life of Pope Clement XIV (Ganganelli). Translated from the French* (London: J. Johnson and J.P. Coghlan, 1776), 75.

[2] Emilia Morelli, *Tre profili: Benedetto XIV, Pasquale Stanislao Mancini, Pietro Roselli* (Rome: Edizioni dell'Ateneo, 1955), 3. On *Il Pasquino*, see Francis Haskell and Nicholas Penny, *Taste and the Antique: The Lure of Classical Sculpture, 1500–1900*, 5th edn. (New Haven: Yale University Press, 1998 [1981]), esp. 291–6.

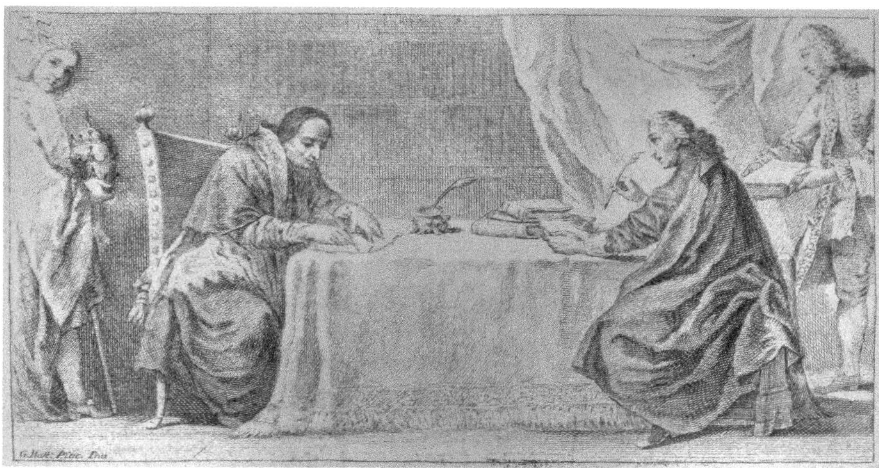

Figure 1.1 Prospero Lambertini (Pope Benedict XIV) portrayed in the act of writing, apparently taking notes over the course of a consultation with a learned man while the symbols of the pontificate are waiting for him, in *SS. Domini nostri Benedicti XIV Dissertationes in omni doctrinae genere selectissimae ex quatuor ejusdem auctoris de Canonizatione Sanctorum libris extractae*..., Venice: Joannes Baptista Albritius, 1751–2, vol. 2, 5.

Montfaucon (who described him as having two souls: one for science and one for society).[3]

Accounts of Lambertini's election to the pontificate equally draw attention to his knowledgeable wit. As the story has it, Lambertini addressed the conclave after months of extended infighting and under the increasing pressure of the summer heat in the following terms: 'Eh! Why should we spend our time discussing and searching? If you want a saint, nominate Gotti; a politician, Aldrovandi; a good man, choose me'—and so he was elected.[4] Drawing attention to Lambertini's personality and humour as crucial features in his being regarded as *papabile* (suitable to become pope), this anecdote took no account of the power games and the instances of infighting and negotiation that resulted in the election of Lambertini as a compromise.[5] Yet, the story became one of the landmarks of the making of

[3] Quotations from Ludwig Freiherr von Pastor, *The History of the Popes: From the Close of the Middle Ages; Drawn from the Secret Archives of the Vatican and Other Original Sources*, trans. E.F. Peeler, vol. 35 (London: Routledge and Kegan Paul, 1949), 205–8, 225, and 486–7. See also Franco Venturi, *Settecento riformatore: Da Muratori a Beccaria*, 2nd edn., vol. 1 (Turin: Einaudi, 1998 [1969]), 109ff. As late as 1970, Renée Haynes' monograph on Lambertini was significantly entitled *Philosopher King*; see Renée Haynes, *Philosopher King: The Humanist Pope Benedict XIV* (London: Weidenfield and Nicolson, 1970). Earlier in the twentieth century, the image of Lambertini as a savant was also reflected in a 'historical comedy' written by the Bolognese playwright Alfredo Testoni, in which Lambertini's knowledgeable wit became an emblem of the spirit of his native city of Bologna; see Alfredo Testoni, *Il cardinale Lambertini: Commedia storica in cinque atti con note* (Bologna: Zanichelli, 1906).

[4] Louis-Antoine de Caraccioli, *Éloge historique de Benoît XIV* (Liège: J. Fr. Bassompière, 1766), 31–3.

[5] On Lambertini's election to the pontificate, see Mario Rosa, *Riformatori e ribelli nel '700 religioso italiano* (Bari: Edizioni Dedalo, 1969), 53–4; Von Pastor, *The History of the Popes*, vol. 35, 1–23.

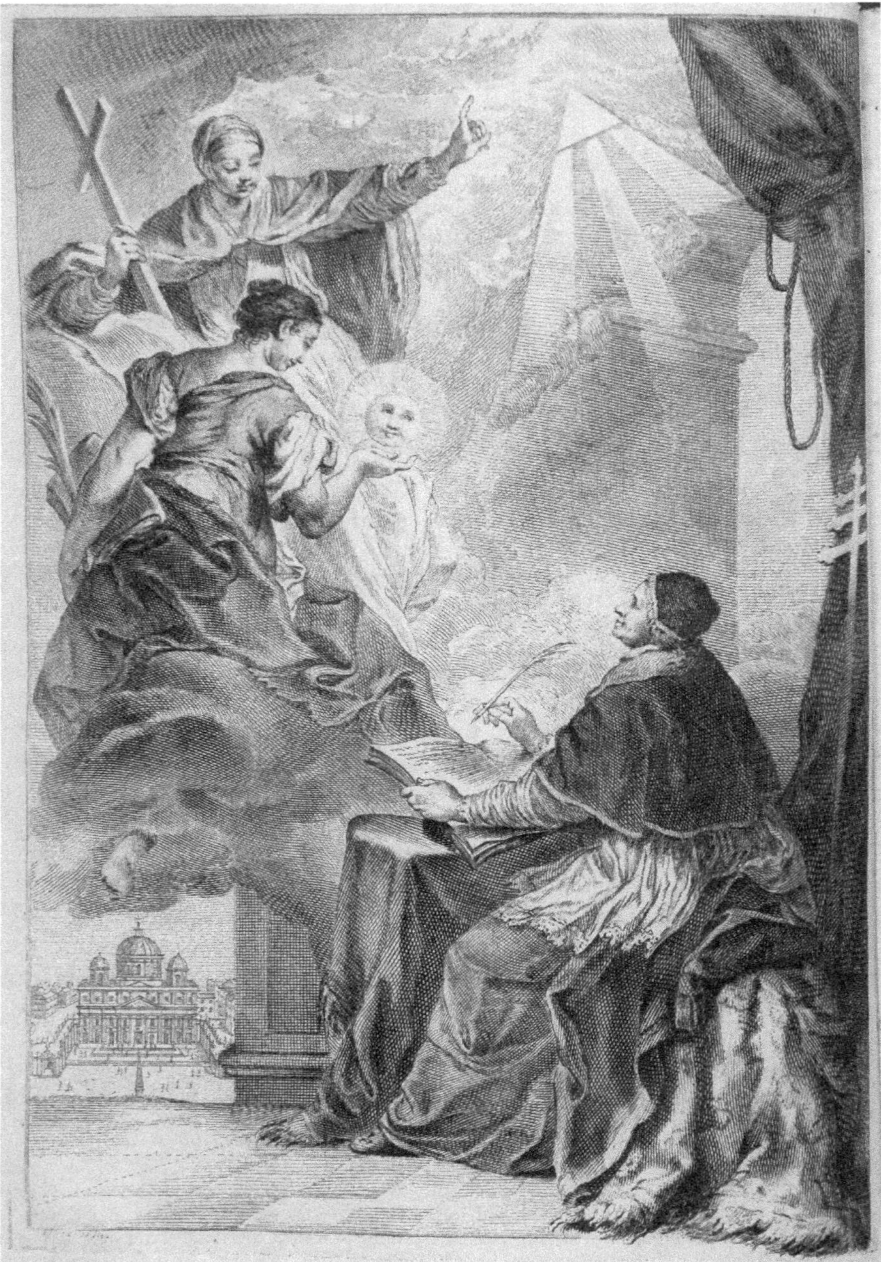

Figure 1.2 Prospero Lambertini (Pope Benedict XIV) portrayed in the act of writing his way to St Peter, in *SS. Domini nostri Benedicti XIV Dissertationes in omni doctrinae genere selectissimae ex quatuor ejusdem auctoris de Canonizatione Sanctorum libris extractae*..., Venice: Joannes Baptista Albritius, 1751–2, vol. 1, frontispiece.

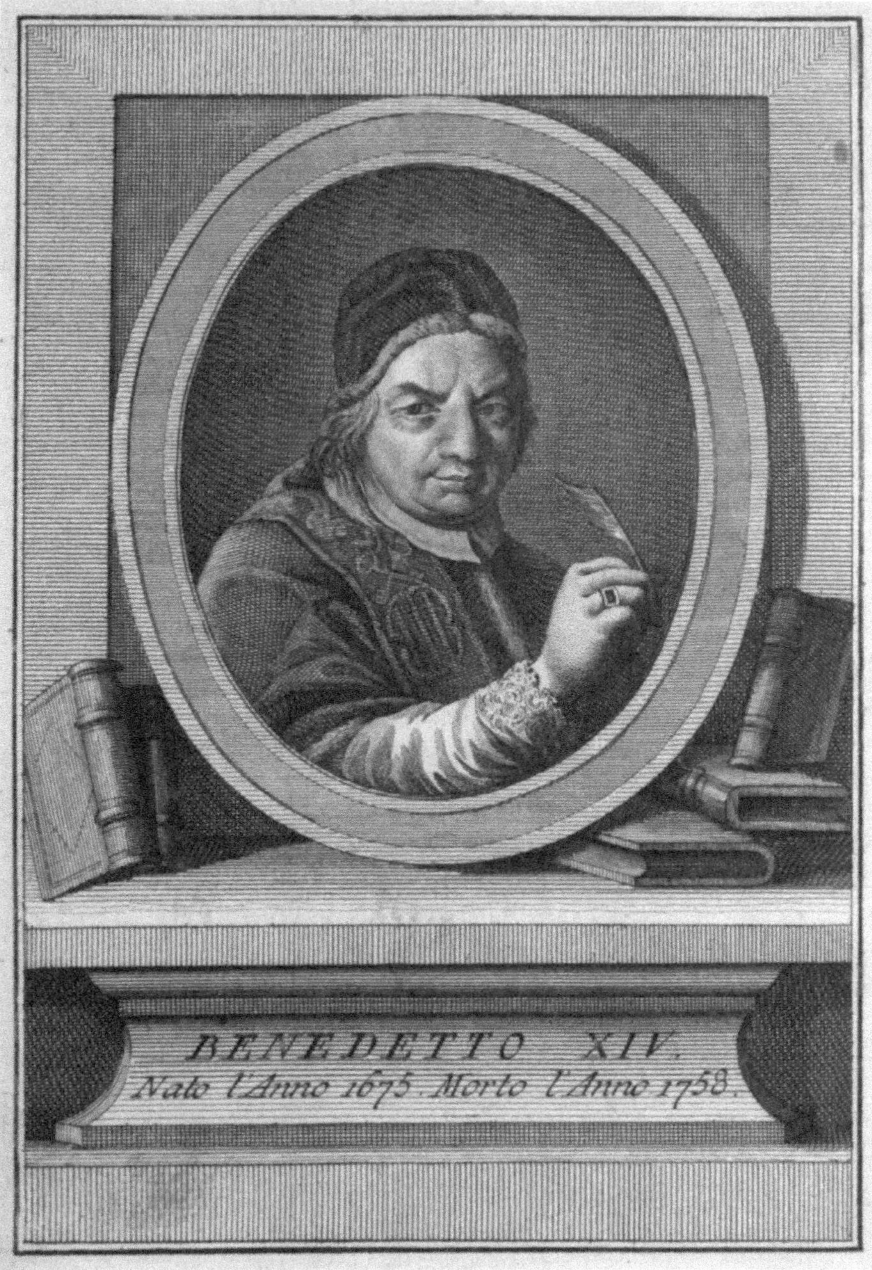

Figure 1.3 Portrait of Prospero Lambertini (Pope Benedict XIV) depicted as wielding a pen in the frontispiece of Louis-Antoine Caraccioli's *Vita del papa Benedetto XIV*, trans. from French, Venice: Simone Occhi, 1783, frontispiece.

Lambertini's public persona. Four days after Lambertini's election to the papacy, the English poet Thomas Gray recorded the episode in a letter to his mother. Gray was then in Florence, travelling on the Grand Tour together with Horace Walpole, and regretted not being in Rome for the coronation of the new pope. As the news of the papal election reached him, Gray reported to his mother that, in his address to the conclave, Lambertini called himself 'a Booby'—but the Italian version (*coglione*), was 'much more expressive and, indeed, not to be translated'; Gray graciously refrained from doing so.[6] In the 1750s, the writer Horace Walpole, son of the former British Prime Minister Sir Robert Walpole, dedicated a poem to Lambertini in which he presented the pope as 'beloved by Papists' and 'esteemed by Protestants'.[7] He also called him 'a Priest, without insolence or interestedness; a Prince, without Favourites; a Pope, without Nepotism; an Author, without Vanity'.[8]

Lambertini's engagement in patronage activities has traditionally been read within the framework established by this image of a learned man, a witty savant, and a conciliatory and moderate pope who was scarcely interested in the privileges and prerogatives proverbially enjoyed by the pontiff. Celebrated as a reformer, a patron of learned women, a supporter of learning and natural inquiry, and a benevolent sovereign, Lambertini has been singled out as a champion of 'the Catholic Enlightenment'. Since the late 1960s, when Bernard Plongeron called for an in-depth study of the dissemination of Enlightenment values in Catholic circles across Europe, the expression 'the Catholic Enlightenment' has been used as an umbrella term referring to various calls for reform, including the promotion of new approaches to natural knowledge within the framework of Catholicism.[9] Providing 'a useful interpretative key to a complex phenomenon that characterized the Christian world in the age of Enlightenment', the expression has been used as convenient shorthand for a diversified movement that purportedly marked a sense of discontinuity with Counter-Reformation orthodoxy.[10] Likewise, Lambertini's role as an advocate of the renewal of liturgy and of the reform of certain devotional

[6] Thomas Gray, *Correspondence of Thomas Gray*, eds. Paget Toynbee and Leonard Whibley, vol. 1 (Oxford: Clarendon, 1935), 173–4 (citations p. 174).

[7] Horace Walpole, *Fugitive Pieces in Verse and Prose* (Strawberry-Hill: n.p., 1758), 218.

[8] Ibid.

[9] The expression 'Catholic Enlightenment' was introduced by Sebastian Merkle in the early twentieth century; see Ulrich L. Lehner, 'Introduction', in Ulrich L. Lehner and Michael Printy (eds.), *A Companion to the Catholic Enlightenment in Europe* (Leiden: Brill, 2010), 3–4. On the Catholic Enlightenment see, for instance, Bernard Plongeron, 'Recherches sur l' "Aufklärung" catholique en Europe occidentale (1770–1830)', *Revue d'histoire moderne et contemporaine*, 16:4 (1969), 555–605; Jeffrey D. Burson and Ulrich L. Lehner (eds.), *Enlightenment and Catholicism in Europe: A Transnational History* (South Bend, IN: Notre Dame University Press, 2014). On the Catholic Enlightenment in the Italian context, see Bernard Plongeron, 'Questions pour l'Aufklärung catholique en Italie', *Il Pensiero Politico: Rivista di Storia delle Idee Politiche e Sociali*, 3:1 (1970), 30–58; Claudio Manzoni, *Il 'cattolicesimo illuminato' in Italia, tra cartesianismo, leibnizismo e newtonismo-lockismo nel primo Settecento (1700–1750): Note di ricerca sulla recente storiografia* (Trieste: Lint, 1992); Mario Rosa, 'Introduzione all'*Aufklärung* cattolica in Italia', in Rosa (ed.), *Cattolicesimo e lumi nel Settecento italiano* (Rome: Herder, 1981), 1–47; Mario Rosa, *Settecento religioso: Politica della ragione e religione del cuore* (Venice: Marsilio, 1999), 116–18 and 149–84; Mario Rosa, 'The Catholic *Aufklärung* in Italy', in Lehner and Printy (eds.), *A Companion to the Catholic Enlightenment in Europe*, 215–50, esp. 215–18.

[10] See Rosa, *Settecento religioso*, 149–84 (citation p. 149); Rosa, 'The Catholic *Aufklärung*'.

practices, his patronage of natural knowledge and anatomical collections, and his support for women who dedicated themselves to natural inquiry, have garnered him a reputation as a prominent figure of the Catholic Enlightenment: 'the Enlightenment Pope'.[11] Not everybody, however, has espoused such a reading. Nuancing the portrayal of Lambertini as a reformer, some scholars have rather stressed the continuity with post-Tridentine values and concerns that characterized his policies and, to some extent, his own reforms.[12] In doing so, they have challenged the picture of the Enlightenment Pope.

This chapter builds on these suggestions to examine Lambertini's patronage of anatomy in the context of his long-term engagement as an assessor of sanctity. In particular, it situates Lambertini's support for anatomy and anatomical displays within the broader historical canvas of post-Tridentine uses of anatomical knowledge as a form of evidence in the process of appraisal and authentication of sanctity.[13] While the complexities underpinning Lambertini's political and cultural course of action and his attitude towards the arts have been the object of scholarly attention, his patronage of visual and material cultures of natural and anatomical knowledge has traditionally been construed in the context of his portrayal as the Enlightenment Pope.[14] In what follows, I suggest reading Lambertini's patronage of anatomical displays against the backdrop of the anatomical interests that he cultivated as part of his long-lasting involvement in the definition of the procedural aspects of saint-making.[15] In particular, I argue that by supporting anatomical collections Lambertini could present and communicate important facets of his *De servorum Dei*—his *magnum opus* on the criteria and procedures that governed beatification and canonization—by other means. Not only did anatomical models unveil the

[11] See, for instance, Giuseppe Cenacchi, 'Benedetto XIV e l'Illuminismo', in Marco Cecchelli (ed.), *Benedetto XIV (Prospero Lambertini): Convegno internazionale di studi storici,* vol. 2 (Cento: Centro Studi G. Baruffaldi, 1981–2), 1077–102; Massimo Mazzotti, 'Maria Gaetana Agnesi: Mathematics and the Making of the Catholic Enlightenment', *Isis*, 92:4 (2001), 657–83; Massimo Mazzotti, *The World of Maria Gaetana Agnesi, Mathematician of God* (Baltimore: Johns Hopkins University Press, 2007); Messbarger, *The Lady Anatomist*, esp. chapter 1. A volume edited by Rebecca Messbarger, Christopher M.S. Johns, and Philip Gavitt, and titled *Benedict XIV and the Enlightenment: Art, Science, and Spirituality* (Toronto: University of Toronto Press, 2016) was published when this book was in production and, to my regret, I have been unable to take it into consideration.

[12] See, for instance, Simon Ditchfield, 'Il mondo della Riforma e della Controriforma', in Anna Benvenuti et al. (eds.), *Storia della santità nel cristianesimo occidentale* (Rome: Viella, 2005), 261–329; Elisabeth Garms-Cornides, 'Storia, politica e apologia in Benedetto XIV: Alle radici della reazione cattolica', in Philippe Koeppel (ed.), *Papes et papauté au XVIIIe siècle: VIe colloque franco-italien; Société française d'étude du XVIIIe siècle, Université de Savoie, Chambéry, 21–22 septembre 1995* (Paris: Honoré Champion, 1999), 145–61; Dacome, 'The Anatomy of the Pope'; Dacome, 'Ai confini del mondo naturale'. For a review of the literature on Lambertini, see Maria Teresa Fattori, 'Introduzione', in Maria Teresa Fattori (ed.), *Le fatiche di Benedetto XIV: Origine ed evoluzione dei trattati di Prospero Lambertini (1675–1758)* (Rome: Edizioni di Storia e Letteratura, 2011), xiv–xxiv.

[13] On the relationship between Lambertini's interest in anatomy, and especially his patronage of anatomical collections, and his involvement in the saint-making process, see Dacome, 'The Anatomy of the Pope'; Dacome, 'Ai confini del mondo naturale'.

[14] On Lambertini's patronage of the arts, see, for instance, Donatella Biagi Maino (ed.), *Benedetto XIV e le arti del disegno: Convegno internazionale di studi di storia dell'arte, Bologna 28–30 novembre 1994* (Rome: Quasar, 1998); Donatella Biagi Maino, 'Arte, scienza e potere: Le risoluzioni di Benedetto XIV per le istituzioni accademiche bolognesi', in Koeppel (ed.), *Papes et papauté*, 27–50.

[15] See Dacome, 'The Anatomy of the Pope'; Dacome, 'Ai confini del mondo naturale'.

inner body for medical practitioners, artists, and lay viewers, they also staged, mediated, and publicized the body of knowledge that was deployed in the delicate task of evaluating the evidence that informed the saint-making process. As such, anatomical models ended up being fashioned as markers of the natural world, and powerful mediators of human nature. I furthermore explore Lambertini's patronage of anatomical displays in light of the peculiar squaring of eighteenth-century approaches to anatomical and antiquarian display with established tenets and dogmas of the Church. In particular, I suggest viewing Lambertini's patronage of collections of anatomical models in Bologna and Christian antiquities in Rome in the context of post-Tridentine concerns about the cult of saints and relics, the vexed question of the definition of the borders of the natural world, and the pontiff's claims of authority and jurisdiction over both the temporal and the spiritual realms.

NEW POPE AND NOVEL PATRON

Lambertini's career as a patron largely coincided with his life as a pope. Although he belonged to an old and established family within the Bolognese aristocracy, by the eighteenth century the Lambertinis were neither particularly powerful nor especially affluent. In this sense, Lambertini's pontificate broke with a long-established tradition according to which the choice of a pope reflected the aspirations of one of the leading Italian families, and, accordingly, perpetuated a distinctively patrician form of patronage.[16] As members of the old and powerful Orsini and Corsini families, Lambertini's predecessors Benedict XIII and Clement XII had carried on this tradition.[17] Conversely, as the descendant of a family that had lost its fortune, Lambertini had to wait to become pope before he could act as a patron. This is not to say that he did not participate in patronage networks before he ascended to the papal throne. Notably, he acted as a broker in the project to create an anatomy room at the Bolognese Institute of the Sciences—a project that he generously sponsored after becoming pope (Plate 4).

A born and bred Bolognese, Lambertini was educated by the Somascan Fathers at the Collegium Clementinum in Rome. In 1694, he graduated in theology and

[16] See Paolo Prodi, *The Papal Prince: One Body and Two Souls. The Papal Monarchy in Early Modern Europe*, trans. Susan Haskins (Cambridge: Cambridge University Press, 1987); Paolo Prodi, 'Carità e galateo: La figura di papa Lambertini nelle lettere al marchese Paolo Magnani (1743–1748)', in Cecchelli (ed.), *Benedetto XIV (Prospero Lambertini)*', 445–71. On early modern papal patronage of medicine and natural knowledge, see, for instance, Elena Brambilla, 'La medicina del Settecento: Dal monopolio dogmatico alla professione scientifica', in Franco della Peruta (ed.), *Storia d'Italia, Annali 7: Malattia e medicina* (Turin: Einaudi, 1984), esp. 46–53; Richard Palmer, 'Medicine at the Papal Court in the Sixteenth Century', in Vivian Nutton (ed.), *Medicine at the Courts of Europe, 1500–1837* (London: Routledge, 1990), 49–78; Findlen, *Possessing Nature*, 349–50; Silvia De Renzi, 'Medical Competence, Anatomy and the Polity in Seventeenth-Century Rome', *Renaissance Studies*, 21:4 (2007), 551–7; Donato and Kraye (eds.), *Conflicting Duties*.

[17] Lambertini's own election to the pontificate followed the Corsini family's failure to maintain its grip on the papacy; see Rosa, *Riformatori e ribelli*, 53–4.

civil and canon law at the University of La Sapienza, and in 1702 he was appointed Consistorial Advocate under the auspices of Pope Clement XI. In 1708, he became promoter of faith for the Congregation of Rites, a juridical body deliberating in matters of liturgy in general, and of beatification and canonization specifically. Between 1718 and 1728, he then acted as secretary of the Congregation of the Council.[18] After becoming the titular archbishop of Theodosia and serving for a period as the archbishop of Ancona, in 1731 Lambertini returned to his hometown as its cardinal and archbishop. Even before then, he had manifested his interest in supporting the Bolognese Institute of the Sciences. As early as 1718, a few years after the Institute's opening, Lambertini expressed his approval for the initiative, which he considered one of the highlights of Bologna, and expressed the hope that he would one day be able to help.[19] Shortly after returning to his native city, he started to visit the Institute on a regular basis. As we saw in the Introduction, during one of these visits he came across two wax models of kidneys made by the artificer Ercole Lelli for the public dissector Lorenzo Bonazzoli and remained deeply impressed (Plate 1).[20] The models had been created after Bonazzoli had found a large anomalous, 'horseshoe' kidney during dissection and reported it to the Academy of the Sciences, which was part of the Institute of the Sciences.[21] The case was considered well worth a visual record. Ercole Lelli was then commissioned to make a cast in wax of the specimen, and to complete two anatomical models displaying both a normally shaped kidney and the horseshoe one, as well as a drawing of the latter.[22] Offering a comparison between a regular and an anomalous kidney, the models encouraged viewers to visually appraise their anatomical differences.[23] Upon seeing them hanging on the Institute's walls, not only did Lambertini launch the idea of an anatomical museum at the Institute of the Sciences, he also became personally involved in its realization. Thanks to his initiative, by the end of 1732 an anatomy room was under construction.[24] The affluent senator Niccolò Aldrovandi was to provide the means to support the initiative and the

[18] See Mario Rosa, 'Benedetto XIV', *Dizionario biografico degli italiani* (*DBI*), vol. 8 (Rome: Istituto della Enciclopedia Italiana, 1966), 393–408; Maria Teresa Fattori, 'Cronologia della vita e delle opera di Prospero Lambertini', in Maria Teresa Fattori (ed.), *Le fatiche di Benedetto XIV*, lv–lxvi. See also Caraccioli, *Éloge historique de Benoît XIV*, 8–9.

[19] ASB, Assunteria d'Istituto, Lettere all'Istituto, n. 2 (1715–24), Letter of 23 July 1718 from Prospero Lambertini in Rome; quoted in Cavazza, *Settecento inquieto*, 235.

[20] Zanotti, 'De anatome in Institutum introducenda', 44.

[21] ASB, Assunteria d'Istituto, Atti, n. 3 (1727–34), 630–2.

[22] Ibid. On Ercole Lelli see, for instance, Michele Medici, 'Elogio d'Ercole Lelli', in *Memorie della Accademia delle scienze dell'Istituto di Bologna*, vol. 7 (Bologna: San Tommaso d'Aquino, 1856), 157–86; Anna Maria Bertoli Barsotti, 'La figura di Ercole Lelli e la nascita del Museo Anatomico', in Raffaele A. Bernabeo (ed.), *Atti del XXXI Congresso internazionale di Storia della Medicina; Bologna, 30 agosto–4 settembre 1988* (Bologna: Monduzzi Editore, 1990), 57–64; C. Forlani, 'Gli strumenti di Ercole Lelli: Analisi storico-comparativa', ibid., 107–14. Susanna Falabella, 'Ercole Lelli', *Dizionario Biografico degli Italiani*, vol. 64 (2005), 332–5.

[23] Francesco Maria Zanotti, 'De iis, quae Instituto jam condito adjuncta sunt', in *De Bononiensi Scientiarum et Artium Instituto atque Academia Commentarii*, vol. 1 (Bologna: Lelio dalla Volpe, 1731), 29.

[24] ASB, Assunteria d'Istituto, Diversorum, busta 10, n. 1, 'Proposte per Statue Anatomiche'. See also Zanotti, 'De anatome in Institutum introducenda', 44.

artist Ercole Lelli the craft.[25] Aldrovandi's untimely death, however, meant that the project was left incomplete and was put on hold until Lambertini relaunched it in 1742, two years after becoming pope.[26]

THE BODY OF THE CHURCH

Lambertini's initial support for the creation of an anatomy room at the Institute of the Sciences was just the beginning of a series of episodes in which he would manifest his interest in anatomical practice. In January 1737, for instance, he famously issued a notification (*Notificazione*) in which he presented the position of the Catholic Church on the subject of anatomy carried out in the university (*pubbliche Scuole*).[27] This notification conveyed Lambertini's reading of Boniface VIII's famous papal bull of 1299, *Detestandae feritatis abusum*, which classed certain practices of dissection, dismemberment, and exhumation as unlawful, and threatened excommunication for those who engaged in them. While some had interpreted Boniface's bull as condemning anatomical dissections altogether, Lambertini maintained that it was not really directed against the study of anatomy. Rather, it targeted the exhumation, disembowelling, and dismemberment of corpses and the boiling of human remains, namely, the practices that had become frequent at the time of the Crusades in order to facilitate distant burial.[28] In fact, Lambertini noticed, after Boniface issued the bull, the study of anatomy continued to be carried out successfully in universities, especially in Bologna.[29] Notably, in his *Anatomia*, which was completed some seventeen years after Boniface's bull, the famous Bolognese anatomist Mondino de' Liuzzi (*c.*1270–1326) admitted having stopped cutting and boiling heads—a practice that allowed for the visualization of the small parts of the ear—out of fear of excommunication. But he also mentioned having dissected two corpses. Thus, although the bull may have partially affected anatomical practice, it did not substantially interfere with its exercise. As Katharine Park has suggested: 'from all available evidence, Boniface's bull and letter were taken as irrelevant by generations of Italian medical professors, private doctors, judges, city councils, and even by later popes, several of whom were themselves embalmed'.[30]

[25] Zanotti, 'De anatome in Institutum introducenda'. See also Medici, 'Elogio d'Ercole Lelli', 173; Bertoli Barsotti, 'La figura di Ercole Lelli e la nascita del Museo Anatomico'.

[26] The details of Lambertini's initiative in 1742 are discussed in Chapter 2.

[27] Prospero Lambertini, 'Sopra la Notomia da farsi nelle pubbliche Scuole …', in *Raccolta di alcune notificazioni, editti, ed istruzioni pubblicate dall'Eminentissimo, e Reverendissimo Signor Cardinale Prospero Lambertini […] pel buon governo della sua diocesi*, vol. 3 (Bologna: Longhi, 1737), 263–8. On Lambertini's notification on anatomy, see Giovanni Martinotti, *Prospero Lambertini (Benedetto XIV) e lo studio dell'anatomia in Bologna* (Bologna: Cooperativa Tipografica Azzoguidi, 1911).

[28] Martinotti, *Prospero Lambertini*, 5–8.

[29] Lambertini, 'Sopra la Notomia'.

[30] See Katharine Park, 'The Criminal and the Saintly Body: Autopsy and Dissection in Renaissance Italy', *Renaissance Quarterly*, 47:1 (1994), 1–33, esp. 10–11 (citation p. 11). See also Katharine Park, 'The Life of the Corpse: Division and Dissection in Late Medieval Europe', *Journal of the History of Medicine and Allied Sciences*, 50: 1 (1995), 111–32; Andrea Carlino, *Books of the Body: Anatomical Ritual and Renaissance Learning*, trans. Anne Tedeschi and John A. Tedeschi (Chicago: University of

Historians of early modern anatomy have equally reappraised the view that Boniface's bull marked anatomy with a particular stigma, and purportedly reflected the Church's stance with regard to the inviolability and integrity of the corpse. They have also noticed how the tradition of sacred anatomy—which was based on the anatomical dissection of individuals who died 'in odour of sanctity' to look for the presence of divine signs in their bodies—long remained a feature of the cult of saints, playing an important part in the relationship between the Church and the medical world.[31] By the time Lambertini issued his notification on 'anatomy in the public schools', the clergy had itself been included among the audiences of anatomical rituals such as the Bolognese public anatomy lesson, which provided a critical stage for the consolidation of medical, civic, and religious powers.[32] As the chief ecclesiastical authority in Bologna, Lambertini himself was no stranger to such rituals. A famous *Insignia degli Anziani* of 1734 visually records his presence in the Bolognese anatomical theatre at the time in which the natural philosopher Laura Bassi (1711–1778)—a recipient of his patronage—made a dramatic appearance in the dissection pit (Plate 5).[33] Portrayed in his characteristic red cardinal's attire on the left-hand side of the picture, here Lambertini stands out among the attendees of the event in the theatre's gallery while sitting next to the Cardinal Legate.

Apart from clarifying the position of the Church in relation to Boniface's bull, Lambertini's notification on anatomy addressed the issue of access to cadavers. In particular, it contained the terms of, as it were, a new contract offered by Lambertini

Chicago Press, 1999), 182–3; Rafael Mandressi, *Le regard de l'anatomiste: Dissections et invention du corps en Occident* (Paris: Éditions du Seuil, 2003), 20ff; Andrew Cunningham, *The Anatomist Anatomis'd: An Experimental Discipline in Enlightenment Europe* (Farnham: Ashgate, 2010), 12–15.

31 See Nancy G. Siraisi, 'Signs and Evidence: Autopsy and Sanctity in Late Sixteenth-Century Italy', in *Medicine and the Italian Universities, 1250–1600* (Leiden: Brill, 2001), 356–80; Gianna Pomata, 'Malpighi and the Holy Body: Medical Experts and Miraculous Evidence in Seventeenth-Century Italy', *Renaissance Studies*, 21:4 (2007), 568–86; Park, *Secrets of Women*; Elisa Andretta 'Anatomie du Vénérable dans la Rome de la Contre-réforme: Les autopsies d'Ignace de Loyola et de Philippe Neri', in Donato and Kraye (eds.), *Conflicting Duties*, 275–300.

32 Ferrari, 'Public Anatomy Lessons'. On the ritual character of early modern anatomical dissection, see Carlino, *Books of the Body*; Andrew Cunningham, 'The End of the Sacred Ritual Anatomy', *Canadian Bulletin of Medical History*, 18:2 (2001), 187–204; Cynthia Klestinec, *Theaters of Anatomy: Students, Teachers, and Traditions of Dissection in Renaissance Venice* (Baltimore: Johns Hopkins University Press, 2011), esp. 17–18.

33 Realized between 1530 and 1796, the *Insignia degli Anziani* provide a unique visual archive of the city's life. Each *Insignia* depicted the most important event that had occurred during the two-month tenure of the city's council of the *Anziani* and chief magistrate (*gonfaloniere di giustizia*); see Giuseppe Plessi (ed.), *Le Insignia degli anziani del comune dal 1530 al 1796: Catalogo–Inventario*, (Rome: Ministero dell'Interno/Pubblicazioni degli Archivi di Stato, 1954). On Laura Bassi, see, for instance, Paula Findlen, 'Science as a Career in Enlightenment Italy: The Strategies of Laura Bassi', *Isis*, 84:3 (1993), 441–69; Paula Findlen, 'The Scientist's Body: The Nature of a Woman Philosopher in Enlightenment Italy', in Lorraine Daston and Gianna Pomata (eds.), *The Faces of Nature in Enlightenment Europe* (Berlin: BWV-Berliner Wissenschafts-Verlag, 2003), 211–36; Gabriella Berti Logan, 'The Desire to Contribute: An Eighteenth-Century Italian Woman of Science', *The American Historical Review*, 99:3 (1994), 785–812; Beate Ceranski, *'Und sie fürchtet sich vor niemandem'. Die Physikerin Laura Bassi (1711–1778)* (Frankfurt: Campus, 1996); Cavazza, 'Dottrici e lettrici'; Marta Cavazza, 'Laura Bassi', *Bologna Science Classics Online*, http://cis.alma.unibo.it/cis13b/bsco3/bassi/bassinotbyed/bassinotbyed.pdf.

to the medical faculty.[34] Much as the public performance of anatomical dissection conveyed moral, religious, and political messages as well as bodily knowledge, the violation of bodily integrity and honour in public anatomy lessons traditionally revolved around the dissection of executed criminals. But executions were not frequent; and the statutes of the University of Bologna also allowed carrying out anatomical dissections on the unclaimed bodies of the poor who died in hospitals and of foreigners, though it restricted the use of the cadavers of the Bolognese.[35] Fashioning himself as the architect of a new deal between Bolognese clergy and the medical faculty, Lambertini remarked that anatomical dissections could be carried out on the cadavers of ordinary individuals—as well as on those of criminals—so long as permission was obtained from the archbishop, namely, from himself. The archdiocese would, in turn, look after obtaining the consensus of the family, guarantee that a priest performed the last rights, and ensure the celebration of funeral rites before dissection and a proper Christian burial for the remains afterwards.[36] Far from turning the management of the dead body over to the medical faculty, Lambertini's notification on anatomy combined instead easier access to cadavers with increased clerical control over anatomists' pursuits. A series of examples appropriately illustrated the terms of the deal. To start with, Lambertini cautioned the medical faculty that in 1697 the appearance in the anatomical theatre of the corpse of a Bolognese man who had suddenly died in the street, had caused the priest of the church of San Michele del Mercato di Mezzo to make such a fuss that the body had to be returned. He similarly recalled that when the scholars of the university tried to pressure the curate of the church of S. Niccolò di S. Felice to obtain the cadaver of a recently buried woman, they did not succeed in their goal.[37] However, when, having snatched the cadaver of a man, the physicians listened to the advice of the diocese's vicar general, they eventually obtained what they wanted. After the wife of the man gave her consent, and the funeral rites were celebrated in the parish church, the corpse was delivered to the '*Signori Scolari*' of the university for the benefit of anatomical knowledge.[38] All in all, the message was clear: anatomy was not at odds with religious precepts, but it had to be subjected to ecclesiastical control. Notably, in the early 1730s, when Lelli was first charged with the task of completing a series of anatomical statues, he turned to Lambertini to seek permission to remove cadavers from the churches and the hospitals of Bologna, promising he would bring back 'in all circumspection and caution' all the parts that had been removed from the holy sites after putting them

[34] Lambertini, 'Sopra la Notomia'.

[35] See Ferrari, 'Public Anatomy Lessons', 59–60 and 87; Park, 'The Criminal and the Saintly Body', 12 and 16.

[36] Prospero Lambertini, 'Motuproprio pel quale s'istituisce in Bologna una Scuola di Chirurgia, e si prescieglie per la prima volta alla carica di Dimostratore delle Operazioni Chirurgiche il Dottore Pietro Paolo Molinelli', in Angelini (ed.), *Anatomie Accademiche*, 524–8.

[37] Martinotti, *Prospero Lambertini*, 7–8. On such forms of resistance, see also Ferrari, 'Public Anatomy Lessons', 60.

[38] See Lambertini, 'Motuproprio pel quale s'istituisce in Bologna una Scuola di Chirurgia'.

'to good use'.[39] On 17 November 1732, he received permission to do so.[40] As Lambertini set off to become a major patron of anatomical and surgical activities, he returned yet again to the subject of access to dead bodies. When, in 1742, he issued a *motu proprio* that sanctioned the establishment of a surgical school in Bologna, he promised easier access to cadavers for teaching purposes and granted the support of the archbishopric to those who had problems obtaining them, under the condition of receiving the approval of the vicar general.[41] Notably, as a document issued by the pontiff on his own initiative, the *motu proprio* reflected Lambertini's personal commitment to support anatomical and surgical practice in Bologna.

Lambertini's notification on anatomy and his *motu proprio* were issued at a time in which, as the anatomist Antonio Cocchi noticed in 1742, dissections of the cadavers of individuals who had died of some disease had for a while been tolerated by the relatives of the deceased.[42] On the other hand, the dissection of the bodies of the Bolognese obtained without the permission of the family continued to be perceived as a noteworthy and troublesome event. When, early in 1754, Paolo Battista Balbi publicly dissected the cadaver of Veronica Scagliarini without the consent of her relatives, the episode was considered well worth recording. The Bolognese chronicler Domenico Maria Galeati reported it in his *Diario* along with other notable events that took place in the city.[43] The following year, on 9 January 1755, at the opening of the anatomical season, Galeati reported a rather different case of anatomical dissection: the story of a man who entered an uninhabited house during the night, was caught, tried to escape from the window, fell in a well, drowned, and ended up on the dissecting table.[44]

Insofar as dissections were carried out on the bodies of criminals, their legitimacy remained unquestioned.[45] Like executions, public dissections of criminals played a part in the moral and political economy of the community.[46] As Giovanna Ferrari has remarked, dissections of criminals reconfirmed the principle that the bodies of offenders belonged to sovereigns who 'could dispose of them from the moment of conviction precisely as they saw fit'.[47] Well into the eighteenth century, warnings about the consequences of crime were expressed through exemplary moral parables

[39] Biblioteca Universitaria di Bologna (henceforth BUB), ms. 90, Lettere di Ercole Lelli al Card. Lambertini e Benedetto XIV, fol. 25r.

[40] Ibid., fol. 26v.

[41] Lambertini, 'Motuproprio pel quale s'istituisce in Bologna una Scuola di Chirurgia', 524–8. See also Luigi Belloni, 'Italian Medical Education after 1600', in Charles Donald O'Malley (ed.), *The History of Medical Education* (Berkeley: University of California Press, 1970), 115.

[42] See Brambilla, 'La medicina del Settecento', 64.

[43] Biblioteca Comunale dell'Archiginnasio di Bologna (henceforth BCABo), ms. B 88, 'Diario e memorie varie dall'anno MDL all'anno MDCCLXXXXVI raccolte e scritte dal Domenico Maria D'Andrea Galeati', vol. 9, 22.

[44] Ibid., 38. [45] Ferrari, 'Public Anatomy Lessons', 60.

[46] See Jonathan Sawday, *The Body Emblazoned: Dissection and the Human Body in Renaissance Culture* (London: Routledge, 1996), chapter 4; Ruth Richardson, *Death, Dissection and the Destitute* (Chicago: University of Chicago Press, 2000), 29, 76–7 and *passim*. See also Peter Linebaugh, 'The Tyburn Riot Against the Surgeons', in Douglas Hay et al. (eds.), *Albion's Fatal Tree: Crime and Society in Eighteenth-Century England* (London: Penguin Books, 1975), 76–7.

[47] See Ferrari, 'Public Anatomy Lessons', 60.

like the one of the man who broke into the house, met his death by falling into a well, and ended up on the dissecting table. Placed at the opposite ends of the moral spectrum, stories about the anatomies of saints equally mediated widely shared moral messages.[48] Conversely, if cases of bodysnatching like that of Veronica Scagliarini became news worth reporting, it was also because the bodies of ordinary individuals who reached the dissecting table without the permission of the family ran the risk of not receiving a proper Christian burial.

The issue was, of course, close to everybody's heart, and particularly so to that of Lambertini, who, as part of his intense activity as the archbishop in Bologna, also reformulated, in more restrictive terms, the rules and rites that governed every aspect of the life of the corpse, from the moment of death to burial. Thus, for instance, Lambertini reiterated that a mass always had to be celebrated for the deceased at the time of burial, and emphasized the importance of psalm singing. The celebration of the mass for the dead had to be granted even to those who could not pay for their funeral, and at least two priests had to accompany the funerary procession and engage in psalm singing. Likewise, he decreed that when a cadaver needed to be transported to the place of burial, the cross had to precede the procession, and both the people on the sides of the cross and those carrying the bier had to hold torches, so that the cortège would be appropriately lit. Accordingly, the habit of burying the cadavers of the rich in a hurry and overnight, with neither proper lighting nor the cross, in order to spare them the insults of the plebs, had to be banned.[49]

Instructions such as these offer a glimpse into the highly regulated and ritualized nature of the handling of early modern corpses. Among the reasons underpinning such control was the Christian creed of resurrection, which prescribed that at the moment of the last judgement the soul would be reunited with the body from which it had been separated by death. Well into the eighteenth century, views of resurrection affected the way in which the body was perceived as an integral part of the person. Accordingly, dead bodies had to be handled properly in order to make sure that at the end of time they could take part in the general resurrection of all dead souls.[50] The incorrupt bodies of saints, which were disseminated in considerable numbers along the Italian peninsula, were largely taken to coincide

[48] On the long history of the association between the criminal and the saintly body, and its relevance for anatomical practice, see Park, 'The Criminal and the Saintly Body', esp. 26–9.

[49] See Prospero Lambertini, 'Sopra il portare i corpi de' defunti alla sepoltura, e Messe da celebrarsi per le anime loro [...]', in *Raccolta di alcune notificazioni, editti, ed istruzioni pubblicate pel buon governo della sua diocesi dall'Eminentissimo e Reverendissimo Signor Cardinale Prospero Lambertini, Arcivescovo di Bologna, ora Benedetto XIV, sommo Pontefice*, 10th edn., vol. 1 (Naples: a spese di Andrea Migliaccio, 1772), 175–83.

[50] On the history of resurrection, see Caroline W. Bynum, 'Material Continuity, Personal Survival, and the Resurrection of the Body: A Scholastic Discussion in its Medieval and Modern Contexts', *History of Religions*, 30:1 (1990), 51–85; Caroline W. Bynum, *The Resurrection of the Body in Western Christianity, 200–1336* (New York: Columbia University Press, 1995); Fernando Vidal, 'Brains, Bodies, Selves, and Science: Anthropologies of Identity and the Resurrection of the Body', *Critical Inquiry*, 28:4 (2002), 930–74; Lucia Dacome, 'Resurrecting by Numbers in Eighteenth-Century England', *Past and Present*, 193 (2006), 73–110.

with the body of resurrection.[51] However, for ordinary individuals the Christian doctrine of resurrection was understood as the story of a body that would change its status and yet maintain its individual characteristics; it would become immortal and incorruptible and nevertheless remain the same. Although the details of such a dramatic transformation were largely left opaque, the creed had a lasting impact on death rituals and the management of the dead body.

In as much as death was an event that affected the whole community, the care of the dead was a duty that called for collective participation.[52] Family members were not alone in handling this responsibility. Congregations and guilds equally expected their members to comply with the rituals that dealt with the deceased from the moment of death to that of burial.[53] Giovanni Manzolini, a Bolognese artist who became one of the protagonists of eighteenth-century anatomical modelling, lived near the small church of San Gabriele in Via dei Giudei. He was a member of the eponymous Congregation, which was known for its oratory, at the time in which this group decided to provide itself with a set of regulations concerning the burial of deceased members. On 25 February 1725, the Congregation was recruiting volunteers to carry the cadavers of fellow members to the graveyard, lead the chanting, and keep the procession away from the troubles that could occur when different congregations competed over the order of precedence within a funeral procession.[54] Franco Fergniani was then charged with the task of carrying the body, and Giovanni Manzolini and Giuseppe Stivani with that of chanting. Thus, before engaging in dissecting cadavers and making anatomical models, Manzolini was dealing with dead bodies by accompanying the corpses of fellow congregates to burial and singing over them.

THE ANATOMY OF THE POPE

When Lambertini's notification on anatomy first appeared in 1737, it was included in a collection of *Notificazioni* that were meant to serve 'the good government of the diocese'. As such it may have looked local in its scope. However, after Lambertini

[51] Bynum, 'Material Continuity'; Bynum, *The Resurrection*; Pomata 'Malpighi and the Holy Body', esp. 585–6.

[52] On the history of the handling of dead bodies, see the classic Robert Hertz, 'Contribution to the Study of the Collective Representation of Death', in his *Death and the Right Hand*, trans. R. and C. Rodney (Aberdeen: Cohen and West, 1960), 27–86; Thomas W. Laqueur, *The Work of the Dead: A Cultural History of Mortal Remains* (Princeton: Princeton University Press, 2015).

[53] On the obligation to participate in the funerals of guild members, see Katharine Park, *Doctors and Medicine in Early Renaissance Florence* (Princeton: Princeton University Press, 1985), 16. On confraternities and congregations in early modern Italy, see Danilo Zardin, 'Le confraternite in Italia settentrionale fra XV e XVIII secolo', *Società e Storia*, 10 (1987), 81–137; Nicholas Terpstra, *Lay Confraternities and Civic Religion in Renaissance Bologna* (Cambridge: Cambridge University Press, 1995); Nicholas Terpstra (ed.), *The Politics of Ritual Kinship: Confraternities and Social Order in Early Modern Italy* (Cambridge: Cambridge University Press, 2000); Christopher F. Black, 'The Public Face of Post-Tridentine Italian Confraternities', *The Journal of Religious History*, 28:1 (2004), 87–101.

[54] ASB, Demaniale, Miscellanea, Compagnia di San Gabriele, 8–6730, 24 February 1725. On the oratory of San Gabriele, see Victor Crowther, *The Oratorio in Bologna (1650–1730)* (Oxford: Oxford University Press, 1999), 40.

was elected to the papacy, it was destined to acquire a much broader significance, well beyond the boundaries of the Bolognese archdiocese. Having supported anatomy by ecclesiastical means as an archbishop, after becoming pope Lambertini could sponsor its practice through the resources of the papal court. His support for anatomy then found expression in an impressive sequence of initiatives that were aimed at promoting anatomical and surgical activities, especially in Bologna. When, in September 1742, Lambertini communicated to the *Assunti* of the Institute of the Sciences (the senators responsible for running it) his intention to revive the project of an anatomy room and to sponsor its realization, they rejoiced at the prospect that the display would bring the Institute the fame it deserved. In the previous month, Lambertini had supported the establishment of a school of surgery in Bologna and had appointed the physician Pier (or Pietro) Paolo Molinelli (1702–1764) as its first chair. Moreover, he had donated a set of surgical instruments to the Bolognese hospital of Santa Maria della Vita for alternate use in anatomical demonstrations both in this hospital and in that of Santa Maria della Morte.[55] Nor was this the end of his conspicuous patronage of anatomical and surgical pursuits in the city. When the anatomical wax modeller Anna Morandi pleaded for his help in 1755, after the death of her husband, it was thanks to the pope's intercession that the Bolognese Senate granted her an annual salary.[56] Again in 1757, just one year before his death, an aging and ailing Lambertini purchased and donated to the Institute of the Sciences the collection of midwifery models that the surgeon Giovanni Antonio Galli had gathered in his residence in order to train midwives and surgeons.[57]

Impressive as they might have been, anatomical collections were not the exclusive focus of papal patronage of natural inquiry in Bologna. Rather, Lambertini's commitment to natural knowledge found expression in a multiplicity of initiatives that were largely aimed at the enlargement and enhancement of the Bolognese Institute of the Sciences. In the years following the opening of the Institute, many had cherished the hope that the new academy would boost the city's reputation as a centre of learning, placing it back on the map of natural knowledge.[58] However, Luigi Ferdinando Marsigli, the Institute's founder, and the city representatives entertained dissimilar views on its function and mission. In the mid-1720s, Lambertini was summoned to mediate between the parties.[59] Yet, Marsigli's

[55] Lambertini, 'Motuproprio pel quale s'istituisce in Bologna una Scuola di Chirurgia'. Lambertini had received the surgical instruments as a gift from the French King Louis XV via his first surgeon, Francois de Lapeyronie (1678–1747).

[56] See ASB, Gabella Grossa, Atti delle Congregazioni (1753–9), I/42, 15 December 1755, fol. 112; ASB, Senato, filza 81, fols. 709r–715v. On Lambertini's support for Morandi, see Chapter 4.

[57] Galli's midwifery collection will be discussed in Chapter 5.

[58] On the perceived decline of the University of Bologna in the seventeenth century, see Ferrari, 'Public Anatomy Lessons'. In his *Travels through Holland, Germany, Switzerland and Italy*, Blainville observed: 'This University once so famous, and by far the most celebrated of all Italy for many ages, is now decayed to an incredible degree and even reduced to nothing'; see [Henry] de Blainville, *Travels through Holland, Germany, Switzerland, and Other Parts of Europe, but Especially Italy*, trans. William Guthrie, vol. 2 (London: printed by W. Strahan for the Proprietor, 1743), 184.

[59] Giorgio Dragoni, 'Marsigli, Benedict XIV and the Bolognese Institute of Sciences', in Judith Veronica Field and Frank A.J.L. James (eds.), *Renaissance and Revolution: Humanists, Scholars, Craftsmen and Natural Philosophers in Early Modern Europe* (Cambridge: Cambridge University Press, 1997), esp. 234–7.

conflict with city authorities ultimately resulted in his decision to leave Bologna in a kind of self-imposed exile.[60] By the early 1730s, the Institute of the Sciences presented a scene of desolation. In 1733, an anonymous letter deplored its 'inaction and decadence': the observatory had taken a very long time to complete, the library was still in progress, the laboratory of chemistry remained largely unused, and foreign visitors seemed to have deserted the place.[61] Having been a keen supporter of the Institute from the outset, once elected to the pontificate Lambertini engaged in tackling some of these problems.

Over the years, the Institute's debt of gratitude to the pope grew in proportion to Lambertini's numerous donations.[62] Alongside the anatomical collections, his gifts included new instruments, an astronomical observatory realized by English artisans, and a collection of optical instruments acquired from the daughter of the late Giuseppe Campani, who had been professor of dioptrics and optics in Rome. Lambertini also made a crucial contribution to the enlargement of the Institute's library, sponsored the production of copies of the most beautiful Florentine and Roman classical statues, and provided support for a number of projects that had been left incomplete. To be sure, not all the gifts that reached the Institute triggered the same degree of enthusiasm. When, in June 1742, Lambertini secured the arrival of an Egyptian mummy donated by Cardinal Alessandro Albani, the gift seemingly generated some uncertainty about its function and location within the Institute. In fact, it kept moving around: some visitors saw the mummy in the room of natural history, others among the antiquities, others still in the anatomy school.[63] When, in October 1754, John Boyle, Earl of Corke and Orrery, visited the Institute and found the Egyptian mummy in the anatomy school, he was taken aback at the sight of its uncovered face: showing a great hole in the place of the nose and two beads in the place of the eyes, the mummy 'smelt excessively strong of spices' and appeared to him 'hideous even to a degree of horror'.[64] Yet, overall the papal gifts generated pride, gratitude, and enthusiasm. The arrival of a

[60] See Cavazza, *Settecento inquieto*; Tripaldi, *Le cere anatomiche*, chapter 1. Marsigli would later return to Bologna where he died in 1730.

[61] ASB, Assunteria d'Instituto, Diversorum, busta 18, n. 11, 'Foglio anonimo sopra l'inazione e decadimento dell'Instituto', read at the Senate on 27 May 1733.

[62] On Lambertini's patronage of the Institute of the Sciences and his support for natural inquiry, see, for instance, Giampaolo Venturi, 'Benedetto XIV e le collezioni universitarie di Bologna', in *Benedetto XIV (Prospero Lambertini)*, vol. 2, 1197–208; Prodi, 'Carità e galateo', ibid., vol. 1, 445–71 (esp. 462–6); Cavazza, *Settecento inquieto*; Walter Tega, 'Papa Lambertini: Una lucida visione dei rapporti fede-scienza', in Andrea Zanotti (ed.), *Prospero Lambertini: Pastore della sua città, pontefice della cristianità* (Bologna: Minerva, 2004), 161–70; Messbarger, *The Lady Anatomist*, chapter 1; Dacome, 'The Anatomy of the Pope'; Dacome, 'Ai confini del mondo naturale'.

[63] John Boyle, Earl of Corke and Orrery, *Letters from Italy, in the Years 1754 and 1755* (London: B. White, 1773), 67; Bibliothèque Nationale de France (henceforth BNF), Site Richelieu-Louvois, Paris, ms. Fr. 7966, Marquis de Dauvet, 'Journal de Voyage. Voyage en Italie, et Lettres Écrites d'Italie', fol. 72r. The mummy's cumbersome and fragile nature generated concern about its transportation and a flurry of correspondence across the Appenines; see, for instance, ASB, Assunteria d'Istituto, Lettere all'Istituto, n. 4 (1734–52), Letters of 13 September 1741, 29 November 1741, and 18 April 1742; ASB, Assunteria d'Istituto, Lettere dell'Istituto, n. 3 (1735–55), Letters of 22 November 1741, 27 June 1742, 17 November 1742, 18 April 1742, 3 June 1742, 23 June 1742, and 12 July 1742.

[64] Boyle, *Letters from Italy*, 67.

number of instruments from the Netherlands gave rise to the hope that, thanks to the pope's gift, the cabinet of physics would offer not only a place of delight and admiration but also a venue for 'all sorts of experiments' that would be carried out to 'universal advantage'.[65] Writing in March 1743 to his cousin and friend Flaminio Scarselli (1705–1776), secretary of the Bolognese legation in Rome, Jacopo Bartolomeo Beccari, first chair of chemistry at the University of Bologna, wished that the Piedmontese, who boasted about their collection of experimental instruments, would visit the Institute so as to appreciate the pope's capacity to promote the sciences and fine arts.[66]

As Lambertini made the Institute of the Sciences one of the primary beneficiaries of his patronage, expectations increased, and so did the responsibilities. Writing again to Scarselli in October 1750, Beccari observed that, insofar as the Institute had been 'little more than the enterprise of a private individual', shortcomings could easily be forgiven in light of the limited resources. However, after 'such a Prince' took over its guidance, even the smallest deficiency was bound to be regarded as a conspicuous fault.[67] More and more was expected from the pope, and yet Lambertini rose to the challenge with further donations. His growing fame as a patron of natural inquiry became a feature of his public persona. Travellers such as John Boyle remarked that Bologna 'is peculiarly fortunate, not only in being a territory of the holy see [*sic*], but in being the birth-place of the present pope, *Benedict* XIV. He is a man of literature, and a great encourager of arts and sciences'.[68] Others similarly reckoned that the magnificent Institute of the Sciences held 'the greater part of its riches because of Benedict XIV's love for his country'.[69] Likewise, providing one of the first occasions on which models of the inner body were on public display in the Italian peninsula, the anatomical collections sponsored by the pope found ever more appreciative viewers among eighteenth-century visitors and foreign travellers. In addition to the Institute of the Sciences' anatomy room, the other anatomical collections that were directly and indirectly supported by Lambertini, namely Anna Morandi's and Giovanni Antonio Galli's, similarly became Grand Tour landmarks and were praised over and over again by both locals and foreigners.

Indeed, by and large the anatomical collections sponsored by Lambertini did fulfil the hope that they would bring about not only a new way of teaching anatomy, but also fame and prestige to the Institute of the Sciences and to the city as a whole. In so doing, they reflected back a fair amount of glory upon their patron.

65 Archivio Segreto Vaticano (henceforth ASV), Segreteria di Stato, Lettere di Particolari, vol. 222 (1743), 'Lettere di Particolari Ecclesiastici e Laici alla *Santità* di Ntro Sig.re PP Benedetto XIV ed al Sig. Card. Silvio Valenti Gonzaga suo Seg.rio di Stato da Gennaio a tutto Giugno 1743', fols. 179v–180v.

66 BUB, ms. 243, Lettere di Jacopo Bartolomeo Beccari a Flaminio Scarselli, Letter of 27 March 1743 from Jacopo Bartolomeo Beccari in Bologna to Flaminio Scarselli, fols. 12r–v.

67 Ibid., Letter of 17 October 1750 from Jacopo Bartolomeo Beccari in Bologna to Flaminio Scarselli, fol. 232r.

68 Boyle, *Letters from Italy*, 64 (original emphasis).

69 [Pierre Jean Grosley], *New Observations on Italy and its Inhabitants: Written in French by two Swedish Gentleman; Translated into English by Thomas Nugent*, 2nd edn., vol. 1 (London: L. Davis and C. Reymers, 1769 [1764]) 130–1.

Lambertini himself contributed to his image as a generous benefactor by emphasizing that his commitment to anatomy was inspired by the desire to promote 'the advancement of the Arts, especially the most useful ones, those most necessary to human society and the preservation of human bodies'.[70] Yet, Lambertini had more than one reason for directing his munificence towards anatomical practice. And by the time he became a key player in the Bolognese anatomical world, he was well acquainted with the importance of anatomical knowledge in the context of one of the institutional pillars of the Roman Catholic Church: the cult of saints.

MODELLING SANCTITY

Saints occupied a central place in Counter-Reformation culture and identity.[71] The verification of claims to sanctity accordingly became a major reason for ecclesiastical concern. As the Church grew wary of cults based on false miracles, the whole process of evaluating and appraising divine election became the object of particular attention. As a consequence, the papacy sought to increase its control over the management of canonization, and simulated sanctity came to be regarded as equal to heresy.[72] Post-dating by a few decades the foundation of the Tribunal of the Holy Office (1542)—which aimed to police heresy—and overlapping with its function and competencies, the Congregation of Rites was established in 1588 with the purpose of securing the authentication of sanctity by means of a juridical body in charge of regulating canonization procedures.[73] In line with its institutional mandate, the Congregation of Rites articulated such procedures under the guise of a legal process.[74] The advocate of the candidate to sanctity provided arguments and proofs in support of the cause for canonization, whereas the promoter of faith raised formal objections (*animadversiones*) about the soundness of the case of sanctity under examination (and thus the promoter of

[70] Lambertini, 'Motuproprio pel quale s'istituisce in Bologna una Scuola di Chirurgia', 524.

[71] See, for instance, Gabriella Zarri (ed.), *Finzione e santità tra medioevo ed età moderna* (Turin: Rosenberg & Sellier, 1991); David Gentilcore, *From Bishop to Witch: The System of the Sacred in Early Modern Terra d'Otranto* (Manchester: Manchester University Press, 1992), esp. chapter 6; Jean-Michel Sallmann, *Naples et ses saints à l'âge baroque (1540–1750)* (Paris: Presses Universitaires de France, 1994); Simon Ditchfield, 'Sanctity in Early Modern Italy', *Journal of Ecclesiastical History*, 47 (1996), 98–112; Ditchfield, 'Il mondo della Riforma e della Controriforma', 261–330; Simon Ditchfield, 'Tridentine Worship and the Cult of the Saints', in Ronnie Po-Chia Hsia (ed.), *The Cambridge History of Christianity*, vol. 6: *Reform and Expansion, 1500–1600* (Cambridge: Cambridge University Press, 2007), 201–24; Simon Ditchfield, 'Thinking with Saints: Sanctity and Society in the Early Modern World', *Critical Inquiry*, 35:3 (2009), 552–84; Giovanna Fiume, *Il Santo Moro: I processi di canonizzazione di Benedetto da Palermo (1594–1807)* (Milan: Franco Angeli, 2002).

[72] See, for instance, Zarri (ed.), *Finzione e santità*; Anne Jacobson Schutte, *Aspiring Saints: Pretense of Holiness, Inquisition, and Gender in the Republic of Venice, 1618–1750* (Baltimore: Johns Hopkins University Press, 2001).

[73] On the relationship between the Holy Office and the Congregation of Rites, see Miguel Gotor, *I beati del papa: Santità, Inquisizione e obbedienza in età moderna* (Florence: Leo S. Olschki, 2002).

[74] See Giuseppe Dalla Torre, 'Santità ed economia processuale: L'esperienza giuridica da Urbano VIII a Benedetto XIV', in Zarri (ed.), *Finzione e santità*, 231; Pierluigi Giovannucci, 'Dimostrare la santità per via giudiziaria', in Fattori (ed.), *Storia, medicina e diritto*, 277–95.

faith was also informally called 'the devil's advocate'). The process presupposed engaging in complex exercises of discernment that aimed at discriminating between true and false signs of sanctity.

As a promoter of faith for the Congregation of Rites, Lambertini was himself charged with the task of assessing the trustworthiness of claims to sanctity. As Louis-Antoine de Caraccioli observed, this was a particularly 'delicate and laborious' task: as well as raising objections that were aimed at verifying the authenticity of sanctity, it necessitated an assessment of the nature of testimony and the reliability of the witnesses. Moreover, it required an appraisal of the evidence concerning individuals who claimed to have received divine inspiration but who may have been unduly 'inclined towards marvels', and could therefore end up confusing the excesses of their own imagination for divine election. Finally, since much was at stake, the promoter of faith had to resist pressures and recommendations, and make no exceptions.[75] Having accumulated substantial experience as a promoter of faith, Lambertini dedicated himself to defining the criteria that guided the appraisal of signs of sanctity. In the mid-1730s, while he was archbishop of Bologna, he sent the press the thick volumes of his *De servorum Dei beatificatione et beatorum canonizatione*, which engaged in the task of ordering, regulating, and defining all aspects of the complex procedures informing canonization processes. While laying out beatification and canonization procedures in all their painstaking complexity, the *De servorum Dei* provided a systematic discussion of the conditions and the criteria that had to be followed in 'evaluating the cause of the servants of God'.[76] The work included material gathered over the years by Lambertini as well as by some of his predecessors. It built on a collection of decrees of canonization that had been originally issued by Urban VIII in 1634 in the papal brief *Coelestis Hierusalem cives*, and was subsequently expanded in 1642 under the title of *Decreta servanda in canonizatione et beatificatione Sanctorum*. Ordering and assessing the complex procedures of beatification and canonization was a massive task that required mastering different areas of knowledge. As Lambertini noticed, had the endeavour been undertaken by himself alone, it would have been unbearable. But luckily he did not have to face it on his own. Indeed, the *De servorum Dei* was the result of Lambertini's extensive reading as well as of his many consultations with legal experts, natural philosophers, physicians, anatomists, and theologians who, as Lambertini himself noticed, had kept him in good company and well informed. Lambertini's engagement as a diligent student ended up being documented visually

[75] Caraccioli, *Éloge historique de Benoît XIV*, 10–11.

[76] Prospero Lambertini, *De servorum Dei beatificatione et beatorum canonizatione*, 4 vols. (Bologna: Longhi, 1734–8). See also the recent edition with an Italian translation that is currently being published by the Libreria Editrice Vaticana (2010–). On the genesis and structure of Lambertini's *De servorum Dei*, see Riccardo Saccenti, 'La lunga genesi dell'opera sulle canonizzazioni', in Fattori (ed.), *Le fatiche di Benedetto XIV*, 3–47; Fattori, 'Il *De servorum Dei beatificatione et beatorum canonizatione* di Prospero Lambertini, papa Benedetto XIV: Materiali per una ricerca', ibid., 121–52; Fattori, 'Le fonti del *De Servorum Dei* e il loro uso nel trattato lambertiniano', in Fattori (ed.), *Storia, medicina e diritto*, 247–75. See also Andrea Zanotti, 'Tra terra e cielo: Prospero Lambertini e i processi di beatificazione', in Zanotti (ed.), *Prospero Lambertini*, 233–53.

in the image that portrays the future pope in the act of taking notes over the course of a consultation with a learned man (Figure 1.1).

ANATOMY AND THE BORDERS OF THE NATURAL WORLD

The establishment of criteria that could guide the identification of true miracles was, of course, central to the whole process of canonization. Taking inspiration from Thomas Aquinas, Lambertini defined a miracle as something that occurred beyond the order of nature.[77] It was a definition through negation, which classed as supernatural those phenomena that could not find explanation in the natural world. As Stuart Clark has put it, the requirement that true miracles 'be "beyond the order of the whole created nature" tied their authentication [...] to an exact understanding of where nature's boundaries actually occurred'.[78] Yet, in the early modern period the borders of the natural (what happens on a regular basis), the preternatural (what is anomalous and takes place rarely and occasionally but still belongs to the natural realm) and the supernatural (what happens through divine intervention only) offered a matter for endless debate.[79] Much as these boundaries were the objects of constant realignment and negotiation, their definition bore significant consequences for the identification of true miracles and, by implication, the verification of sanctity. While the preternatural referred to unusual phenomena that happened within the realm of natural causes (and which included the actions of devils and witches), miracles could only take place outside the natural order, namely, at the level of the supernatural, which specifically pertained to the sphere of the divine.[80]

Anatomy was taken to provide the evidence for what constituted a natural body. As such, it offered a powerful tool for drawing the elusive borders of the natural world. By the mid-eighteenth century, anatomical knowledge had gained a significant role in the saint-making process.[81] As a promoter of faith for the Congregation

[77] Lambertini, *De servorum Dei*, vol. 4/I, esp. chapter 1.

[78] Stuart Clark, *Thinking with Demons: The Idea of Witchcraft in Early Modern Europe* (Oxford: Oxford University Press, 1997), 154.

[79] On the categories of the 'natural', the 'preternatural', and the 'supernatural', see, for instance, Clark, *Thinking with Demons*; Lorraine Daston, 'The Nature of Nature in Early Modern Europe', *Configurations*, 6:2 (1998), 149–72; Silvia De Renzi, 'Resemblance, Paternity and Imagination in Early Modern Courts', in Staffan Müeller-Wille and Hans-Jörg Rheinberger (eds.), *Heredity Produced: At the Cross Road of Biology, Politics and Culture, 1550–1870* (Cambridge, MA: MIT Press, 2007), 61–83.

[80] Clark, *Thinking with Demons*, esp. chapters 10 and 11; Daston, 'The Nature of Nature'.

[81] On the use of medical knowledge in canonization processes, see Joseph Ziegler, 'Practitioners and Saints: Medical Men in Canonization Processes in the Thirteenth to Fifteenth Centuries', *Social History of Medicine*, 12:2 (1999), 191–225; David Gentilcore, 'Contesting Illness in Early Modern Naples: Miracolati, Physicians and the Congregation of Rites', *Past and Present*, 148 (1995), 117–48; Fiume, *Il Santo Moro*, esp. 58–62 and 139–44; Pomata, 'Malpighi and the Holy Body'; Fernando Vidal, 'Miracles, Science, and Testimony in Post-Tridentine Saint-Making', *Science in Context*, 20:3 (2007), 481–508; Fernando Vidal, 'Prospero Lambertini's "On the Imagination and Its Powers"', in Fattori (ed.), *Storia, medicina e diritto*, 297–318; Jacalyn Duffin, 'The Doctor Was Surprised; or, How to Diagnose a Miracle', *Bulletin of the History of Medicine*, 81: 4 (2007), 699–729; Jacalyn Duffin, *Medical Miracles: Doctors, Saints and Healing in the Modern World* (Oxford: Oxford University Press, 2009).

of Rites, Lambertini was well acquainted with the bearing that anatomy had on the authentication of sanctity. While writing his *magnum opus* on canonization, he regularly consulted with physicians, anatomists, and surgeons.[82] When the *Giornale de' Letterati* reviewed his *De servorum Dei*, it pointed to the importance of physicians and surgeons in the evaluation of miracles.[83] Physicians were called on as expert witnesses of the body, and were asked to use their medical and anatomical knowledge to assess the nature of given corporeal phenomena. Lack of a medical explanation gave way to the prospect of supernatural intervention because it discarded the possibility of a natural explanation for extraordinary and apparently miraculous occurrences. Since the bodies of holy individuals could contain the marks of divine intervention inscribed into their flesh, anatomists also inspected the cadavers of those who died in odour of sanctity to assess possible instances of sacred anatomy that provided the evidence of their divine election.[84] The description of such extraordinary anatomies could be included in the lives of aspiring saints as a means of supporting their cult. In the case of Giuseppe da Copertino (1603–1663), the famous 'flying friar', his *Vita* emphasized that upon dissection his pericardium was found to be dry, the ventricles had no blood, and the heart had been desiccated by the flame of divine love.[85] Many agreed that Copertino's striking levitations could not be performed by natural means. Even a man who was typically guarded in such matters like the historian and antiquarian Ludovico Antonio Muratori (1672–1750) recognized the extraordinary character, and in fact divine nature, of Copertino's flights.[86] Copertino was beatified by Prospero Lambertini in 1753, and subsequently canonized in 1768.

Throughout the early modern period, the employment of anatomical expertise in canonization procedures led to the creation of forms of medical authority that

[82] On the use of medical arguments in early modern religious and judicial contexts, see Gentilcore, 'Contesting Illness'; Silvia De Renzi, 'Witnesses of the Body: Medico-Legal Cases in Seventeenth-Century Rome', *Studies in History and Philosophy of Science*, 33:2 (2002), 219–42. See also Michael Clark and Catherine Crawford (eds.), *Legal Medicine in History* (Cambridge: Cambridge University Press, 1994).

[83] *Giornale de' Letterati per l'anno MDCCXLVII* (Rome: Fratelli Pagliarini, 1747), 378. On Lambertini's relationship with the *Giornale de' Letterati*, see Maria Pia Donato, 'Gli "strumenti" della politica di Benedetto XIV (1742–1759)', in Marina Caffiero and Giuseppe Monsagrati (eds.), 'Dall'erudizione alla politica: Giornali, giornalisti ed editori a Roma tra XVII e XX secolo', special issue, *Dimensioni e problemi della ricerca storica*, 1 (1997), 39–61; Saccenti, 'La lunga genesi', 30–1 and 33–4.

[84] On sacred anatomy, see Piero Camporesi, *The Incorruptible Flesh: Bodily Mutilation and Mortification in Religion and Folklore*, trans. T. Croft-Murray (Cambridge: Cambridge University Press, 1988); Luigi Canetti, 'Reliquie, martirio e anatomia: Culto dei santi e pratiche dissettorie fra tarda Antichità e primo Medioevo', *Micrologus*, 7 (1999), 113–53; Siraisi, 'Signs and Evidence'; Katharine Park, 'Relics of a Fertile Heart: The "Autopsy"' of Clare of Montefalco', in Anne L. McClanan and Karen Rosoff Encarnación (eds.), *The Material Culture of Sex, Procreation and Marriage in Premodern Europe* (New York: Palgrave, 2002), 115–33; Park, 'The Criminal and the Saintly Body'; Park, *Secrets of Women*, esp. chapters 1 and 4; Andretta 'Anatomie du Vénérable'.

[85] On Copertino, see Camporesi, *The Incorruptible Flesh*, chapter 3; Catrien Santing, 'Tirami sù: Pope Benedict XIV and the Beatification of the Flying Saint Giuseppe da Copertino', in Andrew Cunningham and Ole Peter Grell (eds.), *Medicine and Religion in Enlightenment Europe* (Aldershot: Ashgate, 2007), 79–100.

[86] Ludovico Antonio Muratori, *Della forza della fantasia umana* (Venice: Giambatista Pasquali, 1745), 77.

were entrenched in the political networks of the papal court.[87] Famous anatomists such as Realdo Colombo (1515?–1559) and Marcello Malpighi (1628–1694) participated in the saint-making process.[88] In the late seventeenth century, Malpighi was involved in the debate over the utility of anatomy after Giovanni Girolamo Sbaraglia (1641–1710), professor of medicine and anatomy at the University of Bologna, disparaged his anatomical techniques and findings and doubted their usefulness.[89] The controversy heated up, eventually leading Malpighi to leave Bologna and relocate to Rome, where he became papal archiater (personal physican to the pope) and pursued a successful medical career at the papal court. Claims about anatomy's uselessness echoed the views of the English physician Thomas Sydenham and the philosopher John Locke, who had co-authored a text in which they stated that

> all that Anatomie can doe is only to shew us the gross and sensible parts of the body, or the vapid and dead juices all which, after the most diligent search, will be noe more able to direct a physician how to cure a disease than how to make a man.[90]

The text was not published, but had wide resonance.[91] Notably, while the issue of anatomy's utility stirred controversy among physicians, anatomy's value and usefulness in the assessment of sanctity remained unquestioned.

Lambertini's own relationship with the medical and anatomical worlds became one of the defining features of his work on canonization. In 1741, shortly after his election to the papacy, Lambertini addressed some of the rules and procedures that governed the participation of medical practitioners in canonization trials. He urged physicians who wrote on miracles either *ad opportunitatem*, or *pro veritate*, to be brief and concise, write no more than one page, and restrain their reasoning to the proposed miracles.[92] He also emphasized that physicians should avoid addressing all the objections of the promoter of faith and limit themselves to the

[87] See for instance Andretta, 'Anatomie du Vénérable'.

[88] The anatomist Realdo Colombo mentioned dissecting Ignatius of Loyola, the founder of the Society of Jesus who was canonized in 1622, in his *De re anatomica libri 15* (1559); see Andretta, 'Anatomie du Vénérable'. On the participation of anatomists and physicians, including Malpighi, in the process of canonization of Caterina Vigri, see *Congregatio Sacrorum Rituum, Coram Sanctissimo Eminentissimo, & Reuerendissimo D. Card. Carpineo Bononiensis Canonizationis B. Catharinae a Bononia Monialis Professae Ordinis S. Clarae, Positio super dubio an et de quibus miraculis constet in casu* (Rome: Ex Typographia Reuerendae Camerae Apostolicae, 1680). See also Pomata, 'Malpighi and the Holy Body'.

[89] On the controversy, see Marta Cavazza, 'The Uselessness of Anatomy: Mini and Sbaraglia versus Malpighi', in Domenico Bertoloni Meli (ed.), *Marcello Malpighi, Anatomist and Physician* (Florence: Leo S. Olschki, 1997), 129–45; Domenico Bertoloni Meli, 'Mechanistic Pathology and Therapy in the Medical *Assayer* of Marcello Malpighi', *Medical History*, 51:2 (2007), 165–80; Domenico Bertoloni Meli, *Mechanism, Experiment, Disease: Marcello Malpighi and Seventeenth-Century Anatomy* (Baltimore: Johns Hopkins University Press, 2011).

[90] See Thomas Sydenham, 'Anatomie', in Kenneth Dewhurst, *Dr. Thomas Sydenham (1624–1689): His Life and Original Writings* (Berkeley: University of California Press, 1966), 85 (original spelling).

[91] See Antonio Cocchi, *Dell'anatomia* (Florence: Gio. Batista Zannoni, 1745), 21–2.

[92] Biblioteca Apostolica Vaticana (henceforth BAV), Miscell. A. 53 (11), 'Nuova tassa e riforma delle spese per le Cause delle Beatificazioni, e Canonizzazioni, e dell'altre spese per la Solennità delle medesime Beatificazioni, e Canonizzazioni, fatta, e pubblicata per ordine di Nostro Signore Papa Benedetto XIV' (Rome: Stamperia della Reverenda Camera Apostolica, 1741), 17–18.

points that concerned their occupation.[93] Their compensation was then set at 30 scudi, regardless of the number of miracles identified. In 1743, the year in which the second edition of his *De servorum Dei* appeared in print, Lambertini completed a list of names of medical practitioners who could be employed for the purpose of saint-making, and included lecturers from the Roman University of La Sapienza, doctors from the College of Physicians and the city, and surgeons who worked in the Roman hospitals.[94]

First published in 1738, the year following Lambertini's notification on 'anatomy in the public schools', Book IV of his *De servorum Dei* was largely dedicated to the role of medical and anatomical knowledge in the saint-making process. Accordingly, it built on the writings and insights of physicians and surgeons and reflected familiarity with the role of medical expertise in the assessment of the borders of the natural realm.[95] Likewise, Lambertini extensively drew on the influential *Quaestiones medico-legales* (1621–51) by the famous seventeenth-century *protomedico* and archiater Paolo Zacchia (1584–1659).[96] Having appeared in print in the earlier part of the seventeenth century, Zacchia's work enduringly provided an authoritative source for dealing with ecclesiastical, medical, civic, and judicial matters.[97] Lambertini largely relied on it in order to assess when healing could be considered miraculous in cases such as blindness, deafness, speechlessness, paralysis, epilepsy, and apoplexy. For instance, drawing on Zacchia's guidelines Lambertini emphasized that miraculous healing had to be sudden, not preceded by bodily evacuation and without relapses. Moreover, where multiple afflictions were involved, it could concern only one of them, even when the patient continued to suffer from the others.[98] As well as building on this body of medico-legal literature, Lambertini also included the insights of contemporary physicians and anatomists such as Antonio Maria Valsalva (1666–1723) and Giambattista Morgagni (1682–1771) into his discussion.[99] A student of Malpighi, a professor of anatomy in Bologna, and an acquaintance of Lambertini, Valsalva was, of course, the celebrated author of *De aure humana tractatus* (1704), the treatise on the anatomy of the ear which became a landmark of Bolognese anatomy. He also assembled an anatomical collection based on dry specimens, which gained reputation in the anatomical world.[100]

93 Ibid. 94 BAV, Miscell. A. 53 (12).

95 On Lambertini's use of medical knowledge, see Jean-Denys Gorce, *L'oeuvre médicale de Prospero Lambertini (Pape Benoît XIV)* (Bordeaux: Destout, 1915); Dacome, 'The Anatomy of the Pope'.

96 Paolo Zacchia, *Quaestiones medico-legales: In quibus omnes eae materiae medicae, quae ad legales facultates videntur pertinere, proponuntur, pertractantur, resolvuntur*, 9 vols. (Rome: Andrea Brogiotti et al., 1621–51).

97 On Zacchia, see Silvia De Renzi, 'La natura in tribunale: conoscenze e pratiche medico-legali a Roma nel XVII secolo', *Quaderni Storici*, 108:3 (2001), 799–822; De Renzi, 'Witnesses of the Body'; Alessandro Pastore and Giovanni Rossi (eds.), *Paolo Zacchia: Alle origini della medicina legale, 1584–1659* (Milan: Franco Angeli, 2008); Jacalyn Duffin, 'Questioning Medicine in Seventeenth-Century Rome: The Consultations of Paolo Zacchia', *Canadian Bulletin of Medical History*, 28:1 (2011), 149–70.

98 Gentilcore, 'Contesting Illness'. 99 Lambertini, *De servorum Dei*, vol. 4.

100 ASB, Assunteria d'Istituto, Diversorum, busta 10, n. 0, 'Museo Anatomico Valsalva'. On the reputation of Valsalva's collection among anatomists, see Domenico Cotugno, 'Iter Italicum

When Lambertini discussed the nature of hearing disorders and their cures in his *De servorum Dei*, he turned to Valsalva's discussion of the cases in which deafness from birth could be cured by surgery to conclude that recovery from this ailment did not necessitate divine intervention. Drawing on contemporary anatomical discussions of the throat and tongue, Lambertini also endorsed the natural character of the cure of a woman who had been mute from birth and had started to speak when she was seventeen after suffering from fever. Likewise, even the case of a woman who had been speechless for years and, having written down her sins for confession, became perfectly eloquent as she was reading her texts in silence by simply moving her lips, did not necessarily point to a miraculous occurrence. In fact, as the physician and naturalist Michael Bernhard Valentini (1657–1729) had put it, fervent devotional eagerness could excite the animal spirits to the point of removing the impediments of speech.[101] These are just a few examples among the many showing how Lambertini relied on anatomical and medical knowledge in order to present cases in which the body could heal itself by natural means, even when it may have appeared to be beyond recovery. Notably, Lambertini was busy pondering and writing about such cases in the period in which he encouraged the creation of an anatomical museum in Bologna. In the same decade, he also published the notification that aimed at clarifying the Church's position on anatomical practice. After becoming pope in 1740, he engaged in the patronage of anatomical collections.[102]

Displaying anatomical knowledge in three dimensions, anatomical models staged an impressive form of evidence about what constituted a natural body. Taken to provide concrete, reliable, and trustworthy embodiments of anatomical features, they exposed the relationship between given physical phenomena and the supposed reality of the state of affairs of the body. In doing so, they also articulated and made publicly available the anatomical insights that underpinned the appraisal and authentication of sanctity, which Lambertini had considered and discussed in his *De servorum Dei*. In 1747, Lambertini remarked that one of the reasons for supporting the creation of an anatomy room at the Institute of the Sciences was the consideration that 'in the public schools and in the houses of lecturers' things were taught in a 'speculative manner', whereas at the Institute they were 'demonstrated and shown practically'.[103] In his view, the anatomy room was meant to complement, rather than replace, dissections.[104] His donation of a set of surgical instruments to the hospital of Santa Maria della Vita was similarly intended to

Patavinum', in Felice Lombardi (ed.), *Le scoperte anatomiche di Domenico Cotugno e il suo 'Iter Italicum Patavinum'* (Naples: R. Licenziato, 1964), 73–5.

[101] Lambertini, *De servorum Dei*, vol. 4/I, chapter 10, 131–3.

[102] BAV, Miscell. A. 53 (11), 17–18.

[103] Prospero Lambertini (papa Benedetto XIV), 'Motuproprio, col quale Ercole Lelli Artefice delle otto Statue Anatomiche, esistenti per liberalità di Nostro Signore nell'Istituto delle Scienze, con altri lavori rappresentanti le parti del Corpo Umano, viene costituito Custode ed Ostensore di dette Statue, e di detti Lavori: ed in oltre de' Capitali di Vetri Diottrici donati essi pure all'Istituto medesimo dalla Santità Sua: come anche de' Torni, che furono dati dal Generale Marsiglj', in Angelini (ed.) *Anatomie Accademiche*, vol. 3, 536.

[104] Ibid., 536 and 539.

ensure that anatomical dissections would be carried out regularly for teaching purposes both in this hospital and in that of Santa Maria della Morte.[105] Discussions as to whether models could effectively replace dissections have accompanied much of the history of anatomical modelling.[106] Two-dimensional anatomical illustrations were regarded as effective teaching tools and memory aids but were often treated as complements to the first-hand experience of anatomical dissection. Conversely, three-dimensional models were considered anatomical embodiments in their own right and could be regarded as potential replacements of the actual body.

Displayed along Grand Tour routes, the anatomy room sponsored by Lambertini presented viewers with the makings of the human body, the most impressive instance of the Creation, and testified to the utility of anatomy in tracing the boundaries of the natural world. Notably, it did so in a public setting. Visitors' access to the Institute of the Sciences was largely filtered on the basis of reputation and letters of recommendation. However, the Institute's displays and activities were public both in the sense that they involved the city's core civic institutions and because they addressed different audiences, including lay visitors and Grand Tour travellers—many of whom wrote about what they saw and in turn mediated its displays to larger publics. Over the course of the eighteenth century, the creation and careful control of public spaces in which natural knowledge was pursued and demonstrated played an important part in the establishment of patterns of trustworthiness and credibility. While unveiling the inner body to different audiences, the anatomical displays of Bologna relied on the models' visual and material features to publicize the body of anatomical knowledge that Lambertini had discussed in his *De servorum Dei* with the purpose of singling out the criteria of verification of sanctity.

Although Lambertini's work on canonization was primarily addressed to the Congregation of Rites, it also reached out to members of the Church who served in local institutions such as bishops, inquisitors, and spiritual guides.[107] The work was also employed in the education of clergymen in ecclesiastical institutions.[108] In 1748, for instance, it became associated with the creation of a chair in liturgy at the Roman College, the purpose of which was to instruct clergymen who were to serve in the Congregation of Rites. The Portuguese Jesuit Emmanuel de Azevedo, who was in charge of editing Benedict XIV's *Opera Omnia* and would publish a synopsis of the *De servorum Dei*, was appointed to the position.[109] The echo generated by Lambertini's work also extended beyond ecclesiastical circles. Together with compendia and synopses, revised, enlarged, and abridged editions of the *De servorum Dei* further contributed to expanding its readership.[110] As a reviewer

[105] Lambertini, 'Motuproprio pel quale s'istituisce in Bologna una Scuola di Chirurgia'.

[106] Well into the nineteenth century, the issue continued to be at the centre of anatomical debate; see Nick Hopwood, 'Artist versus Anatomist, Models against Dissection: Paul Zeiller of Munich and the Revolution of 1848', *Medical History*, 51:3 (2007), 279–308.

[107] Rosa, *Settecento religioso*, 53.

[108] Fattori, 'Introduzione', xxix; Saccenti, 'La lunga genesi', 29–41.

[109] Saccenti, 'La lunga genesi', 31–43.

[110] See, for instance, Nicolas Baudeau, *Analyse de l'ouvrage du Pape Benoit XIV, sur les béatifications et canonisations, Approuvée par lui-même, et dédié au Roi* (Paris: Hardy, 1759); Joseph d'Audierne,

of Lambertini's work put it in the *Giornale de' Letterati* of 1747, on the face of it the subject of canonization may not have looked particularly pertinent to a periodical, yet its readers would be pleased to be offered a compendium that would allow them to familiarize themselves with its offices and procedures.[111] In 1757, the *Assunti* of the Institute of the Sciences similarly welcomed the gift of a 'beautiful synopsy' of the pope's voluminous work and praised its publication as a 'very useful and appropriate thing' that would allow those who might not have the time and ease to read the text in its entirety to acquaint themselves at least with its compendium, and see it all at once 'as in a prospectus'.[112] In the following years, the contents of Lambertini's work also became a matter of discussion in Grand Tour reports, and the abbot Joseph de La Porte (1714–1779) included citations from the text in his *Le voyageur françois*.[113] To be sure, not everybody was as enthusiastic about Lambertini's grand work on canonization. For instance, the writer and traveller Carlo Antonio Pilati (1733–1802) maintained that, although Lambertini's *De servorum Dei* was highly regarded, it did not compare to the comedies of the famous playwright Carlo Goldoni (1707–1793).[114] Still, Pilati's observation shows that the readership of Lambertini's work extended beyond religious circles. Just like its compendia, abridged versions and synopses, the anatomical collections sponsored by Lambertini mediated the body of knowledge presented in the *De servorum Dei* in a way that instructed and impressed different audiences. But why did Lambertini support the presentation of this knowledge in Bologna rather than in Rome?

BOLOGNA AND ROME

On the face of it, Lambertini had a number of reasons to designate Bologna as the centre of his anatomical patronage. For one thing, the fact that he was from Bologna dramatically raised the expectation that once he was elected pope he would do something memorable for the city; and in fact, as we have seen, after his appointment as the local archbishop Lambertini had already encouraged anatomical practice in the city. For another, Bologna had nourished a long and celebrated

Lettres curieuses, utiles et théologiques sur la béatification des serviteurs de Dieu et la canonisation des béatifiés, ou Abrégé du grand Ouvrage du Cardinal Prosper Lambertini, Pape, sous le nom de Benoist XIV, sur la même matière (Rennes: J. Vatar, 1758–64). On the editorial history of the *De servorum Dei*, see Pietro Amato Frutaz, 'Le principali edizioni e sinossi del *De servorum Dei beatificatione et beatorum canonizatione* di Benedetto XIV: Saggio per una bio-bibliografia critica', in Cecchelli (ed.), *Benedetto XIV (Prospero Lambertini)*, vol. 1, 27–90.

111 *Giornale de' Letterati per l'anno MDCCXLVII*, 373.

112 See ASB, Assunteria d'Istituto, Lettere dell'Istituto, n. 4 (1756–65), 12 March 1757; ASB, Assunteria d'Istituto, Lettere all' Istituto, n. 5 (1753–7), Letter of 19 March 1757 from Fulvio Bentivoglio in Rome.

113 Joseph de La Porte, *Le voyageur françois, ou la connoissance de l'ancien et du nouveau monde mis au jour par l'Abbé Delaporte*, vol. 26 (Paris: L. Cellot, 1779), 18ff.

114 Carlo Antonio Pilati, *Voyages en différens pays de l'Europe, en 1774, 1775 et 1776; ou Lettres écrites de l'Allemagne, de la Suisse, de l'Italie, de Sicile et de Paris*, vol. 1 (The Hague: C. Plaat et Comp., 1777), 235.

anatomical tradition and therefore provided an ideal site for its pursuit. Further, as it constituted in effect the northern gate of the Papal States, Bologna was in a particularly felicitous position to present newcomers with an image of the papacy that was in line with the portrayal of Lambertini's pontificate in terms of his patronage of learning and natural knowledge.[115] Indeed, Lambertini's support for anatomy and surgery ended up leaving a strong and enduring mark not only among travellers but also among locals who included the papal gifts among the city's most cherished treasures. In 1778, on the occasion of the religious festival of the Addobbi, during which Bolognese homes and institutions put on public display their most precious art and possessions, the hospital of Santa Maria della Vita decided that the best way to honour the city would be to exhibit the set of surgical instruments that had been donated by the pope.[116]

On the other hand, it is also true that Lambertini himself had asserted that one of the duties of the pope was to maintain the prestige of the Papal States by turning Rome into a model for all other cities' wisdom, science, and the arts.[117] And indeed, despite Charles de Brosses' sardonic remark that in Rome one third of the people were priests, one third did not work, and one third simply did not do anything at all, Rome did enjoy a lively anatomical culture of its own.[118] From the end of the seventeenth century, a flourishing school of anatomy for artists had been associated with the activities of the French Academy in Rome. In 1687, the construction of a new anatomical theatre marked the beginning of the era that linked the fortunes of Roman anatomy with the career of the physician and anatomist Giovanni Maria Lancisi (1654–1720) at the papal court.[119] In the early years of the eighteenth century, Lancisi's rediscovery of Bartolomeo Eustachi's anatomical tables marked an important cultural and political event as well as a pivotal moment

[115] It is worth noting that Lambertini's fashioning of Bologna as the anatomical capital of the Papal States may not have been obvious to everyone: in 1903 the historian of anatomy Robert Ritter von Töply quoted from Lambertini's notification of 1737, but when it came to the sentence 'the study of anatomy has been of much advantage to this city', he added 'Rome' in brackets so as to hint that it had to be the Eternal City. In fact, the notification on anatomy was written while Lambertini was archbishop in Bologna, and it was published as part of a collection concerning the rules of good government of the Bolognese diocese; see Robert von Töply, *Geschichte der Anatomie*, in Theodor Puschmann (ed.), *Handbuch der Geschichte der Medizin,* vol. 2 (Hildesheim: Georg Olms Verlag 1971), 227. See also Martinotti, *Prospero Lambertini*, 5–6.

[116] See Olivier Bonfait, *Les exposition de peintures a Bologne au XVIIIe siécle* (Mémoire de l'Ecole du Louvre, 1990), 157. During the procession of the Santissimo Sacramento it was customary for citizens to display in public their most precious artwork. The procession also offered artists the opportunity to exhibit their work in public settings and along the streets; see BCABo, ms. B 105, Marcello Oretti, *Descrizione delle Pitture che sono state esposte nelle strade di Bologna in occasione degli Apparati fatti [negli anni 1759–1786] per le Processioni del SS. Sacramento che si fanno ogni dieci anni in Bologna.*

[117] Von Pastor, *The History of the Popes*, vol. 35, 182–3.

[118] See de Renzi, 'Medical Competence'; Donato and Kraye (eds.), *Conflicting Duties*.

[119] See Brambilla, 'La medicina del Settecento', esp. 46–53. See also Maria Pia Donato, 'The Mechanical Medicine of a Pious Man of Science: Pathological Anatomy, Religion and Papal Patronage in Lancisi's *De subitaneis mortibus* (1707)', in Donato and Kraye (eds.), *Conflicting Duties*, 319–52; Maria Pia Donato, *Sudden Death: Medicine and Religion in Eighteenth-Century Rome* (Farnham: Ashgate, 2014).

in the history of anatomical representation.[120] In the same period, the establishment of the Biblioteca Lancisiana within the premises of the hospital of Santo Spirito, fulfilled Lancisi's vision of a model of medical education that linked the study of medical and anatomical books in the library with physicians' practice in the hospital. Lambertini himself participated in the activities of the Roman medical and anatomical worlds. He supported the restoration of the anatomical theatre, promoted the enlargement of the hospital of Santo Spirito, and contributed to the establishment of the Accademia Capitolina del Nudo and the reorganization of the Accademia di San Luca, both of which encouraged the study of human anatomy as part of artistic training.[121]

Lambertini's priorities, however, became clear when, a few months after his election to the pontificate, he founded four academies of Christian erudition in Rome, covering subjects including ecclesiastical history, Roman history and antiquities, liturgy and rites, and the Church councils. These academies largely aimed to reconfirm traditional tenets and dogmas of the Church such as the authority of the pontiff, the rights of the Holy See, and the supremacy of Christian over pagan Rome.[122] They held their monthly gatherings on Mondays in the papal residence on the Quirinale, so that the pontiff could easily attend.[123] Later in his pontificate, Lambertini also expressed the intention of furthering the project to establish a museum of Christian antiquities, which had originally been launched by Pope Clement XI with the aim of creating the 'first grand papal museum', a proposal that generated widespread approval.[124] In 1749, the antiquarian Scipione Maffei welcomed the initiative in his *Museum Veronense*, which he dedicated to the pope.[125] Five years later, the prospect of a Christian museum led the antiquarian

[120] See Maria Conforti, 'The Biblioteca Lancisiana and the 1714 Edition of Eustachi's Anatomical Plates, or, Ancients and Moderns Reconciled', in Donato and Kraye (eds.), *Conflicting Duties*, 303–17.

[121] See Silvia Bordini, '"Studiare in un istesso luogo la Natura, e ciò che ha saputo far l'Arte": Il museo e l'educazione degli artisti nella politica culturale di Benedetto XIV', in Biagi Maino (ed.), *Benedetto XIV e le arti del disegno*, 385–94; Giovanna Curcio, 'L'ampliamento dell'ospedale di Santo Spirito in Sassia nel quadro della politica di Benedetto XIV per la città di Roma', ibid., 177–231.

[122] *Notizie delle accademie erette in Roma per ordine della Santità di N. Signore Papa Benedetto XIV* (Rome: Giuseppe Collini, 1740). On Lambertini's academies, see Maria Pia Donato, *Accademie romane: Una storia sociale, 1671–1824* (Naples: Edizioni Scientifiche Italiane, 2000), 86–115. See also the classic Von Pastor, *The History of the Popes*, vol. 35, 183–5; Garms-Cornides, 'Storia, Politica e Apologia in Benedetto XIV', 155–6. On seventeenth- and eighteenth-century views of the primacy and infallibility of the pontiff that preceded the promulgation of infallibility in the First Vatican Council of 1870, see Bruno Neveu, 'Juge suprême et docteur infaillible: Le pontificat romain de la bulle *In eminenti* (1643) à la bulle *Auctorem fidei* (1794)', in *Érudition et religion aux XVIIe et XVIIIe siècles* (Paris: A. Michel, 1994), 385–450; Ditchfield, 'Tridentine Worship and the Cult of the Saints'.

[123] See Giovanni Morello, 'Il "Museo Cristiano" di Benedetto XIV nella Biblioteca Vaticana', in Cecchelli (ed.), *Benedetto XIV (Prospero Lambertini)*, vol. 2, 1120–1.

[124] See Christopher M.S. Johns, *Papal Art and Cultural Politics* (Cambridge: Cambridge University Press, 1993), 33–7.

[125] Scipione Maffei, *Museum Veronense, hoc est, Antiquarum inscriptionum atque anaglyphorum collectio: cui taurinensis adiungitur et vindobonensis: accedunt monumenta id genus plurima nondum vulgata, et ubicumque collecta* (Verona: Typis Seminarii, 1749). See also Morello, 'Il "Museo Cristiano" di Benedetto XIV', 1127–8; Giovanni Morello, 'La creazione del Museo Cristiano', in Biagi Maino (ed.), *Benedetto XIV e le arti del disegno*, 266.

Giovanni Gaetano Bottari to hope that it could make up for the missed opportunity to have a space that could collect and display all the relevant objects of Christian history—such as the instruments of Christian martyrdom, the oil lamps, glasses, vases, terracottas, tools, and utensils—and would then constitute one of the most remarkable marvels of the world.[126]

From the outset, the project of a Christian museum was intended, as Scipione Maffei put it, not only to assist in the recovery of the past but also to prove 'the antiquity of the Christian dogma and the discipline of the Church'.[127] When it opened to visitors, an inscription placed above the entrance eloquently announced that the museum aimed to show 'the splendour of Rome' and 'the truth of the [Catholic] religion'.[128] In fact, by displaying the monuments and specimens of Christian art and history, the museum promised to demonstrate the origins and antiquity of Christian rituals and papal privileges.[129] Its ancient artefacts such as seals, inscriptions, tombstones, and ampoules containing the blood of martyrs, which had been found in the catacombs, were charged with the task of evoking the memory of early Christian history, the idea being that all such specimens and relics provided better testimonies of saints' stories than any written source, codex, or manuscript possibly could.

POWERFUL THINGS

The conclusion that one may be tempted to draw is that Lambertini acted in Bologna as the patron of nature, and in Rome as the sponsor of the past, with Bologna personifying the achievements of the moderns, and Rome celebrating the glories of the ancients. But different as the designs underpinning these projects may have looked, they may in fact be regarded as part of a common agenda. Linking Lambertini's long-standing concerns for the verification of sanctity with his patronage of anatomical and antiquarian displays, this agenda found expression in Lambertini's attitude towards the role of objects and material displays as powerful and reliable sources of evidence about human nature and Christian history. On the one hand, displays of anatomical waxworks participated in the development and dissemination of anatomical knowledge, and enacted an impressive display of the corpus of knowledge that had traditionally contributed to the appraisal of sanctity. On the other hand, the creation of a Christian museum in Rome aimed to provide the material evidence for a historically accurate reconstruction of the Christian past, especially of the lives and deeds of saints and martyrs. Both enterprises had a part to play in Lambertini's lifelong concerns with the assessment of sanctity. Both relied on the evidential power of specimens and artefacts.

[126] Giovanni Gaetano Bottari, *Sculture e pitture sagre estratte dai cimiteri di Roma, pubblicate già dagli autori della Roma sotterranea e ora nuovamente date in luce colle spiegazioni*, vol. 3 (Rome: Niccolò e Marco Pagliarini, 1754), xvii–xxi.

[127] Quoted in Von Pastor, *The History of the Popes*, 219–21.

[128] Ibid., 222.

[129] ASV, Fondo Benedetto XIV, Bolle e Costituzioni, 28, Letter of 22 January 1756, fol. 102.

In a classic article on shifting notions of evidence and changing approaches to the past, Arnaldo Momigliano drew attention to the emergence of a new trend in antiquarianism that over the course of the seventeenth and eighteenth centuries led antiquarians to favour direct contact with past artefacts over literary sources such as the reports of chroniclers and historians.[130] According to Momigliano, this shift was due to a crisis in the reliability of literary evidence and was accompanied by a new kind of antiquarianism that differed from the traditional one in that, for instance, those engaged in it 'preferred travel to the emendation of texts and altogether subordinated literary texts to coins, statues, vases and inscriptions'.[131] Ever since antiquarians and historians such as Ludovico Antonio Muratori drew attention to the view that knowledge of things acquired through the senses enjoyed a higher degree of reliability, a distinction was created between the evidential power of material remains, which were contemporary to past events, and the historical reports that were based on derivative authorities.[132] Because direct experience of material objects not only impressed the eye and the imagination, but also stimulated the approval of reason—as the astronomer and antiquarian Francesco Bianchini put it in his *Istoria universale provata con monumenti*—new practices of inquiry based on direct contact with specimens and artefacts came to be regarded as capable of providing the most reliable insights into the past that one could hope to achieve.[133] Thus advocating the primacy of the senses and encouraging practices that required direct contact with physical objects, the pursuits of antiquarians intersected with the endeavours of those who devoted themselves to natural inquiry and experimental culture in academies such as the Institute of the Sciences. Upon visiting the Institute of the Sciences, the historian Johann Wilhelm von Archenholz (1741–1812) described it as 'a vast collection of what belongs to each science or art in particular', noting that 'it is properly speaking a Cyclopaedia of the senses'.[134] When in the mid-eighteenth century Lambertini became the patron of anatomical

[130] Arnaldo Momigliano, 'Ancient History and the Antiquarian', *Journal of the Warburg and Courtauld Institutes*, 13:3/4 (1950), 285–315. See also Michael H. Crawford and Christopher R. Ligota (eds.), *Ancient History and the Antiquarian: Essays in Memory of Arnaldo Momigliano* (London: Warburg Institute, 1995); Peter N. Miller (ed.), *Momigliano and Antiquarianism: Foundations of the Modern Cultural Sciences* (Toronto: University of Toronto Press, 2007).

[131] Momigliano, 'Ancient History and the Antiquarian', 285.

[132] Ibid., 295–6. See also Ludovico Antonio Muratori, *Delle forze dell'intendimento umano, ossia Il pirronismo confutato* (Venice: Giambatista Pasquali, 1745).

[133] Francesco Bianchini, *La istoria universale provata con monumenti, e figurata con simboli degli Antichi* (Rome: Antonio de' Rossi, 1697), 20–1. Having been nominated by Clement XI 'presidente delle antichità' in 1703, Bianchini actively participated in Clement XI's project to create a museum of Christian antiquities, the Museo Ecclesiastico, which served as inspiration for Benedict XIV's Christian museum. On Bianchini's activities as an antiquarian and an astronomer, see Johns, *Papal Art and Cultural Politics*, chapter 2; Valentin Kockel and Brigitte Sölch (eds.), *Francesco Bianchini (1662–1729) und die europäische gelehrte Welt um 1700* (Berlin: Akademie Verlag, 2005). On the relationship between antiquarianism, empiricism, and medicine in seventeenth-century England, see Craig Ashley Hanson, *The English Virtuoso: Art, Medicine, and Antiquarianism in the Age of Empiricism* (Chicago: University of Chicago Press, 2009).

[134] Johann Wilhelm von Archenholz, *A Picture of Italy*, vol. 1, trans. J. Trapp (London: for G.G.J. and J. Robinson, 1791), 126. On the senses in the eighteenth century see, for instance, Anne C. Vila (ed.), *A Cultural History of the Senses in the Age of Enlightenment, 1650–1800* (New York: Bloomsbury Academic, 2014).

ccollections in Bologna and antiquarian displays in Rome, many were similarly touring the Italian peninsula in search of fresh contact with material remains and physical objects. Following in the footsteps of generations of pilgrims who had preceded them, they responded to the call for proximity and contact with material objects that promised to further their knowledge of both nature and the past.

In supporting notions of authenticity that had been articulated in association with the empowerment of first-hand experience with things, anatomical and antiquarian displays played a distinctive part in Lambertini's claims of authority. Defining how nature and the past should be viewed, they outlined new patterns in the relationship between nature, history, and Christian revelation. In his *De servorum Dei*, Lambertini emphasized that, once the canonization process was completed, the final decision fell to the pope, whose conclusion he took to be incontestable. In 1746, the only ceremony of successful canonization to take place under Lambertini's pontificate was also a celebration of the reliability of the whole process. The event saw the proclamation of five saints. St Peter's Basilica, the centre of Catholic worship, was newly designated as the sole appropriate venue for canonization ceremonies; the decorations were grandiose and the crimson damasks of twenty-nine different churches were added to the Basilica's own magnificent ones (Figure 1.4).

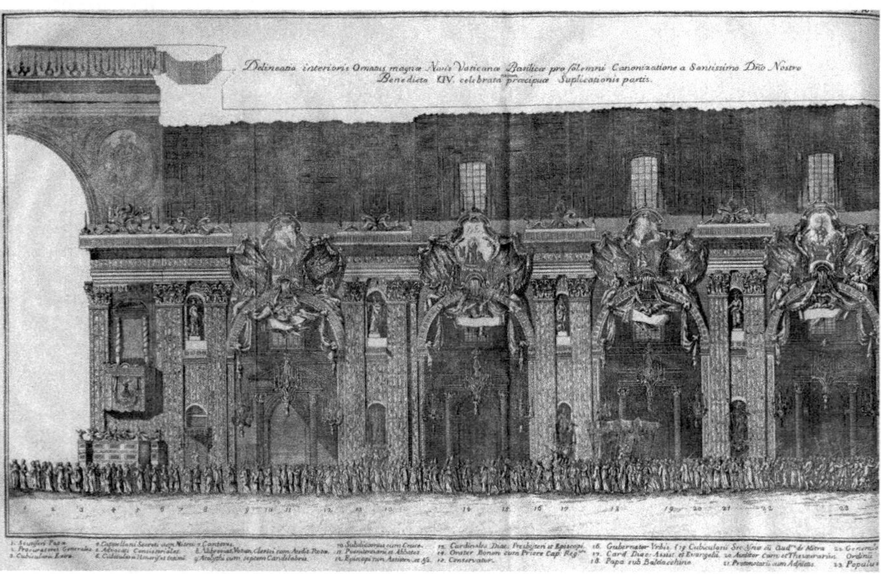

Figure 1.4 Layout of the decorations in the grand nave of St Peter's Basilica for the ceremony of beatification and canonization celebrated by Pope Benedict XIV in June 1746, in Prospero Lambertini (Pope Benedict XIV), *Benedicti XIV, Pont. Opt. Max. olim Prosperic cardinalis de Lambertinis Opera omnia in unum corpus collecta*..., Bassano: Typograhpia Bassanensi, sumptibus Remondini Veneti, 1767, vol. 7.

Read against the foregoing story of Lambertini's patronage of anatomical and natural knowledge in Bologna, and of Christian erudition and antiquities in Rome, such emphasis on the celebration of accomplished beatification and canonization challenges the reading of Lambertini's patronage of anatomical collections as the expression of an 'enlightened' *pape savant* who championed an age of reform. Rather, the imposing ceremony points to the pontiff's involvement in the reorganization of visual and material domains in a way that could support new links between the mapping of the borders of the natural world, the legitimizing role of the relics of the past, and the reliability of saint-making processes, in keeping with the evidence presented via anatomical models, and alongside the pope's claims to jurisdiction over both the temporal and spiritual realms.

2

Artificer and Connoisseur

'LABORIOUS MERE ANATOMICAL BUSINESS'

Ercole Lelli started his career as a harquebus maker and ended it as a connoisseur. As part of the process, he associated his name with the collection of anatomical models sponsored by Benedict XIV for the Bolognese Institute of the Sciences. Some three decades after Lelli's death, in his *Letter to the Society of Dilettanti*, the Irish artist James Barry encouraged the Royal Academy of Arts to adopt Lelli's method of teaching how to draw, which combined the drawing of the nude body with the visual scrutiny of both ancient statues and anatomical models. Barry had been introduced to this method by Giles Hussey, an English artist who had befriended Lelli in Italy. In Barry's view, Lelli's drawing was so 'remarkable for purity and science', and his anatomical figure, even when 'considered independently of the anatomical skill', was 'of so admirable a style as to form and character' that he regretted that Lelli

> had not followed such pursuits and left to others the laborious mere anatomical business of the several wax preparations built upon the skeletons, running into all the infinitesimal details of the gravid uterus, the organs of hearing, vision, and other minute particulars of endless mere observation, upon which so much of his time and attention was thrown away.[1]

Writing at the end of the eighteenth century, Barry regarded Lelli's engagement with the details of anatomical models as a waste of time, something that could have been done just as well 'by inferior characters'.[2] In fact, half a century earlier, anatomical modelling had crucially contributed to Lelli's career and fame in the worlds of natural knowledge and connoisseurship. This chapter follows the making and early viewing of the anatomy room commissioned from Lelli for the Institute of the Sciences. In particular, it explores the creation of a new space of anatomical encounter and reconstructs the bearings that this space had on Lelli's occupational trajectory from harquebus maker to connoisseur. As the anatomy room of the Institute of the Sciences provided one of the earliest occasions for the public display of anatomical models in the Italian peninsula, it also acquired central significance in Lelli's career. In the course of the eighteenth century, the elaboration of a

[1] James Barry, *A Letter to the Dilettanti Society, Respecting the Obtention of Certain Matters Essentially Necessary for the Improvement of Public Taste* [...], 2nd edn. (London: J. Walker, 1799), 125–8. Shortly after the appearance of his *Letter*, in 1799 Barry was expelled from the Royal Academy of Arts.

[2] Ibid., 127–8.

public culture of natural knowledge 'was sustained to a great degree by artisans and craftsmen'.[3] As anatomical models offered a particularly cogent material expression to anatomy's claims and promises, their artificers found themselves at the centre of anatomy's public stage. This chapter reconstructs how, as the primary artificer and demonstrator of the anatomical collection sponsored by the pope, Lelli owed much of his success to his manual and mechanical skills. However, he carefully crafted his public persona as a hands-off connoisseur.

Recent literature has suggested that the anatomy room evoked the moral tone of the public anatomy lesson held in the Bolognese anatomical theatre and was envisioned as a venue for artistic training rather than medical learning.[4] In what follows, I argue that the anatomy room had multiple uses and meanings, and encompassed different vocations that variously contributed to its capacity to serve as a site of knowledge. Commissioned by the pope, and made and demonstrated by an artificer and mechanic who fashioned himself as a connoisseur, the room was employed in the training of both artists and surgeons, and was visited by Grand Tour travellers, *curiosi*, literati, and *personaggi*. Operating as an arena for educating the gaze of artists, surgeons, and antiquarians, it served as a venue for engaging in observational practices that transferred across anatomical, artistic, and antiquarian domains as well as a site of moral warning mediating messages about the transiency of life and evoking the consequences of the Fall. In fact, all these different aspects participated in the fashioning of the anatomy room as a special setting for the display and investigation of human nature.

Different though its meanings may have been, the making and early viewing of the anatomy room ended up being associated with one person, Ercole Lelli, who was entrusted with the task of realizing it and obtained lifetime employment as its custodian and demonstrator. In all of these capacities, Lelli presented himself as a go-between, aptly navigating across anatomical, artistic, and mechanical domains and capable of employing his manual and mechanical skills in a significant array of tasks.[5] Scholars who have explored the role of artisans in early modern domains of natural knowledge have importantly shed light on how famous societies, such as the Royal Society in London and the Academy of the Sciences in Paris, recast the relationships between artisanal knowledge and natural philosophy.[6] Less attention

[3] Larry Stewart and Paul Weindling, 'Philosophical Threads: Natural Philosophy and Public Experiment among the Weavers of Spitalfields', *The British Journal for the History of Science*, 28:1 (1995), 37–62 (citation p. 37).

[4] Messbarger, *The Lady Anatomist*, chapter 1.

[5] On go-betweens, see Schaffer et al. (eds.), *The Brokered World*.

[6] See, for instance, Robert Iliffe, 'Material Doubts: Hooke, Artisan Culture and the Exchange of Information in 1670s London', *The British Journal for the History of Science*, 28:3 (1995), 285–318; Simon Schaffer, 'Experimenters' Techniques, Dyers' Hands, and the Electric Planetarium', *Isis*, 88:3 (1997), 456–83; James A. Bennett, 'Shopping for Instruments in Paris and London', in Smith and Findlen (eds.), *Merchants and Marvels*, 370–98; Liliane Hilaire-Pérez, 'Technology as a Public Culture in the Eighteenth Century: The Artisans' Legacy', *History of Science*, 45:2 (2007), 135–53; Liliane Hilaire-Pérez, 'Technology, Curiosity and Utility in France and in England in the Eighteenth Century', in Bensaude-Vincent and Blondel (eds.), *Science and Spectacle*, 25–42; Smith, *The Body of the Artisan*; Simon Werrett, 'Healing the Nation's Wounds: Royal Ritual and Experimental Philosophy in Restoration England', *History of Science*, 38 (2000), 377–99; Werrett, *Fireworks*.

has been drawn to how eighteenth-century academies rearticulated the relationship between the arts and sciences in the context of the Italian peninsula's widespread artisanal traditions. Here, rich and enduring artisanal cultures, which had developed alongside religious, civic, and courtly rituals and ceremonies, created a particularly fertile terrain for addressing academies' conspicuous demand for 'mindful hands'.[7] Relying on manual skills in endeavours that were aimed at designing their own *raisons d'être* at the crossroads of natural inquiry, experimental culture, and craft, many such academies operated as sites of encounter and exchange—as well as conflict—between artisans and savants.

In this chapter I consider the history of the making and early viewing of mid-eighteenth-century anatomical collections as a significant example of the relationship between artisanal and academic knowledge. I suggest that artificers like Lelli could capitalize on the fluidity of this relationship to present anatomical modelling in ways that could advance the status of their practices and their own role within the world of knowledge and the arts. In particular, following Lelli's engagement in the creation and early viewing of the anatomy room, I reconstruct the story of an artificer whose manifold manual and mechanical skills became critical to his capacity to attract patronage and gain legitimacy in both artistic and anatomical settings. Having entered the Institute of the Sciences as an artist and an anatomical modeller, Lelli ended up engaging in all sorts of activities, thus becoming ever more indispensable to the life of the Institute. As a mechanic, a modeller, an artist, and the demonstrator of several collections, Lelli used his encounters with audiences to publicize his skills and credentials. While fashioning himself as a connoisseur, he also ended up being regarded as a key player in the domain of viewing and visibility that developed alongside the tenet that appreciation of detail could yield true knowledge.[8] Crucial to the success of his undertakings was the presence in the Italian peninsula of a travelling public that integrated anatomical collections, as well as antiquities and curiosities, into Grand Tour itineraries.

LELLI AND THE HARQUEBUS LINCHPIN

Ercole Lelli's entrée into the world of anatomical modelling was preceded by stories about his skilled hands. As a young man, he apprenticed in the workshop of Domenico Brugnoli in Via delle Clavature, one of the narrow medieval streets off Bologna's main square, where he made a name for himself as a harquebus maker.[9]

[7] On 'mindful hands', see Lissa Roberts, Simon Schaffer, and Peter Dear (eds.), *The Mindful Hand: Inquiry and Investigation from the Late Renaissance to Early Industrialization* (Amsterdam: Koninklijke Nederlandse Akademie van Wetenschappen, 2007).

[8] On connoisseurship in the context of early modern natural and medical pursuits, see Cook, *Matters of Exchange*; Hanson, *The English Virtuoso*; Daniela Bleichmar, 'Learning to Look: Visual Expertise across Art and Science in Eighteenth-Century France', *Eighteenth-Century Studies*, 46:1 (2012), 85–111.

[9] Archivio dell'Accademia di Belle Arti di Bologna (henceforth AABAB), Atti dell'Accademia Clementina, 'Ristretto della Vita del defunto sig. Ercole Lelli', vol. 2, fol. 35; BCABo, ms. B 134,

Like many early modern workshops, Brugnoli's shop was a meeting point. Hunters, gunners, and those interested in artillery were habitués of the place where they gathered, chatted, and gossiped. After the marquis Barbazza, Bolognese senator and avid hunter, celebrated English proficiency in the art of working metals, and lamented the lack of refinement of local artefacts, the fourteen-year-old Ercole engineered a hoax. Having secretly made a beautifully carved linchpin, he placed it in an elegant box and passed it on to his accomplice, the *cavalier* Pasi. Upon visiting the workshop, Pasi claimed to have just received a linchpin from London and showed it to his friends. Barbazza called Lelli over to show him its perfect manufacture. When Lelli suggested opening the linchpin, the group was in for a surprise. Upon seeing the name 'Ercole Lelli' engraved in the metal, everybody was amused and full of admiration. Pasi commissioned from Lelli a harquebus that could fit the linchpin.[10]

The story of Lelli's linchpin introduces us to the atmosphere of an early modern artillery workshop, where practitioners, hunters, aristocrats, and connoisseurs gathered around the art of making guns. Here, they gossiped, chatted, exchanged knowledge and expertise, shared views on the state of the art, and enjoyed a good laugh.[11] The episode also draws attention to the role of the artisanal workshop as a site of knowledge, apprenticeship, and patronage—the place of formation of a young talented artificer who had remarkable manual skills. Notably, the event took place in 1714, the year of the inauguration of the Institute of the Sciences.

Luigi Ferdinando Marsigli, the Institute's founder, had been keen to integrate military art into the Institute's experimental agenda.[12] Simon Werrett has observed that as early modern gunners sought to present their engagement in artillery and military arts as a domain of natural inquiry that was suitable for courtly consumption, they articulated the language of artillery in the vocabulary of the liberal arts.[13] Quite naturally, part of their success rested on the extensive employment of European noblemen in the military. Marsigli himself had pursued a military career. Stories of his interest in gathering military as well as natural knowledge during his espionage, diplomatic, and military missions in Ottoman and Habsburg lands appropriately capture his composite identity as a natural inquirer and a military man. While his project to foster experimental culture in Bologna drew on the examples of the French Academy of the Sciences and the Royal Society, his vision for the Institute of the Sciences brought together the fine and the mechanical arts, including gunnery, and experimental knowledge.[14] In 1739, the *Insignia*, which visually recorded the visit of Frederick

Marcello Oretti, *Notizie de' Professori del Dissegno cioè Pittori, Scultori ed Architetti bolognesi e de' forestieri di sua scuola*, vol. 12, 119–24.

[10] Medici, 'Elogio d'Ercole Lelli', 160–1.

[11] On gossip in early modern workshops, see, for instance, Filippo de Vivo, *Information and Communication in Venice: Rethinking Early Modern Politics* (Oxford: Oxford University Press, 2007).

[12] Cavazza, *Settecento inquieto*, esp. chapter 6.

[13] Werrett, *Fireworks*, 35–41.

[14] On gunnery in early modern natural inquiries, see ibid.; Bert S. Hall, *Weapons and Warfare in Renaissance Europe: Gunpowder, Technology, and Tactics* (Baltimore: Johns Hopkins University Press, 1997).

Christian, prince-elector of Saxony and son of the king of Poland, to the Institute, staged a setting where the project was seemingly accomplished: canons and maps of fortifications stood alongside scientific instruments, anatomical models, the school of drawing, and the library, all harmoniously gathered together under the same roof (Plate 6). To be sure, not everybody shared Marsigli's eagerness to integrate the mechanical and the fine arts. The establishment of the Accademia Clementina, the art academy of the Institute of the Sciences, gave expression to the aspiration of a number of Bolognese artists to distinguish themselves from what they regarded as lower level artificers, an agenda that was at odds with Marsigli's own goals.[15] In such a climate, bridging the gap between gun-making and the fine arts was not easy. Lelli himself stumbled into the consequences of this tension when he first tried to set foot into the world of fine arts.

As the story has it, while working in Brugnoli's workshop Lelli sought to befriend the young artists who were apprenticed in the neighbouring atelier of the master painter Giovan Gioseffo Dal Sole (1654–1719) and convince them to teach him how to paint.[16] Yet, when he made a portrait of their teacher and donated it to him, Dal Sole declined the gift and encouraged Lelli to stick to gun-making. In fact, Dal Sole was among the painters who were keen to keep the mechanical and the fine arts apart.[17] Notably, in 1688, he joined the petitioners who requested the establishment of an academy that would sanction the autonomy and the privileges of painters over other artificers. Later on, he supported the foundation of the Accademia Clementina.[18] For his part, unscathed by Dal Sole's dismissal, Lelli continued to work his way into the Bolognese world of fine arts. In 1736, his marriage to Anna Panzacchi, a family member of the well-known painter Maria Elena

[15] Giampietro Zanotti, *Storia dell'Accademia Clementina di Bologna* (Bologna: Lelio dalla Volpe, 1739). See also Massimo Ferretti, 'Il notomista e il canonico', in *I materiali dell'Istituto delle Scienze*, 100–14, esp. 108–10; Stefano Benassi, *L'Accademia Clementina: La funzione pubblica e l'ideologia estetica* (Bologna: Minerva Edizioni, 2004), 85–6.

[16] BCABo, ms. B 134, Marcello Oretti, *Notizie de' Professori del Dissegno*, vol. 12, 119.

[17] See Eugenio Riccomini, *Mostra della scultura bolognese del Settecento: Catalogo* (Bologna: Tamari, 1966), 105; Benassi, *L'Accademia Clementina*, 86–7. As early as 1599, some Bolognese members of the painters' guild, including Ludovico Carracci, had sought to dissociate themselves from the *bombasari*, cotton and wool workers and artificers who made and sold *bambocci*, that is, dolls and three-dimensional figures in materials such as wood, wool, and wax. In 1602, the painters' guild also managed to be separated from the other arts, which meant that whoever exercised the art of painting without being aggregated to the company had to pay a fee, though nothing guaranteed that only painters be aggregated to the guild. The issue was resumed again at the end of the seventeenth century, when a new *Memoriale* submitted by a number of Bolognese painters to the Senate emphasized the role of painting as an activity pertaining to the intellect, rather than to the hand.

[18] Benassi, *L'Accademia Clementina*, 87. Dal Sole may have been among those who remained dissatisfied when the Cardinal Legate and Gonfalonier of Bologna ruled that the *bombasari* belonged to the painters' guild. For their part, painters continued to try to restrict *bombasari*'s activities and their production of paintings, drawings, and figures. As late as 1761, they pleaded to the *Assunti* of the Institute of the Sciences to obtain the right to keep the activities of the *bombasari* in check and thus forbid them from producing sacred images, statues, and bas-reliefs; see ASB, Assunteria d'Istituto, Diversorum, busta 30, n. 16, 'Ricorso degli Accademici Clementini contro gli abusi dei "Formatori" riguardanti la produzione e vendita delle loro statuette e contro le "Perizie" di oggetti artistici operate dai Formatori'. See also Carmen Lorenzetti, 'Tecniche e materiali', in Renzo Grandi et al. (eds.) *Presepi e terrecotte nei Musei Civici di Bologna* (Bologna: Nuova Alfa Editoriale, 1991), 77.

Panzacchi, marked his entrée into one of the notable Bolognese artistic families. And when Maria Elena died the following year, Lelli acted as executor.[19]

By then, Lelli had befriended the Bolognese artist Giampietro Zanotti (1674–1765), who introduced him to the study of anatomy in art. In 1727, Lelli won the prize for painting in the first Marsigli competition that was held at the Accademia Clementina. Along with Giampietro Zanotti, the jury included the artist Angelo Michele Cavazzoni, who had illustrated the tables of both Valsalva's and Morgagni's anatomical works.[20] In the following years, Lelli immersed himself in the study of anatomy. In December 1729, Zanotti famously wrote a sonnet that seemed to hint that Lelli's passion for anatomy was bordering on obsession: 'tell me, Ercolin, what are you up to? I haven't seen you for a long time... I believe you are no longer flaying cadavers just to learn the anatomy, since you already know what a painter should know.'[21] Zanotti warned Lelli about the risks of paying too much attention to anatomy while overlooking other important artistic features, though he encouraged him not to worry about those who disparaged the use of anatomy in art.[22] Over time, Zanotti took a more tentative stand, and in his *Storia dell'Accademia Clementina* (1739) he remarked that artists could acquire sufficient anatomical knowledge without having to dissect.[23] In the meantime, however, Lelli's dedication to anatomy had been praised by Francesco Maria Zanotti, Giampietro's brother and secretary of the Institute of the Sciences, who, in 1731, had celebrated Lelli's engagement in anatomical wax modelling in the *De Bononiensi Scientiarum et Artium Instituto atque Academia Commentarii*.[24] As Zanotti observed, Lelli devoted himself to dissecting and flaying bodily parts so as to reconstruct the origins and progress of muscles. In order to remember what he saw, he made anatomical wax figures of the dissected parts.[25] As we have seen, this is also what he did when he was asked to create a model of the 'horseshoe' kidney found by Lorenzo Bonazzoli (Plate 1).[26] In the following years, Lelli's involvement in the city's anatomical activities continued to grow. In 1732, Giuseppe Ippolito Pozzi, professor of anatomy at the University of Bologna and a member of the Institute of the Sciences, reported to the physician Pier Paolo Molinelli about the anatomical observations he had made with Lelli.[27] In 1734, Lelli famously created, together

[19] ASB, Archivio Boschi, busta 232.

[20] AABAB, Atti dell'Accademia Clementina, vol. 1, 63; Francesco Maria Zanotti, 'De iis, quae Instituto jam condito adjuncta sunt', 29; Giuseppe Gaetano Bolletti, *Dell'origine e de' progressi dell'Istituto delle Scienze di Bologna* (Bologna: Lelio dalla Volpe, 1751), 79.

[21] Giovanni Gaetano Bottari and Stefano Ticozzi, *Raccolta di lettere sulla pittura, scultura ed architettura, scritte da' più celebri personaggi dei secoli XV, XVI, e XVII*, vol. 2 (Milan: Giovanni Silvestri, 1822), 193.

[22] Ibid., 193–8.

[23] Ferretti, 'Il notomista e il canonico', 102 and 103. See also Giampietro Zanotti, *Avvertimenti di Giampietro Cavazzoni Zanotti, per lo incamminamento di un giovane alla pittura* (Bologna: Lelio dalla Volpe, 1756), 74–82.

[24] Zanotti, 'De iis, quae Instituto jam condito adjuncta sunt', 29.

[25] Ibid.

[26] ASB, Assunteria d'Istituto, Atti, n. 3 (1727–34), 631.

[27] Emilio De Tipaldo (ed.), *Biografia degli Italiani illustri nelle scienze, lettere ed arti del secolo XVIII...*, vol. 8 (Venice: Alvisopoli, 1841), 68 (entry on Giuseppe Ippolito Pozzi). On observation in early modern medicine, see Gianna Pomata, 'Observation Rising: Birth of an Epistemic Genre, 1500–1650', in Lorraine Daston and Elizabeth Lunbeck (eds.), *Histories of Scientific Observation*

with the sculptor Silvestro Giannotti, two wooden écorchés for the anatomical theatre, a project for which he claimed to have dissected fifty cadavers (Plate 7). The écorchés replaced the old, moth-eaten caryatis and, in a sense, marked the end of the long gestation of the Bolognese anatomical theatre.[28] By then, Lelli had also started to devote himself to the first project of an anatomical museum launched by Lambertini and was working at a number of anatomical tables that displayed the bones of the human body, 'this being the starting point of anatomy'.[29] A number of anatomical statues were then meant to show 'the origin, progress, insertion, and direction of the fibers of each muscle, so as to acquire knowledge of its use'.[30] As we have seen, the demise of Niccolò Aldrovandi, the sponsor of the initiative, truncated the project in 1734.

In 1739, traces of this early attempt were made visible in the *Insignia* commemorating the visit of Prince Frederick Christian, where one can catch a glimpse of a few anatomical models in the background on the left-hand side of the picture (Plate 6).[31] At that point, however, the unfinished anatomical display looked like a rather modest accomplishment. Upon seeing it in 1738, the mechanic Albertino Reynier, who visited the Institute in order to bring back ideas for the project of a university museum in Turin, was not impressed. Rather, he came to the conclusion that, as far as anatomy was concerned, the Institute did not have much more to offer than the expression of goodwill.[32] In the same period, other visitors praised the Institute's collections but had little to say about its anatomical display.[33] Among them, the savant Charles de Brosses (1709–1777), the first president of the Burgundy parliament, visited the Institute in September 1739 and described it as 'one of the most curious' things in Europe.[34] De Brosses was particularly fond of the room of natural history, where everything 'was disposed in a charming order', in glass cases, and even the smallest specimens had a label, with the name, a small description and 'a reference to the book where one could find the whole history'.[35] In fact, he was so enthusiastic that he concluded that he wished he could take his furniture there and move in. Yet, he mentioned only in passing the 'different kinds of dissected figures, which were contained in glass cases'.[36]

(Chicago: University of Chicago Press, 2011), 45–80; Gianna Pomata, 'A Word of the Empirics: The Ancient Concept of Observation and its Recovery in Early Modern Medicine', *Annals of Science*, 65:1 (2011), 1–25.

[28] See Ferrari, 'Public Anatomy Lessons'.

[29] ASB, Assunteria d'Istituto, Diversorum, busta 10, n. 1, 'Proposte per statue anatomiche'.

[30] Ibid.

[31] Before the initial project of an anatomy room was suspended, Lelli had completed at least two anatomical statues; see ASB, Assunteria d'Istituto, Atti, n. 3 (1727–34).

[32] BCABo, Fondo Speciale *Collezione degli Autografi*, LXV, 17584–754, Letter n. 17587. On the museum in Turin, see Michela di Macco, 'Il "Museo Accademico" delle Scienze nel Palazzo dell'Università di Torino. Progetti e istituzioni nell'età dei Lumi', in Giacomo Giacobini (ed.), *La memoria della scienza: Musei e collezioni dell'Università di Torino* (Turin: Fondazione CRT, 2003), 29–52.

[33] See, for instance, Charles-Nicolas Cochin, *Voyage d'Italie, ou recueil de notes sur les ouvrages de peinture et de sculpture, qu'on voit dans les principales villes d'Italie*, vol. 2 (Paris: Ch. Ant Jombert, 1758), 118.

[34] Charles de Brosses, *Le président de Brosses en Italie, lettres familières écrites d'Italie en 1739 et 1740*, 12th edn., vol. 1 (Paris: Didier et Cie., 1858), 244.

[35] Ibid., 246.

[36] Ibid.

The project of an anatomy room launched by Lambertini was not the first instance of gathering anatomical specimens on the Institute's premises. In the 1720s, the Institute had inherited a collection of dry anatomical preparations that had been completed by Antonio Maria Valsalva.[37] Providing a material complement to his famous anatomical treatise on the ear, the *De aure humana tractatus*, Valsalva's cabinet included dry preparations of the ear, the nerves and arteries, and became renowned among anatomists.[38] Yet, the Institute did not seem to be in a hurry to acquire it. When, shortly after Valsalva's death, his widow Elena Lini was ready to donate 'all the Anatomical Preparations, and the many other Natural and Morbous rarities' that had belonged to her late husband, the Institute did not initially react.[39] Months later, when Lini was about to change residence, she had to urge the Institute's *Assunti* to collect the specimens, lest they be damaged in the move.[40] Once at the Institute, the collection was placed in the tower of the observatory. However, much to everybody's dismay, the specimens rapidly started to show signs of decay. Lelli was then summoned to stop the rot.[41]

Everything was to change when, in September 1742, the Institute of the Sciences received a papal dispatch breaking the news that the pope was keen to resume the project of an anatomical museum. Ten years had passed since the time Lambertini had first suggested creating such a museum at the Institute of the Sciences. Having been elected to the pontificate, Lambertini was now ready to resume the project that he had originally envisioned, this time in his capacity as a powerful patron, personally capable of securing the resources needed to realize it.[42] The *Assunti* were thrilled. Lelli was called back to complete the work he had initiated in the 1730s and submitted a new, enlarged plan.[43] The plan was then sent to the ambassador in Rome who, with a sense of pressing urgency, dispatched it at once to the pope regardless of the stormy weather. With the pope now acting as a willing patron, the whole project of an anatomy room took on a new air of increased expectation and overall grandeur. The hope was that the anatomy room would suffice 'by itself to make the Institute famous'. In fact, 'although Florence, Turin and some other transalpine countries' held some remarkable anatomical cabinets, none of them would equal the degree of accomplishment of the Bolognese plan. Even 'if the project were to be limited to the display of bones and muscles, and were mainly suited for the practical use of surgeons', it promised to ensure the fame of the Institute.[44]

[37] ASB, Assunteria d'Istituto, Diversorum, busta 10, n. 0, 'Museo Anatomico Valsalva'. See also Medici, 'Elogio d'Ercole Lelli', 173–4.

[38] See Cotugno, 'Iter Italicum', 73–5.

[39] ASB, Assunteria d'Istituto, Diversorum, busta 10, n. 0, 'Museo Anatomico Valsalva'.

[40] Ibid.

[41] ASB, Assunteria d'Istituto, Atti, n. 3 (1727–34), 709–10. Lelli saw that some of the specimens showed signs of being worm-eaten. He noticed that oil of turpentine kept the woodworms away and used it to restore the specimens. However, the anatomist Giambattista Morgagni was afraid that the oil of turpentine could harden the preparations and damage them; see Cotugno, 'Iter Italicum', 92.

[42] ASB, Assunteria d'Istituto, Lettere all' Istituto, n. 4 (1734–52), Letter of 15 September 1742.

[43] ASB, Assunteria d'Istituto, Diversorum, busta 10, n. 2. See also Francesco Maria Zanotti, 'De anatome in Institutum introducenda', 44–6.

[44] ASB, Assunteria d'Istituto, Lettere dell' Istituto, n. 3 (1735–55), Letter of 26 September 1742 from the Institute to the ambassador; Ibid., Lettere all'Istituto, n. 4 (1734–1752), Letter from the ambassador of 13 October 1742.

Turin was indeed one of the Institute's main competitors. When, in 1739, the king of Sardinia, Charles Emmanuel III of Savoy, decided to establish a museum for the Royal University, the project included a large anatomy room, gathering both anatomical models from the private cabinets of physicians and surgeons, and some new 'anatomical machines'.[45] The aim was not only to present 'what one could demonstrate on an accurate anatomical sculpture in big, small, or minuscule size', but also to create the conditions for 'a perfect anatomical course', including the display of generation from the egg and the embryo to birth, as well as the development of the human body at different ages. In doing so, anatomical models would save students the 'horror and stench' of anatomical dissection while unveiling the body with 'greater clarity, aptness, and utility' than cadavers could possibly do.[46] The project generated palpable satisfaction, eliciting the conviction that such an anatomical collection could outdo many 'famous museums of Europe' thanks to the 'incredible degree of skill put in the preparation of specimens and the amount of money and time'.[47] In 1742, the *Assunti* of the Bolognese Institute were keen to outdo Turin's plan.

AN ANATOMY ROOM AT THE INSTITUTE OF THE SCIENCES

Nobody thought that it was going to be easy. Not the pope; not the *Assunti*; least of all Lelli. Nor was it going to be cheap. As academicians in Turin observed, one of the reasons why anatomical cabinets were few and far between was the amount of money and time that was involved in their creation.[48] In Bologna, all parties concerned were equally aware that creating an anatomy room was going to be costly and time-consuming. Lelli, the artificer in charge, put conditions in place that were likely to increase the costs even further. Since dissecting cadavers was a proverbially dangerous activity, it required regular intermissions, especially in the summer, and thus the anatomy room would take at least six years to complete.[49] Lelli also asked to continue his work as a coiner at the mint during such intermissions so that he could return to his occupation upon the completion of the anatomy room. Finally, he demanded to be able to count on the assistance of both 'a sculptor capable of working with wax' and a surgeon who would bring bodily parts from the hospital and help with the preparations.[50] It fell on the young surgeon

45 Di Macco, 'Il "Museo Accademico"', 38–39, 46, and 49–50. See also Giacomo Giacobini et al., 'Il Museo di Anatomia umana', in Giacobini (ed.), *La memoria della scienza*, 143.

46 Archivio di Stato di Torino (henceforth ASTo), Corte, Materie Economiche, Istruzione Pubblica, Regia Università di Torino, mazzo 5, fasc. 17, 'Progetto del Magistrato della Riforma de' Studi a' riguardo dello stabilimento d'un Museo'; also quoted in di Macco, 'Il "Museo Accademico"', 49.

47 Ibid. 48 Ibid.

49 Lelli himself had become sick when he was working on the anatomical statues for the anatomical theatre that had been completed in 1734.

50 ASB, Assunteria d'Istituto, Lettere dell'Istituto, n. 3 (1735–55), Letter of 6 October 1742 from the Institute to the ambassador. At the beginning of October, Lelli's plan was sent to the pope along with a drawing of the room to be devoted to anatomy.

Boari to travel back and forth between Lelli's workshop and the hospitals.[51] The chosen sculptor was Filippo Scandellari (1717–1801), who was well known in town for his abilities as a wax sculptor, though the name of the equally renowned wax modeller Domenico Piò also appeared in the early records of the anatomy room.[52] As part of his involvement in the anatomy room, Scandellari would acquire over time 'mechanical cognitions of anatomy' so that he could replace Lelli in case of illness or death.[53]

The new project expanded the initial plan of 1732. Focusing on the anatomy of muscles and bones, which were taken 'to be particularly important for surgery', it included eight anatomical statues and a number of anatomical tables that would introduce viewers to a whole course of anatomy (Plate 4).[54] Two standing wax figures of a naked woman and a naked man (dubbed Eve and Adam), were finished with real teeth and hair, and were meant to display the symmetry and the distinct anatomical sites of the human body while, at the same time, showing the differences between the female and the male body (Plates 8 and 9).[55] A sequence of four écorchés built on natural skeletons was meant to unveil the different muscular layers of the male body (Plates 10–13). Two skeletons, one female and one male, completed the sequence and were also meant to show 'the difference that characterizes the two sexes also in relation to the figure and the layout of some bones' (Plates 14 and 15).[56] Some thirty large tables further presented models of the larynx, the pharynx, the parts of generation, the eye, and the ear, as well as the muscles that could not be displayed on the anatomical statues.

In his initial plan of 1732, Lelli had mentioned that, in his modelling, he followed the anatomical order set out by 'Vesalius, Valverde, Eustachius, and other anatomists, both Ancients and Moderns'.[57] The poses, postures, and general mode of presentation of the écorchés of the anatomy room largely drew on the muscle-men that appeared in these works. In doing so, they also reflected the convention that regarded muscles as characteristic of the male body and demoted the visualization of female muscles as an abuse of anatomical principles in art.[58] Lelli may have based his view that the skeleton was a locus of difference between the female and male body on some of these works. The dating, origins, modes, and motivations of

[51] ASB, Assunteria d'Istituto, Diversorum, busta 10, n. 2; ASB, Assunteria d'Istituto, Lettere dell'Istituto, n. 3 (1735–55), Letter of 20 October 1742 from the Institute to the ambassador.

[52] Carlo Pisarri, *Dialoghi tra Claro, e Sarpiri per istruire chi desidera d'essere un eccellente pittore figurista* (Bologna: Ferdinando Pisarri, 1778), 49.

[53] ASB, Assunteria d'Istituto, Lettere dell'Istituto, n. 3 (1735–55), Letter of 20 October 1742 from the Institute to the ambassador.

[54] ASB, Assunteria d'Istituto, Diversorum, busta 10, n. 2. See also Zanotti, 'De anatome in Institutum introducenda', 45.

[55] ASB, Assunteria d'Istituto, Diversorum, busta 10, n. 2.

[56] Ibid.; Zanotti, 'De anatome in Institutum introducenda'. See also Dacome, '"Un certo e quasi incredibile piacere"', 422–3.

[57] ASB, Assunteria d'Istituto, Diversorum, busta 10, n. 1, 'Proposte per Statue Anatomiche'.

[58] See Girolamo Mercuriale, *De arte gymnastica* (Venice: Junta, 1573). On early modern muscle-men, see Martin Kemp, 'A Drawing for the Fabrica; and Some Thoughts upon the Vesalius Muscle-Men', *Medical History*, 14:3 (1970), 277–88; Stephen Greenblatt, 'Toward a Universal Language of Motion: Reflections on a Seventeenth-Century Muscle Man', in Susan Leigh Foster (ed.), *Choreographing History* (Bloomington: Indiana University Press, 1995), 25–31.

the process of sexualization of the skeleton have been the object of discussion among historians.[59] However, even in the eyes of eighteenth-century viewers, the question was far from settled. Lelli remarked that the female skeleton highlighted the differences between female and male bodies. Yet, when, in 1751, Giuseppe Gaetano Bolletti (1709–1769) published the first comprehensive description of the Institute's collections in his *Dell'origine e progressi dell'Istituto delle Scienze di Bologna*, he referred to the female skeleton in the anatomy room as showing similarities between the sexes.[60] As Bolletti's work informed other writings on Bologna and was shipped home by travellers, the divergence of opinions was only bound to grow.[61]

MAKING MODELS

With a papal mandate, a complete work plan, and the help of a junior surgeon and an artist, Lelli set off to begin work on the anatomy room. It all started with the gathering of the materials, including iron armatures and wires, silk, tallow, trementine, mastic, pigments, pins, varnish, oil of turpentine, and scagliola, as well as, of course, wax, both the wax of the Levant and the lower quality 'sottana' wax.[62] As contemporaries observed, the models of the anatomy room were made of 'soft and durable matter'.[63] When the Neapolitan anatomist Domenico Cotugno visited the Institute of the Sciences in 1765, Lelli shared some insights into the making of the models with him: with the exception of the two wax figures of a woman and a man, the other anatomical statues were built on natural bones. Thus, to begin with, one had to choose the bones of a young and slender body. These had to be pierced, boiled, injected with hot water, boiled again, washed in cold water, exposed to open air and finally coated with white wax before being exposed to the sun and sprinkled with water. The bones were then tied with metals and hooks so as to allow for 'all the possible human movements according to nature'.[64] Being entirely made of wax, the female and male figures ran the risk of melting in the summer and hardening in the winter. However, the écorchés statues 'would live

[59] This point has been articulated in the context of broader discussions on the history of sexual difference; see, for instance, Londa Schiebinger, 'Skeletons in the Closet: The First Illustrations of the Female Skeleton in Eighteenth-Century Anatomy', *Representations*, 14 (1986), 42–82; Thomas W. Laqueur, *Making Sex: Body and Gender from the Greeks to Freud* (Cambridge, MA: Harvard University Press, 1990); Michael Stolberg, 'A Woman Down to Her Bones: The Anatomy of Sexual Difference in the Sixteenth and Early Seventeenth Centuries', *Isis*, 94:2 (2003), 274–99. See also Winfried Schleiner, 'Early Modern Controversies about the One-Sex Model', *Renaissance Quarterly*, 53:1 (2000), 180–91; Helen King, *The One-Sex Body on Trial: The Classical and Early Modern Evidence. The History of Medicine in Context* (Farnham: Ashgate, 2013).

[60] Bolletti, *Dell'origine*, 80.

[61] See, for instance, Ibid., 78; Cesare Orlandi, *Delle città d'Italia e sue isole adjacenti compendiose notizie*, vol. 4 (Perugia: Stamperia Augusta, 1775), 75–6.

[62] ASB, Assunteria d'Istituto, Diversorum, busta 10, n. 1, 'Proposte per statue anatomiche'.

[63] Orlandi, *Delle città d'Italia*.

[64] Cotugno, 'Iter Italicum', 75–6 (citation p. 76). On the preparation of skeletons, see also Anita Guerrini, 'Inside the Charnel House: The Display of Skeletons in Europe, 1500–1800, in Knoeff and Zwijnenberg (eds.), *The Fate of Anatomical Collections*, 93–109.

forever' thanks to their internal metal support.[65] Once the bones were ready, artificers started modelling. Lelli had realized the model of a horseshoe kidney for Bonazzoli through a cast, but the work for the anatomy room was seemingly the result of free modelling. As the artist Carlo Pisarri put it, Lelli would start modelling the muscles on the skeleton with 'ordinary matter', such as hemp, which shaped 'the figure and form'. Giovanni Manzolini, who served for a period as Lelli's main assistant, would subsequently dye the material in a coloured wax that 'imitated the truth' and started modelling it over the skeleton. Lelli would then add the finishing touches.[66]

Ever since the beginning of the work on the anatomy room, Pope Benedict XIV took a vested interest in the process. The marquis Paolo Magnani sent him regular updates from Bologna. On 23 October 1743, the pope was glad to hear from Magnani about Lelli's progress.[67] A couple of weeks later, on 6 November, he again expressed his gratitude for Magnani's interest in the anatomy room and anticipated offering extra compensation to that 'truly special man', that is, Lelli.[68] In 1745, 'cardinals, prelates, clergymen and personalities of different nationalities' started to pay visits to Lelli's residence to admire and monitor the progress of his work.[69] For his part, Lelli relied on his artisanal prowess to ingratiate himself with the pontiff and impress the Institute's *Assunti*. A particularly propitious occasion presented itself in 1746, when the arrival of the mosaic portrait of Pope Benedict XIV in Bologna afforded Lelli the opportunity to put his skills to good use.[70] Lambertini had decided to have the symbols of the papacy prominently displayed within the Institute's premises, and chose to have a mosaic portrait bearing his effigy for the purpose.[71] Weighty and cumbersome, the mosaic travelled from Rome to Ancona by sea. It was then transported on canal boats and, once in Bologna, was carried on a sleigh pulled by eight oxen. Much to everybody's dismay, however, the mosaic reached the Institute in pieces. Charged with the task of restoring it, Lelli also devised a machine that could lift it up. In a dramatic setting of spectacle and suspense, Lelli's machine was set in place in the Institute's main hall. After an audience had gathered in the hall, an eight-year-old girl appeared on the scene and started lifting the mosaic by simply turning a small crank. *Et voilà*, with a *coup de théatre* the weighty mosaic portraying Benedict XIV was lifted and unveiled in the blink

[65] Cotugno, 'Iter Italicum', 76. In his *Dell'origine e de' progressi dell'Istituto delle Scienze*, Giuseppe Bolletti similarly remarked that the models of the anatomy room would 'last a very long time'; see Bolletti, *Dell'origine*, 81.

[66] Pisarri, *Dialoghi*, 48–51 (citations p. 50).

[67] Paolo Prodi and Maria Teresa Fattori (eds.), *Le lettere di Benedetto XIV al marchese Paolo Magnani* (Rome: Herder, 2011), 125.

[68] Ibid., 132.

[69] ASB, Assunteria d'Istituto, Atti, n. 4 (1734–53), 1179 (29 May 1745). See also Lambertini, 'Motuproprio, col quale Ercole Lelli', 536. It is worth noting that at the time of the first project of an anatomy room, there was the plan to allocate a space to Lelli at the Institute of the Sciences; see ASB, Assunteria d'Istituto, Atti, n. 3 (1727–34), 740. However, in the 1740s, Lelli worked on the models in his residence.

[70] ASB, Archivio Salina Bolognini Amorini, cart. 532, Vite dei pittori, 'Vita di Ercole Lelli'.

[71] See Biagi Maino, 'Arte, scienza e potere', in Koeppel (ed.), *Papes et papauté*, 40.

of an eye. The audience applauded the girl and praised the inventor. Lelli stayed on to explain the tricks of the performance.[72] A few months later, he travelled to Rome on a new papal mission.

As part of his growing involvement with the Institute of the Sciences, in 1747 Lambertini decided to acquire Maria Vittoria Campani's prestigious optical cabinet in order to donate it to the Institute. Maria Vittoria was the daughter of the late Giuseppe Campani, who had become renowned for constructing optical instruments. Campani had gathered a collection of optical devices that included instruments for making telescopes and lenses such as the one used by the famous astronomer Giovanni Domenico Cassini (1625–1712) to observe Saturn's satellites from Paris. Lelli was supposed to collect the instruments in Rome and learn how to use them from Maria Vittoria, who was considered an appreciated *professoressa* in her own right.[73] While in Rome, he fulfilled his papal mission, wandered around the eternal city, and drew sketches of its monuments and statues. On 24 June 1747, the Bolognese physician Vincenzo Antonio Menghini (1704–1759) wrote to Lelli and urged him to take advantage of his proximity to the pontiff in order to secure lasting employment.[74] Five years had passed since the beginning of his work on the anatomy room, and only one year remained before the end of the contract. Having reassured the pope about the room's imminent completion, Lelli followed Menghini's advice and asked to be appointed as its custodian and demonstrator for the duration of his lifetime (*vita natural durante*). In a *motu proprio* of 28 November 1747, the pope fulfilled his wishes. He also appointed him as the custodian and demonstrator of both Campani's optical cabinet, and of the room of lathes that Marsigli had left to the Institute with the objective of using them to make guns and cannons.[75] On all accounts, then, the journey was a success: Lelli had travelled to Rome to respond to a papal call and returned to Bologna having secured permanent employment. Before leaving Rome, Lelli donated his sketches of the city's 'most beautiful' statues to Lambertini, and reminded him of the project of expanding the Institute's gallery of statues, a project that the pope himself had entertained in 1744.[76] Back in Bologna, however, things were not going well.

[72] ASB, Archivio Salina Bolognini Amorini, cart. 532, Vite dei pittori, 'Vita di Ercole Lelli'. On Lelli's lifting machine, see also Francesco Maria Zanotti, 'De Senatoribus Instituti Praefectis', in *De Bononiensi Scientiarum et Artium Instituto atque Academia Commentarii*, vol. 3 (Bologna: Lelio dalla Volpe, 1755), 6.

[73] On Campani and his optical cabinet, see Girolamo Tiraboschi, *Storia della letteratura italiana*, vol. 8 (Rome: Luigi Perego Salvioni Stampator Vaticano, 1785), 151ff. See also Silvio A. Bedini, 'The Optical Workshop Equipment of Giuseppe Campani', *Journal of the History of Medicine and Allied Sciences*, 16:1 (1961), 18–38.

[74] BUB, ms. 3882, capsula LVIII, A8, Letter of 24 June 1747 from Vincenzo Antonio Menghini in Bologna to Ercole Lelli. See also Antonio Brighetti, 'Ercole Lelli e le cere bolognesi in carteggi inediti del Settecento', in *La ceroplastica nella scienza e nell'arte*, vol. 1, 207–13.

[75] Lambertini, 'Motuproprio, col quale Ercole Lelli', vol. 3, 537–8.

[76] ASB, Assunteria d'Istituto, Lettere all'Istituto, n. 4 (1734–52), Letter of 12 July 1752 from Fulvio Bentivoglio in Rome. On 'the most beautiful statues', see Francis Haskell and Nicholas Penny, *The Most Beautiful Statues: The Taste for Antique Sculpture, 1500–1900: An Exhibition Held at the Ashmolean Museum from 26 March to 10 May 1981* (Oxford: Ashmolean Museum, 1981).

WAX WARS

When travelling to Rome, Lelli had left behind Giovanni Manzolini who, for a few years, had assisted him on the works for the anatomy room. Manzolini was the son of a shoe-maker (and/or a second-hand dealer) who, as the story has it, refused to pursue his father's occupation and studied first in the workshop and drawing school of Giuseppe Pedretti, and then of Francesco Monti. A print depicting a religious theme, which survives to this day, documents his artistic work.[77] Manzolini's teacher, Francesco Monti, was a staunch opponent of the employment of anatomy in art and wrote 'a venomous comedy' deriding artists' anatomical studies, possibly with the intention of targeting Lelli.[78] Yet, Manzolini became keenly interested in anatomy. Having attended the drawing school of the Accademia Clementina at the same time as Lelli, and having become his neighbour, Manzolini joined Lelli's anatomical workshop.[79] Over the following years, however, issues of rivalry, attribution, and, perhaps, remuneration set Lelli and Manzolini apart. As the working relationship between the two artificers ended amidst bitter reproaches and accusations, Lelli found a new assistant in the clergyman Luigi Dardani, who modelled devotional figures and busts in wax. Once informed about the situation, the pope initially sided with Lelli. On 23 October 1748, he wrote to Magnani that Lelli had done a good job dismissing Manzolini because 'certain clowns, by acting as jesters, try to take over the good dancer, who in order to protect himself has to fire them'.[80] In the same period, Lelli was trying to discredit Anna Morandi, Manzolini's spouse, in the eyes of the pope by delegitimizing the news that she had become an accomplished modeller who made anatomical wax statues that were equal to his own. Marco Antonio Laurenti, archiater to Benedict XIV, reassured him that the pope had downplayed the news of the 'pretend *dottoressa*', and reckoned it to be a matter of gossip.[81] Yet, over time Lelli's lateness in completing the anatomy room made the pope increasingly distressed.[82] Laurenti's letters from Rome became ever more pressing, urging Lelli to drop any other engagement that would distract him from finishing the anatomy room. Laurenti even cautioned Lelli about accepting a prestigious commission from England.[83] In October 1749, Magnani joined the complaints and reprimanded Lelli for giving in to distractions.[84] The pope had declared

[77] See BCABo, G.D.S., *Raccolta stampe di Autori Vari*, cartella XL, n. 12, 'Trinità con i ss. Agostino, Domenico, Petronio e Gregorio' (XVIII century).

[78] See Zofia Ameisenowa, *The Problem of the Écorché and the Three Anatomical Models in the Jagiellonian Library*, trans. Andrzej Potocki (Warsaw: Zakład Narodowy imienia Ossolińskich Wydawnictwo Polskiej Akademii Nauk, 1963), 66. See also Röhrl, *History and Bibliography*, 138.

[79] On Lelli and Manzolini as fellow students at the Accademia Clementina, see Focaccia, 'Anna Morandi Manzolini', in Focaccia (ed.), *Anna Morandi Manzolini*, 40 n. 148.

[80] Prodi and Fattori (eds.), *Le lettere di Benedetto XIV*, 623.

[81] BUB, ms. 3882, capsula LVIII, A5, Lettere autografe di Marco Antonio Laurenti ad Ercole Lelli (1747–52), Letters of 9 and 26 October 1748 from Marco Antonio Laurenti in Rome to Lelli.

[82] Ibid., Letters of 15 January and 29 January 1749 from Rome. The rumour that Lelli was behind schedule had started to circulate in Bologna in 1747, when he was still in Rome; see BUB, ms. 3882, capsula LVIII, A8, Letter of 24 June 1747 from Vincenzo Antonio Menghini in Bologna to Ercole Lelli.

[83] Ibid., A5, Letter of 9 October 1748 from Marco Antonio Laurenti in Rome to Lelli.

[84] Ibid., A7, Letter of 12 October 1749 from Paolo Magnani.

the year 1750 a jubilee year. Flocks of foreigners heading towards Rome were expected to stop in Bologna where papal munificence and support for natural and anatomical knowledge could be showcased to them. Yet, at the beginning of the year, the anatomy room was still incomplete and the pope reached a high point of frustration. Even after completing the anatomy room, Lelli would continue to attract criticism. In the mid-1750s, he was targeted by a group of fellow parishioners of Santa Maria Maddalena who addressed a letter to the pope, describing him as an untrustworthy and mendacious man who had taken credit for the work that had been done by the 'poor Manzolini'. The letter also highlighted that the models made by Lelli after Manzolini had left the workshop were of poor quality and had rapidly cracked and deteriorated, and their colour had faded.[85]

Issues of rivalry, ambition, attribution, and recognition were not, of course, new to early modern artisanal and artistic domains. The proverbially divisive world of artists and artificers was rife with bitter disputes, allegations, reproaches, and rivalry. In the case of anatomical modelling, customary patterns of acrimony were possibly aggravated by the fact that wax's material features made it harder to identify the hand of the maker. As exemplified by the case of Guillaume Desnoües (1650–1735) and Gaetano Giulio Zumbo or Zummo (1656–1701), whose collaboration dramatically ended amid reciprocal accusations, the early history of anatomical modelling was marked by conflicting claims of authorship, reproaches, accusations, and dramatic separations.[86] Although the story of collaboration, crisis, and contention between Lelli and Manzolini unfolded over a relatively short time, its echo dragged on for several decades, stretching well beyond the lifespan of those directly involved, and shaping the memory of the Bolognese world of wax modelling.[87] Letters, local reports, and biographical collections all became apt arenas for battles over claims of authorship and modelling skills. As the attribution of the models became a contested matter, omissions did not pass by unnoticed, accusations started to fly high, and texts seeking to vindicate Manzolini's authorship were set against those that were brought to the fore in Lelli's defence. In 1751, Giuseppe Gaetano Bolletti published a detailed account of the rooms of

[85] BCABo, ms. B 35, n. 48, 'Alla Santità di N.S. Papa Benedetto XIV. Memoriale', fols. 143r–144v. The text was not dated but was written between the contention over Antonio Galli Bibiena's plan for the Bolognese theatre in 1756 and the death of Lambertini in 1758. According to Elio Vassena, the 'Memoriale' may have been written by Marcello Orietti; see Vassena, *La fortuna dei ceroplasti bolognesi*, section on 'Ercole Lelli'. See also Ferretti, 'Il notomista e il canonico', 102 and 122 n. 9.

[86] On Zumbo, Desnoües, and the controversy that ended their collaboration see, for instance, R.W. Lightbown, 'Gaetano Giulio Zumbo—I: The Florentine Period', *The Burlington Magazine*, 106 (1964), 486–96; R.W. Lightbown, 'Gaetano Giulio Zumbo—II: Genoa and France', ibid., 563–9; Antonino Mongitore, *Memorie dei pittori, scultori, architetti, artefici in cera siciliani*, ed. Elvira Natoli (Palermo: S.F. Flaccovio, 1977), 66–73; Maria Luisa Azzaroli Puccetti, 'Gaetano Giulio Zumbo: La vita e le opere', in Paolo Giansiracusa (ed.), *Gaetano Giulio Zumbo* (Milan: Fabbri Editori, 1988), 17–46; Paolo Giansiracusa (ed.), *Vanitas vanitatum: Studi sulla ceroplastica di Gaetano Giulio Zumbo* (Siracusa: Lombardi, 1991); Lemire, *Artistes et mortels*, 28–41; Elena Taddia, 'Corpi, cadaveri, chirurghi stranieri e ceroplastiche: L'Ospedale di Pammatone a Genova tra Sei e Settecento', *Mediterranea*, 6 (2009), esp. 167–74; De Ceglia, 'Rotten Corpses', 418–31.

[87] On the contentious relationship between Lelli and Manzolini, see Ferretti, 'Il notomista e il canonico', 100–15; Mario Fanti, 'Sulla figura e l'opera di Marcello Oretti: Spigolature d'archivio per la storia dell'arte di Bologna', *Il Carrobbio*, 8 (1982), esp. 130–43. See also Messbarger, *The Lady Anatomist*.

the Institute of the Sciences, where he presented Lelli as the sole artificer of the anatomy room.[88] Similarly, a few years later, in 1755, the fourth edition of Carlo Cesare Malvasia's *Le pitture di Bologna*, which charted the Bolognese artistic world, referred only to Lelli as the author of the anatomy room. In 1766, its fifth edition also neglected Manzolini and Morandi, who had by then completed their own anatomical collection and had contributed a number of models to the Institute's midwifery room.[89] Conversely when, in 1769, Luigi Crespi failed to include an entry on Lelli in his supplement to Malvasia's *Felsina pittrice*, and only mentioned him in the entry for Giovanni Manzolini, he triggered noisy discontent among Lelli's pupils and supporters.[90] As polemics continued to rage, in 1778 Carlo Pisarri, Lelli's student, vindicated the image of the two modellers working in harmonious collaboration under Lelli's reassuring guidance. For his part, in 1786 the famous biographer Giovanni Fantuzzi absolved Lelli of the accusation that Manzolini was the only—or at least chief—artificer of the anatomy room.[91]

If the issue of attribution was so contentious, it was also because its consequences reached beyond local dispute and consumption. Works such as *Le pitture di Bologna* offered guidance to Grand Tour travellers and allowed them to both remember what they saw and imagine what they had skipped along their routes. As these texts were shipped back home along with souvenirs and artworks such as paintings, sketches, and the cork models of famous monuments like the Colosseum, they reached well beyond the circle of those who were directly involved in the events. Just like the reports of famous travellers, such as the engraver Charles-Nicolas Cochin, the naturalist Jérôme Richard, and the astronomer Joseph Jérôme Lefrançois de Lalande, this literature offered anatomical modellers a particularly promising source of publicity across the Alps. For local practitioners, appearing or not appearing in such works mattered. When, in 1764, the Philadelphian physician John Morgan (1735–1789), who travelled in Italy after studying medicine at the University of Edinburgh, shipped home both Malvasia's *Le pitture di Bologna* and Bolletti's *Dell'origine e progressi dell'Istituto delle Scienze*, he was likely unaware that he was participating in a controversy.[92]

DANCING AND DISSECTING

Leaving behind a trail of complaints, reprimands, broken collaborations, disappointments, and higher than anticipated monetary investment, the anatomy room was

[88] Bolletti, *Dell'origine*, 78.

[89] See Carlo Cesare Malvasia, *Le pitture di Bologna [...]*, 5th edn. (Bologna: Longhi, 1766), 82. The artist Luigi Crespi noticed the absence of any reference to the midwifery room and, therefore, to Morandi and Manzolini's models in the new editions of these works; see Luigi Crespi, *Felsina pittrice: Vite de' pittori bolognesi*, vol. 3 (Rome: Marco Pagliarini, 1769), 312.

[90] Crespi, *Felsina pittrice*, 307–10.

[91] Giovanni Fantuzzi, *Notizie degli scrittori bolognesi raccolte da Giovanni Fantuzzi*, vol. 5 (Bologna: San Tommaso d'Aquino, 1781–94), 51.

[92] John Morgan, *The Journal of Dr. John Morgan of Philadelphia, from the City of Rome to the City of London* (Philadelphia: J.B. Lippincott, 1907), 239.

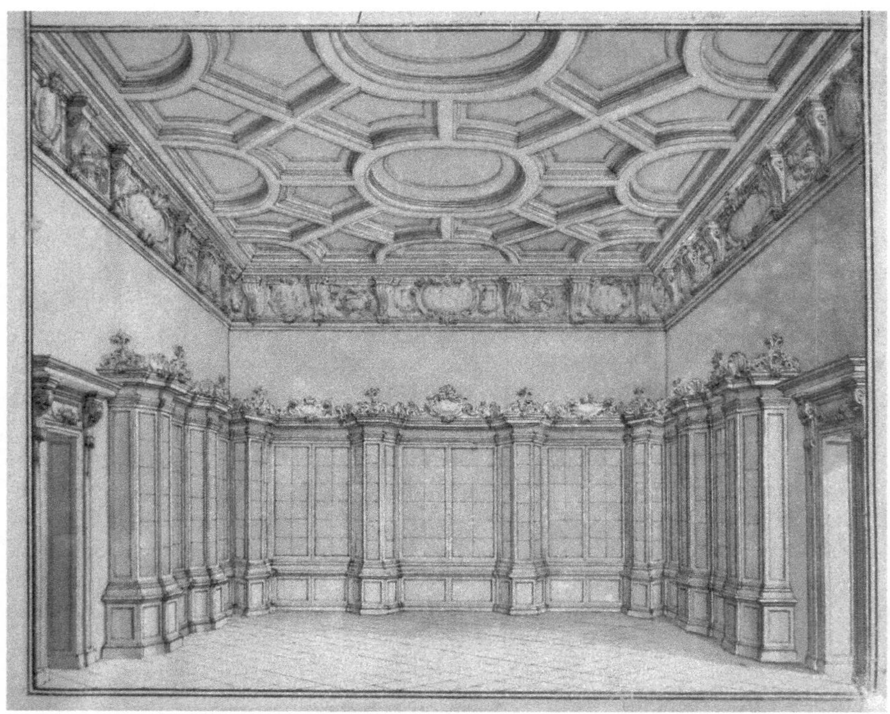

Figure 2.1 Drawing of the anatomy room at the Institute of the Sciences.

finally completed in 1751 (Plate 4).[93] Lelli was ready to start the demonstrations in the elegant space allocated to it (Figure 2.1).[94]

On 17 March 1751, Lelli had added the last anatomical statue.[95] At the end of the year, he wrote to Laurenti to inform him that all the models had been completed.[96] The work delivered by Lelli was then checked against the original plan, and Laurenti could report that everything had been accomplished with the

[93] On the completion of the anatomy room, see BCABo, Fondo Malvezzi de' Medici, cart. 97, n. 6, 'Corrispondenza riguardante i doni di Benedetto XIV all'Istituto delle Scienze', Letter of 17 March 1751 from Sigismondo Malvezzi to Cardinal Millo, Letter of 5 January 1752 from Marco Antonio Laurenti, Letter of 12 January 1752 to Marco Antonio Laurenti; BUB, ms. 3882, capsula LVIII, A5, Lettere autografe di Marco Antonio Laurenti ad Ercole Lelli (1747–52), Letter of 29 December 1751 from Marco Antonio Laurenti in Rome to Ercole Lelli.

[94] ASB, Assunteria d'Istituto, Atti, n. 4 (1734–53), 1282.

[95] BCABo, Fondo Malvezzi de' Medici, cart. 97, n. 6, 'Corrispondenza riguardante i doni di Benedetto XIV all'Istituto delle Scienze', Letter of 17 March 1751 from Sigismondo Malvezzi to Cardinal Millo.

[96] BUB, ms. 3882, capsula LVIII, A5, Lettere autografe di Marco Antonio Laurenti ad Ercole Lelli (1747–52), Letter of 29 December 1751 from Marco Antonio Laurenti in Rome to Ercole Lelli. In the previous months, Lelli had received confirmation of the promise of a lifetime position as the custodian and demonstrator of the anatomy room; see ASB, Assunteria di Studio, Atti, n. 24 (1749–55), fol. 47r.

sole exception of a model of the 'internal ear', which he believed would be finalized by the beginning of the following July.[97] Bologna could now count on a new important venue of anatomical practice in addition to the anatomical theatre, the anatomy rooms of hospitals, and the homes of medical practitioners.[98] As the models of the Institute's anatomy room became part of a culture of public viewing of the inner body, they participated in the creation of new spaces of anatomical encounter that were markedly different from that of the public anatomy lesson.

Originally conceived as a way to return the city to its academic lustre at a time of perceived decline, in mid-eighteenth-century Bologna the public anatomy lesson was still regarded as an important event. It was held in the anatomical theatre, which had been constructed with the purpose of reinstating the decorum of public anatomy as well as 'the splendour, the decoration and the honorific needs of the public schools and the whole city' (Plate 16).[99] Usually performed in a candlelit atmosphere in the cold and humid evenings of the Bolognese winter, the event enacted a highly theatrical and ritualized ceremony that staged 'anatomical dissection amidst the pathos of a baroque drama'.[100] The public anatomy lesson often took place during the carnival period, when the city's inns filled up with visitors who wanted to take advantage of the seasonal entertainments. As in any proper carnival spectacle, viewers were allowed to participate in their costumes and masks, while music accompanied the celebration of the anatomical ritual.[101] Abbot de La Porte noted in his *Le voyageur françois* that wearing masks proved very convenient for women who believed it would be inappropriate to attend the event with their face uncovered.[102]

As one can see in the *Insignia* of 1734 encountered in Chapter 1 (Plate 5), which portrays local heroine Laura Bassi in the anatomical theatre, in mid-eighteenth-century Bologna the public anatomy lesson followed a traditional plot. Here the anatomist Domenico Maria Gusmano Galeazzi (1686–1775) lectures from the cathedra whereas the dissectors and demonstrators attend to the cadaver in the dissection pit.[103] This staging was in keeping with the scholastic scheme of the Latin *disputatio*, where the anatomist in charge of the lecture had 'to answer, in public, questions put to him without prior warning by lectors from various different

[97] BCABo, Fondo Malvezzi de' Medici, cart. 97, n. 6, 'Corrispondenza riguardante i doni di Benedetto XIV all'Istituto delle Scienze', Letter of 5 January 1752 from Marco Antonio Laurenti, Letter of 12 January 1752 to Marco Antonio Laurenti; BUB, ms. 3882, capsula LVIII, A5, Lettere autografe di Marco Antonio Laurenti ad Ercole Lelli (1747–52), Letter of 29 December 1751 from Marco Antonio Laurenti in Rome to Ercole Lelli. The model that still needed to be completed was of Valsalva's preparation of the ear. On Lelli's engagement in the realization of this model, see Medici, 'Elogio d'Ercole Lelli', 175; Cotugno, 'Iter Italicum', 74.

[98] In 1751, Giuseppe Gaetano Bolletti wrote that by focusing on 'the study of Notomy' the anatomy room addressed the only pursuit that was still missing in an Institute that embraced 'almost all arts, and faculties, that are flourishing especially in this period'; see Bolletti, *Dell'origine*, 78.

[99] ASB, Gabella Grossa, Libri segreti, 1/4 (1628–40), 287 (9 October 1637), quoted in Ferrari, 'Public Anatomy Lessons', 75. On early modern anatomical theatres, see Klestinec, *Theaters of Anatomy*.

[100] Dacome, 'Women, Wax and Anatomy', 526.

[101] Ferrari, 'Public Anatomy Lessons'.

[102] De La Porte, *Le voyageur françois*, vol. 26, 43.

[103] Giovanni Martinotti, *L'insegnamento dell'anatomia in Bologna prima del secolo XIX* (Bologna: Cooperativa Tipografica Azzoguidi, 1911), 132. On the staging of the public anatomy lesson, see Ferrari, 'Public Anatomy Lessons'; Carlino, *Books of the Body*; Klestinec, *Theaters of Anatomy*.

disciplines'.[104] Organized well ahead of time, the anatomy lesson was carefully planned in all its aspects, from the appointment of the anatomists to the list of items needed for the event, including the stocks of silk threads, needles, and oil of turpentine. Even the wine, bread, and chocolate for the grave-digger of the hospital of Santa Maria della Morte, and for the students in charge of preparing the cadaver on the morning before the event, were detailed in the planning.[105] The ritualistic meal shared by the anatomists and the civic authorities of the *Anziani* further underscored the ceremony's importance. Yet, at the time in which Bologna gained reputation as a centre of anatomical modelling, its performance hardly lived up to expectations. While the public anatomy lesson was discontinued at the time of the Napoleonic reforms of the university's curricula, the signs of its decline had been all too evident for quite some time.

As Giovanna Ferrari has observed, the *Assunti di Studio*, namely the senators who sat on the *Assunteria di Studio* and supervised the management of the university, were convinced that as long as public anatomy lessons were carried out with due decorum, they 'would restore the university to its ancient splendour'.[106] However, by the mid-eighteenth century, the ceremony had fallen short of expectations. In particular, factors such as the absenteeism of lecturers (who were supposed to attend the public anatomy lesson and raise objections), the habit of attendees to leave before the end of the event, the tendency to skip the argumentation, and students' proverbial noise and unruliness, all seemed to conspire against the smooth unfolding of an event that was meant to secure the university's reputation. On 22 January 1749, for instance, the *Assunti di Studio* noticed that only a scarce number of public lecturers attended the event. The lesson furthermore suffered from a shortage of *argomentanti*, namely, those who were in charge of asking questions that challenged the anatomist's theses.[107] Internal conflicts equally increased the risk of jeopardizing the event as in the case of a dispute between the anatomy professor and the chaplain who was in charge of celebrating mass for the souls of the dissected in the nearby chapel.[108] Over time, the lecturers' absenteeism and the students' rowdiness became unbearable. Growing increasingly concerned, the *Assunti di Studio* intervened to tackle the situation.[109] In January 1761, the secretary of the *Assunteria* was requested to speak to the students' prior about the pressing need to reduce the clamour during the event.[110] One month later, the *Assunti* looked for ways to ensure that the 'argumentation' was carried out on a

[104] See Ferrari, 'Public Anatomy Lessons', esp. 70–1 and 88–9 (citation p. 88). On the role of the disputation in Renaissance anatomy, see also Klestinec, *Theaters of Anatomy*, chapter 3.

[105] BCABo, Fondo speciale Giovanni Antonio, Francesco e Carlo Mondini, cart. VII, n. 1, 'Nota delle spese che si fanno in occasione della pubblica Anatomia ne' Camerini delle Pubbliche Scuole'; ASB, Assunteria di Studio, Atti, n. 25 (1756–77), fol. 35, 27 January 1763.

[106] Ferrari, 'Public Anatomy Lessons', 91.

[107] ASB, Assunteria di Studio, Atti, n. 24 (1749–55), fol. 1v, 22 January 1749.

[108] ASB, Assunteria di Studio, Atti, n. 25 (1756–77), fols. 38v, 41r, 42r–v.

[109] See for instance ASB, Assunteria di Studio, Atti, n. 24 (1749–55), 28 February 1754, 2 April 1754 and 8 January 1755.

[110] ASB, Assunteria di Studio, Atti, n. 25 (1756–77), fol. 22r (5 January 1761).

regular basis.[111] In mid-March, they decided to keep a record of the names of those lecturers who did not attend the 'anatomical function', hoping that this would encourage them to participate and engage in the argumentation.[112] The following November, they further resolved to write down the names of the lecturers who did not stay for at least three quarters of an hour.[113] But even this course of action did not seem to suffice. At the meeting of 18 January 1762, the *Assunti* looked for further measures to monitor lecturers' participation in the argumentation. They also decided to talk to the students' prior to make sure that the students who arrived late would not delay the beginning of the ceremony.[114]

Yet, all these efforts were to no avail. One year later, in January 1763, the *Assunti* returned yet again to the pressing issue of lecturers' participation. This time they urged all the 'Philosophers, Mathematicians and Physicians', no matter whether salaried or honorary, to join the anatomy lesson and contribute to the 'argumentation' for the 'greater decorum of the function'.[115] Still, the sense of incipient chaos did not recede. Two years later, an exasperated group of *Assunti* decided to hire two Swiss guards in case the situation slipped out of control and the regular guards failed to 'execute orders' properly.[116] In January 1769, the anatomist's suggestion not to allow carnivalesque masks in the anatomical theatre on the grounds that they caused disturbance was another sign of persisting concerns.[117] Some of these apprehensions were not new. The attempt to discipline troublesome wearers of masks and raucous students constituted a well-known feature of public anatomy lessons. Nor was the sense of unruliness limited to students. As Ferrari has observed, professors were themselves reluctant to carry out this complex and charged public performance because they feared it could affect their reputation.[118] By the mid-eighteenth century, lecturers' absenteeism and lack of participation, the ever-impending risk of falling short of the expected protocol of 'decorum and modesty', and the ongoing inability to maintain discipline and order, exposed the public anatomy lesson as an increasingly obsolete and pompous ritual, the epitome of old-fashioned and scholastic pedantry.[119] It was a far cry from the imposing, orderly, and well-attended gathering depicted in the *Insignia* of 1734, where Laura Bassi is portrayed while addressing the anatomist in cathedra and lecturing to an attentive and composed audience (Plate 5).[120] Even the hope that the anatomical theatre's impressive architecture would showcase the city's anatomical vitality to foreigners did not seem to bear much fruit. Some travellers did visit the theatre, but they hardly took notice of its activities, and chiefly focused on architectural observations. The antiquarian and travel writer Johann Georg Keyssler (1693–1743), a fellow of the Royal Society whose travelogue was used by Mozart as a guide,

[111] Ibid., fol. 22v (6 February 1761). [112] Ibid., fol. 23r (14 March 1761).
[113] Ibid., fol. 24r (2 November 1761). [114] Ibid., fols. 26r–v (18 January 1762).
[115] Ibid., fol. 34v (8 January 1763). [116] Ibid., fols.53r–v (26 January 1765).
[117] Ibid., no folio number (5 January 1769). [118] Ferrari, 'Public Anatomy Lessons', 88.
[119] Ibid., 91. See also ASB, Assunteria di Studio, Atti, n. 25 (1756–77), fols. 26r–v (18 January 1762). For a different reading, see Messbarger, *The Lady Anatomist*, chapter 1.
[120] ASB, Assunteria di Studio, Atti, n. 25 (1756–77), fol. 22r (5 January 1761) and 3 January 1774 (no folio number).

remarked that the anatomical theatre was 'ornamented with wooden statues of the most celebrated anatomists', and the floor was 'boarded with cypress', but complained that the place lacked 'proper light'.[121] Some visitors praised Lelli's wooden écorchés, but many did not even include the anatomical theatre among the sights worth visiting and recording.[122]

In fact, the very spaces of anatomical practice were themselves undergoing significant changes. While the *disputatio* ran the risk of turning the public anatomy lecture into an obsolete performance, anatomical theatres were seemingly losing the aura of sacred rituality that had been associated with them.[123] In Mantua, for instance, during the carnival period of 1771 some young aristocrats left the local prefect perplexed after asking permission to throw carnival dance parties in the very theatre where the performance of anatomical dissections was just about to begin.[124] In the following years, the theatre ended up being used for operas and dramas as well as for anatomical and experimental performances.[125] In Bologna, anatomists lamented that the anatomical theatre was inadequate to fulfil demands of a closer viewing of the inner body.[126] As early as 1709, Luigi Ferdinando Marsigli had famously complained that the public anatomy lesson was 'noisy and rushed', and that the students could not see what they were shown.[127] In the late eighteenth century, the anatomist Carlo Mondini (1729–1803), who in 1782 replaced Luigi Galvani as professor of anatomy, was still complaining about the impracticalities of viewing dissection in a theatre where the distance of the dissecting table from the cathedra and the students' benches made it difficult to see.[128]

Lighting also became an issue. While public anatomy lectures were celebrated at nighttime amidst the flickering light of candles, the display of anatomical models required a properly lit setting. Ever since the project of an anatomy room was discussed at the Institute of the Sciences, the issue of light stood out as an important factor that had to be considered when planning the display of the models. During the first project of an anatomy room, in May 1734 Niccolò Aldrovandi required

[121] Johann Georg Keyssler, *Travels through Germany, Bohemia, Hungary, Switzerland, Italy, and Lorrain: Giving a True and Just Description of the Present State of Those Countries; Carefully Translated from the Second Edition of the German,* 2nd edn., vol. 3 (London: A. Linde and T. Field, 1756–7), 123.

[122] *Dictionnaire historique et géographique portatif de l'Italie*, vol. 1 (Paris: Lacombe, 1775), 162. As Ferrari has observed, 'the very structure of the seventeenth-century anatomy theatre was largely an outcome of the demands of the dispute' and, in fact, 'instead of revolving around its original central point, the dissecting table, the new theatre clearly had two focuses. The dissecting table was, as it were, counterbalanced by the cathedra from which the anatomy professor propounded and defended his theses'; see Ferrari, 'Public Anatomy Lessons', 76.

[123] On anatomy as a ritual, see Chapter 1 n. 32.

[124] Archivio di Stato di Milano (henceforth ASM), Fondo Studi, parte antica (henceforth p.a.), cartella 11: 3, 'Feste di ballo nel teatro scientifico'.

[125] Ferrari, 'Public Anatomy Lessons', 87.

[126] ASB, Studio, Università unite, Titolo II, Musei e stabilimenti scientifici, busta 462. See also Ferrari, 'Public Anatomy Lessons', 93.

[127] Luigi Ferdinando Marsigli, 'Parallelo dello Stato Moderno dell'Università di Bologna con l'altre di là de' monti (1709)' (BUB, Fondo Marsili, ms. 630), quoted in Ettore Bortolotti, 'La fondazione dell'Istituto e la riforma dello Studio di Bologna', in *Memorie intorno a L.F. Marsili* (Bologna: Zanichelli, 1930), 410–11.

[128] ASB, Studio, Università unite, Titolo II, Musei e stabilimenti scientifici, busta 462. See also Ferrari, 'Public Anatomy Lessons', 93.

that the anatomical statues he had sponsored be allocated a more luminous room.[129] Notably, light was itself a focus of study at the Institute, and replicas of Newton's experiments on light were performed on its premises. One of the rooms of physics was assigned to 'the Newtonian system of light' and dedicated to the performance of such experiments. The physics rooms also included optical instruments, mirrors, prisms, lenses, magic lanterns, and microscopes.[130] Charged with the task of making both lenses and coloured anatomical waxworks, Lelli was no doubt aware of the central place occupied by light amidst the Institute's undertakings. The very decision to locate the anatomy room near the room assigned to 'the Newtonian system of light', and on the upper floor of the Institute, was perhaps driven by considerations related to visibility and the study of light.[131] For sure, proper lighting allowed for the appreciation of detail, which, as we shall see, lay at the centre of models' functions as tools for the training of viewers' eyes.

'THE GREATEST ANATOMIST IN EUROPE'

Providing a more intimate ambiance to the encounter with human anatomy, anatomical models encouraged a close and detailed viewing of the inner body. In doing so, they could build on the well-established tradition of private teaching sessions.[132] Held in the houses of dissectors and professors and in hospitals' anatomy rooms, private sessions often introduced students to the anatomy of bodily parts that were not presented in the public anatomy lesson.[133] For instance, as well as serving as a dissector in the public anatomy lesson, Lorenzo Bonazzoli also demonstrated for smaller groups of students the bodily parts that were not shown in the anatomical theatre, such as the muscles, foetus, and parts of generation, which also ended up figuring prominently in anatomical collections.[134] Allowing for a closer interaction between students and teachers, private teaching sessions were traditionally taken to provide valuable experience for students. They furthermore played a significant part in the making of medical careers. Physicians and surgeons, including Giovanni Antonio Galli, Luigi Galvani, and Pier Paolo Molinelli, offered private lessons at different stages of their careers, and whenever they submitted

[129] ASB, Assunteria d'Istituto, Atti, n. 4 (1734–53), 810.

[130] Bolletti, *Dell'origine*, 71–7; Giuseppe Angelelli, *Notizie dell'origine, e progressi dell'Instituto delle Scienze di Bologna e sue accademie* (Bologna: Nell' Instituto delle Scienze, 1780), 112.

[131] On the location of the anatomy room on the upper floor of the Institute of the Sciences, see Angelelli, *Notizie dell'origine*, 206.

[132] On private anatomy teaching, see Cynthia Klestinec, 'A History of Anatomy Theatres in Sixteenth-Century Padua', *Journal of the History of Medicine and Allied Sciences*, 59:3 (2004), 375–412; Klestinec, *Theaters of Anatomy*, esp. chapter 5. In his *motu proprio* of 28 November 1747, Lambertini himself linked the practice of private teaching sessions with the establishment of an anatomy room at the Institute of the Sciences; see Lambertini, 'Motuproprio, col quale Ercole Lelli', 536.

[133] Private teaching sessions were associated with an academic tradition that, dating back to the early days of the university, allowed students to choose their own professors and receive instruction in small groups.

[134] ASB, Assunteria di Studio, Requisiti dei Lettori, busta 32, fasc. 34, 'Requisiti del Dott.e Lorenzo Ant.o Bonazzoli'.

promotion requests to the university they highlighted their role as teachers in such settings. Just as private lessons, anatomical displays allowed for the detailed observation of bodily parts. One of the purposes of such a close viewing was surgical training. As one can read in the inventory of the Institute's anatomy room, a number of tables were meant to show 'all the separate bones that make the skeleton' and accordingly convey an understanding and explanation of luxations.[135]

Both students and lay viewers frequented the anatomy room, though apparently without much overlap. Upon visiting the Institute, John Boyle noticed that there was a 'picture-gallery, but no painters', and 'an anatomy-school, but no surgeons'.[136] Another British traveller, Christopher Hervey, similarly noticed in October 1761 that in the Institute all that seemed 'to be wanting were the students, but I suppose that there are times when they appear, however I saw nobody'.[137] Yet, as Lelli explained to Cotugno in 1765, the anatomy room had been realized for the benefit of both artists and, in the summer, dissectors.[138] Other records related to Lelli's demonstrations in the anatomy room similarly point to its use as a site of teaching. In his *motu proprio* of 1747 Pope Benedict XIV had deliberated that Lelli would demonstrate the models of the anatomy room, but would be no professor. As a consequence, he would not have to show up at the Institute on the days in which 'the professors need to be in their rooms'.[139] However, in his article 'on the Institute's professors' of 1755 Francesco Maria Zanotti highlighted in the *Commentarii* that in practice Lelli was a professor 'even more so than the others'.[140] After Lelli died in March 1766, and was replaced by Luigi Galvani, the position of the demonstrator of the anatomy room was officially transformed into a professorship. Galvani was then charged with the task of demonstrating anatomy to students and scholars (*studiosi*) from Lent to May or June, or when Giovanni Antonio Galli offered his course on the 'art of obstetrics' in the midwifery rooms.[141] By the early 1770s, training on the Institute's anatomy and midwifery models became a noteworthy credential for applicants to the position of assistant surgeon in the hospital of Santa Maria della Morte in Bologna.[142]

As well as being used as a site of anatomical teaching, the anatomy room also fulfilled the expectation that its models would attract the attention and admiration

[135] ASB, Assunteria d'Istituto, Diversorum, busta 10, n. 2. [136] Boyle, *Letters from Italy*, 68.

[137] Christopher Hervey, *Letters from Portugal, Spain, Italy and Germany in the Years 1759, 1760 and 1761*, vol. 3 (London: Printed by J. Davis for R. Faulder, 1785), 450.

[138] Cotugno, 'Iter Italicum', 76. According to Lambertini, the anatomy room was meant to provide a space for the close study of bones and muscles ('Miology' and 'Osteology') for the benefit of 'painters and sculptors' and of 'various surgical operations'. As such, it was meant to complement the public anatomy lesson; see Lambertini, 'Motuproprio, col quale Ercole Lelli', 536.

[139] Lambertini, 'Motuproprio, col quale Ercole Lelli', 535–40.

[140] See Francesco Maria Zanotti, 'De Professoribus Instituti', in *De Bononiensi Scientiarum et Artium Instituto atque Academia Commentarii*, vol. 3 (Bologna: Lelio dalla Volpe, 1755), 8–10.

[141] ASB, Assunteria d'Istituto, Atti, n. 6 (1761–75), fol. 76v. On the same occasion, the *Assunti* also decided to provide a table and some benches for the classes held in the anatomy room; see ibid., fol. 79r. Galli's collection will be discussed in Chapter 5.

[142] See, for instance, the applications for the position of assistant surgeon at the hospital of Santa Maria della Morte in ASB, Ospedale di Santa Maria della Morte, Serie VII/22, including the Letter of March 1774 from Stefano Barberini in Cesena.

of travellers and lay viewers, thus contributing to the fame of the Institute. In 1759, the connoisseur and artist Jean-Claude Richard, Abbé de Saint-Non (1727–1791), undertook a tour of Italy together with fellow artist Jean-Honoré Fragonard (1732–1806), cousin of the anatomist Honoré Fragonard and a student at the French Academy in Rome. Upon visiting the Institute of the Sciences, he praised the anatomy room for displaying one of its finest collections.[143] Again, in 1767, the Polish count and diplomat Michal Mniszech (1742–1806) remarked in his diary that the anatomy room was 'perhaps the most complete and most beautiful collection of its kind in Europe'.[144] As Lelli regularly opened the crystal glass of 'the beautiful custom-made cases' and demonstrated the models to different audiences, he found himself in a particularly favourable position to display his own anatomical skills. In doing so, he could capitalize on his encounters with travellers and illustrious visitors. The benefits of such encounters became clear when Richard de Saint-Non wrote in his travel diary that Lelli was 'undoubtedly the greatest anatomist in Europe'.[145] The Scottish engraver Robert Strange, who travelled in Italy in 1760, similarly praised Lelli as 'an ingenious artist and an excellent anatomist'.[146] Likewise, when the literatus Giuseppe Baretti addressed the criticism that Grand Tour writers such as Samuel Sharp and Tobias Smollett had reserved for Italian peoples and manners, he referred to Lelli as one of the 'painters, statuaries, architects and engravers' who 'are looked upon as tolerably ingenious in their several ways, even by some of the English lords and gentlemen who do us the honour to visit our country'.[147]

Many more mentioned Lelli in their reports, expressing appreciation for his anatomical work. Notably, they did so at a time during which the rumour that Lelli may not have been the sole artificer of the anatomy room had started to spread in Bologna. In the same period, Lelli also became a more or less overt target of those who disapproved of their fellow artists' engagement with anatomy. The painter Luigi Crespi, for instance, scorned an age in which artists spent much time learning about the abstrusities of anatomical language when this would normally be the business of 'physicians, surgeons, and philosophizers' (*filosofanti*).[148] Still, if Lelli's involvement in anatomical activities precipitated ironical comments, his growing anatomical fame allowed him to build an extensive network

[143] See, for instance, Jean-Claude Richard de Saint-Non, *Panopticon italiano: Un diario di viaggio ritrovato, 1759–1761* (Rome: Elefante, 1986), 86.

[144] Biblioteca di Archeologia e Storia dell'Arte (Rome), ms. 35 C, 'Journaux des voyages par le Comte Michel Mniszech', 206. See also Bronisław Biliński, 'Bologna nel ritrovato manoscritto "Journaux des Voyages" di Michele Mniszech (1767)', in Riccardo Casimiro Lewanski (ed.), *Laudatio Bononiae: Atti del Convegno storico italo-polacco svoltosi a Bologna dal 26 al 31 maggio 1988 in occasione del Nono Centenario dell'Alma Mater Studiorum* (Bologna: Università degli Studi di Bologna/Warsaw: Istituto Italiano di Cultura di Varsavia, 1990), 367.

[145] Saint-Non, *Panopticon italiano*, 86.

[146] Robert Strange, *An Inquiry into the Rise and Establishment of the Royal Academy of Arts: To Which is Prefixed a Letter to Earl of Bute* (London: E. and D. Dilly; J. Robson, and J Walter, 1775), 27.

[147] Giuseppe Marco Antonio Baretti, *An Account of the Manners and Customs of Italy: With Observations on the Mistakes of Some Travellers, with Regard to That Country*, vol. 1 (London: T. Davies, L. Davis; and C. Rymers, 1768), 225–6.

[148] Crespi, *Felsina pittrice*, vol. 3, 159. See also Dacome, 'Waxworks', 30.

of influential acquaintances. For instance, his friendship with prominent literati such as the savant and traveller Francesco Algarotti and the well-known anatomist and antiquarian Giovanni Bianchi from Rimini (1693–1775) helped him to increase his renown.

When, in 1756, Algarotti returned to Bologna, the city where he had studied, he was a well-known cosmopolitan savant. Famously nicknamed by Voltaire 'le cigne de Padoue', he had published a number of writings, including several editions of his famous *Newtonianism for the Ladies*, corresponded with countless savants, and sat at the table of the powerful. He had been the chamberlain of Frederick the Great in Potsdam and an envoy of Augustus III, king of Poland and elector of Saxony, for whom he drew up the plan for the enlargement of the royal gallery in Dresden and made recommendations for its art collection.[149] While in Bologna, Algarotti participated in the cultural life of the city and cultivated social relations. He also befriended Lelli, with whom he shared views on the significance of anatomy in art and supported him in local contentions. In fact, Algarotti was not the only prominent savant to figure in Lelli's carefully constructed web of illustrious acquaintances. Among others, Lelli also consorted with Giovanni Bianchi, known as Janus Plancus, who had studied in Bologna, and regularly visited the city where he maintained amicable relations with many colleagues and friends. Bianchi included in his *De Conchis* plates of marine specimens that had been engraved by Carlo Pisarri on the basis of Lelli's drawings.[150] He and Lelli also corresponded during the latter's sojourn in Rome.[151] Over the years the two developed ever more amicable ties, exchanged letters and books, and engaged in conversations on anatomical subjects.[152] Bianchi also entrusted some of his friends to Lelli on account that he 'had made so much progress that he could be counted among the first men of our age, in anatomy and in many other beautiful and useful arts no less than in sculpture'.[153] On 26 October 1755, Bianchi visited Lelli in the company of his nephew Girolamo. On this occasion, Lelli discussed 'anatomical matters' with Bianchi, showed him a book of wrestlers printed in Leiden, and introduced Girolamo to some anatomical figures in wax.[154] Two days later, on 28 October, Bianchi visited the anatomy room at the Institute of the Sciences, and remained deeply impressed.

[149] Francis Haskell, *Patrons and Painters: Art and Society in Baroque Italy* (New Haven: Yale University Press, 1980), 350–1.

[150] See Giovanni Bianchi, *De Conchis minus notis liber: cui accessit specimen aestus reciproci maris superi ad littus portumque Arimini* (Venice: J.B. Pasquali, 1739).

[151] See Biblioteca Civica Gambalunga (Rimini), Fondo Gambetti, Lettere autografe al Dott. Giovanni Bianchi, fasc. Ercole Lelli, Letters of 22 June, 4 July, 26 July, and 29 July 1747 from Ercole Lelli in Rome. See also Brighetti, 'Ercole Lelli e le cere bolognesi', 208–10.

[152] Biblioteca Civica Gambalunga (Rimini), Fondo Gambetti, Lettere autografe al Dott. Giovanni Bianchi, fasc. Ercole Lelli, Letter of 15 January 1756 from Ercole Lelli in Bologna; Giovanni Bianchi, *Viaggio, 1755, 1756, 1757, 1758, 1759, 1762, 1763* (Edizioni digitali del CISVA, 2007), 8, 10, and 61. See also Biblioteca Civica Gambalunga (Rimini), Fondo Gambetti, Lettere autografe al Dott. Giovanni Bianchi, fasc. L.M. Caldani, Letter of 4 October 1758 from L.M. Caldani.

[153] See BUB, ms. 3882, capsula LVIII, A11, Letter of 12 May 1745 from Giovanni Bianchi in Rimini to Ercole Lelli. See also, ibid., Letter of 6 June 1749 from Giovanni Bianchi in Rimini to Ercole Lelli.

[154] Bianchi, *Viaggio*, 8 and 10.

While Lelli's anatomical fame continued to grow, he became ever more indispensable to the Institute's life. As he put his manual and mechanical skills at the service of all sorts of tasks, he acted as a versatile factotum capable of addressing many of the demands of an academy that was in constant need of adroit hands. In 1756, Lelli devoted himself to new anatomical pursuits and worked with the anatomist Tommaso Laghi to perfect the art of anatomical injection by employing a new liquid and a new siphon.[155] Lelli was furthermore consulted on the coining of the Institute's medals, restored Valsalva's anatomical specimens, and was commissioned to make lenses and binoculars, as well as a bust of Marsigli. Moreover, he devised an optical theatre, was called to supervise the relocation of the military room, and became a key player in the purchase and display of copies of the 'most beautiful' statues of Rome and Florence.[156] In 1755, Francesco Maria Zanotti remarked that Lelli seemed to be born with a talent for all things, having distinguished himself in making statues and machines, as well as in the fields of anatomy and optics.[157] Likewise, when Domenico Cotugno visited Bologna in 1765, he was keen to meet Lelli for his reputation as 'a man renowned for his many activities' and 'distinguished in mechanical works'.[158] As a result of his manifold skills, Lelli could also count on ever more power and responsibility at the Institute. In the summer of 1757, the surgeon and man-midwife Giovanni Antonio Galli lamented that 'nothing is done at the Institute' without Lelli's advice and approval.[159] By then, Lelli had started his own transformation from artificer and mechanic into connoisseur. As part of the process, he fashioned the anatomy room into a privileged venue for training the gaze of the connoisseur.

BODIES, MODELS, AND STATUES

Although eighteenth-century Bologna was regarded as a city that 'abunded in wits', few liked to engage 'themselves in the investigation of antiquity'.[160] Still, since the time of its inauguration, the Institute of the Sciences could count on a gallery of casts of ancient statues.[161] After travelling to Rome and devoting himself to

[155] Tommaso Laghi, 'De perficienda injectionum anatomicarum methodo', in *De Bononiensi Scientiarum et Artium Instituto atque Academia Commentarii,* vol. 4/I (Bologna: Lelio dalla Volpe, 1757) 120–32, esp. 121–3. See also Medici, 'Elogio d'Ercole Lelli', 164. As we shall see in Chapter 7, injections were used in the production of anatomical preparations that unveiled inner bodily parts through the injection of embalming materials.

[156] See, for instance, ASB, Assunteria d'Istituto, Atti, n. 4 (1734–53), 1350 (13 November 1753); ibid., n. 5 (1754–60), 5, 21, 34 (1 February, 5 April, 20 June 1754).

[157] Zanotti, 'De Professoribus Instituti', 8. See also *Novelle letterarie, pubblicate in Firenze nell'anno MDCCLV,* vol. 16 (Florence: Stamperia della SS. Annunziata, 1755), 794.

[158] Cotugno, 'Iter Italicum', 73.

[159] BUB, ms. 72, Corrispondenza Letteraria dell'abate Flaminio Scarselli, Letters of 20 August 1757 and 20 December 1758 from Gian Antonio Galli in Bologna to Flaminio Scarselli.

[160] Getty Research Institute, Los Angeles, Special Collections, Collections of Letters from Italian Intellectuals on Cultural and Academic Subjects (1610–1822), ms. 980033, vol. 3, 203, Letter of 1 December 1734 from Bologna (not signed).

[161] See Donatella Biagi Maino, 'Luigi Ferdinando Marsili e le arti del disegno: La nuova visione del mondo', in Donatella Biagi Maino (ed.), *L'immagine del Settecento da Luigi Ferdinando Marsigli a Benedetto XIV* (Turin: Umberto Allemandi, 2005), 30–1.

the study of antiquities, Marsigli had secured the arrival in Bologna of the plaster casts of some famous ancient statues, such as the Farnese Hercules, the Laocoön, the Belvedere Torso, the Apollo Belvedere, the Venus de' Medici, and the Borghese Gladiator.[162] After taking on the expansion of the Institute of the Sciences, Pope Benedict XIV had entertained the idea of enlarging the gallery of statues.[163] Yet, by the time Lelli pleaded with the pope to implement the project, Lambertini had changed his mind. Too many among the projects he had sponsored at the Institute had gone astray, especially those associated with Lelli. Frustrated and disgruntled, the pope maintained that the response to his munificence had been less than satisfactory: the anatomy room had ended up being more time-consuming and expensive than anticipated, not even 'a pair of glasses' had resulted from his gift of optical instruments to the Institute, and the lathes had been languishing in idleness.[164] Furthermore, substantial amounts of money and resources had been wasted during work on the library. Lambertini was not impressed.

In the summer of 1752, he declared himself unwilling to embark on a new project that ran the risk of generating further disappointment, and would in fact distract Lelli from adding the final touches to the anatomical tables that still needed to be completed.[165] When, the following September, Fulvio Bentivoglio, the Bolognese ambassador to Rome, informed Lambertini that the experiments in the Institute's observatory had been suspended, it looked like the line of the pope's patience had been crossed.[166] However, when, in 1753, the Venetian nobleman and abbot Filippo Vincenzo Farsetti (1703–1774) asked the pontiff for permission to make plaster casts of the most beautiful statues of Rome and committed himself to donate a copy of each cast to the Institute, Lambertini reversed his decision.[167] Discussions about the project were resumed, and practicalities such as the location of the statues at the Institute were addressed.[168] As part of the deal, Bologna was to be provided with fifty plaster casts of the most beautiful statues of Rome and 'other foreign cities'.[169] Lelli was charged with the task of supervising the production and transportation of the casts to the Institute. He also had to ensure that, following the pope's wishes, once the statues reached their destination, they would replicate the disposition of those displayed at the French Academy in Rome.[170]

[162] Ibid., 30–1 and 34–5.

[163] Donatella Biagi Maino, 'La rifondazione dell'Accademia in età benedettina', in Biagi Maino (ed.), *L'immagine del Settecento*, 90.

[164] ASB, Assunteria d'Istituto, Lettere all'Istituto, n. 4 (1734–52), Letter of 12 July 1752 from Fulvio Bentivoglio in Rome to the Institute.

[165] Ibid.; ASB, Assunteria d'Istituto, Lettere dell'Istituto, n. 3 (1735–55), Letter of 19 August 1752 from the Institute to the ambassador.

[166] ASB, Assunteria d'Istituto, Lettere all'Istituto, n. 4 (1734–52), Letter of 13 September 1752 from Fulvio Bentivoglio in Rome to the Institute.

[167] BCABo, ms. B 134, Marcello Oretti, *Notizie de' Professori del Dissegno*, vol. 12, 120. See also [Grosley], *New Observations*, vol. 1, 130.

[168] Some even maintained that it was thanks to the sketchbook that Lelli had donated to the pope in Rome back in 1747 that the enlargement of the gallery of the statues had been made possible at all; see Biagi Maino, 'La rifondazione dell'Accademia', 90.

[169] ASB, Lettere all'Istituto, n. 5 (1753–7), Letter of 31 January 1756 from Filippo Farsetti in Venice to the Institute. See also Haskell, *Patrons and Painters*, 83; Haskell and Penny, *Taste and the Antique*, 85.

[170] ASB, Assunteria d'Istituto, Lettere all'Istituto, n. 4 (1734–52), Letter of 12 July 1752 from Fulvio Bentivoglio in Rome to the Institute.

Opened to the public in 1755 in the family palace on the Grand Canal in Venice, Farsetti's collection included casts of classical statues, cork copies of antique monuments, and a large number of terracotta models of the artworks of seventeenth- and eighteenth-century masters. Offering one of the most notable assemblages of casts and copies of ancient sculpture in Europe, the collection became a favourite destination for travellers and connoisseurs. As the story has it, it was also the place where the young Antonio Canova took his first steps in the world of sculpture. For his part, Lelli took advantage of his new role as the broker in charge of the Institute's casts. He cultivated his relationship with the influential Farsetti and donated to him a copy of his own anatomical statuette.

As early as 1752, Lelli had envisioned a new method of teaching for the school of drawing ('Scuola del Nudo') that relied on an enlarged gallery of statues at the Institute of the Sciences.[171] In particular, Lelli's method combined traditional candlelit night sessions, during which a nude human model was drawn from life, with daytime sessions. These sessions could rely on daylight to link the study of ancient statues and the drawing of the nude body with the scrutiny of anatomical detail from the models of the anatomy room. The length of study would then end up being almost doubled, and the school's calendar would be such that following the period of the usual candlelit night sessions (which ran from 'All Saints' day to Easter'), from 'Easter to May' the students could 'observe, study, and copy' the models of ancient Greek statues so as to appreciate the 'exactness of proportions', 'beauty of ideas', and 'variety of characters'.[172] Studying the statues during springtime would also help to contain the costs of hiring a model because, at this time, 'the season was not yet warm enough to have a man pose naked for two hours without a fire'. Finally, in June and July, students could combine the study of the nude body with the 'observation and study' of the anatomical models of the anatomy room so as to 'discover and rectify the mistakes' that they could have made 'while drawing the nude' from life.[173] As Lelli noticed, the students themselves were eager to scrutinize the models of the anatomy room for this purpose. The room then became a special venue of visual training and verification where students could rely on the models' anatomical details to correct the mistakes made in the process of drawing from life. While doing so, they also honed their visual skills.[174]

[171] Benassi, *L'Accademia Clementina*, 217.

[172] ASB, Archivio Ranuzzi, Archivio del Co: Giuseppe Segni, N. Carte relative all'Accademia Clementina. On Lelli's new curriculum for the school of drawing, see also Benassi, *L'Accademia Clementina*, 217–19.

[173] Benassi, *L'Accademia Clementina*, 217–19.

[174] On visual training and its histories, see Anne Secord, 'Botany on a Plate: Pleasure and the Power of Pictures in Promoting Early Ninenteenth-Century Scientific Knowledge', *Isis*, 93 (2002), 28–57; Lorraine Daston and Peter Galison, *Objectivity* (New York: Zone Books, 2007), 331; Daniela Bleichmar, 'Training the Naturalist's Eye in the Eighteenth Century: Perfect Global Visions and Local Blind Spots', in Cristina Grasseni (ed.) *Skilled Visions: Between Apprenticeship and Standards* (Oxford: Berghahn Books, 2007), 166–90, esp. 175; Daniela Bleichmar, *Visible Empire: Botanical Expeditions & Visual Culture in the Hispanic Enlightenment* (Chicago: University of Chicago Press, 2012), esp. chapter 2; Bleichmar, 'Learning to Look'; Erna Fiorentini (ed.), *Observing Nature—Representing Experience: The Osmotic Dynamics of Romanticism, 1800–1850* (Berlin: Reimer Verlag, 2009); Daston and Lunbeck (eds.), *Histories of Scientific Observation*; Berkowitz, 'The Beauty of Anatomy', esp. 267–8; Mary Terrall, *Catching Nature in the Act: Réaumur and the Practice of Natural History in the Eighteenth Century* (Chicago: University of Chicago Press, 2014).

Lelli's involvement in the enlargement of the gallery of statues and in the school of drawing marked a time in which he could fulfill his aspiration to be regarded as an accomplished artist and a connoisseur.[175] Having first served as the prince of the Accademia Clementina in 1746, he was appointed again to the position both in 1753 and in 1763.[176] In 1758, his request of affiliation to the Royal Academy of Painting, Sculpture and Architecture in Parma found a favourable response.[177] Two years later, he became a member of the Accademia del Disegno in Florence.[178] As his fame crossed the Alps, he obtained affiliation to the Academy of Liberal Arts in Augsburg.[179] In 1759, Lelli was appointed director and custodian of the gallery of the statues at the Institute of the Sciences.[180] In 1760, the school of drawing started its summer activities.[181] Algarotti helped publicize Lelli's method in the second edition of his *Saggio sulla pittura*, where he praised both the models of the anatomy room and Lelli's school of drawing.[182] Before its publication, on 21 March 1763, Algarotti sent a draft of the text to Lelli, informing him that he would find in it several tokens of admiration for his work. However, he also feared that the controversies that had developed in Bologna around Lelli's persona had taken a toll on his friend's chance for recognition and was afraid that 'all the good things that we will say' would remain '*vox clamantis in deserto*' ('a voice crying out in the desert').[183] In fact, Algarotti's passages on Lelli did not go unnoticed. After the English translation of the second edition of his *Essay on Painting* appeared in London in 1764, the echo of Lelli's skills reached out to new audiences. In 1778, Algarotti's praise of Lelli also appeared in the *Encyclopædia Britannica*'s entry for painting, thus offering the Bolognese modeller lasting, if posthumous, consecration.[184]

THE STRIPPING OF THE STATUES

Lelli maintained that the aim of the art of drawing was to acquire 'a clear idea of the mechanical construction of the human body'.[185] His school of drawing

[175] On the arrival of the statues in Bologna, see ASB, Assunteria d'Istituto, Lettere dell'Istituto, n. 4 (1756–65), Letter of 19 November 1757 from the Institute to the ambassador. See also Biblioteca Reale (Turin), Var. 266, Lettere di Francesco Lodovico Berta, Bibliotecario della Regia Università, Lettera 26, Letter of 21 June 1754 from Felice Durando di Villa in Bologna.

[176] Falabella, 'Ercole Lelli'.

[177] Lelli was affiliated here as *accademico associato libero*; see ASB, Carte di Famiglie Bolognesi, Acquisto Succi, 'Lelli Ercole', busta 4, n. 23.

[178] Archivio di Stato di Firenze, 'Giornale di Deliberazioni e Decreti dell'Accademia del Disegno di Firenze dal 1755 al 1771', Filza 21, fol. 24.

[179] Medici, 'Elogio d'Ercole Lelli', 185.

[180] ASB, Assunteria d'Istituto, Atti, n. 5 (1754–60), 20 April 1759.

[181] See Benassi, *L'Accademia Clementina*, 218–19.

[182] Francesco Algarotti, *Saggio sopra la pittura*, 2nd edn. (Livorno: Marco Coltellini, 1763), 24ff. For a comparison of the first edition of 1756 and the second edition of Algarotti's *Saggio sopra la pittura*, see Biagi Maino, 'La rifondazione dell'Accademia', 88.

[183] Francesco Algarotti, *Opere del conte Algarotti*, vol. 10 (Venice: Carlo Palese, 1794), 157–8.

[184] *Encyclopædia Britannica, or, a Dictionary of Arts, Sciences, &c.* [...], 2nd edn., vol. 8 (Edinburgh: J. Balfour et al., 1781), 5801 (entry for 'Painting').

[185] BCABo, ms. B 1562, Ercole Lelli, 'Compendio Anatomico per uso delle Arti del Disegno di Ercole Lelli Bolognese Pittore, Scultore e Disegnatore Famosissimo'. On the art of drawing and its history, see

accordingly aimed to accomplish this idea through the integrated observation of anatomical models, classical statues, and natural bodies. But if the anatomy room could be turned into a site of truthful knowledge, it was also because anatomy itself was considered capable of retrieving corporeal flawlessness. With a display that took viewers from skeletons to musclemen and whole human figures, and back, the anatomy room unfolded as a familiar narrative of bodily layering and unlayering. At the same time, it also developed along the lines of a well-known drama. Naked, ashamed, and distressed, the statues of the anatomy room presented visitors with an anatomical dramatization that evoked the consequences of the Fall: while acquiring knowledge about anatomy, viewers were called to mourn the condition of mortality affecting post-lapsarian humanity.[186] The two skeletons holding sickles further resonated with the traditional imagery of the *memento mori*, evoking the ephemerality of things.[187] By the mid-eighteenth century, stories of the Fall had extensively populated anatomical literature, staging a recognizable narrative of transience and mortality that helped to orchestrate audiences' affective responses. Since the medieval period, medicine itself had been regarded 'as a divine gift given as a remedy for the debility natural to fallen man, a formulation that enhanced the standing of medicine by insisting on the lasting physical consequences of the Fall'.[188] Discussions of Adam's own physical nature referred with increasing frequency to medical knowledge in order to discuss pre- and post-lapsarian workings of the body.[189] Linking the starting point of anatomical investigation with the origins of human creation, Eve and Adam were themselves well-known tropes of early modern anatomical representation. As such, they also constituted familiar figures for Bolognese citizens. As devotees and visitors approached the main portal of the basilica of San Petronio, the main church of Bologna, they encountered the figures of Eve and Adam portrayed in full anatomical glow in the relief panel representing their expulsion from the Garden of Eden sculpted by the fifteenth-century Sienese artist Jacopo della Quercia (Plate 17).

By dubbing the female and male statues of the anatomy room Eve and Adam, viewers could similarly associate its display with narratives of the Fall.[190] However, transience and mortality were not the only motifs evoked by the anatomy room.

Ann Bermingham, *Learning to Draw: Studies in the Cultural History of a Polite and Useful Art* (New Haven: Yale University Press, 2000).

[186] Early modern representations of Eve and Adam were themselves regarded as expressions of the motif of the *memento mori*; see Sawday, *The Body Emblazoned*, 73ff.

[187] Messbarger, *The Lady Anatomist*, chapter 1. On the display of skeletons in early modern Europe, see Guerrini, 'Inside the Charnel House'.

[188] See Nancy G. Siraisi, *History, Medicine, and the Traditions of Renaissance Learning* (Ann Arbor: University of Michigan Press, 2007), 28. See also Chiara Crisciani, 'History, Novelty, and Progress in Scholastic Medicine', *Osiris*, 6 (1990), 118–39, esp. 120–5.

[189] Joseph Ziegler, 'Medicine and Immortality in Terrestriak Paradise', in Peter Biller and Joseph Ziegler (eds.), *Religion and Medicine in the Middle Ages* (York: York Medieval Press, 2001), 201–42. On biblical metaphors of knowledge in early modern Europe, see also Jim Bennett and Scott Mandelbrote, *The Garden, the Ark, the Tower, the Temple: Biblical Metaphors of Knowledge in Early Modern Europe* (Oxford: Museum of the History of Science in association with the Bodleian Library, 1998); Röhrl, *History and Bibliography*, 80.

[190] See, for instance, Morgan, *The Journal of Dr. John Morgan*, 44.

If it's true that anatomy participated in the moral economy of a fallen humanity, anatomical representation also provided enduring testimony to the parameters of lost bodily perfection. Humanity may have been subjected to unrelenting decline, but many saw anatomical knowledge as a resource for reverting the effects of the Fall and retrieving pre-lapsarian perfection. Lelli himself was among those who maintained that anatomical representation had the capacity to recover bodies' lost flawlessness.[191] In his *Compendio*, he remarked that anatomy was the source of a 'second nature' that allowed artists to amend nature's faulty models, and thus turn its offspring from objects of reprehension into 'objects of admiration'.[192] Nor was Lelli alone in envisioning anatomy as a medium of corporeal perfection. In his *Saggio sopra la pittura*, Francesco Algarotti similarly highlighted anatomy's role in recovering the human body's original faultlessness. He observed that while it had become very difficult to find bodies that were well formed in all their parts, anatomy had the capacity to repair physical imperfections. Building on medical and antiquarian views that linked bodily prowess with physical fitness, Algarotti further noticed that the legs of dancers were quite well developed and that Venetian gondoliers could count on well-built arms and back, but the ancient youth exercised all the muscles and thus instantiated models of perfection that remained unparalleled.[193] Like many contemporaries, and most famously the antiquarian Johann Joachim Winckelmann (1717–1768), Algarotti maintained that classical statues bore testimony to such accomplishments.[194] Classical sculpture similarly defined the parameters for judging the beauty and perfection of the models of the anatomy room: when, in the mid-1740s, Francesco Maria Zanotti announced the completion of the female and male wax figures in the Institute's *Commentarii*, he remarked that the statues were so beautiful that they emulated the zeal of ancient sculptors.[195]

[191] See Roger French, *Dissection and Vivisection in the European Renaissance* (Aldershot: Ashgate, 1999), 74. Instruments such as the microscope were similarly regarded as capable of recovering the pre-lapsarian body; see Simon Schaffer, 'Regeneration: The Body of Natural Philosophers in Restoration England', in Christopher Lawrence and Steven Shapin (eds.), *Science Incarnate: Historical Embodiments of Natural Knowledge* (Chicago: University of Chicago Press, 1998), 83–120.

[192] BCABo, ms. B 1562, Lelli, 'Compendio ', 4 and 6. After Lelli's demise, a version of his writing was published as Ercole Lelli, *Anatomia esterna del Corpo Umano per uso de' Pittori, e Scultori delineata, ed incisa da Ercole Lelli* (Bologna: Cattani e Nerozzi, n.d.).

[193] Algarotti, *Saggio sopra la pittura*, 26–7. As Nancy Siraisi has remarked, 'early modern humanists, antiquarians, and physicians shared an interest not only in the physique of ancient humanity but also in ancient physical culture'; see Siraisi, *History, Medicine, and the Traditions*, 42. When the physician Girolamo Mercuriale brought together antiquarianism and medicine in his *De arte gymnastica* (1569), an erudite reconstruction of the physical exercises practised by the ancients, he drew on a variety of ancient and contemporary textual sources and material remains (ruins, inscriptions, coins) to shed light on the activities that shaped ancient bodies to perfection; see Nancy G. Siraisi, 'History, Antiquarianism and Medicine: The Case of Girolamo Mercuriale', *Journal of the History of Ideas*, 64:2 (2003), 231–51.

[194] Johann Joachim Winckelmann famously drew a correlation between the well-exercised bodies of the Greeks and 'the strong and manly contours which the masters then imparted to their statues without any exaggeration or excess'; see Johann Joachim Winckelmann, *Reflections on the Imitation of Greek Works in Painting and Sculpture*, trans. Elfriede Heyer and Roger C. Norton (La Salle, IL: Open Court, 1987), 7.

[195] Zanotti, 'De anatome in Institutum introducenda', 46.

Of course, discussions on the anatomical perfection of ancient statues were not new to the world of anatomy. Much of early modern anatomy viewed classical sculpture as a privileged site for the study and visualization of bodily proportions. Ever since excavations in sixteenth-century Rome led to the resurfacing of famous ancient statues such as the Gladiator, the Apollo, the Belvedere Torso, the Farnese Hercules, and the Laocoön—namely, in Plinius' own words, the most beautiful statues of the ancient world—a wave of enthusiasm swept across artistic, antiquarian, and medical worlds, triggering not only a new season in the history of antiquarianism but also a new trend in medical and anatomical representation.[196] As we have seen, Vesalius referred to the canon of the Greek sculptor Polykleitos as the model of a perfectly proportioned human body.[197] His inclusion in the *Fabrica* of the frame of the statue of the Belvedere Torso to show visceral anatomy was less an exercise in medical erudition than an effective strategy of communication aimed at enhancing the image and status of anatomy.[198] Well into the eighteenth century, classical sculpture continued to offer anatomy the makings of a canonical body and a powerful source of intellectual and social prestige. For one thing, linking anatomical practice with classical sculpture granted anatomy an enduring connection with the prestige of antiquarian culture.[199] For another, it shifted attention away from the bloodiest aspects of anatomical dissection and placed the classical tradition at the centre of the definition of a universal bodily norm. While taking the anatomical body away from the physical context of death and decomposition, the anatomical statues displayed at the Institute of the Sciences similarly re-naturalized bodily features through a classicizing sculptural language. As Michael Baxandall has observed, early modern medicine 'trained a physician to observe the relations of member to member of the human body as a means to diagnosis, and a doctor was alert and equipped to notice matters of proportion in painting too'.[200] The study of proportions and symmetry in classical statues equally informed anatomical pursuits. As Francesco Algarotti observed in his *Saggio sopra la pittura*:

> the study of anatomical things needs to be accompanied by the study of symmetry. For knowing the various parts of the body, and their functions, without knowing the order and proportions between them and their relation to the whole body, would amount to knowing nothing. The Greek sculptors distinguished themselves for the correct symmetry in the structure of bodily members as well as for anatomical science, and among them Polykleitos acquired great renown for his statue of the Canon, whereby artificers could measure each part of the human body as taken from a perfect example.[201]

[196] Haskell and Penny, *The Most Beautiful Statues*.

[197] On the canon of Polykleitos, see Mandressi, *Le regard de l'anatomiste*, 133–4; Kusukawa, *Picturing the Book of Nature*, 213–15.

[198] See Glenn Harcourt, 'Andreas Vesalius and the Anatomy of Antique Sculpture', in 'The Cultural Display of the Body,' special issue, *Representations*, 17 (1987), 28–61. See also Kusukawa, *Picturing the Book of Nature*, 214ff.

[199] See Harcourt, 'Andreas Vesalius'; Mario Biagioli, 'Scientific Revolution, Social Bricolage, and Etiquette', in Roy Porter and Mikuláš Teich (eds.), *The Scientific Revolution in National Context* (Cambridge: Cambridge University Press, 1992), 11–54.

[200] Michael Baxandall, *Painting and Experience in Fifteenth-Century Italy: A Primer in the Social History of Pictorial Style*, 2nd edn. (Oxford: Oxford University Press, 1988), 39.

[201] Algarotti, *Saggio sopra la pittura*, 45.

The anatomical statues displayed at the Institute of the Sciences were similarly praised for their symmetry. Zanotti remarked that in the statues of Eve and Adam, 'symmetry, the harmony and agreement of their parts' was 'so great that they, amazingly', drew 'the eyes by this alone'.[202] While doing so, they also provided a privileged locus for the study of human proportions that catered to medical and anatomical as well as artistic and antiquarian practices of observation and visual training.[203]

LEARNING TO LOOK

As Malcolm Baker has put it, 'the ability to look at, appreciate and discuss sculpture was one of those accomplishments that was learned and practised above all by young men on the Grand Tour'.[204] But learning to look was not easy. Rather, it demanded the development of an attentive, mediated, and comparative gaze that could transcend the appearance of irrelevant things and accordingly discern and appreciate visual features that could yield truthful knowledge.[205] A series of activities were meant to support this complex act of contemplation by encouraging the acquisition of particular visual skills. For instance, in order to instruct the eyes of artists and connoisseurs a number of art academies, such as the Accademia di San Luca in Rome, organized night candlelit viewings that were meant to highlight the details and fleshy character of the muscles of ancient statues.[206] Many equally saw in the scrutiny of classical sculptures the basis for understanding anatomy and acquiring an anatomical eye. In 1787, for instance, Johann Wolfgang von Goethe wrote in Rome that 'the continual examination of the ancient statues' stimulated 'a more perfect understanding' of anatomy and the human frame. He reported seeing in the hospital of Santo Spirito a beautiful écorché and remarked that, in keeping with the example of the ancients, the human skeleton was studied 'not merely as an artistically arranged series of bones, but rather for the sake of the ligaments with which life and motion are carried on'.[207] By then, the practice of scrutinizing ancient sculpture in order to look for the details of anatomical perfection had been

[202] Zanotti, 'De anatome in Institutum introducenda', 46.

[203] On observation in the histories of science and medicine, see Daston and Lunbeck (eds.), *Histories of Scientific Observation*. See also Siraisi, 'History, Antiquarianism, and Medicine'; Siraisi, *History, Medicine, and the Traditions*, 42–55; Gianna Pomata and Nancy G. Siraisi (eds.), *Historia: Empiricism and Erudition in Early Modern Europe* (Cambridge, MA: MIT Press, 2005).

[204] Malcolm Baker, 'Viewing Canova's Sculpture', *Object* (Leeds, 1994). As Chloe Chard has put it, the viewing of 'the famous classical sculptures in Rome and Florence' were 'established components of a tour to Italy', and thus became an integral part of the topography of the Grand Tour; see Chloe Chard, 'Nakedness and Tourism: Classical Sculpture and the Imaginative Geography of the Grand Tour', *Oxford Art Journal*, 18:1 (1995), 14–28 (citation p. 16).

[205] On the training of the eye, see n. 174 above.

[206] Hester Lynch Piozzi, *Observations and Reflections Made in the Course of a Journey through France, Italy, and Germany*, vol. 1 (London: A. Strahan and T. Cadell, 1789), 429. See also Jon Whiteley, 'Light and Shade in French Neoclassicism', *Burlington Magazine*, 117:873 (1975), 768–73.

[207] Johann Wolfgang von Goethe, *Goethe's Travels in Italy: Together with his Second Residence in Rome and Fragments on Italy*, trans. A.J.W. Morrison and Charles Nisbet (London: George Bell and Sons, 1892), 154.

shared by antiquarians, surgeons, and physicians alike. As we have seen, the Institute of the Sciences' anatomy room was itself part of a viewing circuit that integrated the drawing of the nude body with the scrutiny of the casts of 'the most beautiful statues' and the observation and study of anatomical models. It defined a space where the detailed anatomical rendering of the models allowed students to hone their visual skills. A classic example of the effort required by the connoisseur's act of looking is represented in Joseph Wright of Derby's famous painting 'Candlelight viewing of the Gladiator' (1765). This kind of effort is also captured by William Pether's mezzotint version of the painting 'Three Persons Viewing the Gladiator by Candlelight', where three men scrutinize and collectively witness ancient bodily perfection through a small copy of the statue of the Gladiator (Figure 2.2).

Peter De Bolla has suggested that in Wright of Derby's image 'the viewers are learning how to look with sculptural form, educating the eye either through the pencil, as in the young man sketching, or in the comparative movement of the gaze between the drawing of the statue and the sculpture itself'.[208] As the painting was

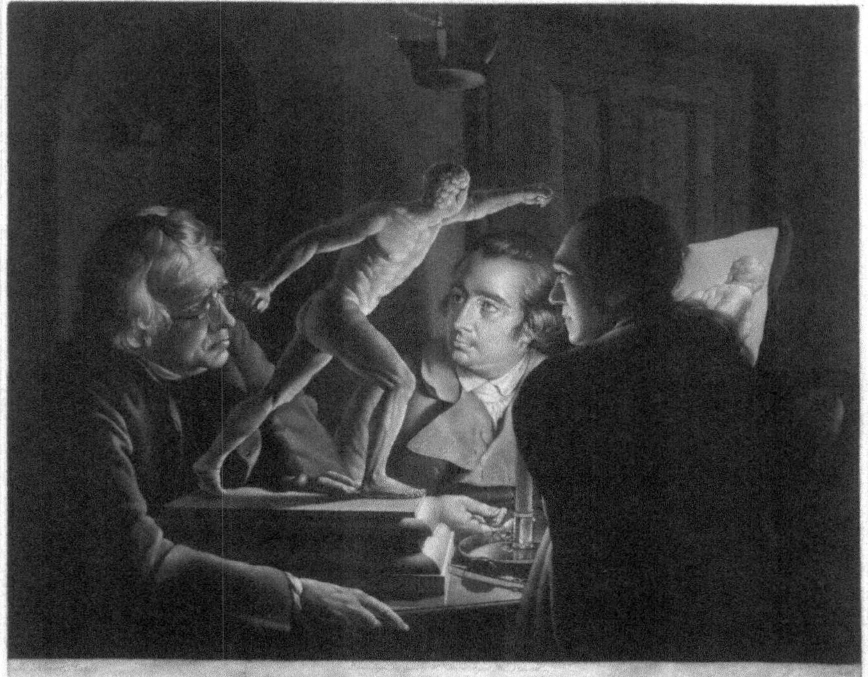

Figure 2.2 William Pether, 'Three Persons Viewing the Gladiator by Candlelight' (1769), after Joseph Wright of Derby's oil painting, 'Candlelight Viewing of the Gladiator' (1765); mezzotint in black on off-white laid paper, image/plate: 48.2 cm × 55.5 cm, sheet: 48.9 cm × 56.5 cm.

[208] Peter De Bolla, *The Education of the Eye: Painting, Landscape and Architecture in Eighteenth-Century Britain* (Stanford: Stanford University Press, 2003), 69.

put on display in London's public exhibition, it educated, in turn, viewers' eyes by turning them into the witnesses of an exemplary act of looking.[209]

In his self-portrait, Lelli similarly portrayed himself as engaged in an exemplary act of looking (Plate 18). As an anatomist, artificer, mechanic, modeller, and demonstrator, Lelli crossed back and forth between the world of making and the realm of gazing. Yet, in his self-portrait he represented himself as a wigged connoisseur caught in the intense, unblinking scrutiny of his own anatomical statuette. First completed in the early 1730s, Lelli's statuette enjoyed remarkable fortune and ended up appearing 'in almost all artists' quarters'.[210] It was copied in different materials and entered the economy of polite sociability and rituals of gift exchange. By including the statuette in his self-portrait, Lelli implicitly referred to his own role as its maker. Yet, he did not depict himself as an artificer. In fact, in the portrait little remains of Lelli's identity as the maker who was praised for his manual skills and mechanical abilities. Even Lelli's hands, which were instrumental to his career, slip out of sight, hidden behind the lush red cloth that wraps his arms. Instead, Lelli presents himself as a connoisseur. Just like in 'Three Persons Viewing the Gladiator by Candlelight', he is rapt in the contemplation of the statuette's perfect anatomy. One may argue that by presenting himself as a hands-off observer, Lelli distanced himself from the manual world of anatomical modelling which had made him famous. Standing against an anonymous dark background, he stripped his persona of any reference to the local circumstances that characterized that world. As the portrait invited viewers to witness, and indirectly participate in, Lelli's exemplary act of looking, it taught them how to use their eyes in a way that could transcend local contingencies and reconnect with lost anatomical flawlessness.

In fact, in mid-eighteenth-century Bologna, wax modelling was a locally rooted practice. Being associated with local religious ceremonies, theatrical processions, devotional practices and displays, the world of funerary rituals and effigies, and the cult of holy individuals, it was largely carried out by nuns and artificers like the *bombasari*, that is, those artists that the members of the Accademia Clementina had attempted to push to the margins of the artistic world.[211] Before becoming Lelli's assistant in the making of the models for the anatomy room, the wax modeller Scandellari had himself lamented the attempt to create a divide between the affiliates of the Accademia Clementina and the other Bolognese artificers.[212]

[209] Ibid.

[210] Pisarri, *Dialoghi*, 48–9. See also ASB, Assunteria d'Istituto, Atti, n. 6 (1761–75), fol. 141, 22 December 1771. The statuette became a well-known token of Lelli's art well into the nineteenth century. A few years after the death of Lelli, the Accademia Clementina donated a copy in bronze to the Imperial Academy in St Petersburg, which reciprocated by sending minerals, marbles, and precious stones from Russian caves. Moreover, when the Bolognese painter Anna Mignani died in 1846, she left to the Art Academy (formerly Accademia Clementina) 'a small anatomy in wax by Ercole Lelli'; see 'Sessione della domenica 11 Aprile 1847', in *Atti della Pontificia Accademia di Belle Arti in Bologna per la distribuzione de' premi dell'anno 1847* (Bologna: Tipografia Camerale alla Volpe, 1848), 20.

[211] See footnotes 17 and 18 above.

[212] BCABo, ms. B 134, Marcello Oretti, *Notizie de' Professori del Dissegno*, vol. 12, 119–24 and 299–304.

The world of wax modelling was furthermore inhabited by female as well as male artificers, such as the famous Anna Morandi, who engaged in the production of both anatomical and religious waxworks, and nuns like Laura Chiarini (1684–1762) who created devotional waxworks.[213] At a time in which Morandi ended up becoming Lelli's rival, and a potential obstacle on his way to celebrity, Lelli sought to carve a place for himself in Grand Tour culture as a connoisseur, and portrayed himself engaged in defining a realm of exact viewing.

As Ann Bermingham has suggested, the refinement of looking and the accomplishment of the connoisseur's gaze was largely a prerogative of Grand Tour masculinity.[214] Although, especially from the 1740s, ever more women travelled on the Grand Tour, and shared routes, guides, and experiences with their male companions, connoisseurship largely remained a preserve of the male elite.[215] When, in 1798, Barry wrote to the Society of Dilettanti to encourage the Royal Academy to adopt Lelli's plan for the study of drawing, he addressed this public. Founded as a convivial dining club in 1732, the Society consisted of an elite group of British upper-class men who had travelled on the Grand Tour and proclaimed themselves arbiters of taste on the basis of the study of antiquities.[216] When Barry lamented Lelli's engagement in the world of anatomical modelling, and praised his accomplishments in the domains of art and connoisseurship, his words reflected Lelli's own self-fashioning strategies and his construction of a public image that downplayed his identity as a maker while emphasizing his persona as a connoisseur.

In fact, as the story of the anatomy room shows, anatomical models played a significant part in the visual economy of the Grand Tour. Lelli participated in this visual culture not only through the creation of anatomical models, but also through his involvement in optical pursuits such as the realization of a 'new, rare and never seen before optical pictorial theatre', as well as the making of lenses and binoculars. Lenses lay at the centre of eighteenth-century mocking of connoisseurship's reliance on detail. Caricatures equally portrayed connoisseurs as inseparable from their magnifying lenses. Yet, the fashion of optical devices like optical theatres provided a new way of grappling with issues of representation and spectatorship by luring and training the eyes of viewers with illusory spectacles that unveiled the limits of deception. Lelli's optical theatre showed some '1500 mutations', including 'moving pictures' of architecture and landscapes, and portraits of 'illustrious painters and poets', both ancient and modern.[217] In the late 1760s, the theatre was

[213] The story of Laura Chiarini will be discussed in Chapter 4.

[214] See Ann Bermingham, 'The Aesthetic of Ignorance: The Accomplished Woman in the Culture of Connoisseurship', *Oxford Art Journal*, 16:2 (1993), 3–20.

[215] Chloe Chard, 'Effeminacy, Pleasure and the Classical Body', in Gillian Perry and Michael Rossington (eds.), *Femininity and Masculinity in Eighteenth-Century Art and Culture* (Manchester: Manchester University Press, 1994) 143 and 156–7; Sweet, *Cities and the Grand Tour*, 32ff.

[216] See Bruce Redford, *Dilettanti: The Antic and the Antique in Eighteenth-Century England* (Los Angeles: Getty Research Institute, 2008); Jason M. Kelly, *The Society of Dilettanti: Archaeology and Identity in the British Enlightenment* (New Haven: Yale University Press, 2009).

[217] See *Foglio ordinario*, 31, 2 August 1768, 'Napoli, 2 Agosto'; *Gazzetta Toscana*, 4, January 1769, 'Firenze, 28 Gennaio'. On the long history of optical devices as means for defining spectatorship and the realm of visibility, see Charlotte Bigg, 'The Panorama, or La Nature a Coup d'Oeil', in Fiorentini (ed.), *Observing Nature*, 73–95.

taken on a tour around the Italian peninsula and underwent great success at courtly gatherings in several cities such as Naples. In Bologna, it was on display in Luigi Guidotti's library shop. The shop was located steps away from Brugnoli's artillery workshop, where Lelli had apprenticed, and next to the public schools of the Archiginnasio, which housed the anatomical theatre. Here, Lelli's optical theatre lured viewers to a very different kind of performance, a show that was in line with what audiences could expect in the anatomy room, but marked a substantial hiatus from the spectacle one could see in the nearby anatomical theatre. Just like anatomical models, optical theatres redesigned the borders between the seen and the unseen in terms of an ideal of exact visibility that relied on the appreciation of detail. In doing so, both anatomical models and optical theatres worked as visual tools and memory aids, evoking the absent and overcoming the ephemeral while training the eye to look in a way that promised to yield true knowledge.

3

Anatomy, Embroidery, and the Fabric of Celebrity

SPREADING THE NEWS

In the late 1740s, Anna Morandi was likely unaware that she had become the target of gossip. As we saw in Chapter 2, Ercole Lelli was afraid that the news of a skilful woman who made anatomical wax statues in Bologna had reached the pope, and he tried to dismiss it.[1] In 1740 Morandi had married into anatomy by taking as her husband the artist Giovanni Manzolini, who had then assisted Lelli in the work on the anatomy room.[2] At the time of Lelli's attempt to discredit her, Morandi was working with her husband on their own collection of anatomical models. In the following years, she became renowned as one of the protagonists of the city's golden age of anatomical modelling. This chapter turns to the anatomical collection of Anna Morandi and Giovanni Manzolini to explore the place that these two artificers crafted for themselves in the world of anatomical practice. Completed by an artistic couple, displayed in a domestic setting, demonstrated by a woman, and accessible to different audiences, Manzolini and Morandi's anatomical collection developed into a very special site of making and knowing. It defined a domestic space where the display and viewing of anatomical models affected the life of their makers, and where a woman like Morandi could advance claims to knowledge and become a transnational celebrity. Of course, Morandi was neither the first nor the only Italian woman to participate in the world of natural knowledge and gain fame. As is well known, during Morandi's lifetime, women such as Laura Bassi and Maria Gaetana Agnesi (1718–1799) became renowned icons of knowledge, and famously benefited from the patronage of Pope Benedict XIV.[3] As a by-product of the city's attempt to create an honourable tradition that could support, justify, and celebrate women's presence in the world of learning,

[1] BUB, ms. 3882, capsula LVIII, A5, Lettere autografe di Marco Antonio Laurenti ad Ercole Lelli (1747–52), Letters of 9 and 26 October 1748 from Marco Antonio Laurenti to Ercole Lelli.

[2] On the contentious relationship between Lelli and Manzolini, see Chapter 2.

[3] On Lambertini's patronage of learned women see, for instance, Findlen, 'Science as a Career'; Paula Findlen, 'Calculations of Faith: Mathematics, Philosophy, and Sanctity in 18th-Century Italy (New Work on Maria Gaetana Agnesi)', *Historia Mathematica*, 38 (2011), 248–91; Ceranski, *'Und sie fürchtet sich vor niemandem'*; Cavazza, 'Dottrici e lettrici'; Berti Logan, 'Women and the Practice', 506–35; Messbarger, 'Waxing Poetic'; Messbarger, *The Lady Anatomist*, chapter 1; Dacome, 'Women, Wax and Anatomy'; Mazzotti, 'Maria Gaetana Agnesi'; Mazzotti, *The World of Maria Gaetana Agnesi*; Dacome, 'Ai confini del mondo naturale'.

commemorative stories of learned women from the heyday of the university started to circulate in Bologna.[4] In 1739, the lawyer Alessandro Macchiavelli went as far as to forge documents to fabricate the story of Alessandra Giliani, the mythical young female assistant of the anatomist Mondino de' Liuzzi.[5] When, a decade later, Jacopo Bartolomeo Beccari tried to convince Maria Gaetana Agnesi to move to Bologna to take up the professorship offered to her by the pope, he emphasized that 'since ancient times Bologna had listened to people of your sex lecturing from the *pubbliche catedre*' (public chairs).[6] In this climate, it would have been hard for Lelli to arrest the rumour that a skilled woman made anatomical models in the city. In fact, the story continued to spread. As the cabinet of Morandi and Manzolini was included among the attractions of the Grand Tour, news of Morandi's anatomical skills acquired a whole new level of amplification. Joining reports about the other Italian learned women who dedicated themselves to natural knowledge, accounts of Morandi's anatomical proficiency appeared in venues as diverse as periodicals, travel diaries, and academic reports, thus enticing different audiences' imagination about women's participation in the world of anatomy.

Historical evidence about Morandi's life points to social origins that were more modest than those of other accomplished women such as Agnesi and Bassi.[7] At a time in which social status played a key role in defining the opportunities that were available to women, Morandi's background would have put her at a disadvantage in seeking recognition as a learned woman. Yet, in the mid-eighteenth century the idea that a woman of humble origins could become learned was not unthinkable. And by the time the news of Morandi's anatomical skills started to circulate in Bologna, the celebrated playwright Carlo Goldoni had already exposed theatregoers to the character of a learned woman from an unprivileged background. First presented in Venice in 1744, Goldoni's 'comedy of character' *La donna di garbo* staged the figure of Rosaura, the 'daughter of a poor laundress', as a learned woman who was conversant with a variety of 'sciences' ('*scienze*'). When critics objected that he had made the character of a woman appear too erudite and knowledgeable, Goldoni replied that they would be disproved 'by all those sage and learned Ladies, who are admired these days mainly in Bologna, and in Venice, and in all the other parts of Italy where I have been, and finally in all Europe'.[8] When detractors

[4] Joseph Jérôme Lefrançois de Lalande, *Voyage en Italie [. . .]. Second Edition corrigée & augmentée*, 2nd edn., vol. 2 (Paris: Desaint, 1786), 352. On stories of medieval learned women circulating in eighteenth-century Bologna, see Marta Cavazza, 'Between Modesty and Spectacle: Women and Science in Eighteenth-Century Italy', in Findlen, Wassyng Roworth, and Sama (eds.), *Italy's Eighteenth Century*, 281; Paula Findlen, 'Listening to the Archives: Searching for the Eighteenth-Century Women of Science', in Paola Govoni and Zelda Alice Franceschi (eds.), *Writing about Lives in Science: (Auto) Biography, Gender, and Genre* (Göttingen: V&R Unipress, 2014), 87–116, esp. 103–4.

[5] Alessandro Macchiavelli, *Effemeridi sacro-civili perpetue bolognesi* (Bologna: Lorenzo Martelli, 1739), 40–1. On Macchiavelli's story of Giliani, see Franco Bacchelli, 'Mondino de' Liuzzi', *Dizionario Biografico degli Italiani*, vol. 65 (Rome: Istituto della Enciclopedia Italiana, 2005), 309–14; Findlen, 'Listening to the Archives', 103.

[6] Biblioteca Ambrosiana (Milan), ms. O 201 sup, fol. 46v.

[7] See Berti Logan, 'Women and the Practice', 512.

[8] Carlo Goldoni, 'Lettera dell'Autore allo Stampatore', in *La donna di garbo*, in *Le commedie del dottore Carlo Goldoni* (Venice: Giuseppe Bettinelli, 1753), vol. 1, 22–3.

thought it even more unlikely for a woman to be learned if she were poor, Goldoni responded that 'intellects cannot be measured either by birth or by blood, and even a woman of humble conditions, who has the possibility to study and the talent to learn, can educate herself, become learned, and grow into a *Dottoressa*'.[9] Thus, on the stage of the mid-eighteenth-century theatrical imagination, even poor women could become learned. A few years later, Morandi, a woman of seemingly humble origins, became famous thanks to her mastery of anatomical knowledge and her modelling skills. Like Rosaura, Morandi pursued much of her knowledge within the domestic environment.

In recent years, historians have drawn attention to the domestic setting as a crucial arena in the development of early modern natural knowledge. They have shed light on the role of the home as a particularly felicitous site for experimental pursuits whose laborious engagements involved female as well as male household members.[10] The home was also the place where the quotidian and the mundane met the world of health and sickness, birth and death, and where women participated in knowledge-making processes by translating bodily care into health practices, recipes, and advice.[11] In the case of Morandi, the domestic setting provided a venue where she could not only dedicate herself to anatomical pursuits as a fully engaged member of the anatomical household but also become a public figure and a celebrity. This chapter explores how Morandi and Manzolini's anatomical home worked as a complex, multi-functional, and porous space of production, presentation, consumption, and commercialization of anatomical knowledge, which served both private and public functions.

The issue of the conceptualization of private and public spaces of knowledge has, of course, been at the centre of much historical debate. The discussion has partly developed in response to Jürgen Habermas' famous account of the emergence in the eighteenth century of the 'public sphere' as a domain that presupposed 'a strict separation of the public from the private realm'.[12] While taking on Habermas' account, scholars have emphasized the contingent, unstable, and variable

[9] Ibid.

[10] Steven Shapin, 'The House of Experiment in Seventeenth-Century England', *Isis*, 79:3 (1988), 373–404; Deborah E. Harkness, 'Managing an Experimental Household: The Dees of Mortlake and the Practice of Natural Philosophy', *Isis*, 88:2 (1997), 247–62; Rob Iliffe and Frances Willmoth, 'Astronomy and the Domestic Sphere: Margaret Flamsteed and Caroline Herschel as Assistant-Astronomers', in Lynette Hunter and Sarah Hutton (eds.), *Women, Science and Medicine, 1500–1700* (Stroud: Sutton Publishing, 1997), 235–65; Gadi Algazi, 'Scholars in Households: Refiguring the Learned Habitus, 1480–1550', *Science in Context*, 16:1/2 (2003), 9–42; Monika Mommertz, 'The Invisible Economy of Science: A New Approach to the History of Gender and Astronomy at the Eighteenth-Century Berlin Academy of Sciences', trans. Julia Baker, in Judith P. Zinsser (ed.), *Men, Women, and the Birthing of Modern Science* (DeKalb: Northern Illinois University Press, 2005), 159–78; Terrall, *Catching Nature*, esp. chapter 2.

[11] See, for instance, Montserrat Cabré, 'Women or Healers? Household Practices and the Categories of Health Care in Late Medieval Iberia', *Bulletin of the History of Medicine*, 82:1 (2008), 18–51; Leong, 'Making Medicines'; Leigh Whaley, *Women and the Practice of Medical Care in Early Modern Europe, 1400–1800* (Basingstoke: Palgrave Macmillan, 2011), chapter 8; Cavallo and Storey, *Healthy Living*.

[12] Jürgen Habermas, *The Structural Transformation of the Public Sphere: An Inquiry into a Category of the Bourgeois Society*, trans. T. Burger and F. Lawrence (Cambridge, MA: MIT Press, 1989), 175–6.

character of notions of the public and the private, and have accordingly offered more nuanced narratives of how spaces inscribed and mediated power and gender relations.[13] Building on Michael McKeon's characterization of the relationship between the private and the public as a 'distinction without separation', Elizabeth Cohen has remarked that in early modern Italy

> both inside and outside houses, spaces often served multiple purposes and might be occupied by diverse people going about various businesses. Some spaces were more private, others more public, and behaviour adjusted accordingly.[14]

The domestic setting has been equally regarded as a fluid private-cum-public space of agency for women who were engaged in natural and medical pursuits.[15] What follows draws attention to Morandi and Manzolini's artisanal home as a site of making and knowing where family life intersected with the anatomical workshop and its practices. Here, some of the couple's engagements, such as dissection and modelling, were pursued out of sight and delimited a secluded space of withdrawal within the anatomical home. Conversely, other activities, such as demonstrations, were open to audiences and defined a venue of anatomical encounter where the models were displayed and presented to viewers through Morandi's impressive performances.

Over the course of the eighteenth century, artisans' workshops and cabinets catered to an increasing demand for anatomical and natural knowledge. In so doing, they defined sites of display, knowledge, and conversation that were alternative to both the institutional sphere of the academy and the salon.[16] Frequently ordered, commercially oriented, and usually accessible by the public, they differed from cabinets of curiosities held in patrician households, though members of the aristocracy looking for materials for their collections remained the 'best-paying

[13] On the responses of historians of the sciences to Habermas see, for instance, Mary Terrall, 'Public Science in the Enlightenment', *Modern Intellectual History*, 2:2 (2005), 265–76; Golinski, *Science as Public Culture*; Bensaude-Vincent and Blondel (eds.), *Science and Spectacle*. Studies of how eighteenth-century notions of private and public life affected women's lives and gender relations include Amanda Vickery, 'Golden Age to Separate Spheres? A Review of the Categories and Chronology of English Women's History', *The Historical Journal*, 36:2 (1993), 383–414; Lawrence Klein, 'Gender and the Public/Private Distinction in the Eighteenth Century: Some Questions about Evidence and Analytic Procedure', *Eighteenth-Century Studies*, 29:1 (1995), 97–109; Mary Terrall, 'Gendered Spaces, Gendered Audiences: Inside and Outside the Paris Academy of Sciences', *Configurations*, 3:2 (1995), 207–32; Susan Dalton, *Engendering the Republic of Letters: Reconnecting Public and Private Spheres in Eighteenth-Century Europe* (Montreal and Kingston: McGill-Queen's University Press, 2003); Nussbaum, *Rival Queens*; Engel, *Fashioning Celebrity*. For a follow-up of the discussion in the context of 'the spatial turn', see Beat Kümin and Cornelie Usborne, 'At Home and in the Workplace: A Historical Introduction to the "Spatial Turn"', *History and Theory*, 52:3 (2013), 305–18.

[14] Elizabeth S. Cohen, 'Miscarriages of Apothecary Justice: Un-separate Spaces for Work and Family in Early Modern Rome', *Renaissance Studies* 21:4 (2007), 480–504.

[15] Harkness, 'Managing an Experimental Household'; Mommertz, 'The Invisible Economy of Science'; Cohen, 'Miscarriages of Apothecary Justice', 482.

[16] See, for instance, Bennett, 'Shopping for Instruments in Paris and London'; Hilaire-Pérez, 'Technology as a Public Culture'; Hilaire-Pérez, 'Technology, Curiosity and Utility'; Bernadette Bensaude-Vincent and Christine Blondel, 'Introduction: A Science Full of Shocks, Sparks and Smells', in Bensaude-Vincent and Blondel (eds.), *Science and Spectacle*; Larry Stewart, 'The Laboratory, the Workshop and the Theatre of Experiment', ibid., 11–24.

customers'.[17] While intersecting and overlapping with the domestic spaces of family life, Manzolini and Morandi's anatomical home similarly expanded the venues of anatomical pursuit through a space that was at the same time curious, instructive, domestic, commercial, and both useful and delightful. This chapter considers its role as a site of anatomical inquiry where instances of natural, moral, and social order were lodged both in the collection and in its makers' family life. Likewise, it examines Manzolini and Morandi's domestic setting as a site where the world of maternity and the largely female practices of sewing and needlework could be recast as the correlates of a new relationship between women and anatomy that could naturalize their presence in the anatomical world.[18]

UN/ORDINARY HOUSEHOLDS

Accounts of Anna Morandi's life normally start at the point when she married into anatomy by taking Giovanni Manzolini as her spouse. Not much is known about her life before this event.[19] As Gabriella Berti Logan observed, Morandi spent part of her youth with her mother Rosa Giovannini and her brother Lazzaro in a household that had no servants, a sign that the family could not rely on the comforts of a middling estate.[20] Furthermore, Morandi benefited from the system of charity designed to pay for the dowries of young women who came from needy families.[21] Dowries were, of course, essential assets for early modern Italian women. In order to make sure that even underprivileged women could be granted one, the city of Bologna relied on a complex system of charity that involved various constituencies and patrons, such as *confraternite*, parishes, patrician families, and the university.[22] In some cases, benefactors chose their protégée. In others, dowries were dispensed on the basis of a lottery system among deserving unmarried women. A number of Bolognese patrician families were actively engaged in this endeavour. A banking institution, the Monte del matrimonio, was set up to collect the funds, granting

[17] Bensaude-Vincent and Blondel, 'Introduction', 5.

[18] Of course, the domestic setting was not an exclusive site for women to engage in anatomical practice. As we saw in Chapter 2, since the early days of the university, anatomical dissections and private teaching sessions had been regularly carried out in the homes of Bolognese anatomists, surgeons, and dissectors. Lelli himself worked on the models of the anatomy room in his residence. Nor were women precluded from accessing public spaces of anatomical pursuits.

[19] According to some of her contemporaries and, in particular, Luigi Crespi, Morandi was a woman 'without education' ('*senza letteratura*') and 'disheartened ("*disanimata*") by the lack of necessary comfort'; see Crespi, *Felsina pittrice*, vol. 3, 310. For a reading that offers an alternative interpretation, see Messbarger, 'Re-Membering a Body of Work'.

[20] Berti Logan, 'Women and the Practice', 512 n. 12.

[21] See ASB, Ufficio del Registro, Libro delle copie 351, fols. 603r–604r. On the system of charity dispensing dowries to the needy women of Bologna, see Isabelle Chabot and Massimo Fornasari, *L'economia della carità: Le doti del Monte di Pietà di Bologna (secoli XVI–XX)* (Bologna: Il Mulino, 1997); Mauro Carboni, *Le doti della 'povertà'. Famiglia, risparmio, previdenza: il Monte del Matrimonio di Bologna (1583–1796)* (Bologna: Il Mulino, 1999).

[22] See *Notizia delle Doti, che annualmente si dispensano in Bologna a Zitelle povere Cittadine, o del Territorio dalli quì sotto notati Personaggi, Parrocchie, Confraternite, e Università, per direzione alle Concorrenti nel formare li lor memoriali* (Bologna: n.p., 1761).

some interest until the marriage and the withdrawal of the bride's savings from the bank. First as a child, and again upon reaching the 'marriageable age', Anna Morandi benefited from this system of charity. The completion of her dowry took a long time and required the intervention of different benefactors, including the patrician family of the Malvasia—which contributed the largest sum.[23] In 1739 the dowry was finally completed, consisting of the sum of 292.7 lire along with a number of objects including six golden medals, a ring with rubies, six linen shirts, twelve handkerchiefs, and a vest in black damask.[24] These assets became the property of Manzolini, and on 24 November 1740 Anna and Giovanni were married in the church of San Nicolò degli Albari.[25] As eighteenth-century sources have it, Anna and Giovanni had met while studying under the painters Giuseppe Pedretti and Francesco Monti.[26] Before becoming an anatomical modeller, Giovanni had worked in Bologna as a painter, focusing on making copies of the works of the old masters. Anna also painted copies of the old masters as well as *vari quadri storiati* (paintings narrating a story with a historical, religious, or mythological theme), which one could find in the houses of Bolognese collectors.[27] However, not much is known about Morandi's artistic life before she dedicated herself to the creation of anatomical models.

Throughout the early modern period, Bologna was home to a remarkable number of accomplished female artists, including the famous Properzia de' Rossi (*c.*1490–1530), Lavinia Fontana (1552–1614), and Elisabetta Sirani (1638–1665). Even the famous female saint of Bologna, Caterina Vigri (1413–1463), known as *La Santa* and canonized in 1712, was a renowned painter as well as a poet and musician.[28] As such, she 'was crucial in shaping Bolognese views of women artists and their self-imagery'.[29] In the late seventeenth century, Carlo Cesare Malvasia (1616–1693), who wrote on the lives of Bolognese artists in his *Felsina pittrice*, a work that also served as a catalogue for art dealers and collectors, maintained that the conspicuous number of women artists constituted one of the city's most memorable accomplishments.[30] When, in 1769, Luigi Crespi added a supplementary volume to Malvasia's

[23] In 1720, when Morandi was a child, a Luigia Giacomi deposited the first instalment; see Archivio Storico del Monte del Matrimonio (Bologna), serie archivistica *Giornale*, Giornale E (1711–26), Numero di corda 37.6, fol. 295 (Posta Terza: 5 February 1720). In 1736, the aristocratic Malvasia family, which was long engaged in the allocation of dowries to needy women, added a substantial amount.

[24] ASB, Ufficio del Registro, Libro delle copie 351, fols. 603r–604r; ASB, Atti dei notai, Giuseppe Monari, 5/11 (1740). See also Archivio Storico del Monte del Matrimonio (Bologna), Campioncelli (1739–45), Reg. 1739, 111.77; ibid., Reg. 1740, 111.78; ibid., Serie Depositi, filza (1711–20), 126.6; ibid., Serie Depositi, filza (1732–43), 126.8; ibid., Giornale E (1711–26), 37.6, fol. 295; ibid, Giornale G (1739–49), 37.8, fol. 67.

[25] Archivio Arcivescovile di Bologna (henceforth AAB), Par. San Nicolò degli Albari, *Liber Matrimoniorum*, 35/4, fol. 15r (24 November 1740).

[26] Fantuzzi, *Notizie degli scrittori bolognesi*, vol. 6, 113.

[27] BCABo, ms. B 133, Marcello Oretti, *Notizie de' Professori del Dissegno*, vol. 11, 227.

[28] Pomata, 'Malpighi and the Holy Body', 570.

[29] Babette Bohn, 'Female Self-Portraiture in Early Modern Bologna', *Renaissance Studies*, 18:2 (2004), 239–86 (citation p. 240).

[30] On the use of Malvasia's work as a catalogue for collectors, see Olivier Bonfait, 'Il valore della pittura: L'economia del mecenatismo di Pompeo Aldrovandi', in *Arte a Bologna. Bollettino dei Musei Civici d'Arte Antica* (Bologna: Nuova Alfa, 1990), vol. 1, 83. See also Bohn, 'Female Self-Portraiture in Early Modern Bologna', 239.

work, he similarly dwelt upon the achievements of the female artists of Bologna. Echoing contemporary discussions over women's education and entitlement to learning, Crespi emphasized that, if properly educated, women had the potential to outdo men. 'Were women to be introduced from a young age to the liberal arts and scientific studies', he remarked, many would be 'excellent, and prevail over many male professors thanks to their being patient, diligent, attentive, and not so distracted as men mostly are'.[31] The volume counted at least thirty-five women artists who had been active in Bologna, including Anna Morandi. Many among them had been initiated into the world of art through their families, often via a male relative.[32]

While Anna Morandi's entrée into the anatomical world seemingly followed her marriage to Giovanni Manzolini, Morandi was related, through a female family member, to the Sienese painter Galgano Perpignani, who at the time was active in Bologna.[33] A friend of Ercole Lelli and a pupil of Giovan Gioseffo Dal Sole, on 1 February 1747 Perpignani served as a witness in the baptism of Morandi and Manzolini's daughter Marianna Teresa.[34] Since witnesses at baptisms were normally chosen from among family members, friends, patrons, and acquaintances, Perpignani's presence seemingly points to the ties forged by the couple with the local artistic community. Next to the family, neighbourhood relations also facilitated the introduction of Morandi to the world of anatomy. Having lived for a period in Manzolini's residence near the church of San Gabriele, in 1744 the couple moved to Ca' San Petronio in Borgo della Paglia (or Borgo Paglia), within the parish of Santa Maria Maddalena, in the vicinity of the Institute of the Sciences.[35] In doing so, the two artificers became the neighbours of Ercole Lelli, who was at the time working in his residence on the models of the anatomy room for the Institute.[36] When, in 1745, Lelli searched for a new assistant to work on this commission, he did not have to look far given that Manzolini and his family had conveniently settled in the same building.

Much as early modern domestic settings were spaces of porous interaction between private and public domains, they extended beyond the physical premises of the home to include the whole building, its surroundings, the neighbourhood,

[31] Crespi, *Felsina pittrice*, vol. 3, 246, entry for the eighteenth-century painter Lucia Casalini Torelli.

[32] For an analysis of how kinship relations governed women's participation in the activities of early modern artisanal workshops, see Sandra Cavallo, *Artisans of the Body in Early Modern Italy: Identities, Families, and Masculinities* (Manchester: Manchester University Press, 2007).

[33] On Perpignani's kinship relation with Anna Morandi, see Leonardo de' Vegni, 'Lettera preliminare in cui alquanto discorresi del celebre Ercole Lelli al Ch. Sig. Cav. Onofrio Boni', *Memorie per le belle arti*, vol. 4 (Rome: Pagliarini, 1788), vi.

[34] AAB, Registri Battesimali della Cattedrale, 200, fol. 27r. See also BCABo, ms. B 890, Baldassarre Carrati, Battesimi donne (1740–9), 91.

[35] AAB, Stati delle Anime della ex-Parrocchia di San Donato (1740–9); Archivio Parrocchiale di Santa Maria Maddalena (Bologna), cart. 4, Stati delle Anime (1724–51).

[36] Archivio Parrocchiale di Santa Maria Maddalena (Bologna), cart. 4, Stati delle Anime (1724–51); AAB, Archivio Parrocchiale di San Pietro, cart. 71, Stati delle Anime (1723–79), Lib. 8 (1737–57).

the parish, and its congregations.[37] That the neighbourhood constituted an essential point of reference for early modern life is no novelty for social historians.[38] Yet, historians of science have largely overlooked its significance as a realm of patronage, knowledge production, gossip, and exchange.[39] For artificers like Morandi and Manzolini, the neighbourhood constituted an important site of bonding and socialization, leading to the establishment of relationships that ended up marking their lives, practices, and occupations. The very story that led to the creation of Morandi and Manzolini's collection of anatomical models may also be regarded as a story of neighbourly ties gone wrong. As the relationship between Lelli and Manzolini deteriorated, the latter parted company with Lelli, and he and his family looked for a new home.[40] By the spring of 1747, Manzolini, Morandi, and their children had left Ca' San Petronio and moved to Palazzo Pichi, in the same parish neighbourhood of Santa Maria Maddalena, where the couple continued to work together on their own anatomical collection.[41] Here, amidst artistic amity turned into rivalry, neighbourly acrimony and solidarity, epistolary gossip and marital support, Anna Morandi made her entrée on the historical stage of anatomical modelling.

ANATOMICAL HOMES

Within months of their break with Lelli, Morandi and Manzolini were gaining a reputation in town as proficient modellers. While Lelli was still behind in his work on the anatomy room and was receiving fresh reproaches from Rome, Morandi and Manzolini were enjoying increasing appreciation from members of the Institute of the Sciences, much to Lelli's dismay.[42] In 1749, the surgeon Pier Paolo Molinelli commissioned preparations of the ear from Giovanni Manzolini as well as a clay cast of the womb of a woman who had died in childbirth. As the story has it, Morandi subsequently made a 'much more accurate and detailed' copy of the latter model in wax.[43] The following year, Molinelli's pupil and colleague, the surgeon Giovanni Antonio Galli commissioned a number of midwifery models from

[37] As Elizabeth Cohen has put it, in early modern Italy 'clear thresholds seldom separated family from outsiders, or men from women', see Cohen, 'Miscarriages of Apothecary Justice', 482.

[38] See, for instance, Riitta Laitinen and Thomas V. Cohen (eds.), *Cultural History of Early Modern European Streets* (Leiden: Brill, 2009).

[39] Among the exceptions, see Cavallo, *Artisans of the Body*.

[40] Archivio Parrocchiale di Santa Maria Maddalena (Bologna), cart. 4, Stati delle Anime (1724–51); AAB, Archivio Parrocchiale di San Pietro, cart. 71, Stati delle Anime (1723–79), Lib. 8 (1737–57).

[41] Archivio Parrocchiale di Santa Maria Maddalena (Bologna), cart. 4, Stati delle Anime (1724–51).

[42] BUB, ms. 243, Lettere di Jacopo Bartolomeo Beccari a Flaminio Scarselli, Letter of 18 September 1749 from Jacopo Bartolomeo Beccari in Bologna to Flaminio Scarselli, fols. 173r–175v. See also Focaccia, 'Anna Morandi Manzolini', 41.

[43] Crespi, *Felsina pittrice*, vol. 3, 307; Michele Medici, 'Elogio di Giovanni, e di Anna Morandi coniugi Manzolini', *Memorie della Accademia delle Scienze dell'Istituto di Bologna*, vol. 8 (Bologna: San Tommaso d'Aquino, 1857), 7.

the couple in order to use them in the teaching sessions that he offered in his residence.[44] Meanwhile, Morandi and Manzolini worked on creating their own collection of anatomical models, which included dry preparations of the parts of the human body that could be preserved as well as wax models of the parts that were subject to decay.[45] By the spring of 1752, the couple had moved again, settling this time in the Casa del Seminario, near the metropolitan cathedral of San Pietro, where they continued to expand their collection and present it to viewers.[46]

News of Morandi and Manzolini's anatomical collection travelled rapidly along the city's narrow alleys and swiftly spread around town. Created and displayed outside the boundaries of the Institute of the Sciences, the modellers' cabinet was more easily accessible than the Institute's anatomy room. While the Institute of the Sciences filtered admission, Manzolini and Morandi's anatomical home expanded the spaces of anatomical inquiry by making the display of the inner body widely available. Developed as the impressive creation of an artisanal household, where the spaces of family life overlapped with those of anatomical practice, the collection participated in shaping new arenas of production and consumption of bodily knowledge. Carefully arranged around the modellers' home, it also staged an intimate connection between the domestic setting and the orderly display of anatomical parts. Upon entering the house, viewers crossed the threshold of corporeal integrity and accessed an arena where they could link their own spatial experience of the collection with the acquisition of knowledge about the body.[47] In 1755, when Francesco Maria Zanotti praised the cabinet in the Institute's *Commentarii*, people had already started flocking in large numbers to the Casa del Seminario where they could admire the models and attend Morandi's anatomical demonstrations.[48] We can imagine the anatomist Giovanni Bianchi as one of them, arriving in Bologna on his way back to Rimini from the Bagni di Pisa where he had studied spa waters, and being curious and eager to visit a cabinet that had already gained local standing.

MODELLING AND MOTHERING

Being in contact with many Bolognese colleagues and friends, including Ercole Lelli, Bianchi was well acquainted with the city's activities and events. When, in September 1754, he stopped in Bologna to visit his friend the naturalist Ferdinando Bassi and headed towards the residence of Morandi and Manzolini, he might have

[44] Galli's collection will be discussed in Chapter 5.

[45] Giovanni Bianchi, 'Lettera del Signor Dottor Giovanni Bianchi di Rimino scritta da Bologna ad un suo amico di Firenze', *Novelle letterarie, pubblicate in Firenze*, 15 (1754) 708–11, esp. 711.

[46] AAB, Archivio Parrocchiale di San Pietro, cart. 71, Stati delle Anime (1723–79), Lib. 8 (1737–57), 'Descrizione dell'Anime nella Pasqua del cor[rent]e anno 1752'.

[47] On the spatial experience of anatomical displays, see Thomas Schnalke, 'Casting Skin: Meanings for Doctors, Artists, and Patients', in de Chadarevian and Hopwood (eds.), *Models*, 207–41, esp. 211.

[48] Francesco Maria Zanotti, 'De re obstetricia', in *De Bononiensi Scientiarum et Artium Instituto atque Academia Commentarii*, vol. 3 (Bologna: Lelio dalla Volpe, 1755), 87–9.

already known what to expect. Yet, as he entered the modellers' home, he remained deeply impressed. While still in Bologna, on 21 September 1754 he completed a glowing report of his visit to the couple's collection, and sent it to his friend Giovanni Lami, editor of the *Novelle letterarie*, for publication in the periodical.[49] Here Bianchi drew attention to how the display provided special insight into the human body. He placed Anna Morandi side by side with the famous Bolognese natural philosopher Laura Bassi and turned to the language of wonder to talk about this other remarkable Bolognese woman.[50] Offering one of the earliest occasions in which a report of Morandi's anatomical activities appeared in a widely read periodical, the article imparted to Morandi and the couple's cabinet a whole new level of visibility.

Faced with the task of reporting on his extraordinary encounter with this 'prodigy in a woman' who 'took no disgust in dissecting', modelled bodily parts, and demonstrated anatomy to viewers, Bianchi turned to a familiar narrative that cast motherhood as the measure of a woman's talents.[51] By the time Bianchi visited the collection, Morandi had given birth to eight children, though only Giuseppe and Carlo survived to adulthood.[52] In his article, Bianchi observed that being still young, Morandi gave birth frequently and, right after the delivery, went back to the dissecting table and resumed the production of anatomical models and preparations.[53] By engaging in all such endeavours, Morandi was, in Bianchi's view, valuable to humanity with regard to both 'the synthetic and the analytic methods': on the one hand, she produced anatomical knowledge through the dissection of cadavers; on the other hand, she created new, fully formed anatomies through motherhood. By commending Morandi as a mother, an anatomist, and a modeller, Bianchi provided one of the rhetorical devices that made it possible to describe her as a trustworthy medical practitioner and a praiseworthy public figure.[54] Alternating the creation of new bodies through generation with the production of anatomical knowledge through dissection, Morandi embodied both the wonders of generation and anatomy's promise to unveil its secrets. Moreover, what was peculiar to Morandi was the fact that she participated in the realm of anatomical knowledge

[49] Bianchi, 'Lettera del Signor Dottor Giovanni Bianchi'. [50] Ibid., 710.

[51] Ibid., 711. While lauding the painter Sofonisba Anguissola, for instance, Giorgio Vasari had linked Anguissola's skills in depicting human beings with women's capacity to bear children; see Fredrika H. Jacobs, 'Woman's Capacity to Create: The Unusual Case of Sofonisba Anguissola', *Renaissance Quarterly*, 47:1 (1994), 74–101.

[52] BCABo, ms. B 876, Baldassarre Carrati, *Battesimi* (1740–50), 38, 73, 117, and 222; BCABo, ms. B 877, Baldassarre Carrati, *Battesimi* (1751–62), 29; BCABo, ms. B 890, Baldassarre Carrati, *Battesimi-Donne* (1740–9), 77 and 91; BCABo, ms. B 891, Baldassarre Carrati, *Battesimi-Donne* (1750–61), 8. See also AAB, Registri Battesimali della Cattedrale, 194, fol. 202r; ibid., 196, fol. 59v; ibid., 199, fol. 4v; ibid., 200, fol. 27r; ibid., 201, fol. 45v; ibid., 202, fol. 298v; ibid., 205, fol. 85v; ibid., 250, fol. 285v.

[53] Bianchi, 'Lettera del Signor Dottor Giovanni Bianchi', 711.

[54] Ibid. An anonymous sonnet in Bolognese dialect similarly celebrated the wedding of Laura Bassi and the physician Giuseppe Veratti by relating Bassi's promise as a creator of natural knowledge with the anticipation of her generation of babies; see BCABo, ms. B 3634, 105, 'Sonetto in occasione delle nozze della Sig.ra Dottoressa e Lettrice Pubblica Sig.ra Laura Bassi col Sig.re Dott.re Verati'. My thanks to Marta Cavazza for drawing my attention to this sonnet. On the sonnet and its context, see Findlen, 'The Scientist's Body', 212–13.

precisely by replicating bodies, and this could in turn mirror the representation of her mothering body as a modelling body.[55]

A great deal of the literature on the history of anatomy has focused on dissecting practices and their representation. Yet, much as dissecting and unlayering the body led to the acquisition of anatomical knowledge, early modern anatomists, such as Lorenzo Bellini (1643–1704), regarded anatomy as a realm of inquiry that was equally concerned with how 'to make and maintain a man'.[56] Even John Locke and Thomas Sydenham's derogatory remarks about anatomy's failure to elucidate how 'to make a man' (as well as how 'to cure a disease'), reflected, however negatively, contemporaries' views that anatomy could potentially provide insight into the principles of physical creation.[57] Making anatomical models and creating new human anatomies through generation could then be regarded as cognate activities. Bianchi drew attention to both of them by linking Morandi's pregnancies with her anatomical activities. In doing so, he turned her childbearing into a public event that blurred the intimate setting of family life with Morandi's public presentation of the inner body.

The story of the accomplished Bolognese anatomist rapidly crossed the Alps, breaking the news of the mothering anatomist to transnational audiences. In January 1755, a few months after Bianchi visited her collection, the French *Annonces, affiches, et avis divers* published a note on Morandi which opened by observing that in Italy the appetite for science was stronger than ever, constantly gaining more ground even among women.[58] In the same month, the Flemish *Gazette van Gendt* also reported on Morandi.[59] Both periodicals echoed Bianchi's portrayal of Morandi and presented her along with the famous learned women Maria Gaetana Agnesi and Laura Bassi. Both also paraphrased Bianchi's observation concerning Morandi's virtues as a mother and an anatomist, and the association between Morandi's maternal body and her anatomical skills. The article in the *Annonces* further concluded that, by combining the production of new citizens with 'her learning from the dead for the preservation of the living', Morandi was particularly worthy of praise 'with regard to the domains that are of particular interest to humankind'.[60] As Bianchi's article linking Morandi's endeavours in anatomy with her childbearing was echoed across the Alps, it also defined some of the features that ended up characterizing Morandi and Manzolini's anatomical practice and display: the couple's dedication to dissection as well as to modelling, the fashioning of Morandi's anatomical activities in association with motherhood and family life, anatomy's promises about the possibility of recreating the fabric of the body, and the role of Morandi as the demonstrator of the collection. Bianchi also shed light on the peculiarity of Morandi and Manzolini's residence as a place that was, at the same time, a family home, a venue of sociable interaction, a site of

55 See Dacome 'Women, Wax and Anatomy', 530.

56 Lorenzo Bellini, *Discorsi di Anatomia*, vol. 2/II and III (Florence: Francesco Moüke, 1741–4), 78.

57 Sydenham, 'Anatomie', 85.

58 *Annonces, affiches, et avis divers*, 3, 15 January 1755, 11; ibid., 6, 20 January 1755, 46.

59 *Gazette van Gendt*, 9, 30 January 1755, unpaginated (report from Bologna of 12 January 1755).

60 *Annonces, affiches, et avis divers*, 3, 15 January 1755, 11.

anatomical display and demonstration, and an abode where women could dissect bodies, make anatomical specimens and bear children, and, in so doing, contribute to the betterment of society.

ANATOMY LIKE EMBROIDERY

Regardless of whether they side with Lelli or Manzolini, eighteenth-century biographers largely agree in their portrayal of Giovanni Manzolini as 'melancholic', 'pusillanimous', 'afflicted', and 'of hypochondriacal temperament'.[61] Similarly, they concur in their depiction of Anna Morandi as the loving, industrious, eager, and diligent spouse who carefully managed 'the domestic affairs', and in fact was so dedicated to her husband that she studied and practised anatomy in order to help him.[62] Bianchi observed that having learned to dissect from her husband, Morandi cut up bodies 'like any expert dissector'.[63] Contemporaries equally highlighted over and over again the extraordinary and heroic character of Morandi's engagements with anatomical dissection. As early as 1754, Francesco Maria Zanotti remarked that Morandi was a 'beautiful and ingenious woman' who handled decomposing cadavers strenuously, and in order 'to ensure that falsehoods would not be passed on to posterity' did not shy away from the unpleasant work.[64] Luigi Crespi further observed that Morandi controlled her revulsion for cadavers and started dissecting in order to support her melancholic husband.[65] Likewise, the antiquarian and biographer Marcello Oretti (1714–1787) reported that when the Holy Roman Emperor visited Morandi in 1769, he expressed his great esteem 'for a lady who had done so many studies on cadavers and parts that were so repugnant to delicate women'.[66]

According to Bianchi, Morandi was 'the first woman who attended to practical anatomy with so much propriety'.[67] In fact, even in Bologna she was not, strictly speaking, the first woman to do so. The famous *Insignia* of 1734 (Plate 5), which depicts Laura Bassi participating in a public anatomy lecture, shows that Bassi was well versed in anatomy, which she had studied under the guidance of Gaetano Tacconi (1689–1782), professor of medicine and philosophy at the University of Bologna.[68] Being an important public figure, Bassi continued to be associated with the Bolognese anatomical world and regularly attended public anatomy lessons.[69] When Charles-Marie de La Condamine visited the Institute of the Sciences in

[61] See Crespi, *Felsina pittrice*, vol. 3, 307 and 309; Fantuzzi, *Notizie degli scrittori bolognesi*, vol. 6, 113–14.

[62] Crespi, *Felsina pittrice*, vol. 3, 309. See also Galvani, *De Manzoliniana supellectili*.

[63] Bianchi, 'Lettera del Signor Dottor Giovanni Bianchi', 710.

[64] Zanotti, 'De re obstetricia', 89.

[65] Crespi, *Felsina pittrice*, vol. 3, 309. See also Gaetano Giordani, *Articolo di biografia a lode dell'Anna Morandi Manzolini, celebre anatomica* (Bologna: Nobili e Comp., 1835), 7–8.

[66] BCABo, ms. B 133, Marcello Oretti, *Notizie de' Professori del Dissegno*, vol. 11, 228.

[67] Bianchi, 'Lettera del Signor Dottor Giovanni Bianchi', 711.

[68] Fantuzzi, *Notizie degli scrittori bolognesi*, vol. 1 (1781), 384–5 and vol. 7 (1789), 60.

[69] On Bassi's participation in public anatomy lectures, see Findlen, 'Science as a Career'.

1756, and saw 'the ample anatomical collections and preparations, natural and artificial', he met Bassi there and described her as 'one of the professors of anatomy'.[70] His observation makes one wonder whether she might have been the 'very learned and eloquent woman' who, at the end of January 1751, demonstrated the anatomical models of the Institute of the Sciences to Carl Jörg, who was touring the Italian peninsula with the Count Palatine Friedrich Michael von Zweibrücken.[71] Nor was Morandi, of course, the only woman who made a name for herself in Europe as an accomplished anatomical practitioner. In France, Marie Marguerite Bihéron (1719–1795), a contemporary of Morandi, acquired renown as an anatomist, a modeller, and a demonstrator.[72] Many more engaged in anatomical pursuits.

For women like Morandi and Bihéron who dedicated themselves to anatomical modelling, the mid-eighteenth century proved to be a particularly favourable period. For one thing, their work could build on the long-standing tradition of expertise in wax modelling that included a number of renowned women, both lay and religious, such as the nun Caterina de Julianis in Naples (1695–1742) and Anna Fortino (1673–1749) in Palermo.[73] For another, they devoted themselves to anatomical modelling at a time in which anatomy was included among the realms of knowledge that women were invited to join. The *Insignia* portraying Laura Bassi in the pit of the Bolognese anatomical theatre visually marked the entrée of a woman anatomist into the city's anatomical temple (Plate 5). At the same time, anatomical modelling also became part of a widespread culture of natural inquiry that reached out to lay audiences, including women, beyond universities, academies, and anatomical theatres.[74] Women were accordingly addressed as consumers, producers, and mediators of anatomical knowledge, and stories about their growing interest in anatomy began to spread. In France, for instance, Stéphanie Félicité Ducrest de St-Aubin, known as Madame de Genlis (1746–1830), famously narrated in her *Mémoires* the story of the young Countess de Coigny who became so fond of anatomy that she never travelled without a cadaver in the carriage so as to keep herself busy with its

[70] Charles-Marie de La Condamine, 'Extrait d'un journal de voyage en Italie', in *Histoire de l'Académie Royale des Sciences, Année 1757* (Paris: Imprimerie Royale, 1762), 401.

[71] Friedrich Leist, *Pfalzgraf Friederich Michael von Zweibrücken und das Tagebuch seiner Reise nach Italien* (Munich: Buchner, 1892), 77. For a different reading, which identifies Morandi as the woman who demonstrated at the Institute, see Vassena, *La fortuna dei ceroplasti bolognesi*, section on 'Anna Morandi Manzolini'; Messbarger, *The Lady Anatomist*, 92.

[72] On Bihéron, see Haviland and Parish, 'A Brief Account', esp. 60–2; Lemire, *Artistes et mortels*, 80–5; Georges Boulinier, 'Une femme anatomiste au siècle des Lumières: Marie Marguerite Bihéron (1719–1795)', *Histoire des sciences médicales*, 35:4 (2001), 411–23; Adeline Gargam, 'Marie-Marguerite Biheron et son cabinet d'anatomie: une femme de science et une pédagogue', in Isabelle Brouard-Arends and Marie-Emmanuelle Plagnol-Diéval (eds.), *Femmes éducatrices au siècle des Lumières* (Rennes: PUR, 2007), 147–56; Dacome, '"Une dentelle"'.

[73] On Anna Fortino, see Mongitore, *Memorie dei pittori*, 42–3. On women wax modellers, see Marjan Sterckx, 'Pride and Prejudice: Eighteenth-Century Women Sculptors and their Material Practices', in Jennie Batchelor and Cora Kaplan (eds.), *Women and Material Culture, 1660–1830* (Basingstoke: Palgrave Macmillan, 2007), 86–102, esp. 92–98.

[74] On eighteenth-century women's participation in public culture of natural knowledge, see Sutton, *Science for a Polite Society*; Patricia Fara, *Pandora's Breeches: Women, Science and Power in the Enlightenment* (London: Pimlico, 2004).

dissection during the journey.[75] Madame de Genlis was herself interested in anatomy and took anatomy lessons from Marie Marguerite Bihéron. Since Genlis was conversant with anatomy and medicine, and knew how to perform bloodletting, the Countess de Coigny liked to engage her in anatomical conversations. According to Genlis, however, the young countess' passion for anatomy was excessive, and in fact it ended up causing her untimely death.[76] Another friend of the Countess de Coigny, Madame de Voyer d'Argenson, manifested a keen interest in anatomical practice and attended anatomical dissections.[77] Other stories included that of the dogaressa Pisana Corner Mocenigo in Venice who devoted herself to anatomy, receiving the praises of both the Venetian physician and *protomedico* Giandomenico Santorini and the famous anatomist Giambattista Morgagni.[78] Notably, the dogaressa's spouse, Alvise Giovanni Mocenigo, commissioned from Morandi a copy of her anatomical models of the senses.

Women's growing enthusiasm for anatomy and anatomy's increasing inclusion of women did not develop in isolation. At a time of intense discussions over the nature of childbearing, the realms of generation and pregnancy became themselves a major focus of anatomical inquiry. As a consequence, women were invited to acquire knowledge of the anatomy of their own bodies so as to contribute to the prosperity and well-being of society.[79] In the decades preceding Bihéron's and Morandi's rise to fame, a number of voices had emphasized that there was a need to introduce women to the study of anatomy and natural knowledge. In order to make such study more appealing, some had stressed that learning anatomy and philosophy was no more difficult than practising embroidery, sewing, and needlework.[80] In his *De l'egalité des deux sexes* (1673) the Cartesian philosopher François Poullain de la Barre (1647–1723?) observed that 'the sciences of reasoning demand less intelligence [*esprit*] and time than learning needlework and upholstery'.[81] The following year, in *De l' éducation des dames* (1674) he further remarked: 'it isn't as hard to become a Philosopher as it is to become an Upholsterer'.[82] Focusing specifically on the dangers of childbirth and the benefits of anatomy, in 1709 the physician Bernard de Mandeville (1670–1733), author of the famous/infamous *Fables of the Bees*, equally encouraged women to devote themselves to anatomical pursuits on account that 'the study of anatomy

[75] Stéphanie Félicité Ducrest de St-Aubin, Madame de Genlis, *Mémoires inédits de Madame la comtesse de Genlis, sur le dix-huitième siècle et la révolution françoise depuis 1756 jusqu'à nos jours*, vol. 1 (Paris: Ladvocat, 1825), 308–9.

[76] Ibid., 308.

[77] Sophie Delhaume, 'Interférences du discours scientifique dans la correspondance conjugale de Madame de Voyer d'Argenson (1734–1783) comme contribution à la représentation épistolaire de la femme d'esprit', in Gargam (ed.), *Femmes de science*, 135–42.

[78] Pompeo Molmenti, *La dogaressa di Venezia* (Turin: Roux and Favale, 1884), 358–9.

[79] Such calls continued well into the eighteenth century; see Maerker, *Model Experts*, chapter 2.

[80] See Estelle Cohen, '"What Women At All Times Would Laugh At": Redefining Equality and Difference, circa 1660–1760', *Osiris*, 12 (1996), 121–42.

[81] François Poullain de la Barre, *De l'égalité des deux sexes: Discours physique et moral, où l'on voit l'importance de se défaire des préjugéz* (Paris: Jean Du Puis, 1673), 106.

[82] François Poullain de la Barre, *De l'éducation des dames pour la conduite de l'esprit dans les sciences et dans les moeurs: Entretiens* (Paris: Jean du Puis, 1674), 241.

and the inward government of our bodies' was 'as diverting and fully of as much use, as the contriving, and making the best order'd, and most exact piece of fillegrew [*sic*] work'. It was, in fact, also much less time consuming.[83]

By the time Mandeville likened anatomical practice to the making of 'fillegrew work', the body itself had come to be regarded as a complex piece of embroidery in its own right. In the late seventeenth century, the anatomist Lorenzo Bellini represented the human body as a kind of divine embroidery and dwelled upon the complex, minute, warp-knitted fabric of muscles, nerves, veins, and arteries.[84] Well into the eighteenth century, the language of embroidery and needlework continued to inform discussions on human anatomy. The British physician James Keill (1673–1719), for instance, noticed that the ramifications of veins and arteries 'make a most agreeable embroidery and delicate network'.[85] Dictionaries similarly pointed to the very 'beautiful embroidery' of bodily vessels.[86] Likewise, when, in 1764, the abbot and antiquarian Cesare Orlandi added an allegory of 'Anatomy' to Cesare Ripa's *Iconologia*, the popular early modern repertoire of allegorical subjects, he remarked that anatomy was aimed at discovering 'the internal and external fabric [*tessitura*]' of the human body.[87] While highlighting corporeal features such as complexity and intricacy, the framing of anatomy in terms of fabric promised to shed light on the body's material properties, such as softness and solidity, and it helped to defy its proverbial opaqueness. Not surprisingly, representations of the human body as a complex piece of fabric entered the material culture of anatomy. In an eighteenth-century model of the human arm portrayed as a third-class lever, a skein of silk was used to portray the muscle, thus highlighting the close connection between corporeal texture and textiles (Plate 19). The midwifery models created and used by Angélique-Marguerite Le Boursier du Coudray, known as Madame du Coudray (*c.*1712–1794), were also made out of cloth (Plate 20). Similarly, the anatomical modeller Marie Marguerite Bihéron made use of fabrics in the making of her wax models. In particular, she employed textiles covered by a coat of wax to represent the muscles, linen and silk to depict bodily membranes, and strings or threads to show nerves or vessels.[88]

[83] Bernard Mandeville, *The Virgin Unmask'd: Or, Female Dialogues Betwixt an Elderly Maiden Lady, and her Niece*, 2nd edn. (London: Printed and sold by G. Strahan, W. Mears, and F. Stagg, 1724 [1709]), 111. On the analogy between anatomical practice and needlework, see Dacome, '"Une dentelle"'.

[84] Bellini, *Discorsi di Anatomia*. See also Antonio Cocchi, 'Prefazione', in ibid., xxx–xxxi.

[85] James Keill, *The Anatomy of the Human Body Abridg'd; or A Short and Full View of All the Parts of the Body*, 7th edn. (London: John Clarke, 1723), 20–1. On the use of metaphors of embroidery and textiles to account for the fibrous body, see Hisao Ishizuka, '"Fibre Body": The Concept of Fibre in Eighteenth-century Medicine, *c.*1700–40', *Medical History*, 56:4 (2012), 562–84.

[86] See, for instance, Ephraim Chambers, *Ciclopedia, ovvero Dizionario universale delle arti e delle scienze [. . .]. Tradotto dall'Inglese, e di molti Articoli accresciuto da Giuseppe Maria Secondo in otto tomi*, vol. 6 (Naples: n.p., 1752), 102 (entry for 'membrana').

[87] Cesare Orlandi, 'Anatomia', in Cesare Ripa, *Iconologia del cavaliere Cesare Ripa, perugino; notabilmente accresciuta d'immagini, di annotazioni, e di fatti dall'Abate Cesare Orlandi*, vol. 1 (Perugia: Piergiovanni Costantini, 1764–1767), 127–30 (citation p. 128). Notably, Orlandi dedicated the work to Raimondo di Sangro, the prince of San Severo, whose anatomical display will be the subject of Chapter 7. Orlandi praised him for his works in experimental philosophy and his hydrostatic, pneumatic, and pyrotechnical inventions.

[88] Archives Nationales, Paris, 242 AP/1, Dossier 5, Fonds Docteur Auzoux. See also Dacome, '"Une dentelle"'; Marieke M.A. Hendriksen, 'The Fabric of the Body: Textile in Anatomical Models and Preparations, ca. 1700–1900', *Histoire, médecine et santé*, 5 (2014), 21–31.

Depictions of the human body as an exquisitely complex and divinely embroidered fabric added to the calls for women to participate in the anatomical world on the grounds that anatomy was no more difficult than needlework. In early modern Europe, spinning, weaving, and sewing were among the activities that shaped female identities. As Raffaella Sarti has put it, early modern women 'spun and spun and spun'.[89] Bologna itself was known for the production and trade of silk, and in 1750 an *Insignia* that portrayed women at work in a silk factory mediated views of gender and social order, as well as promises of prosperity for the city (Plate 21). Morandi's own self-portrait in wax drew on the repertoire that linked anatomy with the world of needlework (Plate 22).[90] Completed after the death of her husband Giovanni, the self-portrait depicts Morandi in the act of dissecting a brain. It was displayed together with the models of the collection and her wax portrait of her husband. As Morandi's dissecting hand is portrayed in a gesture that could be mistaken for a sewing hand, here the realm of needlework is superimposed over that of anatomical practice (Plates 23 and 24).[91] Early modern representations of the crafts and the trades of Bologna depicted sewing women in a characteristic gesture that was similar to the one performed by Morandi in the portrait. The same gesture can also be observed in an eighteenth-century illustration in which a woman sitting at a table with her companions is engaged in sewing (Figure 3.1).

By inscribing her self-portrait into a domain that evoked the practice of needlework, Morandi could redeploy the exact and controlled gesture of the embroiderer as an anatomical gesture. In doing so, she could portray herself as legitimately entitled to unravel the complex and minute embroidery of the human fabric with due precision.[92] In a similar manner, through her self-portrait Morandi could also construct a public image that corroborated her claims to anatomical expertise by evoking those virtues of diligence, patience, and attention, which, according to Crespi, characterized female identity and could lead educated women 'to prevail over the male professors'.[93] Later pictures of the self-portrait similarly situated Morandi's anatomical gesture in the realm of needlework (Figure 3.2). Even the complex interweaving of Morandi's own elaborate dress could evoke the anatomical intricacy of corporeal fabric, and the anatomist's capacity to both unravel and recreate it.

References to needlework equally marked comments on Morandi's skills, framing her accomplishments with either positive or negative connotations. In 1777, Luigi Galvani emphasized that Morandi's achievements were all the more remarkable

[89] See Raffaella Sarti, *Europe at Home: Family and Material Culture, 1500–1800*, trans. Allan Cameron (New Haven: Yale University Press, 2004), 192. It is worth noting that embroidery and, in general, needlework were not exclusively female activities.

[90] See Peiffer, 'L'âme, le cerveau et les mains'; Dacome, 'Waxworks'.

[91] Dacome, 'Waxworks'. For a different account, which dismisses the suggestion that Morandi's self-portrait is evocative of the world of needlework, see Messbarger, *The Lady Anatomist*, 77.

[92] On the persistence of embroidery metaphors into twentieth-century neurosurgery, see Delia Gavrus, *Men of Strong Opinions: Identity, Self-Representation, and the Performance of Neurosurgery, 1919–1950* (PhD Thesis, University of Toronto, 2011), chapter 3.

[93] Crespi, *Felsina pittrice*, vol. 3, 246.

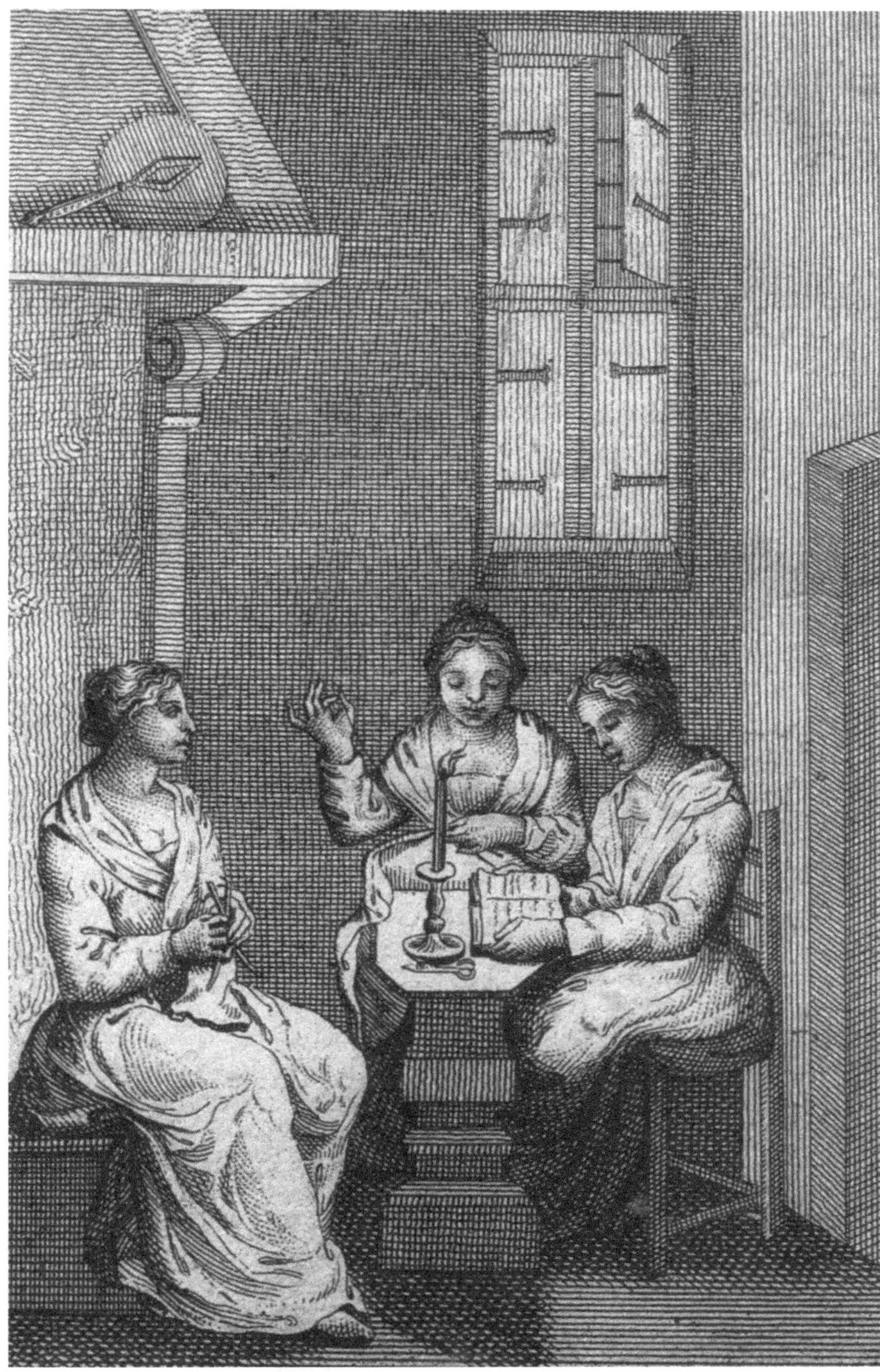

Figure 3.1 Three women reading, sewing, and knitting in a domestic setting. The woman who is sewing displays a gesture typically associated with needlework, XVIII century; engraving.

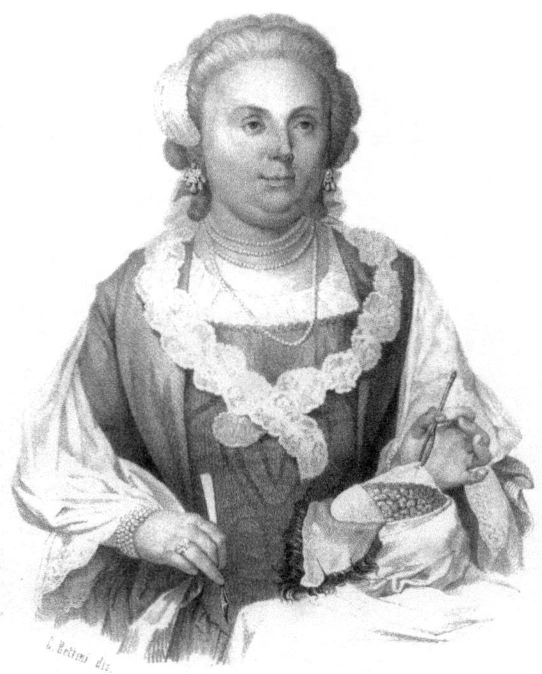

Figure 3.2 Portrait of Anna Morandi Manzolini, in Michele Medici, 'Elogio di Giovanni, e di Anna Morandi coniugi Manzolini', in *Memorie della Accademia delle Scienze dell'Istituto di Bologna*, 8, 1857. Morandi's portrait evokes the features of her self-portrait and similarly situates her anatomical gesture within the realm of needlework.

because she had wandered away from the path of sewing and weaving, which lay at the centre of women's lives.[94] Some ten years later, in 1788, the Sienese architect Leonardo de' Vegni, a pupil of Lelli, employed the language of sewing and embroidery in a derogatory fashion. Returning again to the issue of the rivalry between Lelli and Morandi, de' Vegni reported having been told by the artist Galgano Perpignani that it was because of jealousy towards Lelli (who thanks to papal intercession had grown from harquebus maker into a lecturer) that some had invested much in 'teaching, translating and explaining books' to Morandi, thus transforming a 'lace maker' ('*orditrice di veli*') into a 'lecturer and savant' ('*Lettrice e Accademica*').[95] Ultimately, however, by drawing on the visual vocabulary of needlework, the self-portrait acted as an embodied personification of anatomy and its promises. Presenting anatomy as an art that enjoyed the same level of complexity and precision as embroidery and needlework, it also drew attention to the domestic setting as an arena where women could practise anatomy (as well as needlework), and where the uncontrollable and bloody aspects of anatomical dissection could be

[94] Galvani, *De Manzoliniana supellectili.*

[95] De' Vegni, 'Lettera preliminare', vi.

put under control by the orderly and intimate context of unveiling the complex, intricate, and beautiful fabric of the inner body.

THE BEAUTY OF ANATOMY

As Francesco Maria Zanotti observed in the Institute's *Commentarii* of 1755, Manzolini and Morandi's home was decorated 'with parts of the human body', which were 'prepared with admirable art and displayed very elegantly'.[96] Art historians have drawn attention to the eighteenth-century Bolognese custom of covering the walls of domestic spaces with paintings that served as adornments.[97] In Manzolini and Morandi's residence, anatomical models took the place of paintings as wall decorations. Hanging vertically, models of different bodily parts, including the limbs, the senses, the chest, and the heart were presented to standing viewers, just like paintings and bas-reliefs would normally do. Viewers liked what they saw. Many found Manzolini and Morandi's anatomical models pleasing to the eye. When, in 1777, Luigi Galvani delivered a speech in honour of Anna Morandi, he highlighted how the beauty of her models was functional to the creation and acquisition of anatomical knowledge. He noticed that there was nothing 'gloomy and putrid' about her models. Rather, being 'beautiful and elegant', the models were bound to stimulate in viewers 'an incredible pleasure'; so great a pleasure, in fact, that they would convince many to undertake the study of anatomy.[98] While praising the elegance of Morandi's models, Galvani pointed to the role of beauty in the making of eighteenth-century anatomical knowledge. Beauty did indeed play a significant part in the way anatomical visualization was carried out in the Italian peninsula. Johann Wolfgang von Goethe, for instance, noticed that whereas in the German lands even '*the sorriest picture of the muscles*' generated anatomical interest, 'in Rome the most exquisite parts would not even be noticed, unless as helping to make a noble and beautiful form'.[99]

Morandi and Manzolini's own models inscribed parameters of beauty such as symmetry, order, proportion, and *variatio*, which had come to inform anatomical as well as artistic representation and architecture.[100] A sense of orderly beauty characterized some of the models in the couple's collection. For instance, in the tables of the eye the anatomy of the eye is revealed through sequences arranged in a geometrical, clockwise layout around an octagonal table (Plates 25 and 26). Here, viewers could follow the unfolding of the anatomy of the eye, and appreciate its beauty while, at the same time, experiencing the movement of their own eyes.[101] In other cases,

[96] Zanotti, 'De re obstetricia', 89. [97] Bonfait, *Les exposition de peintures*.

[98] Galvani, *De Manzoliniana supellectili*, 48. On the continuing significance of beauty in early nineteenth-century anatomical pursuits, see Berkowitz, 'The Beauty of Anatomy'.

[99] Goethe, *Goethe's Travels*, 154 (original emphasis).

[100] See, for instance, Ermenegildo Pini, *Dell'architettura: Dialoghi* (Milan: Marelliana, 1770). On the role of symmetry in illustrations of nature, see Emma C. Spary, 'Scientific Symmetries', *History of* Science, 42 (2004), 1–46, esp. 10 and 16.

[101] The tables also allowed Morandi to display her anatomical discoveries such as the termination of the oblique muscles of the eye.

such as in one of the tables of the larynx, the core presentation of the larynx and adjacent anatomical parts lie at the centre of the composition while other related parts are displayed at its sides (Plate 27). Another established category of beauty—that of *variatio*—characterized the presentation of the models of the hands, where one hand expressed serenity and the other was depicted as contracted in pain (Plate 28).[102]

As we observed in Chapter 2, rowdy scenes, a tense atmosphere, and problems of public order had become defining features of public anatomy lessons. By contrast, while taming the risk of excessive affective responses to the unveiling of the flesh, the orderly beauty of Morandi and Manzolini's collection created the conditions for new forms of anatomical sociability. Displaying and demonstrating handsomely crafted and well-arranged bodily parts, the models reassuringly encapsulated and mediated the beauty and order of human nature. Their symmetrical arrangements, harmony of colours, elegant choreographies, and graceful gestures similarly kept the messiest and bloodiest aspects of anatomical dissection at bay. While doing so, they allowed for sociable encounters that were properly framed within the intimate atmosphere of the domestic setting. In the blurring of the public-cum-private spaces of the anatomical home, audiences gathered around the beautiful models and offered controlled affective responses that were in line with the demands of polite exchange. On the other hand, while Morandi and Manzolini transformed their residence into a site of anatomical sociability, they also used their home to dedicate themselves to proverbially impolite practices of anatomical dissection that remained out of sight.[103] By the mid-eighteenth century, the custom of pursuing anatomical activities at home was well established. As the sixteenth-century artist and historian Giorgio Vasari famously noted in his *Vite*, the artist Bartolomeo Torri kept 'in his rooms and under his bed members and pieces of men that poisoned the house'.[104] In eighteenth-century Bologna, the habit of keeping bodily parts at home received institutional blessing after anatomical modellers, as well as 'professors of medicine' and 'professors of surgery and anatomy', were granted permission 'to keep parts of fresh cadavers in their homes'.[105] In the case of Morandi and Manzolini, anatomical dissections defined a space of withdrawal within the anatomical home. However, these activities were not secretive. On the contrary, during her anatomical encounters Morandi emphasized over and over again her familiarity with dissection. In doing so, she could highlight her anatomical expertise and assure viewers about the accuracy and trustworthiness of the models on display. And, indeed, as a hands-on practitioner in search of legitimation in the anatomical world, she had good reasons for doing so.

[102] On *variatio*, see for instance, Pini, *Dell'architettura*, 33.

[103] On anatomical practice's impolite aspects, see, for instance, Anita Guerrini, 'Anatomists and Entrepreneurs in Early Eighteenth-Century London', *Journal of the History of Medicine and Allied Sciences*, 59:2 (2004), 219–39.

[104] Vasari, *Le vite*, vol. 3 (part III/vol. 2), 387.

[105] BCABo, Fondo speciale Giovanni Antonio, Francesco e Carlo Mondini, cart. VIII, n. 3, 'Note, appunti e discorsi. Richieste di clienti', 'Ragione per le quali i professori di Medicina, e molto più quelli di Chirurgia ed Anatomia abbisognano del privilegio di poter tenere in casa propria parti fresche di umani cadaveri'.

ANATOMISTS, NOT CHARLATANS

While the question of the utility of anatomy had stirred controversy in the late seventeenth and early eighteenth centuries, by the mid-eighteenth century anatomy had come to be regarded as an important aspect of sound medical pursuits. In 1745, the anatomist Antonio Cocchi claimed that anatomical knowledge helped to identify the sites of ailments.[106] A decade later, the Modenese physician Antonio Morandi joined the conversation with a dissertation discussing anatomy's capacity to serve as a solid foundation for medicine.[107] As reported in the *Novelle letterarie*, in his view a practitioner 'who did not have perfect knowledge of anatomy was more properly called an empiric, or a charlatan, rather than a physician'.[108] Anatomy could then help to determine proper medical pursuits. By fashioning themselves as practitioners who were busy dissecting as well as modelling, Morandi and Manzolini could highlight their experience as consummate anatomists and accordingly dispel possible doubts about their role and status in the medical world. In fact, it seems possible to situate the activities of the couple in the context of the diversified world of early modern medical practice.[109] As this world was defined by systematic negotiations among different practitioners and healing groups, accusations of inadequacy flew around the various camps. Morandi's emphasis on her familiarity with anatomical dissection and her claims to anatomical expertise could shelter the couple's activities from becoming the target of similar accusations.

Morandi and Manzolini's own network of friends and acquaintances included medical practitioners such as the apothecary Paolo Andrea Parenti, who did not have a university degree yet made a name for himself in eighteenth-century medical circles. Son of an apothecary and nephew of a doctor, Parenti received medical training in the family. In 1723, he was appointed surgeon and apothecary at the Bolognese hospital of Santa Maria della Vita. Over the following years, he studied tirelessly 'the works of the most renowned physicians', and published books on remedies in both Italian and Latin.[110] Parenti's activities in the hospital included attending to patients on a daily basis, listening to judges and physicians, and preparing remedies for different ailments. Parenti also entered patronage circles and

[106] Cocchi, *Dell'anatomia*, 24–6.

[107] Antonio Morandi, 'Dissertazione terza del Signor Dottore Antonio Morandi: Se la perfetta cognizione dell'Anatomia sia il fondamento più sodo, su cui si possa, e si debba assicurare il corpo intiero della Medicina', in *Saggi di Medicina degli Accademici Conghietturanti di Modena*, vol. 1 (Carpi: Nella stamp. del pubbl. per Francesco Torri, 1756), 43–71.

[108] *Novelle letterarie, pubblicate in Firenze*, 18 (1757), 103.

[109] On medical pluralism in early modern Italy see, for instance, David Gentilcore, *Healers and Healing in Early Modern Italy* (Manchester: Manchester University Press, 1998); David Gentilcore, *Medical Charlatanism in Early Modern Italy* (Oxford: Oxford University Press, 2006); Gianna Pomata, *Contracting a Cure: Patients, Healers and the Law in Early Modern Bologna*, trans. Gianna Pomata with the assistance of Rosmarie Foy and Anna Taraboletti-Segre (Baltimore: Johns Hopkins University Press, 1998).

[110] On Paolo Andrea Parenti, see Fantuzzi, *Notizie degli scrittori bolognesi*, vol. 6, 286–8 (citation p. 286); Antonio Lombardi, *Storia della letteratura italiana nel secolo XVIII* (Modena: Tipografia Camerale, 1828), vol. 2, 84. Paolo Andrea Parenti's books include his *Trattato di medicamenti spettanti alla chirurgia* (1739) and his *De dosibus medicamentorum* (1761). On early modern surgeons who authored books and treatises, see Cavallo, *Artisans of the Body*, chapter 1.

engaged in correspondence with prominent physicians with whom he exchanged letters, remedies, and books. In 1755, he dedicated his *Trattato di medicamenti spettanti alla chirurgia* to the papal archiater Marco Antonio Laurenti. All these activities, Fantuzzi noted, earned Parenti the esteem of the professors of the College of Physicians.[111] Parenti was also personally acquainted with Morandi and referred to her in his writings as the example of an illustrious patient to whom he had dispensed a remedy for headache (*cephalalgia*).[112] On 15 April 1752, he was also a witness at the baptism of Morandi and Manzolini's son Petronio Gaetano Vincenzo, a fact that points to the couple's ties to other local medical practitioners who did not have a university degree, but gained reputation in the Bolognese medical world.[113] As Gianna Pomata has observed, after Benedict XIV sponsored the establishment of a professorship in surgery in Bologna in 1742, a generation of university-educated surgeons was seeking to extend their realm of practice to manual activities that had traditionally pertained to the domain of practitioners who did not hold a university degree.[114] Still, for a period, skilled practitioners such as Parenti, Morandi, and Manzolini remained at the centre of the Bolognese medical world. Thanks to their anatomical skills, Morandi and Manzolini actively participated in the training of this new generation of surgeons who received university education.

Morandi's and Manzolini's familiarity with dissection and their expertise as meticulous observers of the inner body were corroborated by their ownership of a set of anatomical instruments, which included knives, scalpels, saws, scissors, siphons, a special visor to protect against the stench of cadavers and, notably, two microscopes fitted with a number of lenses.[115] By the mid-eighteenth century, lenses and microscopes had become landmarks of the fashioning of anatomy as an experimental domain of knowledge.[116] In 1764, Cesare Orlandi presented the allegory of anatomy in Cesare Ripa's *Iconologia* as a matron wearing glasses in order to carefully observe and distinguish between the smallest parts of the human body. Moreover, he portrayed the woman as working in a room where microscopes were gathered along with sketches, ampoules, and anatomical instruments (Figure 3.3).[117]

Similarly relying on the use of microscopes, Manzolini and Morandi could frame their anatomical practice within the tradition of microscopic anatomy

[111] Fantuzzi, *Notizie degli scrittori bolognesi*, vol. 6, 286–8.

[112] Paolo Andrea Parenti, *Dosium tum ad simplicia, tum ad composita medicamenta spectantium index* (Venice: Apud Petrum Valvaselsem, 1761), 253.

[113] AAB, Registri Battesimali della Cattedrale, 250, fol. 85v.

[114] Gianna Pomata, 'Barbieri e comari', in *Cultura popolare nell'Emilia Romagna: Medicina, erbe e magia* (Milan: Silvana Editorale, 1981), 161–83.

[115] ASB, Archivio Ranuzzi, Scritture diverse spettanti alla Nobil casa Ranuzzi, 1769–73, Lib. 124, fasc. n. 21.

[116] See Cunningham, *The Anatomist Anatomis'd*. On microscopy in the eighteenth century, see Catherine Wilson, *The Invisible World: Early Modern Philosophy and the Invention of the Microscope* (Princeton: Princeton University Press, 1995); Jutta Schickore, *The Microscope and the Eye: A History of Reflections, 1740–1870* (Chicago: University of Chicago Press, 2007); Marc J. Ratcliff, *The Quest for the Invisible: Microscopy in the Enlightenment* (Farnham: Ashgate, 2009).

[117] Orlandi, 'Anatomia', 127–8.

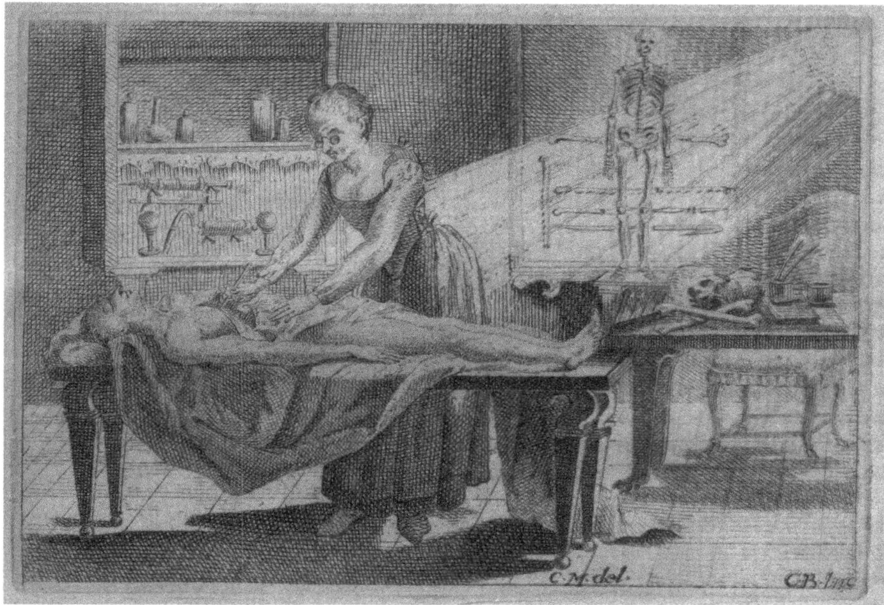

Figure 3.3 'Anatomia': Allegory of anatomy added by Cesare Orlandi to Cesare Ripa's famous *Iconologia*. It portrays anatomy as a 'matron' wearing glasses to observe the details of the inner body, in Cesare Ripa, *Iconologia del cavaliere Cesare Ripa, perugino; notabilmente accresciuta d'immagini, di annotazioni, e di fatti dall'Abate* Cesare Orlandi, Perugia: Piergiovanni Costantini, 1764, vol. 1, 127.

inaugurated by Marcello Malpighi.[118] Some of their models, such as that of the tongue, presented enlarged anatomical details (Plate 29). They incorporated such details while presenting perfected bodily forms, and this is worth noting. While the making of idealized representations has often been regarded as the result of reduced attention to detail, Morandi and Manzolini's models displayed gross anatomy in a way that integrated the presentation of a corporeal norm with the display of bodily details.[119] As Jérôme Richard noticed, Manzolini and Morandi's wax models presented all the parts of the human body, especially the most delicate ones like the

[118] On Malpighi and the use of the microscope in anatomical practice see, for instance, Meli, *Mechanism, Experiment, Disease*. On Manzolini and Morandi's use of the microscope, see Dacome, 'Waxworks', 31; Messbarger, *The Lady Anatomist*, 58, 123 and 143. On the role of the microscope in the production of early modern anatomical illustrations, see Nuria Valverde, 'Small Parts: Crisóstomo Martínez (1638–1694), Bone Histology, and the Visual Making of Body Wholeness', *Isis*, 100:3 (2009), 45–80.

[119] On detail as a feature of complexity and its role in early modern idealized anatomical images, see Valverde, 'Small Parts', 510 and 536. For a different account of the relationship between detail and the ideal in the visual culture of early modern antiquarian and natural knowledge, see Stephanie Moser, 'Making Expert Knowledge through the Image: Connections Between Antiquarian and Early Modern Scientific Illustration', *Isis*, 105:1 (2008), 58–99.

eye and the ear, with the 'greatest detail and luminous precision'.[120] Focus on detail elicited a sense of complexity that involved both the elaborate composition of the body and the modellers' own ability to grasp and represent it. Highlighting bodily detail on the models could thus support Morandi and Manzolini's claims about their capacity to map the human body down to its minutest parts, unravel its fabric, and accordingly use anatomy to tackle ongoing corporeal uncertainties.[121]

Claims to anatomical expertise marked salient moments in the couple's rise to anatomical renown. In keeping with the custom of complementing public anatomy lessons with the demonstration of bodily parts that could not be shown in the anatomical theatre, Manzolini examined the anatomy of the ears of a man who had hearing and speech impairments and whose head had been partially dissected by the anatomist Domenico Gusmano Galeazzi in a public anatomy lesson. He then presented an account of his examination at the Academy of the Sciences, where he concluded that people who were unable to hear did not speak because they did not have the experience of sound.[122] Episodes such as this show that although Morandi and Manzolini's collection largely presented idealized bodily parts, the modellers also reflected on anatomical anomalies and their capacity to affect bodily and sensory experience.

First-hand familiarity with dissection also led the artificers to engage in discussions on the nature of anatomical representation. In another dissertation read at the Academy of the Sciences, Manzolini questioned the accuracy of some of the tables completed by the artist Angelo Michele Cavazzoni for Valsalva's *De aure humana tractatus*, such as the illustration of the cochlea.[123] In the following years, others similarly expressed doubts about Valsalva's and Cavazzoni's approach to the representation of the anatomy of the ear. Upon visiting Bologna in 1765, for instance, the Neapolitan anatomist Domenico Cotugno, himself the author of a treatise on the anatomy of the ear, was particularly eager to see Valsalva's anatomical preparation 'of the whole organ of hearing', having long waited to view

[120] Jérôme Richard, *Description historique et critique de l'Italie, ou Nouveaux mémoires sur l'etat actuel de son gouvernement, des sciences, des arts, du commerce, de la population & de l'histoire naturelle*, 2nd edn., vol. 2 (Paris: Saillant et al., 1769), 118–19.

[121] It is worth noting that the couple's collection included dry specimens that likely presented individualized bodily features as well as wax models that presented idealized corporeal forms; see Bianchi, 'Lettera del Signor Dottor Giovanni Bianchi', 711. As Carin Berkowitz has observed, eighteenth-century anatomical displays encompassed a variety of approaches to representation. As such, they differed from atlases that, as suggested by Lorraine Daston and Peter Galison, maintained a primary focus on idealized forms; see Berkowitz, 'Systems of Display'. On images in scientific atlases, see Lorraine Daston and Peter Galison, 'The Image of Objectivity', *Representations*, 40 (1992), 81–128; Daston and Galison, *Objectivity*.

[122] Archivio dell'Antica Accademia delle Scienze, Reg. Atti, G. Manzolini, 'Osservazioni sopra le Orecchie, e le parti inservienti all'articolazione della voce fatte in un cadavero che vivendo era Muto e Sordo a Nativitate', 4 March 1751. See also Raffaele A. Bernabeo and I. Romanelli, 'Considerazioni di Giovanni Manzolini (1700–1755) sull'anatomia dell'orecchio in condizioni normali e patologiche', in *Atti del XXVII° Congresso Nazionale di Storia della Medicina, Estratto* (Capua: n.p., 1977).

[123] Archivio dell'Antica Accademia delle Scienze, Reg. Atti, G. Manzolini, 'Sopra l'orecchio', 16 April 1750'; Giovanni Manzolini, 'Dissertazione del Sig: Manzolini, letta nell'Accademia dell'Instituto li 16 Aprile 1750', in Bernabeo and Romanelli, 'Considerazioni di Giovanni Manzolini'. See also Messbarger, *The Lady Anatomist*, 85–8.

'such a marvel'.[124] However, when he begged Lelli to show him the preparation, Lelli hesitated. In fact, when Cotugno finally saw the specimen, he remained disappointed: the specimen looked nothing like what he had expected.[125] Lelli explained that he had tried to finish the preparation that he thought was based on Cavazzoni's drawing in Valsalva's book, but had not succeeded. He had then turned to Cavazzoni who told him that, in fact, in the *De aure humana* he had drawn the figure 'of the whole organ of hearing' by using different anatomical preparations that were brought together in the drawing. As a consequence, in the case of the cochlea the drawing did not present the actual bone, but the space contained within it. This was why the cochlea's canals appeared 'separated, thus disagreeing with what happens in nature'.[126] Cavazzoni also explained to Lelli that he had made the drawings for Valsalva by following the anatomist's request to draw on the basis of 'a reconstruction of the intellect' rather than 'an imitation of nature'. However, Cavazzoni added, Valsalva did not clearly explain what he meant and rather encouraged him to fill 'the gaps on the basis of the fantasy'.[127]

Manzolini's and Cotugno's reactions to Valsalva's approach to anatomical representation point to the risk that reconstructing anatomies in the imagination could result in idiosyncratic outcomes. By the mid-eighteenth century, such risk had been at least partly mitigated by the creation of a conspicuous pictorial repertoire that had been made available through anatomical books. From the moment Lelli was charged with the task of realizing a collection of anatomical models at the Institute of the Sciences, he requested access to anatomy books. While Morandi and Manzolini emphasized their familiarity with anatomical dissection as the basis of the accuracy of their models, they created their anatomical collection in line with the canon articulated by this well-established bookish tradition of anatomical illustration. They themselves amassed a sizable anatomical library which included many well-known books, both in Latin and in Italian, by prominent anatomists and surgeons such as Caspar Bauhin, William Cowper, Georges de La Faye, Bernardino Genga, Guido Guidi, Marcello Malpighi, Jean-Jacques Manget, François Mauriceau, Giambattista Morgagni, Antonio Maria Valsalva, Juan Valverde, Andreas Vesalius, Johann Vesling, and Jacques-Bénigne Winslow.[128] By the mid-eighteenth century, the visual repertoire that Morandi and Manzolini found in their books had come to define a set of shared conventions for visualizing the inner body. Appealing to this visual grammar allowed them to avoid situations in which, as in the case of the tables in Valsalva's book, anatomical representation generated in the imagination could run the risk of being unintelligible to others. As Sachiko Kusukawa has suggested with regard to Vesalius' pictorial enterprise, in the early modern period anatomical illustrations had come to articulate a cogent form of visual argumentation that could support

124 Cotugno, 'Iter Italicum', 73–5 and 92.

125 Ibid., 75. 126 Ibid., 74. 127 Ibid.

128 BUB, ms. 2193, 'Inventari dei Libri e Ferri inservienti allo Studio Anatomico'; ASB, Archivio Ranuzzi, Scritture diverse spettanti alla Nobil Casa Ranuzzi (1769–1773), Lib. 124, fasc. n. 21. See also Raffaele A. Bernabeo, 'La libreria scientifica di Anna Morandi Manzolini', in Armaroli (ed.), *Le cere anatomiche bolognesi*, 36–9.

anatomy's status and claims to universality.[129] Drawing on the pictures they found in their anatomical library, Morandi and Manzolini could transfer some of these claims to their own anatomical collection. While channelling and training the point of view of the observer, this visual repertoire also defined how the internal body should be viewed and represented in order to train and educate the anatomical eye.

In the course of the eighteenth century, anatomical displays were taken to directly address the senses and accordingly convey knowledge to viewers at a glance.[130] At the same time, the appreciation of anatomical detail required thorough training to develop skills related to exact viewing and mediated observation of bodily parts.[131] Anatomical anthologies such as Jean-Jacques Manget's *Theatrum Anatomicum* (1716–17), which was included in Morandi and Manzolini's library, could serve as tools of visual instruction. Highlighting specific anatomical features and postures, they educated the eyes of students and practitioners. Morandi and Manzolini took inspiration from this corpus and integrated it into their own anatomical practice. Their models accordingly inscribed, articulated and, in turn, displayed similar conventions of anatomical visualization. Indeed, if we look at Morandi and Manzolini's models side by side with the illustrations of some of their anatomical books, it would be easy to recognise patterns of continuity in the way the inner body was presented and viewed both on the page and in the cabinet.[132] In a setting that partly relied on the non-verbal communication of anatomical knowledge but still valued the authority of bookish culture, the pictorial world of anatomical treatises informed reliable and truthful observations and representations of the body. Later in the century, accounts of the famous anatomical wax models at La Specola in Florence would highlight 'both the explicit reference to authoritative representations from classic anatomy textbooks and the use of real bodies and body parts as support for models' claims to accuracy'.[133] In the previous decades, the Bolognese modellers had similarly relied on both the visual canon of anatomy and the dissection of cadavers to advance their own claims to anatomical expertise.

ARTISTS AND ANATOMISTS

At a time in which, as Giambattista Morgagni lamented, there was a scarcity of 'real anatomical discoveries', anatomical modellers found themselves at the centre

[129] Kusukawa, *Picturing the Book of Nature*.

[130] See, for, instance, [Felice Fontana], *Saggio del Real Gabinetto di Fisica e di Storia naturale di Firenze* (Rome: Giovanni Zempel, 1775), 29–30.

[131] On the difference between the spectacular character of images of nature and their role as tools of visual training in eighteenth-century botany, see Bleichmar, *Visible Empire*, 46–7.

[132] See Dacome, 'Waxworks'.

[133] See Anna Maerker, 'The Anatomical Models of la Specola: Production, Uses and Reception', *Nuncius*, 21:2 (2006), 295–321 (citation p. 298); Mazzolini, 'Plastic Anatomies and Artificial Dissections', 43–70.

of the anatomical world.[134] By the 1770s, the claims of the Bolognese anatomical modellers were being widely endorsed. When, in 1761, Domenico Cotugno suggested that the labyrinth of the ear was filled with liquid, the anatomist Giovanni Bianchi wondered what 'the anatomy professors of Bologna', and especially Ercole Lelli, had to say.[135] Ever since the publication of Valsalva's *De aure humana* in 1704 the anatomy of the ear had turned into a point of interest for the Bolognese anatomical community.[136] Reactions to Cotugno were protective of that tradition. For one thing, the anatomist Tommaso Laghi remarked that he had never observed what Cotugno claimed to have seen. For another, Germano Azzoguidi turned to the authority of the modellers to report that Ercole Lelli and Anna Morandi, who had worked extensively on the ear, had assured him of 'having never found any liquid in the labyrinth', except for the case of three people who were deaf from birth.[137] In his *Observationes ad uteri constructionem pertinentes* (1773), Azzoguidi further recalled that he regularly entertained anatomical conversations with Morandi and turned to her authority in his dispute with the French physician Jean Astruc (1684–1766). Astruc had claimed that there were venous appendages and lacteal vessels situated in the womb. Azzoguidi considered Astruc's suggestion 'false and unreal' on account of the observations of anatomists, such as Anna Morandi, who had 'gained much fame as the result of her incredible ability in dissecting cadavers' and in the art of making anatomical preparations in wax.[138] Had the venous appendages existed, Azzoguidi remarked, Morandi would have seen them.

In fact, at first gaining anatomical credibility had not been easy for Morandi. As we have seen, in September 1754 Giovanni Bianchi commended Morandi's anatomical prowess in dissecting cadavers 'like any expert dissector'.[139] However, when, a few months later, Morandi and Manzolini offered an anatomical opinion that was in contrast with his own, he dismissed their judgement on the grounds that they were 'no surgeons'.[140] It is worth recalling here some of the highlights of the story, as the incident draws attention to anatomical modellers' claims to knowledge based on their multifaceted engagements with the anatomical world. After Carlo Serra, a physician from the city of Cesena, entered into an argument with Giovanni Bianchi over a suspected carious bone, the bone was first taken to Padua

[134] Giambattista Morgagni and Francesco Maria Zanotti, *Carteggio tra Giambattista Morgagni e Francesco M. Zanotti* (Bologna: Zanichelli, 1875), 511–12.

[135] BUB, ms. 233, vol. 7, Lettere di Giovanni Bianchi (6 February 1751–29 December 1761), Letter of 8 December 1761 from Rimini, fols. 458v–459r.

[136] See Messbarger, *The Lady Anatomist*, 85. It is worth noting that the anatomy of the ear did not exclusively attract the interest of Bolognese anatomists. For instance, as we shall see in Chapter 7, in the mid-eighteenth century the Palermitan anatomist Giuseppe Mastiani also made anatomical models of the ear.

[137] BCABo, Fondo Speciale *Collezione Autografi*, IV, 1091–123, Letter of March 1762 (n.d.) from Germano Azzoguidi in Bologna to Leopoldo Marco Antonio Caldani.

[138] Germano Azzoguidi, *Observationes ad uteri constructionem pertinentes* (Bologna: Josephus Longhi, 1773), 35–7.

[139] Bianchi, 'Lettera del Signor Dottor Giovanni Bianchi', 710.

[140] Biblioteca Civica Gambalunga (Rimini), Fondo Gambetti, Lettere autografe al Dott. Giovanni Bianchi, fasc. Manzolini (Anna Morandi e Giovanni). On this episode, see Messbarger, *The Lady Anatomist*, 95–8. See also Dacome, 'Women, Wax and Anatomy', 545.

and presented to Morgagni. It then travelled to Bologna and was shown to the city's most prominent anatomists and physicians such as Galeazzi, Laghi, Beccari, Galli, and Molinelli who agreed that it was carious or worm-eaten. Following the advice of Beccari and Molinelli, the anatomists Galeazzi and Laghi went with Serra to Morandi and Manzolini's residence. They asked the modellers whether they could observe any caries in the bone and invited them to make an 'exact drawing' of it. Although Morandi and Manzolini reckoned that drawing was not one of their main occupations, they drew the bone and were happy with the result. The drawing corroborated the view that the bone was carious and invalidated that of Bianchi. Bianchi was not pleased and disparaged the modellers on the grounds that, since they were not surgeons, they could not really judge.

Bianchi's comments triggered reactions from Morandi and Manzolini, who replied with two letters. In the first, dated 15 April 1755, the modellers protested that they spent 'day and night' carrying out anatomical dissections, and reminded Bianchi that academies across Europe displayed their models for the instruction of students.[141] The following month, the couple wrote a new letter in which they emphasized that they had dissected 'hundreds and hundreds of cadavers' and had preserved the bones for their preparations. While doing so, they had come across many bones of *infrancessati* (i.e. individuals affected by the French disease), a disease that was taken to be mainly present in the Roman hospital of the Incurabili but, as the modellers noticed, was evident in many Bolognese cadavers.[142] The letters were signed with the names of both modellers, and the second one preceded Manzolini's death only by a couple of weeks.

Providing one of the few paper trails left behind by the couple, these documents bring into focus several important aspects of the artificers' anatomical life. In particular, they draw attention to the role of anatomical drawing as a particularly efficacious tool of observation and a form of anatomical evidence in its own right. Moreover, they shed light on the diversified world of anatomical practice where the couple acted as a unit of production of anatomical knowledge not only through dissection and modelling, but also through observation and drawing. The letters also highlight the fashioning of the modellers' home as a landmark of anatomical practice in the city and the confidence of the modellers, linking their expertise as observers and illustrators with their experience as consummate anatomists. Finally, Morandi and Manzolini's letters to Bianchi offer a further example of the modellers' familiarity with morbid anatomy alongside their focus on an idealized bodily norm in their wax modelling practice. Perhaps also thanks to the two letters, Bianchi changed his mind. Some months later, in a letter of 22 November 1755 to his friend Ferdinando Bassi, Bianchi expressed his greatest admiration for the Bolognese anatomical modellers. In particular, he emphasized that anatomy seemed to be, at the time, better cultivated by 'painters than by physicians', and

[141] Biblioteca Civica Gambalunga (Rimini), Fondo Gambetti, Lettere autografe al Dott. Giovanni Bianchi, fasc. Manzolini (Anna Morandi e Giovanni), Letter of 15 April 1755 from Anna Morandi Manzolini and Giovanni Manzolini in Bologna.

[142] Ibid., Letter of 24 May 1755 from Anna Morandi Manzolini and Giovanni Manzolini in Bologna.

referred specifically to the work of Ercole Lelli, and that 'of Manzolini and his wife', whom, Bianchi noted, he had not seen for some time.[143] Indeed, Manzolini had died the previous June, leaving Morandi to manage the anatomical home and engage in its various activities alone: carrying out dissections, making models, and introducing viewers to the collection through impressive and spectacular demonstrations.

WITH A 'LEARNED AND BEAUTIFUL HAND'

Manzolini and Morandi had engaged together in anatomical dissections and the making of models. However, even before Manzolini's demise, Morandi had seemingly been in charge of the demonstrations that introduced visitors to the collection.[144] At a time in which women were addressed as particularly well-suited mediators of natural knowledge, Morandi appeared at the forefront of the anatomical home, making the ghastly business of dissection palatable for polite audiences. In his *Wilhelm Meisters Wanderjahre*, Johann Wolfgang von Goethe pointed to the intrinsic theatricality of anatomy: he emphasized that theatre performance was analogous to anatomy in that it gave special exposure to the various parts of the body.[145] Anatomical displays offered particularly cogent examples of the performance of this corporeal drama. While mastery of the complex language of anatomy supported Morandi's claims to anatomical expertise, her capacity to dramatize this language into a striking performance boosted her celebrity status. Indeed, after word about Morandi's models and demonstrations crossed the Alps, her anatomical collection became a Grand Tour landmark. When a physician from Brussels visited the cabinet in September 1755, he noticed that Morandi imparted 'anatomy lessons to young students by way of a new method and admirable connaissances', and remained deeply impressed.[146] In the following years, many more visitors attended Morandi's performances and were equally enthralled. Viewers appreciated Morandi's eloquence and raved about her 'exhaustive and clear' demonstrations and 'very clear, native and pure' idiom.[147]

To many, the opportunity to be exposed to the complex language of anatomy in a way that could directly address the senses provided a refreshing departure from the abstruse and pedantic character of the public anatomy lesson that was carried out in Latin in the anatomical theatre. As in an Adamitic process of recreation of the human body, much of early modern anatomy focused on naming. Proper command of the anatomical vocabulary constituted a distinctive sign of anatomical

[143] BUB, ms. 233, vol. 7, Lettere di Giovanni Bianchi (6 February 1751–29 December 1761), Letter of 22 November 1755 from Giovanni Bianchi to Ferdinando Bassi, fols. 111v–112r.

[144] Bianchi, 'Lettera del Signor Dottor Giovanni Bianchi', 711. See also Dacome, 'Waxworks'.

[145] Johann Wolfgang von Goethe, *Wilhelm Meisters Wanderjahre*, in *Sämtliche Werke: Briefe, Tagebücher und Gespräche*, ed. Gerhard Neumann and Hans-Georg Drewitz, vol. 10 (Frankfurt am Main: Deutcher Klassiker Verlag, 1989), 600–1.

[146] 'Journal de voyage d'un médecin bruxellois de Munich à Rome en 1755', ed. Charles Terlinden, *Bulletin de l'Institut historique belge de Rome*, 23 (1944–6), 135.

[147] Zanotti, 'De re obstetricia', 88–9.

expertise. When Luigi Crespi wanted to target his fellow artists' excessive enthusiasm for anatomy, he scorned an age in which artists indulged in the use (and abuse) of anatomical language. He lamented that one of the main criteria to judge the 'ability of professors' was their capacity to master the most abstruse anatomical terminology. This included talking profusely about 'osteology, and sarcology', 'tunics, membranes, and fibres like the nervous ones', 'filaments that constitute the muscles', and from time to time come up with 'the cartilages as bending or plastic', and surely never to mention bodily extremities unless

> with the anatomical name of limbs in general, and in particular of scapula, clavicle, humerus, cubit, carpal, metacarpal, femur, tibia, fibula, tarsal, metatarsal, and all the other anatomical names.[148]

Morandi and Manzolini mastered this complex anatomical vocabulary and displayed their models together with labels that referred to the relevant bodily parts as described in Morandi's lecture notes.[149] In her demonstrations, however, Morandi turned this bookish anatomical lexicon into a dazzling theatrical experience that stimulated viewers' senses and affects. Having scorned the abstrusities of anatomical language, Crespi observed that Morandi was 'so knowledgeable' and 'talked, explained and instructed' with so much eloquence that students never tired of listening to her.[150] Hardly so much perspicuity, Francesco Maria Zanotti emphasized, could be found in an anatomist.[151]

Over the course of the eighteenth century, public performances and demonstrations played a fundamental part as sites of production and legitimation of natural and anatomical pursuits. Morandi's demonstrations equally provided a crucial venue for constructing her image as an accomplished anatomist and gaining status as a celebrity. Upon attending Morandi's demonstration of the models of the eye and the ear, Jérôme Richard observed that Morandi was 'really respectable for her talents', 'had *esprit* and liveliness', and accounted for her operations 'like the best of anatomical demonstrators'.[152] The Scottish traveller William Patoun similarly noted that she read 'a lecture as well as Hunter or Monro'.[153] Building on the long-standing topos of the 'anatomist anatomized', demonstrations superimposed the anatomist's own body on the anatomies displayed in the collection.[154] In April 1758, Giampietro Zanotti highlighted how Morandi's own 'learned and beautiful hand' accompanied her 'beautiful modes of reasoning' while introducing viewers to wax replicas of bodily parts.[155] As reports of her performances started to appear

148 Crespi, *Felsina pittrice*, vol. 3, 159.

149 Johann Jacob Volkmann, *Historisch-kritische Nachrichten von Italien [. . .]*, vol. 1 (Leipzig: Caspar Fritsch, 1770), 391–2. On Morandi's lecture notes, see Focaccia (ed.), *Anna Morandi Manzolini*; Messbarger, *The Lady Anatomist*.

150 Crespi, *Felsina pittrice*, vol. 3, 308.

151 Zanotti, 'De re obstetricia', 89.

152 Richard, *Description historique*, vol. 2, 119.

153 William Patoun, 'Advice on Travel in Italy', in John Ingamells (ed.), *A Dictionary of British and Irish Travellers in Italy, 1701–1800* (New Haven, Yale University Press, 1997), xliv.

154 On the tradition of the anatomized anatomist, see for instance, Sawday, *The Body Emblazoned*, 110ff.

155 BCABo, ms. B 256, Rime di Giampietro Cavazzoni Zanotti; also quoted in Crespi, *Felsina pittrice*, vol. 3, 308.

in the press, they fuelled the interest of many who became 'curious to judge her talents by themselves' and started to visit her collection in ever growing numbers.[156] To viewers, the sight of Morandi standing next to her models and engaging in eloquent, clear, erudite, and pleasant conversation, as Bianchi, Zanotti and many others witnessed, became memorable.

Since the mid-eighteenth century, women played an ever more important part in shaping the culture of the Grand Tour as both spectators and performers.[157] Innumerable women including savants, *salonnières*, artists, philosophers, mathematicians, translators, improvisers, and poets populated the routes of the Grand Tour. In some cases, as Chloe Chard has suggested, travelling women were themselves transmuted 'into tourist attractions'.[158] The anatomical demonstrations of women anatomists such as Bihéron and Morandi became a must-see for travellers heading to Paris or Bologna, and some compared their cabinets in their travel diaries.[159] The fact that a woman demonstrated the workings of the inner body added to the effect of marvel, and turned Morandi into a rarity and a curiosity in her own right.[160] Demonstrations also offered Morandi a felicitous arena for advancing claims to knowledge and negotiating her place in the world of learning. When, in the early 1770s, the Bolognese anatomist Petronio Ignazio Zecchini triggered polemics over women's intellectual capacities, his colleague Germano Azzoguidi defended women's learning by referring to the demonstrations of the two famous women of Bologna (Bassi and Morandi): not only did these women generate the greatest respect and admiration in everybody who met them, they also managed to convince all those who entered into a dispute with them to change their mind.[161] Demonstrations equally provided Morandi with the opportunity to highlight her experience as a skilled anatomist and to inform viewers about her familiarity with anatomical dissection. In September 1755, she revealed to one visitor that she received a regular supply of cadavers from the hospital of Santa Maria della Morte, and that by then she had dissected something like one thousand corpses.[162] Jérôme Richard similarly reported having been told by Morandi that the study of the anatomy of the eye alone had necessitated the dissection of thirty heads.[163] Such claims amazed and enticed both visitors and readers of travel literature. Years after Morandi's death, travellers still recalled that

156 Richard, *Description historique*, vol. 2, 118.

157 Findlen, Wassyng Roworth, and Sama (eds.), *Italy's Eighteenth Century*; Chard, *Pleasure and Guilt*; Sweet, *Cities and the Grand Tour*, 32ff.

158 See Chloe Chard, 'Women who Transmute into Tourist Attractions: Spectator and Spectacle on the Grand Tour', in Amanda Gilroy (ed.), *Romantic Geographies: Discourses of Travel, 1775–1844* (Manchester: Manchester University Press, 2000), 109–26.

159 See, for instance, Johan Jakob Ferber, *Travels through Italy, in the Years 1771 and 1772*, trans. R.E. Raspe (London: L. Davis, 1776), 74.

160 Bianchi, 'Lettera del Signor Dottor Giovanni Bianchi'.

161 [Germano Azzoguidi], *Lettres de Madame Cunégonde écrites de B [. . .] à Madame Paquette à F*, in Paul Mengal (ed.), *Giacomo Casanova: Lana Caprina; Une controverse médicale sur l'utérus pensant à l'Université de Bologne en 1771–1772*, trans. Roberto Poma (Paris: Honoré Champion, 1999), 122. The context of Zecchini's polemics and Azzoguidi's response will be discussed in Chapter 6.

162 'Journal de voyage d'un médecin bruxellois', 135.

163 Richard, *Description historique*, vol. 2, 119.

Morandi had become 'famous for her ability to make anatomical waxworks and her public anatomy lectures'.[164]

In addition to providing sites for displaying oratorical skills and for advancing claims to knowledge, demonstrations also offered a venue for publicizing the collection to potential acquirers. While highlighting the usefulness of the models as an introduction to the anatomy of the human body, they served as advertisements of the accomplishments of their artificers. In 1755, the article presenting Morandi and her collection in the *Annonces, affiches, et avis divers* promised to further expand the commercial aspirations of the cabinet.[165] As Colin Jones has suggested, in the mid-eighteenth century the *affiches* served as a widely read venue for medical advertising.[166] Here, news about Morandi's cabinet appeared amidst miscellaneous advertisements concerning, for instance, the rent of houses, the trade of paintings, the sale of porcelain ware and bijous, and the spectacles of the *comédie italienne*. In doing so, it reached out to a readership that was well acquainted with a dynamic and diversified world of commerce and consumption. Indeed, some of Morandi and Manzolini's models travelled along the routes that informed the grand circulation of artefacts, specimens, curiosities, and luxury goods. When, in 1754, Bianchi introduced Morandi to the readership of the *Novelle letterarie*, he noted that she had already received commissions from the king of Sardinia, the king of Naples, and the king of Poland, as well as other *personaggi*.[167]

After Manzolini passed away in 1755, Morandi also expanded the scope of her demonstrations through an impressive medium of self-representation. By realizing the wax portraits of herself and her husband, she enriched the collection with two new powerful self-advertising tools (Plate 30). Having survived to this day, Morandi's wax portraits provide complex insights into the self-representation of anatomical modellers who became exceptionally famous. Displayed along with the collection, the wax portraits reflected the modellers' aspirations about their standing both in the city and in the anatomical world. The literature has mainly focused on Morandi's self-portrait perhaps because it is just so striking. Yet, considering the two portraits together allows us to appreciate how Morandi carefully constructed her and her husband's public identity as an anatomical couple. Indeed, as the portraits introduced viewers to the household's anatomical practice, they embodied many of the features that accompanied Morandi's rise to fame: from the emphasis on observation to claims of anatomical expertise, from polite sociability to self-advertising and the acquisition of celebrity status, and from domesticity and family life to the complex world of anatomical dissection, modelling, and demonstration in the multifunctional spaces of the anatomical home.

164 See, for instance, Juan Andrés, *Cartas familiares del Abate D. Juan Andrés a su hermano D. Carlos Andrés*, vol. 1 (Madrid: Don Antonio de Sancha, 1786), 20.

165 *Annonces, affiches, et avis divers*, 6, 20 January 1755, 42–6.

166 See Colin Jones, 'The Great Chain of Buying: Medical Advertisement, the Bourgeois Public Sphere and the Origins of the French Revolution', *American Historical Review*, 101:1 (1996), 13–40.

167 Bianchi, 'Lettera del Signor Dottor Giovanni Bianchi', 711.

WIGS, COLLARS, AND 'DESPERATE PHYSIOGNOMIES'

Realized after the death of Giovanni Manzolini, Morandi's self-portraits were displayed along with the anatomical collection. Complementing Morandi's demonstrations, they allowed Morandi to give expression to the artificers' multifaceted engagement with anatomy. Unlike Lelli, who in his self-portrait concealed his hands, Morandi's portraits depicted the modellers as anatomists busy dissecting. In doing so, they also gave Morandi the opportunity to bring anatomical dissection to the forefront of the anatomical home while keeping its most gruesome aspects at bay. In particular, Morandi depicted herself as a matron wearing an elegant dress and jewels and holding anatomical instruments in her hands while dissecting a brain (Plates 22–4 and 30). At the same time, she portrayed her late husband in the act of dissecting a heart, while sporting a black doctoral gown (Plates 30 and 31). With its reclined eyes, wrinkled forehead, and nervous fingers, Giovanni's portrait presents physiognomic features that echo both early modern portrayals of melancholic learned men and contemporaries' accounts of the modeller as a hypochondriac. Historians have suggested that eighteenth-century medical portraiture played a part in redefining the identity of anatomists and surgeons according to codes of respectability that linked the culture of conversation with that of medical learning.[168] Morandi's portraits may be regarded as an attempt to address both aspirations. Being displayed alongside the models of the collection, the portraits staged an anatomical demonstration within the demonstration that was performed by Morandi for visitors and, at the same time, advertised her own modelling skills. Mirroring, doubling, re-enacting and replacing the modellers's engagement with anatomical dissection, they duplicated Morandi's anatomical practice and blurred the borders between the maker and the sitter. In doing so, the portraits also highlighted the role of the artificer as a mediator between the inner body and its spectators.[169]

Marta Cavazza has suggested reading the portraits as displaying some kind of specialization that was internal to the couple. Realized at a time in which the philosophical and medical doctrines advanced by anatomists, such as Thomas Willis, emphasized the significance of the brain over that of the heart, in Cavazza's view Morandi's choice to present herself in the act of dissecting a brain pointed to 'her own contribution to a deeper knowledge of the nervous system (meant to suggest the interrelation of senses, the nerves, and the brain)'.[170] Presenting Morandi busy dissecting a brain, her self-portrait also drew attention to the significance of touch in the world of knowledge.[171] Her raised eyes could equally speak to the primacy

[168] Ludmilla Jordanova, 'Medicine and Genres of Display', in Lynne Cooke and Peter Wollen (eds.), *Visual Display: Culture Beyond Appearances* (New York: The New Press, 1995), 202–17. See also Ludmilla Jordanova, *Defining Features: Scientific and Medical Portraits, 1660–2000* (London: Reaktion Books in association with The National Portrait Gallery, 2000).

[169] See Jordanova, *The Look of the Past*, 179.

[170] Marta Cavazza,'Women's Dialectics or the Thinking Uterus: An Eighteenth-Century Controversy on Gender and Education', in Daston and Pomata (eds.), *The Faces of Nature*, 237–57 (citation p. 244).

[171] See San Juan, 'The Horror of Touch', 441.

of touch over sight (Plate 22). Miriam Focaccia and Rebecca Messbarger have construed the presence of the heart in the portrait of Giovanni Manzolini in reference to contemporary debates on the notion of irritability famously articulated by the Swiss physician Albrecht von Haller (1708–1777).[172] As is well known, Haller regarded sensibility as a correlate of the nerves' capacity to react to stimuli and transmit sensation, and irritability as the property of muscles fibres to contract when stimulated. By the time debates on his views developed in Bologna in the late 1750s, Manzolini had passed away. Yet, other anatomical modellers joined the conversation. At the end of September 1758, for instance, the anatomical modeller Ercole Lelli sat down with the anatomist Giovanni Bianchi and the physician Leopoldo Marco Antonio Caldani (1725–1813), a supporter of Haller's theory who would succeed Giambattista Morgagni as the chair of anatomy at the University of Padua, to converse about 'anatomical matters' and in particular the implications of Haller's views of 'insensibility'.[173]

As much as they spoke to medical debates on the nature and role of nerves and fibres, Morandi's portraits also echoed the affective choreography that was ingrained in the culture of sensibility, and that found expression in the largely female cultures of the salon and conversation.[174] Just like the models of the collection, the portraits transformed the proverbially impolite setting of anatomical dissection into a resource of learning that was in line with the codes of polite sociability and could appeal to many, both inside and outside the medical world.[175] Morandi's own self-portrait dressed up in luxury the effort of dissecting, thus addressing the audiences that normally frequented salons, theatres, and courtly demonstrations. Notably, it did so at a time in which wax mannequins were employed to advertise fancy clothing to fashionable buyers.[176] When, in 1764, Cesare Orlandi portrayed anatomy as a matron who personified the discipline's 'excellence and antiquity', he remarked that the woman's black dress was supposed to express the terror inspired by death

[172] See Focaccia, 'Anna Morandi Manzolini'; Messbarger, *The Lady Anatomist*, 103. On the Bolognese debate over irritability, see Marta Cavazza, 'La ricezione della teoria halleriana dell'irritabilità nell'Accademia delle Scienze di Bologna', *Nuncius*, 12 (1997), 359–77; Marco Bresadola, 'Medicine and Science in the Life of Luigi Galvani (1737–1798)', *Brain Research Bulletin*, 46:5 (1998), 367–80, esp. 371–3. See also Miriam Focaccia and Raffaella Simili, 'Luigi Galvani, Physician, Surgeon, Physicist: From Animal Electricity to Electro-Physiology', in Harry A. Whitaker (ed.), *Brain, Mind, and Medicine Essays in Eighteenth-Century Neuroscience* (New York: Springer, 2007), 145–58.

[173] See Bianchi, *Viaggio*, 61.

[174] On sensibility and its cultures see, for instance, G.J. Barker-Benfield, *The Culture of Sensibility: Sex and Society in Eighteenth-Century Britain* (Chicago: University of Chicago Press, 1992); John Mullan, *Sentiment and Sociability: The Language of Feeling in the Eighteenth Century* (Oxford: Clarendon Press, 1988); Anne C. Vila, *Enlightenment and Pathology: Sensibility in the Literature and Medicine of Eighteenth-Century France* (Baltimore: Johns Hopkins University Press, 2006). See also Christopher Lawrence, 'The Nervous System and Society in the Scottish Enlightenment', in Barry Barnes and Steven Shapin (eds.), *Natural Order: Historical Studies of Scientific Culture* (London: Sage, 1979), 19–49. On the eighteenth-century culture of conversation as a largely female culture, see Benedetta Craveri, *The Age of Conversation*, trans. Teresa Waugh (New York: The New York Review of Books, 2006).

[175] For a different characterization of anatomical demonstration in eighteenth-century London, see Guerrini, 'Anatomists and Entrepreneurs'.

[176] See, for instance, Daniel Roche, *The Culture of Clothing: Dress and Fashion in the Ancien Régime*, trans. Jean Birrell (Cambridge: Cambridge University Press, 1996), 474–5.

and the gloomy nature of anatomical dissection. Her shambolic hair further pointed to the horror that is naturally invoked by 'such a necessary and yet cruel carnage', because it is all too appropriate 'that nature should resent its own undoing' (Figure 3.3).[177] Conversely, little of this anatomical drama transpires in Morandi's self-portrait. While the Marquis de Sade felt the urge to cover his nose at the sight of Zumbo's wax models of putrefying corpses, nothing in Morandi's portrait invoked the visor that belonged in her anatomical toolkit to protect her from the stench of cadavers.[178] Not a single drop of blood appears in the scene, and what Orlandi described as the horror of anatomy is firmly kept at bay. Rather, Morandi's serene countenance, the ringed puffy hands, pink dress, fluffy lace, and jewels all contribute to the effort of presenting anatomy as a polite activity and Morandi as its reassuring personification.

Thus, just like the models, Morandi's wax portraits offered a reassuring image of anatomy and covered a number of different functions: they highlighted the modellers' engagement with anatomical dissections and possibly pointed to a division of labour within the couple; they brought anatomical dissection to the forefront of the anatomical home and mediated it to different audiences while situating the modellers' activities in the context of family life. Finally, the portraits also presented a memento of Morandi's dedication to her late husband and a means to perpetuate the memory and the fame of the couple as anatomists, modellers, and demonstrators. The hope of being remembered by posterity drove the ambitions and the actions of many early modern individuals.[179] Morandi's wax portraits promised the long-lasting fulfilment of such aspirations. As we shall see in Chapter 6, her self-portrait became a landmark of the modeller's accomplished celebrity, and ended up being copied and duplicated in its own right, thus contributing to the perpetuation of her fame. Taken together, the wax portraits also acted as signatures, reasserting the modellers' authorship over the collection at a time in which some of the foreign visitors who crucially contributed to its fortune seemed to be somewhat confused about its makers' identity.[180]

In fact, although the portraits gave expression to Morandi and Manzolini's complex and carefully constructed anatomical identities, they did not manage to shield the couple's memory from the risks of equivocation. As we have seen, family life played an important part in framing Morandi's anatomical persona both in terms of her accomplishments and her portrayal as a mother and an anatomist who could both unravel and knit together the fabric of the human body. As travellers echoed this focus on the couple's domestic life, and placed it at the centre of Morandi's

[177] Orlandi, 'Anatomia', 127–9 (citation p. 128).

[178] See Donatien Alphonse François, marquis de Sade, *Voyage d'Italie*, in *Oeuvres complètes du Marquis de Sade*, ed. Gilbert Levy, vol. 16 (Paris: Cercle du livre précieux, 1967), 152. On Morandi's tools, see BUB, ms. 2193, 'Inventari dei Libri e Ferri inservienti allo Studio Anatomico'; ASB, Archivio Ranuzzi, Scritture diverse (1769–73), Lib. 124, fasc. n. 21.

[179] Galvani evoked the importance of being remembered by posterity in the speech he pronounced in honour of Morandi; see Galvani, *De Manzoliniana supellectili.*

[180] On the role of early modern self-portraiture as a form of signature, see Evelyn Lincoln, 'Invention and Authorship in Early Modern Italian Visual Culture', *DePaul Law Review*, 52:4 (2003), 1093–119.

transformation from local practitioner into transnational celebrity, a degree of confusion ended up accompanying her rise to fame. While family life became a feature of Morandi's public identity, in the stories that circulated in print the details of her household also became the object of misunderstanding, so much so that Morandi mistakenly ended up being presented as the spouse of her lifelong rival.

It is true that the Grand Tour was instrumental in putting the Bolognese modellers on the map of anatomical knowledge, fashion them as accomplished anatomists, and boost their celebrity. Yet, while providing a particularly receptive and enthusiastic audience, it also led to the proliferation of stories that the modellers could only partially control. Multiple encounters, short visits, lunches, dinners, gatherings, masquerades, sightseeing, spectacles, conversations, long uncomfortable carriage rides, and all kinds of adventures and commitments overloaded Grand Tour travellers with information, and tested their memories. Thus, while in Bologna the contention between Lelli and the couple Morandi and Manzolini continued to engage acolytes into the late eighteenth century, travellers brought home a different story altogether. When, in July 1764, the Philadelphian physician John Morgan, who himself had made anatomical preparations, visited the Institute of the Sciences, he left the building convinced that its 'most elegant Adam & Eve done in wax' had been completed 'by ye celebrated *Signora Manzaline*'.[181] In his detailed report of his meeting with Morandi, the abbé Richard similarly presented her as Lelli's widow and the latter as the father of her children and the man represented by her portrait.[182] Others followed in the same vein. Upon visiting the midwifery room of the Institute of the Sciences in 1767, the Polish count and diplomat Mnizech confused Lelli and Manzolini and attributed to the former the models of the midwifery room that Manzolini and Morandi had completed for the surgeon Giovanni Antonio Galli.[183] The second edition of Lalande's famous *Voyage* equally accredited the models of Galli's midwifery room to Ercole Lelli and 'Madame Manzolini'.[184] After Morandi's collection was purchased by the Institute of the Sciences in 1776 and joined Lelli's models on its premises, the risk of confusion was only bound to grow. Indeed, in his *Tour through Italy* (1791), the naturalist Thomas Martyn, who was professor of botany at the University of Cambridge, reported having seen in the Institute of the Sciences the 'figures of the human body, and its parts finely executed in wax by Ercole Lelli and his wife Anna Mansolini'.[185] Again, when in 1793 the military surgeon René-Nicolas Desgenettes proposed the creation in France of a collection of anatomical waxworks like the one he had seen in Florence, he paired Lelli and Anna Morandi as the authors of both the models of Galli's midwifery collection and the models of the Institute of Science.[186] No matter how

[181] Morgan, *The Journal of Dr. John Morgan*, 97. On Morgan's anatomical preparations 'by corrosion', see Académie Nationale de Médecine (Paris), ms. 41 (41), Letter of 19 May 1764 from John Morgan in Rome, fols. 63r–v (original emphasis).

[182] Richard, *Description historique*, vol. 2, 118.

[183] See Biblioteca di Archeologia e Storia dell'Arte (Rome), ms. 35 C.

[184] Lalande, *Voyage en Italie*, vol. 2, 67 and 86.

[185] See Thomas Martyn, *The Gentleman's Guide in his Tour through Italy: With a Correct Map, and Directions for Travelling in that Country* (London: G. Kearsley, 1787), 106.

[186] See Desgenettes, 'Réflexions générales'.

attentively Morandi crafted and staged her public image, how carefully she attended to it, inscribed it into her self-portrait and the portrait of her husband, and integrated it into her encounters with viewers, she managed to maintain only partial control over it in her rise to celebrity.

At the local level, however, things took yet another turn. After Morandi's death, her self-portrait and her portrait of her husband continued to leave a strong impression on viewers and became powerful mementos of the defunct couple, preserving the memory of the artificers and acting as simulacra of the makers of the collection. Quite inevitably, they also ended up being caught in polemics, partly reflecting the animosity that had marked the lives and activities of Lelli, Manzolini, and Morandi. In a series of letters presumably written in the 1770s, Giovanni Lodovico Bianconi (1717–1781), physician to the court of Saxony and brother of Carlo, Lelli's pupil and friend, scorned Luigi Crespi, who in his *Felsina pittrice* had taken sides against Lelli, for his clumsy drawing of Morandi's portrait. He also dwelt upon Morandi's portraits of herself and her husband, confessing to having become amazed and obsessed after looking at one after the other for the whole day; unable to stop thinking about them, everywhere he turned, and anywhere he looked, he saw 'those wigs', 'those collars', 'those desperate physiognomies'.[187]

[187] The letters were published posthumously in 1802. See Bianconi, *Lettere del consigliere Gian Lodovico Bianconi*, 11–12.

4

Women, Wax, and Anatomy

THE FLUID WORLD OF WAX

Only a couple of weeks had elapsed since the day Morandi and Manzolini had signed the letter to Bianchi highlighting their anatomical abilities, when, in early June, Manzolini died of 'hydropsy of the chest' and a liver attack.[1] In contemporary chronicles, Giovanni's fate was reworked into the story of a skilful man whose lack of recognition brought him to ill-health and death.[2] Morandi was left with two children to face the hardship of widowhood and the task of preserving the vocation and memory of her deceased husband. Early modern widowhood could occasionally open up new spaces of agency for women. However, it also carried a heavy social and economic weight, often bringing about loss of property and economic uncertainty.[3] Indeed, insecurity and hardship loomed over the early days of Morandi's widowhood. In order to face them, Morandi sought the support of the Bolognese system of charity and asked to have her eldest son Giuseppe admitted to the orphanage of San Bartolomeo di Reno, which offered maintenance and education to orphaned boys.[4] In early modern Bologna, leaving children in charity institutions was not easy. Plagued by a constant shortage of funds and resources, orphanages were wary of the ever-present risk of overcrowding.[5] As a consequence, they were particularly careful in the selection of children, and requests of admittance were often accompanied by 'recommendations made by noble and qualified people'. When Morandi sought to have her son admitted to the orphanage, one of the admission clauses stipulated that parents be 'of good reputation' (*'di chiara fama'*). On 16 November 1755, eight out of nine *Assunti* of the orphanage voted in support of Giuseppe's acceptance, yet it took almost a whole year before he was

[1] AAB, Archivio Parrocchiale di S. Pietro, cart. 35, 'Morti', 42; Crespi, *Felsina pittrice*, vol. 3, 307.

[2] Crespi, *Felsina pittrice*, 307–10.

[3] On widowhood in early modern Europe, see Olwen Hufton, *The Prospect Before Her: A History of Women in Western Europe, 1500–1800* (London: HarperCollins, 1995), chapter 6; Maura Palazzi, 'Solitudini femminili e patrilignaggio: Nubili e vedove fra Sette e Ottocento', in Marzio Barbagli and David I. Kertzer (eds.), *Storia della famiglia italiana, 1750–1950* (Bologna: Il Mulino, 1992), 129–58; Sandra Cavallo and Lyndan Warner (eds.), *Widowhood in Medieval and Early Modern Europe* (New York: Longman, 1999).

[4] ASB, Orfanotrofio di San Bartolomeo, Filze e Congregazioni, busta n. 9, fasc. 3 ('Libri degli Atti dei Governatori, 1720–1761'), 'Memoriali di Giuseppe Manzolini e Carlo Cauedagna con rescritti fauorevoli', fols. 85r–v; ASB, Orfanotrofio di San Bartolomeo, Statuti-Ammissioni, busta n. 2, Campione dei Putti (1646–1810), fol. 26v. See also Richard, *Description historique*, vol. 2, 142–4.

[5] See Nicholas Terpstra, *Abandoned Children of the Italian Renaissance: Orphan Care in Florence and Bologna* (Baltimore: Johns Hopkins University Press, 2005).

eventually admitted on 3 October 1756.[6] By then, Morandi's life had taken a new dramatic turn.

When her husband died in 1755, Morandi had already established herself as an accomplished anatomist, modeller, and demonstrator. Yet, becoming a widow meant that she had to renegotiate her place in the city as a skilled practitioner and a public figure. Several months after her husband's death, Morandi sought and obtained the patronage of Pope Benedict XIV, an event that was to boost her reputation and increase the visibility and value of her collection.[7] The pope's intercession in Morandi's favour was a sign that Lelli's attempt to discredit her had not achieved much. In fact, as Benedict XIV stood out as both an eager patron of anatomical practice and a committed supporter of accomplished women, Morandi could carve out a place for herself within the patronage strategies of the papal court. This chapter focuses on the circumstances surrounding Lambertini's support for Morandi.

As we saw in Chapter 1, ever since returning to Bologna as the local archbishop, Lambertini had been keen to sponsor anatomical displays. While he was busy writing his monumental work on beatification and canonization, he relied on anatomy as a veritable tool for assessing sanctity's ambiguous and elusive signs. Shifting perspective from the pope's patronage of anatomical collections to his support for a woman who made anatomical models, this chapter further explores Lambertini's patronage of anatomy in light of his ongoing concerns for the verification of sanctity. In particular, while situating the pope's sponsorship of Morandi in the context of his long-lasting engagement with the procedural aspects of saint-making, it reads Lambertini's support for this accomplished anatomical modeller against the backdrop of his long-term preoccupation with the verification of the claims of mystical women in matters of vision, apparition, and revelation.

During the Renaissance, living saints, especially women mystics, were widely venerated, and became the sought-after recipients of courtly patronage.[8] By the seventeenth century, however, growing preoccupations with false and simulated sanctity led to increased concerns about the authenticity of claims of divine inspiration.[9] Still, the causes of aspiring saints continued to pile up. As a promoter of faith for the Congregation of Rites, Lambertini ended up being personally involved in the evaluation of many such cases and developed a reputation as an exacting and uncompromising assessor of sanctity.[10] At the same time, he also

[6] ASB, Orfanotrofio di San Bartolomeo, Statuti-Ammissioni, busta n. 2, Campione dei Putti (1646–1810), fols. 5 and 26; ASB, Orfanotrofio di San Bartolomeo, Filze e Congregazioni, busta n. 9, fasc. 3 ('Libri degli Atti dei Governatori, 1720–1761'), 'Memoriali di Giuseppe Manzolini e Carlo Cauedagna con rescritti fauorevoli', fols. 85r–v and 113v–114v (citations on fols. 85v and 114v).

[7] ASB, Governo Misto, Senato, Filza 81, fols. 709r–715v.

[8] Gabriella Zarri, *Le sante vive: Profezie di corte e devozione femminile tra '400 e '500* (Turin: Rosenberg & Sellier, 1990).

[9] As the need to scrutinize claims of inspiration grew ever more pressing, aspiring saints ran the risk of being charged with heresy and having their cases investigated by the Inquisition rather than by the Congregation of Rites; see Zarri (ed.), *Finzione e santità*; Gotor, *I beati del papa*; Schutte, *Aspiring Saints*.

[10] In 1627, a papal decree established that the evaluation of the claims of individuals who had died in odour of sanctity could only start fifty years after their death. On seventeenth-century visionary and

became renowned for his support of learned women. As Massimo Mazzotti has observed, in the course of the eighteenth century 'the Church was looking for new, charismatic figures who could promote the new ideals of civil devotion and lay sainthood. Centered on social utility, these ideals contrasted bluntly with the baroque models of mystical and visionary sainthood'.[11] First as a promoter of faith and then as pontiff, Lambertini became a chief interpreter of this trend, and ended up being the celebrated patron of accomplished women such as Maria Gaetana Agnesi, Laura Bassi, and Anna Morandi, who dedicated themselves, respectively, to mathematics, natural knowledge, and anatomy. At a time in which claims of visionary inspiration were fashioned as the potential correlate of an unruly imagination, Agnesi, Bassi, and Morandi offered exemplary cases of women's capacity to subject themselves to a discipline of learning that could keep their minds in check. In doing so, they could present an alternative to mystical women's models of spiritual guidance, and contributed to elaborate the model, as Mazzotti has put it, of 'a new female mind'.[12] Thanks to her engagement with anatomical dissection, observation, and modelling, Morandi provided a particularly cogent example of a woman who not only had control over her senses and imagination, but also created artefacts that unveiled their workings. Thus, she also contributed to expanding the range of meanings associated with the making, display, and viewing of waxworks.

While focusing on the circumstances surrounding Lambertini's patronage of Morandi, this chapter also considers the place of anatomical waxworks in the diversified culture of wax that characterized Bologna. By the time the city became a capital of anatomical modelling, waxworks had been at the centre of a variety of practices and rituals. Taken to be capable of embodying and mediating the holy as well as the demonic, they became the target of campaigns that were aimed at regulating devotional practices related to the cult of saints. In the same period, wax also became a privileged means of portraying bodily parts in anatomical collections. This chapter explores the relationship between mid-eighteenth-century anatomical and devotional displays and their affective bearings. On the one hand, it investigates how anatomical collections inscribed patterns of continuity and discontinuity between rituals of adoration based on the veneration of holy objects and practices of knowledge that relied on the proximity of things. On the other hand, it considers how anatomical wax models offered a view of wax that was alternative to the perception of its indiscriminate use in devotional practices. Further, it examines how anatomical modelling played a part in redefining the meaning of wax from a substance that was traditionally considered a medium of supernatural and preternatural domains into a marker of the natural world. This process did not amount, of course, to the disappearance of wax from other realms. Rather, waxworks continued to act as malleable cultural artefacts that moved across religious,

mystical women whose candidacy to sanctity was considered in the early eighteenth century, see Adriano Prosperi, *Tribunali della coscienza: Inquisitori, confessori, missionari* (Turin: Einaudi, 1996), 455ff; Rosa, *Settecento religioso*, chapter 2.

11 Mazzotti, *The World of Maria Gaetana Agnesi*, 140.

12 Ibid., chapter 7.

artistic, medical, and magical domains. Yet, as the stories of Lambertini's patronage of anatomical waxworks and of Morandi's practice of anatomical wax modelling show, much was invested in the attempt to keep these domains separate, regulate their borders, and transform wax into a material that could help to draw the boundaries of the natural world. Crucial to this attempt was the rearticulation of rites of adoration based on proximity to things into practices of knowledge and, in particular, the refashioning of the act of worshipping waxworks into an act of learning.

PLEADING WITH THE POPE

For Morandi, the months of mourning that followed the death of her husband were also months of frenzy. Not only did she try to consign her son Giuseppe to the care of the orphanage of San Bartolomeo, she also continued her demonstrations for viewers and foreigners, and took steps to address a plea for help to Pope Benedict XIV. Having been publicly celebrated by Giovanni Bianchi in the *Novelle letterarie* as 'a prodigious woman' and 'the first woman who attended to practical anatomy with so much propriety', months after her husband's demise Morandi took up her pen and addressed the pope.[13] In particular, she drew the pope's attention to her predicament as a needy anatomical demonstrator, and the widow of a man who 'had laboured for many years in the anatomical works', had dedicated himself to the realization of the anatomical statues in wax of the Institute of the Sciences, and had carried out anatomical teaching for the public benefit of students, but who had died without 'any suitable remuneration'.[14] Emphasizing that she had equally devoted herself to similar efforts, Morandi begged the pontiff to grant her 'some annual income' so that she could carry on her work with more confidence (*coraggio*) to 'the advantage and honor of the homeland' without being distracted by the urgent needs of the family. She further mentioned that she had received offers to work abroad, but would rather stay in her hometown.[15]

At a time when flocks of Italian artists and artisans found employment and accommodation in princely courts abroad, the possibility that a skilled artificer like Morandi might leave her hometown in search of fortune, and take along her creations, was not an unlikely prospect.[16] Indeed, Morandi's words touched a sensitive chord, and the pope intervened promptly. On 19 November 1755, Lambertini wrote to the Bolognese Cardinal Legate and the *Assunti di Studio e Gabella* and encouraged them to oblige her request. On 12 December, the matter was discussed at a meeting of the *Assunteria di Studio* (the Senate committee in charge of supervising the management of the university). Senator Isolani and Signor Cospi were assigned the tasks of negotiating with the *Congregazione di Gabella Grossa* (the body in charge of financing the University of

[13] Bianchi, 'Lettera del Signor Dottor Giovanni Bianchi', 711.

[14] ASB, Governo Misto, Senato, Filza 81, fols. 709r–715v.

[15] Ibid.

[16] On Italian artists and artisans in eighteenth-century London and Paris, see, for instance, John Brewer, *The Pleasures of the Imagination: English Culture in the Eighteenth Century* (New York: Farrar, Straus and Giroux, 1997); Werrett, *Fireworks*, chapter 5.

Bologna) and obtaining from the professors of the *Assunteria di Studio* 'certificates that proved the abilities of the beseecher in her occupation', as well as an estimate of the resources that were to be allocated.[17] A committee of *Assunti di Studio* was thus established with the goal of verifying Morandi's talent in anatomical dissections, wax modelling, and demonstrations, 'which she had continued to carry out after her husband's demise'. The physician Jacopo Bartolomeo Beccari assured the *Assunti* of the merits of Morandi's collection. It was acknowledged that everybody praised Morandi's art, but there was not enough demand to allow her to make a living. As a consequence, the pope's recommendation was well worth pursuing.[18] Morandi's plea was read on 15 December 1755 at a meeting of the *Assunteria di Buon Governo, e Studio.*[19] On the same occasion, it was announced that the *Congregazione di Gabella Grossa* could address the request of the pontiff by contributing an annual salary of 300 lire on the condition that Morandi would not leave the city and that she would conduct anatomical demonstrations 'for the public advantage' whenever the *Assunti* asked her to do so.[20] On 27 February 1756, the Senate's offer was finalized.[21]

In the following weeks, Morandi asked for and obtained access to cadavers of the hospital of Santa Maria della Morte.[22] The concession was in line with both the notification on anatomy that Lambertini had issued in 1737 and the *motu proprio* with which, in 1742, he had established a school of surgery.[23] As we have seen, in these documents Lambertini had sought to facilitate practitioners' access to hospital cadavers under the condition of first obtaining the permission of the bishopric, thus ensuring the control of the Church over anatomical practice. In the following years, however, things did not necessarily go according to plan. In particular, due to 'numerous disorders' occurring in the anatomy room of the hospital of Santa Maria della Morte, from 7 April 1752 access was severely restricted in an attempt to ban improper use of the space.[24] It was resolved that the key could no longer be given to anyone—including the professors of medicine—without the approval of the hospital's *Assunti*. Nor could any anatomical operation

[17] ASB, Assunteria di Studio, Atti, n. 24 (1749–55), 12 December 1755; BCABo, ms. B 2383, Estratti storico-artistici dall'Archivio del Reggimento (oggi Legazione) in Bologna, Raccolti negli Anni 1841–1848 da Michelangelo Gualandi, 135 (entry n. 2124). On the role of the *Gabella Grossa* in financing the University of Bologna, see Paul F. Grendler, *The Universities of the Italian Renaissance* (Baltimore: Johns Hopkins University Press, 2002), 14. On the history of the relationship between the city and the university, see Gian Paolo Brizzi, 'Lo Studio di Bologna tra *orbis academicus* e mondo cittadino', in Prosperi (ed.), *Storia di Bologna*, vol. 3/II, 5–113.

[18] ASB, Governo Misto, Senato, Filza 81, fols. 709r–715v.

[19] ASB, Gabella Grossa, Atti delle Congregazioni (1753–9), I/42, fols. 112r–v.

[20] Ibid. See also ASB, Senato, Partiti, n. 39, fols. 2v–3r; ASB, Governo Misto, Senato, Filza 81, fols. 709r–715v.

[21] ASB, Senato, Partiti, n. 39, fols. 2v–3r.

[22] BCABo, Fondo speciale Giovanni Antonio, Francesco e Carlo Mondini, cart. VIII, n. 3, 'Note, appunti e discorsi. Richieste di clienti', 'Richiesta all'Ospedale di S.Maria della Morte dell'Amm.re C.o Vittori per procurar cadaveri alla Anna Manzolini'.

[23] Lambertini, 'Motuproprio pel quale s'istituisce in Bologna una Scuola di Chirurgia', 526.

[24] ASB, Ospedale di Santa Maria della Morte, Atti di Congregazione, Serie II/12, 'Libro Settimo delle Congregazioni dello Spedale della Morte', 27 April 1750–15 April 1755, fol. 36r, 'Decreto per la stanza anatomica dello Spedale, 7 Aprile 1752'.

be carried out in the room without the presence of at least one of them. Likewise, no part of the cadavers could be removed from the room. Further measures included a prohibition on utilizing human fat unless requested to do so by the hospital's administration.[25] Yet, thanks to Lambertini's intervention, Morandi could circumvent all of these constraints. Even before receiving papal support, she told visitors who attended her demonstrations that cadavers from the hospitals of Bologna were sent to her every month.[26] However, after the papal intercession the supply of hospital cadavers was made official. As of 6 March 1756, the *Assunti* of the hospital of Santa Maria della Morte had to make sure that Morandi could 'obtain all she needed in terms of parts of the human body'.[27] For her part, Morandi joined the *Unione di Sant'Anna*, a congregation created within the hospital's church for the purpose of engaging in charitable activities, such as dispensing dowries by lottery to poor young women and assisting the sick.[28] As mentioned in Chapter 3, Morandi had managed to amass her dowry thanks to the support of local charity networks. As her renown as a public figure and the recipient of papal patronage continued to grow, Morandi joined a tradition of patronage and charitable activities that included both patrician and accomplished women, such as Laura Bassi, who was personally involved in helping underprivileged women to gain access to dowries.[29]

FRIVOLOUS MINDS AND FUTILE THINGS

When Pope Benedict XIV responded to Morandi's request for support, he had already made a name for himself as a patron of learned women.[30] Ever since returning to Bologna, he had supported the career of the natural philosopher Laura Bassi and significantly contributed to the process that consecrated her as a transnational icon of female learning.[31] Moreover, after the mathematician Maria

[25] Ibid. [26] 'Journal de voyage d'un médecin bruxellois', 135.

[27] BCABo, Fondo speciale Giovanni Antonio, Francesco e Carlo Mondini, cart. VIII, n. 3, 'Note, appunti e discorsi. Richieste di clienti', 'Richiesta all'Ospedale di S.Maria della Morte dell'Amm.re C.o Vittori per procurar cadaveri alla Anna Manzolini'.

[28] I have not been able to identify the exact date on which Morandi joined the *Unione di Sant'Anna*. However, she had certainly done so by 1760. On the *Unione di Sant'Anna*, see ASB, Ospedale di S. Maria della Vita, Serie VII/3, 'Miscellanee di memorie diverse: sec, XII–XVIII'; ASB, Ospedale di Santa Maria della Morte, Serie VIII/35, 'Miscellanea contenente fascicoli e carte sciolte, secc. XVII–XVIII'; ASB, Ospedale di S. Maria della Vita, Serie VIII/37, 'Miscellanea contenente fascicoli e carte sciolte, secc XVII–XVIII'.

[29] In March 1747, for instance, Bassi interceded with Flaminio Scarselli, secretary of the Bolognese legation in Rome, on behalf a young woman who was from a large, poor family, 'without a mother', and who was 'very virtuous' and suited for a religious life, but whose dowry was insufficient to allow her to become a nun in the Bolognese convent of the Corpus Domini founded by Caterina Vigri; see BUB, ms. 72, vol. 6, Letter of 22 March 1747 from Laura Bassi to Flaminio Scarselli. On the history of women's patronage networks, see Lucia Ferrante, Maura Palazzi, and Gianna Pomata (eds.), *Ragnatele di rapporti. Patronage e reti di relazione nella storia delle donne* (Milan: Rosenberg & Sellier, 1988).

[30] On Lambertini's patronage of learned women, see Chapter 3, n. 3.

[31] Findlen, 'Science as a Career'; Ceranski, *'Und sie fürchtet sich vor niemandem'*; Marta Cavazza, 'Laura Bassi', *Bologna Science Classics Online*, http://cis.alma.unibo.it/cis13b/bsco3/bassi/bassinotbyed/bassinotbyed.pdf.

Gaetana Agnesi sent him a copy of her *Istituzioni analitiche* (1748), in 1750 the pope supported her appointment to an honorary lectureship in mathematics at the University of Bologna with a proposal that lifted the requirement of having completed a doctorate, to which even the famous mathematician and astronomer Giovanni Domenico Cassini had been subjected.[32] Some six years later, Lambertini responded favourably to Morandi's request for help. By then, the learned women of Bologna had been elected to represent a novel season in which the city aspired to regain standing in the world of learning.[33] Occupying a significant place in the munificence that Lambertini directed towards his native city, these women supported the effort to promote the image of the papacy as a source of patronage of natural knowledge. They also played a part in the attempt to mark a point of discontinuity with baroque visionary mysticism.

In a famous letter to Agnesi, Lambertini manifested his eagerness to give women the opportunity to express their 'knowledge [*scienze*] and talents', and encouraged them to educate other women to demonstrate that they were 'as deserving as men' when they engaged in intellectual activities.[34] In the same document, he also highlighted the benefits of 'reflective thinking' to counter the risk that the soul might become frivolous if it is 'occupied with trifles'.[35] In 1783, Louis-Antoine Caraccioli published part of this letter in his biography of Lambertini, thus turning the missive into a manifesto of the pope's policies towards learned women and a token of the mythology surrounding Lambertini's persona.[36] In previous decades, Lambertini's patronage of learned women had offered compelling examples of how learning could provide a powerful resource for keeping the mind in check. Notably, the pope's support for accomplished women took place at a time of widespread concerns for unwarranted claims of divine inspiration.

VISIONS AND THE NATURE OF THE IMAGINATION

By the late seventeenth century, the claims of mystical women had fallen under the scrutiny of both religious and medical judgement, inspiring extensive debates about the nature of visions, apparitions, and revelations. Elena Brambilla has reconstructed the complex intellectual and theological threads that led the Church to approach claims of demonic possession and divine revelation as the potential expressions of an unruly imagination that had to be subjected to medical scrutiny.[37] In a related manner, she has suggested reading the support for women's learning expressed by some famous eighteenth-century savants in the context of an attempt

[32] ASB, Assunteria di Studio, Atti, 24 (1749–55), fol. 26r (3 July 1750).

[33] See Findlen, 'Science as a Career'; Ceranski, *'Und sie fürchtet sich vor niemandem'*; Cavazza, 'Dottrici e lettrici'.

[34] Louis-Antoine Caraccioli, *La vie du pape Benoît XIV, Prospero Lambertini* (Paris: Rue et Hôtel Serpente, 1783), 104–5.

[35] Ibid., 105. [36] Ibid., 104–5.

[37] Elena Brambilla, *Corpi invasi e viaggi dell'anima: Santità, possessione, esorcismo dalla teologia barocca alla medicina illuminista* (Rome: Viella, 2010).

to expose the elusive nature of mystical claims and devotional excesses.[38] In June 1723, for instance, the physician and naturalist Antonio Vallisneri (1661–1730), who was professor of medicine at the University of Padua, expressed his support for women in a session of the Paduan Accademia dei Ricoverati. Here, in his capacity as the academy's prince, he proposed to discuss the question 'whether women ought to be admitted to the study of the sciences and the noble arts', concluding that, indeed, they should.[39] According to Brambilla, on this as well as on other occasions, Vallisneri's support for women's learning was related to his attempt to promote a new model of female authority that could counterbalance that of visionary women and aspiring saints.[40] Lambertini similarly engaged in promoting a model of female learning that could offer guarantees about women's ability to keep their thoughts in check. The matter had far-reaching implications. As we saw in Chapter 1, the definition of the criteria that governed the verification of sanctity played an important part in Lambertini's ecclesiastical career and patronage policies. As Caraccioli observed in his biography of Lambertini, one of the key tasks of the promoter of faith was to appraise the cases of individuals who claimed to have received divine inspiration but were in fact at risk of confusing the excesses of their own imagination for divine election.[41] In keeping with this pursuit, Lambertini engaged in the investigation of the hazy borders between seeing and imagining, and warned that mystical claims had to be examined and assessed with particular care.

As Stuart Clark has suggested, in the early modern period changing accounts of the senses and the imagination gave way to an age of visual uncertainty. As confidence in the trustworthiness of sight was being eroded, debates on the power and possibilities of visual resemblance reflected a widespread sense of crisis in the reliability of the eye.[42] Preoccupations about visual uncertainty intersected with concerns about the workings of the imagination.[43] Well into the eighteenth century, the imagination was conceptualized in visual terms as a faculty that mediated between the senses and the brain. However, it could also work as an internal sense that produced images that were not necessarily rooted in the experience of the external world. As such, it was regarded as a compelling, potentially disruptive, and intrinsically illusory force that had the power to gain free rein over the mind.

Lambertini was well aware that the imagination could act as an agent of illusion, and concluded Book 4 of his *De servorum Dei* with a chapter that examined its

[38] Brambilla, 'La medicina del Settecento', 91. On Vallisneri's support of women's learning, see Antonio Vallisneri, 'Introduzione del Signor Antonio Vallisneri [...] al Problema da lui proposto, il dì 16 Giugno 1723, mentr'egli era Principe dell'Accademia de' Ricovrati: Se le Donne si debbano ammettere allo Studio delle Scienze, e delle Arti nobili', in *Discorsi accademici di vari autori viventi intorno agli Studi delle donne* (Padua: Stamperia del Seminario presso Giovannni Manfrè, 1729), 1–5. See also Rebecca Messbarger and Paula Findlen (eds.), *The Contest for Knowledge: Debates over Women's Learning in Eighteenth-Century Italy* (Chicago: University of Chicago Press, 2005), 67–101.

[39] Vallisneri, 'Introduzione del Signor Antonio Vallisneri'.

[40] Brambilla, 'La medicina del Settecento'.

[41] Caraccioli, *Éloge historique de Benoît XIV*, 10–11.

[42] Stuart Clark, *Vanities of the Eye: Vision in Early Modern European Culture* (Oxford: Oxford University Press, 2007).

[43] Ibid., 46.

nature and power.[44] Here, for instance, he addressed contemporary discussions of the maternal imagination to endorse the view that the imagination of the mother could affect the appearance of the unborn.[45] He also maintained that the imagination had the power to affect feelings, and could both cause and cure disease and soothe pain.[46] However, he ruled out the possibility that the imagination could act at a distance on a different body. Likewise, he argued that the phenomenon that led the body of a victim to bleed in proximity of the murderer could not be explained in terms of the imagination.[47] Nor could the imagination account for the appearance of stigmata.[48] Wary of the power of the imagination, Lambertini also addressed the issue of its illusory capacity, and warned against the risks of failing to distinguish between divinely inspired visions and a disorderly imagination. Accordingly, he expressed particular caution in the evaluation of claims related to visions, revelations, ecstasy, and apparitions.

Visions and revelations lay at the basis of claims of divine inspiration. But they were inherently ambiguous. All too often their manifestations looked dangerously close to symptoms of ailments such as epilepsy, apoplexy, and frenzy; so similar, in fact, that they could be easily confused. As a consequence, evaluating claims of divine inspiration was not easy, and discerning their nature necessitated complex operations of interpretation of uncertain signs and elusive phenomena. As a promoter of faith for the Congregation of Rites, Lambertini was wary that claims of inspiration could disguise false or simulated sanctity. Drawing on an established tradition of interpretation of the signs of the divine presence in mystics, in his *De servorum Dei* he set out to outline the criteria that would make it possible to tackle uncertainty and distinguish between divine inspiration, demonic possession, and a disorderly imagination.[49] He cautioned that bodily expressions such as screaming, grimaces, contortions of face and limbs, the rolling of the eyes, paleness, stammering, confused speech, and mourning were utterly inappropriate to the manifestation of the divine. Just like the clouding of the mind and loss of memory, such behaviours had to be regarded as manifestations of nervous disorder or demonic possession, rather than as indications of divine inspiration. Likewise, discussing the role of feeling in deciphering the authenticity of inspiration, Lambertini turned to a well-established theological tradition to conclude that while a sensation of

[44] Lambertini, *De servorum Dei*, vol. 4/I, chapter 33, 461–84. On Lambertini's account of the imagination, see Vidal, 'Prospero Lambertini's "On the Imagination and Its Powers"', 297–318. As Fernando Vidal has noted, Lambertini used the notions of imagination and fantasy interchangeably, and claimed to be interested in their effects rather than in philosophical discussions on their nature. On early modern views of the imagination, see Claudia Swan, 'Eyes Wide Shut: Early Modern Imagination, Demonology, and the Visual Arts', *Zeitsprünge. Forschungen zur Frühen Neuzeit*, 7:4 (2003), 560–81.

[45] Lambertini, *De servorum Dei*, vol. 4/I, chapter 33, esp. 468ff.

[46] See Vidal, 'Prospero Lambertini's "On the Imagination and its Powers"', 312.

[47] On this phenomenon, see Ferrari, 'Public Anatomy Lessons', 101.

[48] On Lambertini's account of stigmata, see Vidal, 'Prospero Lambertini's "On the Imagination and its Powers"', 307–8.

[49] Lambertini, *De servorum Dei*, vol. 3, chapters 49–53, 686–764. On Lambertini's views on visionary mystics, see Mario Rosa, 'Prospero Lambertini tra "regolata devozione" e mistica visionaria', in Zarri (ed.), *Finzione e santità*, 521–50; Rosa, *Settecento religioso*, chapter 2, esp. 52–3; Brambilla, *Corpi invasi*, 233–6.

inner joy turned into sadness was the mark of diabolic visions and apparitions, an initial feeling of horror that transformed itself into inner sweetness revealed the presence of the divine.[50] Further elaborating on long-lasting medical accounts of the female body, he observed that women were particularly prone to 'vehement thoughts and affects' because their more humid constitution and their soft and malleable bodies made them more impressionable. As a consequence, they were more inclined to see 'what they wish to see', and their claims of divine revelation had to be examined with particular care.[51] In general, 'sick and delirious' persons, 'those who are afflicted with melancholy', and those who are stirred 'by vehement thoughts and feelings', could easily end up seeing 'what does not exist', and believe that it comes from heaven.[52]

HEATING UP PEOPLE'S HEADS

Lambertini's activities and deliberations as an assessor of sanctity largely echoed the views that he articulated in his *De servorum Dei*. And while he ended up being acclaimed as the munificent patron of learned women, his career as an evaluator of sanctity was characterized by a series of 'grand refusals' that involved a number of famous mystical women. A well-known incident occurred in 1727, when Lambertini was serving as a promoter of faith for the Congregation of Rites. In this capacity, he contributed to the decision to turn down the case of Marguerite-Marie Alacoque, a nun in the monastery of the *Visitation* at Paray-le-Monial in France whose revelations had triggered the cult of the Sacred Heart of Jesus. This cult highlighted the humanity of the incarnated God and was often associated with an image of the suffering Jesus holding a bleeding heart.[53] After becoming pope, in the mid-1740s Lambertini was faced again with the case of a mystic nun, Crescentia (Maria Crescentia Höss), from the Franciscan monastery of Kaufbeuren, in the diocese of Augsburg, who had built a large following in the wake of her visions of the holy spirit appearing in the guise of a boy whose head was surrounded by tongues of fire. As news of Crescentia's visions and cult reached Rome, an episcopal committee was set up to assess the matter. In 1745, the papal brief *Sollicitudini Nostrae* dismissed the case.[54] In the same period, the famous case of the seventeenth-century visionary nun Maria d'Agreda—whose cause for beatification was reopened in the mid-1740s, and its discussion involved both Lambertini and Ludovico Antonio Muratori—generated much noise, and ended with the Church's cautious invitation to further investigate the mystic's claims and writings.[55] Notably, the power of

[50] On this tradition, see Clark, *Vanities*, 222ff.

[51] Lambertini, *De servorum Dei*, vol. 3, chapter 51, 726.

[52] Ibid., 725–6.

[53] See Rosa, *Settecento religioso*, 17ff. On the cult of the Sacred Heart of Jesus, see Scott Manning Stevens, 'Sacred Heart and Secular Brain', in David Hillman and Carla Mazzio (eds.), *The Body in Parts: Fantasies of Corporeality in Early Modern Europe* (New York: Routledge, 1997), 263–82; Ottavia Niccoli, *La vita religiosa nell'Italia moderna: Secoli XV–XVIII* (Rome: Carocci, 1998), 178–9.

[54] See François Boespflug, *Dieu dans l'art: Sollicitudini Nostrae de Benoît XIV (1745) et l'affaire Crescence de Kaufbeuren* (Paris: Editions du Cerf, 1984); Rosa, *Settecento religioso*, 58–60.

[55] Rosa, *Settecento religioso*, 52 and 61ff; Brambilla, *Corpi invasi*, 236.

d'Agreda's visionary experience extended beyond the religious environment. In the summer of 1755, having been jailed in the *Piombi*, the famous prison in the doge's palace in Venice, the savant and adventurer Giacomo Casanova came across d'Agreda's *Mystical City of God*. At first he was dismissive, but ended up being captivated by the book—identifying himself with the inspired woman and giving in to the power of the imagination expressed in the text.[56]

Lambertini's reputation as a harsh castigator of mystical women filtered into his biographies. For instance, Louis-Antoine Caraccioli exposed readers to stories about the pope's lack of patience for mystical claims, and recalled the episode in which he had mandated the incarceration of a woman who was accused of heating up 'the head' of 'simple and credulous people' by simulating divine inspiration, and ordered for her to be taken around the streets of Rome like a criminal, as a form of public humiliation.[57] Narratives of Lambertini's intransigent attitude towards mystical women intersected with anecdotes about his engagement in policing the devotional world that was steeped in the visual culture of baroque mysticism. Caraccioli again reported that Lambertini had stormed off in rage when a clergyman approached him with the portrait of a saint, asking him to apply an indulgence to the image in order to transfer its blessing to everything that touched it.[58] Moreover, as the story has it, in a rare case of Catholic iconoclasm, after becoming pope Lambertini ordered the demolition of twelve baroque statues which were located in the Borrominian niches of the church of the University of Rome, and which he had seen and despised ever since he was consistorial advocate, maintaining that they spoiled the beauty of the church.[59]

POLICING DEVOTION

As is well known, in the early modern period the cult of saints was carried out through a wealth of holy paraphernalia that captivated the senses.[60] Images, amulets, crowns, relics, devotional figures, and objects were widely circulated in order to promote the veneration of those who died in odour of sanctity. The result was, as Simon Ditchfield has put it, a 'synaesthetic', and '*kinetic, multimedia* experience, a mobile *gesamtkunstwerk* in which art, architecture, sculpture, word, music, and print were deployed to move heart and soul through eye and ear'.[61] The adoration of relics and sacred images loomed high on the list of items that informed Protestant criticism of the Roman Catholic Church. But even within the Roman Catholic world, attitudes towards devotional practices based on relics and holy images were not uniform.[62] After Pope Urban VIII secured the control of the

[56] Rosa, *Settecento religioso*, 69–72.

[57] Caraccioli, *La vie du pape Benoît XIV*, 122–4.

[58] Ibid.

[59] See Venturi, *Settecento riformatore*, 112–13; Filippo Maria Renazzi, *Storia dell'Università degli studi di Roma*, vol. 3 (Rome: Pagliarini, 1805), 200.

[60] On early modern devotional practices related to the cult of saints and their involvement of different senses, see Ditchfield, 'Il mondo della Riforma e della Controriforma', esp. 269ff.

[61] Ditchfield, 'Thinking with the Saints', 552–84, esp. 554, 563, and 576.

[62] Ditchfield, 'Il mondo della Riforma e della Controriforma'.

Inquisition over the production and use of images, the management of the world of devotion remained somewhat torn between, on the one hand, the stated centrality of relics and sacred images and, on the other hand, the need to control and police the production, dissemination, and consumption of these popular means of devotion.[63] Studies in the history of holy objects have largely focused on the medieval and early modern periods, namely, the periods in which the production, consumption, movement, and traffic of such objects became an integral part of the life of communities, and they were turned into a crucial medium of political, economic, and ecclesiastical power.[64] Yet, well into the eighteenth century sacred objects continued to represent an essential part of the life of the Italian peninsula. Enjoying holy, and sometimes healing, powers they remained a ubiquitous presence in both urban and rural settings, and played an important part in both local and transregional politics. Many participated in this widespread culture of devotion.[65] Yet, when associated with mystical visions and claims of divine inspiration, devotional objects could also raise concerns. For instance, in the case of Crescentia of Kaufbeuren discussed above, the mystic nun was acquitted of the charge of simulating sanctity, but a clear condemnation was issued against the use of the devotional images and objects, including oils, crowns, and amulets, which had proliferated as part of her cult.[66]

Lambertini's attitude towards visions, revelations, the effects of the imagination, and devotional practices were partly echoed in the works of Ludovico Muratori, who authored a series of popular writings, including his *Della forza della fantasia umana* ('On the Power of Human Imagination', 1745), and *Della regolata divozion de' cristiani* ('On the Regulated Devotion of Christians', 1747).[67] In his *Della forza della fantasia umana*, Muratori built on Lambertini's discussion of the imagination to suggest that during ecstasy the mind retracted from the senses in order 'to contemplate internally only the ideas and images gathered in the imagination'.[68] Since such ideas and images could be considered either a product of the imagination or a sign of divine inspiration, understanding the nature of contemplation was crucial to the assessment of mystical claims.[69] For Muratori, just as for Lambertini, female fantasy was particularly lively, making women prone to see the signs of divine inspiration in any instance of contemplation, regardless of its actual nature. Women's imagination was also

[63] Ibid.

[64] See, for instance, Patrick Geary, 'Sacred Commodities: The Circulation of Medieval Relics', in Appadurai (ed.), *The Social Life of Things*, 169–91; Alexandra Walsham (ed) *Relics and Remains* (Oxford: Oxford University Press, 2010); Caroline Walker Bynum, *Christian Materiality: An Essay on Religion in Late Medieval Europe* (New York: Zone Books, 2011); Cynthia Hahn, *Strange Beauty: Issues in the Making and Meaning of Reliquaries, 400–circa 1204* (University Park: Pennsylvania State University Press, 2012).

[65] Notably, in 1742 Alessandro Macchiavelli published a book on 'the most worshipped, prodigious and famous images of the Virgin Mary' that were venerated in Bologna. In the book he claimed that a number of Bolognese citizens and literati helped him by volunteering information about these images. This information should be taken with some caution, however, as Macchiavelli developed a reputation as a forger; see Alessandro Macchiavelli, *Avviso sopra la stampa della serie istorica delle più divote, prodigiose, e celebri immagini dell'intatta madre di Dio, Maria Vergine Santissima, che nella città di Bologna si venerano* (Bologna: Bartolomeo Borghi negli Orefici, 1742), 28–9.

[66] See Rosa, *Settecento religioso*, 59–60.

[67] See Venturi, *Settecento riformatore*, 147ff.

[68] Muratori, *Della forza della fantasia umana*, 71ff (citation p. 71).

[69] Ibid., chapter 9.

particularly susceptible to the power of devotional objects as shown in the incidents that occurred in the church of San Marco in Venice or in the Duomo of Milan, where the display of relics generated 'the screaming, yelling, and crying of plebeian women who thought to be divinely possessed, and this was accompanied by the twisting of their body and rolling of their eyes'.[70] Just like Lambertini, Muratori maintained that such manifestations were the expression of disturbances of the imagination rather than genuine divine inspiration.

During Lambertini's pontificate, an inquiry that was meant to inform the pope's proposal to promote a reform of religious holidays (*feste di precetto*) pointed to the proliferation of devotional practices related to the cult of saints.[71] The response was an attempt to regain control over the world of devotion as well as to reform the calendar and celebration of festivities. The proposal generated much discussion and prompted ecclesiastical controversy. Muratori, who wholeheartedly supported the project of reform, was disappointed when the pope abandoned the initiative in 1748.[72] The previous year, under the pseudonym Lamindo Pritanio, Muratori had published his *Della regolata divozion de' cristiani*, which offered the template for his campaign advocating a reform of devotional practices. Here, Muratori had called for the dismissal of practices such as the unreasonable cult of holy images, the use of grandiose machineries, statues, and costumes in religious processions, and the wearing of relics and amulets in place of ornaments.[73] Likewise, he had expressed concern for the risks of idolatry embedded in the adoration of sacred images and objects, and had included devotional waxworks among the targets of his call for the regulation of religious practices.[74]

Occupying a special place in the dissemination of the cult of saints, wax had traditionally been regarded as a material that enjoyed special agency and mediated complex boundaries among natural, preternatural, and supernatural domains. One of the reasons why wax figures were so compelling was that they acted not only as representations, but also as replicas that could embody the power and life of the original.[75] Wax's very material properties, its capacity to melt, solidify, and change shape, characterized it as a particularly well-suited medium for crossing the borders of the natural world.[76] Famously, in the early modern period wax figures and wax dolls were employed in magic spells and charms. In his *La piazza universale di tutte le professioni del mondo* (1585), Tomaso Garzoni referred to sorcerers who used wax figures to induce 'crazy love and disordered hatred'.[77] In seventeenth-century Bologna, love spells that involved the preparation of wax statues

[70] Ibid., 91. [71] See Venturi, *Settecento riformatore*, 136–61.

[72] Ibid., esp. 158–60; Niccoli, *La vita religiosa*, 201–2.

[73] Lamindo Pritanio, pseud. [Ludovico Antonio Muratori], *Della regolata divozion de' cristiani* (Venice: Giambattista Albrizzi & Gir., 1747), 343.

[74] Ibid., 332.

[75] See Julius von Schlosser 'History of Portraiture in Wax', in Panzanelli (ed.), *Ephemeral Bodies*, 171–314; Panzanelli, 'Compelling Presence'.

[76] Dacome, 'Women, Wax and Anatomy'.

[77] Tommaso Garzoni, 'De' Maghi incantatori, o venefici, o malefici, o negromanti largamente presi, et prestigiatori, e superstitiosi, e strie', in *La piazza universale di tutte le professioni del mondo*, vol. 1, ed. Giovanni Battista Bronzini (Florence: Leo S. Olschki, 1996), 515.

and the melting of wax fell under the scrutiny of the Inquisition.[78] Well into the eighteenth century, wax modelling continued to be at the centre of practices that generated ecclesiastical and political concern. As Sabina Loriga has observed, a series of witchcraft trials held in Turin in the 1710s and 1720s focused on the uncontrolled production of statues and wax dolls of the royal family. And when Antonio Boccalaro was accused of plotting to make a wax figure of the sovereign in order to melt it and, as a consequence, kill him, the situation ended badly: Boccalaro was hanged and quartered as an example to others.[79]

As well as providing a privileged medium for magic spells and charms, wax was used in devotional practices related to the world of healing, such as the offering of ex-votos and, in particular, the creation of anatomical wax votives.[80] Wax also played a part in fertility rituals, as in the famous case of the offering of wax figures of Priapus in Isernia.[81] Likewise, it featured in devotional practices related to the Agnus Dei. The Agnus Dei was a medallion made from the wax of Easter candles and impressed with the figure of Jesus as the lamb. It was blessed by the pope, and subsequently employed in exorcisms as well as religious practices that were meant to avert evil.[82] Veneration of the Agnus Dei became so popular that in the mid-seventeenth century a papal decree sought to regulate its cult and put an end to its inappropriate uses.[83] Yet, the adoration of the Agnus Dei remained widespread. In 1721, *La comare levatrice*, Sebastiano Melli's popular text dedicated to the training of midwives, recommended parturient women to carry a devotional object like the Agnus Dei at the time of delivery.[84] When, in his *Della regolata divozion de' cristiani*, Muratori criticized the excessive employment of wax in religious rituals, he included the Agnus Dei among the many objects, such as images of saints, medals, crowns, cordons (*cordoni*), relics, and 'similar other instances of devotion', which ran the risk of making religion look 'overly dressed'.[85]

[78] Alessandra Fioni, 'L'Inquisizione a Bologna: Sortilegi e superstizioni popolari nei secoli XVII–XVIII', *Il Carrobbio*, 18 (1992), 142.

[79] Sabina Loriga, 'A Secret to Kill the King: Magic and Protection in Piedmont in the Eighteenth Century', in Edward Muir and Guido Ruggiero (eds.), *History from Crime*, trans. Corrada Biazzo Curry et al. (Baltimore: Johns Hopkins University Press, 1994), 88–109.

[80] As we saw in the Introduction, wax votives represented bodily parts affected by accidents and illnesses in order to invoke or acknowledge divine intervention.

[81] See William Hamilton and Richard Payne Knight, *An Account of the Remains of the Worship of Priapus, Lately Existing at Isernia, in the Kingdom of Naples [...]* (London: T. Spilsbury, 1786). See also Giancarlo Carabelli, *In the Image of Priapus* (London: Duckworth, 1996); Whitney Davis, 'Wax Token of Libido: William Hamilton, Richard Payne Knight, and the Phalli of Isernia', in Panzanelli (ed.), *Ephemeral Bodies*, 107–29.

[82] In the mid-seventeenth century, the use of wax objects in devotional practices had become so popular that a papal decree was aimed at regulating the cult of the *Agnus Dei*. On the *Agnus Dei*, see Vincentio Bonardo, *Discorso intorno all'origine, antichita et virtu degli Agnus Dei di cera benedetti* (Rome: Vincentio Accolti, 1586). On the use of *Agnus dei* in exorcisms, see Wellcome Library, London, ms. 4250, fol. 15.

[83] ASV, Arm. Misc. IV–V, n. 5, 'Editto per li Agnus Dei e Reliquie'.

[84] Sebastiano Melli, *La comare levatrice istruita nel suo ufizio secondo le regole più certe, e gli ammaestramenti più moderni* (Venice: Gio. Battista Recurti, 1721), 218 and 259.

[85] Pritanio [Muratori], *Della regolata divozion de' cristiani*, 347–8. See also Dacome, 'Women, Wax and Anatomy', 541.

WAXWORKS AND THE INVISIBLE HAND

In order to further explore how Lambertini's patronage of a woman like Morandi, who dedicated herself to anatomy and wax modelling, may be read in the context of discussions and concerns related to visionary claims and the unregulated veneration of devotional objects, it is worth drawing some attention to the story of the Bolognese nun and wax modeller Laura Chiarini. A contemporary of Morandi, Chiarini was a nun in the Bolognese monastery of San Pietro Martire whose capacity to work wax down to perfect likeness was taken to be the outcome of divine inspiration.[86] Chiarini made votive figures in wax such as cribs and images of saints. Moreover, she contributed to the tradition of devotional wax figures of holy babies (such as baby Jesus and baby Saint Anne, the mother of the Virgin Mary), which were displayed publicly on special occasions. In doing so, she participated in a devotional trend that overtly addressed female devotees by drawing on the imagery of maternity and childbearing. Contemporaries offered words of praise for her work and she befriended Maria Clementina Sobieska (1702–1735), the spouse of the exiled Stuart King James III, who became a great admirer of her artistic talent.[87] The Bolognese antiquarian Marcello Oretti remarked that, had Chiarini 'studied under the direction of a good professor, she would have become very famous', but she preferred to dedicate herself to the tasks and offices of the convent. Still, although she had apparently received no training, Chiarini was so quick, so good, and so much at ease in modelling wax that she surprised 'artificers and professors'.[88] In fact, while modelling, Chiarini seemed to be following an invisible divine hand that realized the very thing she was about to model. Her hagiographers viewed this ability as a measure of her divine inspiration, something that equalled her other extraordinary performances, such as her apparent levitation when going down the stairs.[89] Indeed, Chiarini was thought capable of working miracles and gained a reputation for holiness.

Chiarini's life was recorded in writing, and testimonies were gathered to support her cause. The anatomist Domenico Gusmano Galeazzi was called to testify and described how, just before her death, Laura miraculously healed a nun who suffered from long and incurable infirmity. He concluded that the healing could not have taken place 'by any natural or human means' and rather occurred 'through supernatural and divine help'.[90] In 1762, Chiarini died in odour of sanctity. Eight days after she was buried, her cadaver was exhumed and found incorrupt, fragrant, and 'palpable as if she were alive'.[91] Winning over the stiffness of death and acquiring some of the very features of lifelikeness that characterized

[86] ASB, Demaniale, Domenicane di San Pietro Martire, 45-2019, 'Scritture concernenti la vita, e la morte di Suor Maddalena Laura Catterina Chiarini', 24–6.

[87] BCABo, ms. B 133, Marcello Oretti, *Notizie de' Professori del Dissegno*, vol. 11, 304–5.

[88] Ibid.

[89] ASB, Demaniale, Domenicane di San Pietro Martire, 45-2019, 'Scritture concernenti la vita, e la morte di Suor Maddalena Laura Catterina Chiarini', 24–6.

[90] Ibid.

[91] BCABo, ms. B 133, Marcello Oretti, *Notizie de' Professori del Dissegno*, vol. 11, 304–5.

her waxworks, Chiarini's own body became the evidence of the authenticity of her inspiration.[92] The Bolognese wax modeller Filippo Scandellari—one of the artificers involved in the making of the anatomy room at the Institute of the Sciences—was asked to take a death mask, and made her portrait in wax. Yet, extraordinary as Laura Chiarini's performances in life and after death may have been, at a time of widespread preoccupation with the proliferation of mystical claims, her inspired, visionary practice of wax modelling could also raise concerns. As a matter of fact, Chiarini did not become a saint and the record of her life and extraordinary deeds remained buried in the archives of the monastery of San Pietro Martire.[93]

When considered together, the stories of Chiarini and Morandi shed light on the diverse cultures of wax and wax modelling that coexisted in mid-eighteenth-century Bologna. Chiarini's performances as a wax modeller, her visionary capacity, and divinely inspired waxworks pointed to a model of inspiration that the Church was keen to put under close scrutiny. Conversely, Morandi's activities as an anatomist and a trustworthy modeller of nature who claimed to have gained all her knowledge from engaging her senses correctly, instantiated an example of female accomplishment that met with Lambertini's approval and support. Unlike the religious woman Chiarini, whose extraordinary abilities as a wax modeller were associated with her inspired visions, the artificer Morandi emphasized her experience as a skilled observer.[94] The status and nature of her waxworks were then markedly different from Chiarini's. While Chiarini's waxworks were purportedly created as the outcome of visionary inspiration, Morandi's anatomical wax models were the result of the training of her senses through anatomical dissection, observation, and the study of anatomical books. Depicting the wax modeller in the act of dissecting a brain, Morandi's own self-portrait in wax (Plate 22) re-dressed with new meanings a practice that, as in the case of Chiarini, supported the cult of individuals who died in odour of sanctity. In doing so, it turned the genre of the wax portrait, which accompanied claims to sanctity, into a striking exemplification of Morandi's achievements as a woman who mastered anatomical knowledge and knew how to keep her senses in check.

IMPRESSING THE SENSES

Understanding the workings of the senses and the imagination was crucial both to the verification of the authenticity of visionary claims and to keeping at bay devotional excesses related to the cult of holy things. It is worth recalling that in the famous *Insignia* of 1734, Laura Bassi was depicted in the Bolognese anatomical

92 As we have seen, during the early modern period, the material properties of softness, malleability, and palpability were regarded as characteristic features of life and associated with the representation of lifelikeness. In dead bodies, they could be regarded as signs of holiness and supernatural intervention. For a discussion of the relevance of bodily features such as softness and suppleness in the canonization trial of Caterina Vigri, see Pomata, 'Malpighi and the Holy Body'.

93 See ASB, Demaniale, Domenicane di San Pietro Martire, 45-2019, 'Scritture concernenti la vita'.

94 See Chapter 3.

theatre while offering an anatomical discussion of the eye (Plate 5).[95] By creating anatomical models of the eyes, ears, hands, nose, and tongue, Morandi could similarly display a thorough and intimate knowledge of the senses. Notably, her anatomical notebook opened with the anatomy of the eye.[96] This was then followed by the anatomy of the other senses: the ear, the nose, the tongue and, finally, the hands. In his *De servorum Dei* Lambertini himself discussed the nature and workings of the senses in the context of their relationship with the imagination. Endorsing the view that the imagination mediated between the senses and the brain through a web of nerves, he maintained that images were first impressed on the senses and, thanks to animal spirits, were carried along the nerves to the brain. Since the brain was made of soft and spongy matter, the images collected by the senses were impressed upon dimples and folds, and were then stored in the imagination and in the memory. The liveliness of these impressions depended on the depth of the traces left by images on the matter of the brain. While the substance of the brain was not altered in the process, the risk of misunderstanding the nature of such images rested in this process' contingencies and modalities, which could lead some people to see 'what they wish to see' and, on this basis, claim to be the recipients of divine revelation.[97]

The idea that the workings of the senses and the imagination, and in fact of knowledge as a whole, were equivalent to modelling and impressing wax tablets, was, of course, a long-lasting topos of the philosophical literature. While this view had ancient roots, and was discussed and dismissed by Plato in the *Theaetetus*, the idea was effectively revisited by early modern philosophers to discuss the nature of learning and the relationship between the senses, the imagination, the nerves, and the soft matter of the brain.[98] Lambertini himself relied on such discussions to expose the physical processes that governed the imagination.[99] Needless to say, wax itself constituted a particularly well-suited medium for giving visual and material expression to such accounts of the workings of the senses and the imagination. Likewise, anatomical waxworks could provide a felicitous means for visualizing the process of impressing images of the senses on the brain. In doing so, they promised to create imitations of nature that could guarantee resemblance and offered reassurances about the possibility of restoring confidence in the role of visual representation. Not surprisingly, Morandi's series of the senses became one of the most appreciated sections of the modeller's collection and the object of prestigious commissions.[100]

[95] Martinotti, *L'insegnamento dell'anatomia*, 132.

[96] See BUB, ms. 2193; Focaccia (ed.), *Anna Morandi Manzolini*, 99ff.

[97] Lambertini, *De servorum Dei*, vol. 3, chapters 49–53, 686–764; ibid., vol. 4/I, chapter 33, 461–84. See also Dacome, 'Women, Wax and Anatomy'.

[98] See, for instance, René Descartes, *Meditations on First Philosophy: With Selections from the Objections and Replies*, ed. John Cottingham (Cambridge: Cambridge University Press, 1996), 20–2; John Locke *An Essay Concerning Humane Understanding: In Four Books*, 5th edn. (London: Awnsham and John Churchill, 1706), 61, 75, 79, 80, 147, 197, 215, 256.

[99] Lambertini, *De servorum Dei*, vol. 3, chapters 49–53, 686–764; ibid., vol. 4/I, chapter 33, 461–84.

[100] See Bianchi, 'Lettera del Signor Dottor Giovanni Bianchi', 711; Archivio Storico dell'Università di Torino, Spese, XII, c. 3, 'Registro mandati, Tomo VIII', fols. 17–18.

The reasons underpinning the long-lasting success of Morandi's models of the senses are, of course, manifold. Throughout the early modern period, discussions about the nature of the senses intersected with ongoing concerns about their unstable and illusory character.[101] Since the senses played a central part in the formation of ideas, many of Morandi's contemporaries continued to worry about their reliability.[102] Visualizing the anatomy of the senses spoke to one of the burning topics of the day. While John Locke, champion of the tenet that ideas were based on sensation and perception, had denied the value of anatomy, Morandi's models inscribed the view that the workings of the senses were rooted in bodily anatomy. In her lecture notes and demonstrations, Morandi referred to the actual experience of the senses as well as to their anatomical shape. In doing so, she provided viewers with a key to appreciate the anatomical basis of their sensations and accordingly trust their own sense experience. In the famous example of the model of the hands, for instance, she described one hand as resting serenely on a surface that is soft and tender, and therefore inducing an 'amiable and sweet sensation'.[103] Conversely, the other hand was presented as being stung by thorns and therefore contracted in pain (Plate 28). As Rose Marie San Juan has noticed, Morandi's sequence of dissected arms equally revealed 'the ways the sense of touch works from the inside of the body'.[104]

By the time Morandi represented the senses in wax, the theme of the five senses had also come to define an established representational trope mediating moral warnings about the transient character of sensory life and calling for proper employment of the senses while cautioning against potential misuse. Depicting the acts of listening to music, gazing at mirrors, tasting food and drink, sniffing, and touching things, countless paintings, sculptures, drawings, and prints instructed viewers on how to use the senses correctly and manage them in an appropriate way.[105] In early modern Bologna, the well-known engraver Giuseppe Maria Mitelli (1634–1718) portrayed the acts of seeing, tasting, smelling, hearing, and touching along with the external anatomies of eyes, mouths, noses, ears, and hands depicted from different viewpoints, just as anatomical treatises would normally do (Figure 4.1).

Similarly elaborating on anatomical and artistic representations of the eyes, ears, hands, mouth, and nose, Morandi's models of the senses could draw on an established tradition that represented the senses as moral mementos and instructed and disciplined viewers' sensory experience. As Morandi investigated the anatomy of the body, replicated it in wax, and presented it to viewers, she also offered an

[101] See, for instance, Clark, *Vanities*.

[102] On the cultural setting in which the importance of the senses was discussed in eighteenth-century Italy, see, for instance, Vincenzo Ferrone, *Scienza, natura, società: Mondo newtoniano e cultura italiana nel primo Settecento* (Naples: Jovene, 1982).

[103] BUB, ms. 2193, 'Preparazione Anatomica della Mano', fols. 50r–51v. See Maurizio Armaroli, 'Le cere anatomiche bolognesi del Settecento', in Maurizio Armaroli (ed.), *Le cere anatomiche bolognesi*, 59; Messbarger, 'Waxing Poetic', 90–2; Dacome, 'Women, Wax and Anatomy', 548; San Juan, 'The Horror of Touch', 444.

[104] San Juan, 'The Horror of Touch', 444.

[105] See Sylvia Ferrino-Pagden (ed.), *I cinque sensi nell'arte: Immagini del sentire* (Milan: Leonardo Arte, 1996).

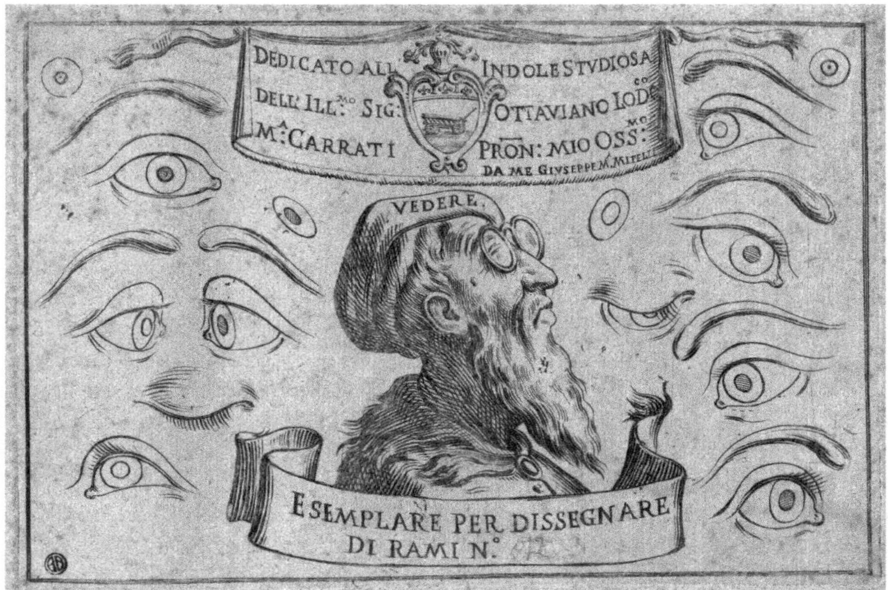
DEDICATO ALL INDOLE STVDIOSA
DELL' ILL.MO SIG. OTTAVIANO LODE
M.CARRATI PRON: MIO OSS.MO
DA ME GIVSEPPE M. MITELLI
VEDERE.
ESEMPLARE PER DISSEGNARE
DI RAMI N.°

Figure 4.1 Giuseppe Maria Mitelli, 'Vedere' ('Seeing'), from the series of the five senses; etching, 15.7 cm x 22.8 cm, Albo D 130, tav. 1.

exemplary case of a woman who not only enjoyed thorough knowledge of the senses, but also had the capacity to instruct audiences about their workings. In a sonnet dated 27 April 1758 and dedicated to Morandi, Giampietro Zanotti focused precisely on Morandi's demonstrations of the models of the senses: he emphasized Morandi's extraordinary skills in replicating 'those minute fibers, through which a visual object is seen and a sound is heard' and explaining their workings with eloquence and intelligence (*ingegno*).[106] Lambertini was to die about a week later, but the support he had offered to Morandi had borne fruit.

KEEPING THINGS SEPARATE

It is worth emphasizing that Lambertini's concern for devotional excesses did not amount, of course, to a dismissal of the importance and centrality of sacred objects. Quite the opposite: in the same period in which he was involved in supporting anatomical collections and natural knowledge, Lambertini was equally engaged in choreographing important religious events in Bologna and securing the cult of its relics and sacred objects. In January 1736, for instance, he drew on antiquarian sources to reconstruct the history of the skull of St Anna from its origins in

[106] BCABo, ms. B 256, Rime di Giampietro Cavazzoni Zanotti; also quoted in Crespi, *Felsina pittrice*, vol. 3, 308.

Constantinople to its transfer first to France and then to Bologna.[107] In doing so, he reassured the Bolognese about the authenticity of the relic preserved in the city, and encouraged its cult. Even after becoming pope and moving to Rome, Lambertini continued to orchestrate, from a distance, the public presentation and display of devotional objects in his home town. In the summer of 1743, shortly after commissioning the anatomy room for the Institute of the Sciences, he discussed with his long-term correspondent, Bolognese Canon Pier Francesco Peggi, details of the transportation of the head of St Petronius, the patron saint of Bologna, in an imposing procession that would take the relic from the church of Santo Stefano to the city's main church of San Petronio.[108]

Attention to the details of the public display and management of holy objects intersected with concerns about the possibility of sacred images being mismanaged and abused. Precisely because holy things were taken to possess special powers, their display required compliance with specific social, cultural, and political norms. While archbishop in Bologna, Lambertini dedicated one of his many notifications 'for the good government of the diocese' to the subject. Here he expressed his approval of the custom of the Bolognesi to depict devotional images under street arcades, but urged them to avoid locating holy images of the Virgin Mary, the saints, and the cross in places where they could be mismanaged and soiled by 'human waste'.[109] Again in his notifications, Lambertini introduced new regulations concerning the display and procession of holy images, such as the famous icon of the Madonna di San Luca, which was believed to protect the city, and was transported every year from neighbouring Mount Guardia to the city in a popular procession.[110]

Even beyond Bologna, attempts to police the making and use of sacred images were widespread, extending to centres of production such as art academies. In 1745, for instance, a series of regulations addressing the Accademia di San Luca in Milan aimed at tackling the 'abuses that had been insensibly introduced in the metropolis with little respect for religion'. Art dealers were accordingly warned not to trade works that had not been approved by the academy, and were forbidden to show painted or sculpted images that had been made against the commandments of 'the Sacred Council of Trent' or the Scriptures. Moreover, images of pontiffs and princes could not be left unattended because this would expose them to mud and dog attacks.[111] In *Della regolata divozion de' cristiani*, Muratori similarly argued

[107] Prospero Lambertini, 'Invito a celebrare un triduo in onor di Sant'Anna nella Chiesa ad essa dedicata, ove si esporrà il di lei sagro Cranio. Esser la medesima Reliquia autentica [...]', in *Raccolta di alcune notificazioni, editti, ed istruzioni* (1772), vol. 1, 248–9.

[108] Franz Xaver Kraus (ed.), *Lettere di Benedetto XIV scritte al canonico Pier Francesco Peggi a Bologna, 1729–1758* (Freiburg: J.C.B. Mohr, 1884), 11–12. Even after Lambertini's death, important religious events and processions of relics in Bologna continued to be associated with his name; see *Diario bolognese, ecclesiastico e civile* (Bologna: Lelio dalla Volpe, 1759–1800).

[109] Prospero Lambertini, 'Sopra le Immagini della Santissima Croce, e de' Santi, che nei muri delle Case si dipingono [...]', in *Raccolta di alcune notificazioni, editti, ed istruzioni* (1772), vol. 2, 77–9.

[110] Mario Fanti and Giancarlo Roversi (eds.), *La Madonna di San Luca in Bologna: Otto secoli di storia, di arte e di fede* (Bologna: Silvana Editoriale, 1993), esp. 104–5.

[111] ASM, Fondo Studi, p.a., cartella 194, 'Accademia di San Luca, Guida ad istanza degli ascritti nell'Accademia della Pittura, Scultura ed Architettura sotto l'invocazione dell'Evangelista S. Luca, in

against the custom of publicly displaying sacred images on the grounds that they could end up being soiled and misused, especially when they appeared on the signs of inns and taverns.[112]

Thus, on the one hand, Lambertini supported theatrical anatomical displays as tools that helped viewers to acquaint themselves with the borders of the natural world. On the other hand, he maintained strict control over the display of holy images and objects, and relied on antiquarian knowledge to assess their authenticity and support their cult. Indeed, Lambertini's active and meticulous involvement in the handling and display of holy objects, and his sustained concern for the verification of their authenticity, offer a more complex picture than his portrayal as the 'Enlightenment pope' who became a patron of natural knowledge and allegedly downplayed the role of relics and other devotional objects.[113] Rather, they point to Lambertini's concern for the role of public displays in staging, celebrating, and safeguarding the authenticity of sacred objects and supporting their cult.[114] As we follow Lambertini's manifold engagements in sponsoring natural and anatomical knowledge at the Institute of the Sciences, becoming the patron of learned women, and choreographing the display of relics, we encounter a pontiff concerned with securing the truthfulness of holy domains, and accordingly turning to the visual and material cultures of natural, anatomical, and antiquarian knowledge in order to define and patrol the borders of natural and sacred realms in a way that could verify and validate that authenticity. Yet, keeping these realms separate was not easy. And no matter how much Lambertini invested in safeguarding their borders, one may wonder whether, to the eyes of contemporaries, the boundaries between them appeared just as sharp.

IN THE PROXIMITY OF KNOWLEDGE

Ludmilla Jordanova has observed that the custom of visiting collections and displays has historically been elaborated in analogy with religious rituality. She has suggested that the very patterns of attribution of authenticity to objects on display may not be dissociated from the religious context, where demands of physical presence and proximity were essential to validating the authenticity of holy objects.[115]

Atti diversi relativi alla istituzione d'un Accademia de Pittori, Scultori, ed Architetti eretta sotto gli auspici di San Luca evangelista', Milan, 13 April 1745.

112 Pritanio [Muratori], *Della regolata divozion de' cristiani*, 338–9.

113 On the literature portraying Lambertini as 'the Enlightenment Pope', see Chapter 1. On the depiction of Lambertini as 'the Enlightenment Pope' campaigning 'against the popular cult of relics and *agnus dei*', see Messbarger, *The Lady Anatomist*, chapter 1, esp. 48.

114 On Lambertini's concern for the cult of saints, see Ditchfield, 'Il mondo della Riforma e della Controriforma'.

115 Ludmilla Jordanova, 'Museums: Representing the Real?' in George Levine, *Realism and Representation: Essays on the Problem of Realism in Relation to Science, Literature and Culture* (Madison: University of Wisconsin Press, 1993), 255–78, esp. 263. On the relationship between the cult of relics and anatomical practice see, for instance, Canetti, 'Reliquie, martirio e anatomia'; Knoeff, 'Touching Anatomy'; Rina Knoeff, 'Ball Pool Anatomy: On the Public Veneration of Anatomical Relics', in Knoeff and Zwijnenberg (eds.), *The Fate of Anatomical Collections*, 279–91.

Religious rituals such as the elevation of the consecrated host during the celebration of the Eucharist similarly informed habits that linked proximity to powerful objects with a special engagement of the senses. Indeed, turning 'a metaphysical moment into an aesthetic artefact' and an 'object of spectatorship' that called for particular visual attention, the elevation of the Host in the Eucharist marked not only important moments in religious processions and celebrations but also, as Florian Nelle has suggested, a sensory and experiential space of knowledge and certainty.[116] Early modern preachers occasionally complained that during the mass people would leave the church to chat or hang out in the local *osteria*, only to return in haste to attend the elevation of the Host. This was in fact regarded as a unique moment in which, thanks to visual attention and concentration, one could hope to enter a distinct form of communication with the divine and plead for special protection.[117] In 1734 Lambertini intervened on this matter in his capacity as the archbishop of Bologna, and included the regulation of the cult of the Eucharist in his intense regulatory agenda. In particular, he sought to strike a compromise between the Bolognese habit of displaying the Eucharist every day for public, 'visible and adorable' veneration, and the more restrictive directives of the Church, while at the same time increasing the archbishop's power and control over this popular devotional practice.[118]

As Anna Maerker has observed, in late eighteenth-century Florence the Grand Duke Pietro Leopoldo sought to ensure the success of the newly founded Royal Museum, including its conspicuous anatomical collection, by policing 'alternative venues for learning, such as itinerant shows and religious spectacles'. In doing so, he made 'his new Museum of Physics and Natural History quite literally the only show in town'.[119] Conversely, in eighteenth-century Bologna anatomical displays regularly intersected with religious and civic events, and complemented them as part of the theatrical spectacles that infused the city's public life. The *Diario bolognese*, a publication that chronicled the life of the city in the late eighteenth century, allows us to catch a glimpse of how Bologna's public culture of anatomy cohabited with the city's many religious ceremonies, as well as with its civic fairs and festivals, all of which established strong ties among piety, politics, learning, and commerce. Initiated by the famous printer Lelio dalla Volpe, the *Diario* provided a useful source of information for both locals and travellers. Joseph Jérôme de Lalande referred to it in his famous *Voyage d'un François en Italie*.[120] Browsing through its pages, readers could come across information about events such as the public anatomy lesson, the appointment of university professors and anatomical

[116] Florian Nelle, 'Eucharist and Experiment: Spaces of Certainty in the 17th Century', in Helmar Schramm, Ludger Schwarte, and Jan Lazardzig (eds.), *Collection, Laboratory, Theater: Scenes of Knowledge in the 17th Century* (Berlin: Walter de Gruyter, 2005), 316–37 (citation p. 328).

[117] Niccoli, *La vita religiosa*, 40. Prolonged elevation lay at the basis of the popularity of the Bolognese procession of the Corpus Domini.

[118] See Prospero Lambertini, 'Sopra l'Esposizione del SS. Sagramento dell'Eucaristia [...]', in *Raccolta di alcune notificazioni, editti, ed istruzioni* (1772), vol. 1, 138–46.

[119] Maerker, *Model Experts*, 38–9 and 186–7.

[120] Joseph Jérôme Lefrançois de Lalande, *Voyage d'un François en Italie, fait dans les années 1765 et 1766*, vol. 2 (Venice: Desaint, 1769), 111.

modellers, the visit of the Holy Roman Emperor Joseph II, as well as information about religious ceremonies, processions, and the relics displayed around town, including the skull of St Anna, 'the fleshy thigh' ('*la coscia con carne*') of St Innocence, the jaw bone of St Apollonia, the clavicle of St Francis and, most famously, the incorrupt body of Caterina Vigri, *La Santa*.[121]

Vigri was the 'only local candidate to sanctity whose canonization proceedings were successfully concluded in this period'.[122] Her own incorrupt body was in many ways an anatomical, if holy and healing, specimen.[123] Gianna Pomata has reconstructed how, as part of her process of canonization, Vigri's body was subjected to anatomical inspection, and features such as suppleness were carefully examined in order to investigate whether her state of incorruption could be considered truly lifelike, and therefore miraculous.[124] In the course of the eighteenth century, the chapel of the church of the Corpus Domini in which *La Santa* was displayed became the venue for civic gatherings and social events. Since Vigri was the patroness of the Accademia Clementina, its members regularly paid visits to her relic.[125] When Elisabetta Farnese, queen of Spain, visited Bologna in 1727, she gave audience to the noble women of the city in the chapel displaying Vigri's body, rather than in the theatre, as in fact a queen would have normally been expected to do.[126] After Vigri's canonization, the whole process of care and maintenance of the precious relic became more demanding. In 1752, the keeper of *La Santa* complained to a traveller that he had been forced to cut Vigri's nails every week and her hair on a monthly basis for some thirty years.[127] In the late 1770s, the traveller Rinaldo de Rinaldis observed that Vigri's body was 'incorruptible and nearly self-standing', it had 'tender flesh' and was dressed and washed regularly, and the water was then distributed among devotees.[128]

BOLOGNA'S WAX CULTURES

In the case of wax, its cultural-cum-physical plasticity seemed to make the task of keeping things separate look particularly arduous. Waxworks were ubiquitous in eighteenth-century Bologna, being displayed in academies, cabinets, and churches, as well as in domestic and institutional settings, and being paraded along the streets in theatrical processions. Although anatomical wax models became a landmark of

[121] *Diario bolognese, ecclesiastico e civile.*

[122] Pomata, 'Malpighi and the Holy Body', 568. As we saw in Chapter 3, Vigri was canonized in 1712.

[123] On Vigri's healing power and the anatomical investigation of her body, see Gianna Pomata, 'Practicing between Earth and Heaven: Women Healers in Seventeenth-Century Bologna', *Dynamis*, 19 (1999), 119–43; Pomata, 'Malpighi and the Holy Body'.

[124] Pomata, 'Malpighi and the Holy Body'. As a promoter of faith for the Congregation of Rites, Lambertini was involved in Vigri's canonization trial.

[125] AABAB, Atti dell'Accademia Clementina, vol. 1, 176.

[126] ASB, Archivio Isolani, Lettere di casa, Letter of 24 June 1727 from Claudia Isolani.

[127] British Library, Add ms. 19739, M. Housset, *Observations sur les Voyage d'Italie* (1752), 122–3.

[128] Rinaldo de Rinaldis, *Memorie del viaggio in Italia (1779–1780)*, ed. Pier Giorgio Sclippa (Pordenone: Accademia di San Marco, 2000), 82.

the refashioning of wax as a particularly suitable medium for the representation of the natural world, they were hardly created and viewed in isolation. No matter whether their purpose was devotional, anatomical, ceremonial, or ornamental, waxworks shared modes of making and inscription techniques, conventions and styles of representation, rhetorical motifs and parameters of beauty. In doing so, they also elicited affective responses that transferred across different domains of wax modelling. As a meticulous and perceptive observer of the eighteenth-century Bolognese art world, Marcello Oretti inventoried and described the conspicuous production of religious, anatomical, and artistic waxworks that were disseminated around town at the time of the development of anatomical collections. His writings offer a felicitous point of entry into the variety of wax genres that were on display for viewers: from religious waxworks to anatomical wax models, and from the wax portraits of individuals who died in odour of sanctity to those of renowned Bolognese citizens.[129]

Artificers like Morandi participated in this diversified culture of wax, and transferred practices, skills, and styles across religious, civic, and anatomical domains. Although she became famous for her anatomical models, Morandi also produced devotional waxworks, and her contemporaries recalled her wax figure of the crucifix with Mary Magdalene among her most noteworthy creations.[130] In some of Morandi and Manzolini's anatomical waxworks, the stylistic choices underpinning the gestures and postures of bodily parts were in line with the conventions characterizing the display of devotional statues, relics, and ex-votos.[131] In Plate 32, for instance, the model of the foot evoked the mode of presentation of the same bodily part in ex-votos, though it also reveals a painstaking attention to anatomical detail that was aimed at the instruction of surgeons (Plates 32 and 33). Further aspects shared by anatomical and devotional waxworks included the use of fabric to frame the bodily parts on display, a technique that was commonly adopted in the presentation of relics and holy objects in order to demarcate the space of the sacred and direct devotees' gaze and attention. Many of Morandi and Manzolini's anatomical waxworks were similarly framed by drapery that defined the space of viewing. In some cases, even specific details of the wax figures could end up shifting across devotional and anatomical domains. A notable example is the wax sculpture of the *Sacra Famiglia* made by the wax modeller Angelo Piò, characterized by the gesture of Mary's hand lifting the fabric to unveil the baby Jesus and the intense feeling of joy and marvel that leads Joseph to rest a hand on his breathless chest

[129] See, for instance, BCABo, mss. B 123–135, Marcello Oretti, *Notizie de' Professori del Dissegno cioè Pittori, Scultori ed Architetti bolognesi e de' forestieri di sua scuola*; BCABo, ms. B 106, Marcello Oretti, *Diario Pittorico nel quale si descrivono le Opere di Pittura e tutto ciò che accade intorno alle belle Arti in Bologna*.

[130] BCABo, ms. B 133, Marcello Oretti, *Notizie de' Professori del Dissegno*, vol. 11, 227–8.

[131] See Bianchi, 'Femminea natura'; San Juan, 'The Horror of Touch', 444. Dating back to the medieval period, the devotional and artistic tradition of the Lamentation, which portrayed grieving figures gathered around the body of Jesus, gave lasting artistic expression to the whole gamut of feelings of suffering and sorrow. In Bologna, it found its most famous example in Niccolò dell'Arca's *Compianto sul Cristo morto*, realized in clay for the Church of Santa Maria della Vita in the fifteenth century.

(Plates 34 and 35).[132] Here the gesture of the hand uncovering the divine birth could be juxtaposed with that of Morandi's hand supposedly holding the scalpel in her self-portrait (Plate 24). In both cases, the two women are engaged in acts of unveiling that could generate wonder. Yet, the purposes of their gestures were no doubt different. While Mary's hand in the *Sacra Famiglia* exposes the miracle of the incarnation, Morandi's dissecting hand reveals the marvellous order and harmonious intelligence of the divine creation.

As is well known, early modern anatomy was taken to provide a particularly advantageous point of entry into the perfection of God's handiwork. Faced with the wondrous complexity of the inner body, nobody could fail to appreciate the exactness of the divine design.[133] As we observed in Chapter 3, anatomists like Bellini envisioned the human body as a kind of complex and flawless divine embroidery. The very beauty of early modern anatomical visualizations was taken to reveal nature's underlying order and divine intelligence.[134] Thus, while devotional waxworks generated veneration because they embodied holiness and allowed devotees to enter into close proximity to the divine, anatomical wax models elicited a sense of marvel because they revealed the complexity, beauty, and order of the Creation. The transformation of waxworks from objects of adoration into sources of anatomical knowledge and markers of the natural world presupposed re-contextualizing wax modelling and its stylistic apparatus from the realm of local religious practice to that of natural order through the well-arranged sequences of the anatomical display.

Indeed, order stood out as one of the features that, in the eyes of viewers, characterized both Morandi's collection and her demonstrations. In 1754 Giovanni Bianchi described how Morandi guided visitors through the display in an orderly manner. He noticed that, to start with, Morandi showed the human bones in differently aged skeletons. She then demonstrated the muscles of arms and legs that she had completed in wax over natural human bones. Finally, she turned to the eye, the ear, the nose, 'the organ of speech and other parts', some of which she preserves dry, and others she has replaced with models 'formed in wax with natural colouring, admirably explaining the location and use of these parts'.[135] When, in 1767, the Polish diplomat and traveller Count Michal Mniszech, visited Morandi's cabinet, he was similarly impressed by 'the greatest precision and order' that characterized her demonstrations.[136] As the collection expanded to include new models, its sequences of anatomical specimens continued to shape ideas of natural order.[137] In 1769, Luigi Crespi highlighted how Morandi's demonstrations reflected natural order 'in the formation of bones, starting from a

[132] On Angelo Piò's *Sacra Famiglia*, see Riccomini, *Mostra della scultura bolognese*, 93.

[133] This is what the artist Louise-Élisabeth Vigée Le Brun concluded after visiting the anatomical collection of La Specola; see Vigée-Lebrun, *Souvenirs*, vol. 1, 237.

[134] See, for instance, Martin Kemp, 'Style and Non-Style in Anatomical Illustration: From Renaissance Humanism to Henry Gray', *Journal of Anatomy*, 216:2 (2010), 198.

[135] Bianchi, 'Lettera del Signor Dottor Giovanni Bianchi', 710–11.

[136] Biblioteca di Archeologia e Storia dell'Arte (Rome), ms. 35 C.

[137] For a discussion of Morandi's models of the parts of generation, see Messbarger, *The Lady Anatomist*, chapter 6.

one-month-old unborn ("*aborto*") to a thirty-year-old adult, followed by the demonstration of foetuses ("*feti*") in the egg, and then all the male parts of generation, and many other very superb demonstrations'.[138] Over the course of the eighteenth century order was, of course, a ubiquitous notion that served a moral, social, and political as well as natural agenda.[139] By displaying and demonstrating anatomy through well-arranged sequences of bodily parts, Morandi's collection embodied and manifested the order and complexity of human nature. Her demonstrations further contributed to turning the collection's corporeal narrative into an enticing performance that addressed the senses and touched the chords of affect in a controlled way. After attending her demonstration, viewers left her residence 'all filled with admiration for her divine talents'.[140]

WAX EFFIGIES

Continuities and discontinuities in the meaning and values of wax modelling found cogent expression in the development of mid-eighteenth-century Bolognese wax portraiture. It is worth recalling that in the same period in which the city fashioned itself as a capital of anatomical waxworks, wax portraiture was also booming.[141] Drawing some attention to this particular genre of wax modelling can further add to our understanding of the city's rich and composite culture of wax. Notably, wax portraiture played a part in the city's rituals of self-celebration at a time of heightened aspirations in the world of learning. Moreover, it participated in promoting new notions of female renown that were in line with Lambertini's own attempt to support new models of female authority and guidance. As we saw in Chapter 3, Morandi's self-portrait and her portrait of Giovanni Manzolini expanded the couple's anatomical collection and staged an anatomical demonstration within the demonstrations carried out by Morandi. In the same period, ever more wax portraits of renowned Bolognese individuals started to appear in patrician houses across the city.

[138] Crespi, *Felsina pittrice*, 310.

[139] As Emma Spary has observed, practices of ordering were not the inevitable course of the unveiling of nature but rather omnipresent social, moral, and political acts, which stretched 'into the manufacture of dictionaries, encyclopaedias, and projects for the reform of language, and even into the naturalist's own workspace'; see Emma C. Spary, *Utopia's Garden: French Natural History from Old Regime to Revolution* (Chicago: University of Chicago Press, 2001), 81. See also Lorraine Daston and Katharine Park, *Wonders and the Order of Nature, 1150–1750* (New York: Zone Books, 1998).

[140] 'Journal de voyage d'un médecin bruxellois', 135.

[141] On eighteenth-century wax portraits in Bologna, see *Mostra del Settecento bolognese* (Bologna: Mareggiani, 1935); Andrea Emiliani, 'Ritratti in cera del '700 bolognese', *Arte Figurativa*, 44 (1960), 28–35; Riccomini, *Mostra della scultura bolognese*; Antonia Nava Cellini, *La scultura del Settecento* (Turin: UTET, 1982), 113–32; Stefano Tumidei, 'Terrecotte bolognesi di Sei e Settecento: Collezionismo, produzione artistica, consumo devozionale', in Renzo Grandi et al. (eds.), *Presepi e terrecotte nei Musei Civici di Bologna* (Bologna: Nuova Alfa Editoriale, 1991), 36–7, and 21–51; Vassena, *La fortuna dei ceroplasti bolognesi*; Andrea Daninos, 'Wax-Figures in Italy: Outline for a Story Yet to be Written', in Daninos (ed), *Waxing Eloquent*, esp. 23–7.

The genre of wax portraiture was not, of course, new to the eighteenth century. Throughout the early modern period, wax portraiture had pervaded political as well as artistic landscapes, playing an important part in the rituals related, among other things, to the 'sacralization of royalty' and 'the construction of absolutism'.[142] In Renaissance Florence, for instance, wax was widely used in civic and religious ceremonies, conferring on the ruling Medici family 'a new sense of history and dynastic importance'.[143] Needless to say, wax effigies also played an important part in the world of saint-making. As in the case of Laura Chiarini, wax portraits acted as tributes that preserved the memory of individuals who died in odour of sanctity and promoted their cult. Along with images, relics, and statues, they provided visual and material complements to the genre of the lives of saints, and helped to make candidates to sanctity renowned: if a cause for canonization turned out to be successful, the effigy of a newly proclaimed saint could offer a particularly felicitous medium for disseminating her cult.[144] In the 1730s, Filippo Scandellari, the maker of Chiarini's wax portrait, took credit for the revival of making naturalistically coloured figures in wax.[145] In 1742, he completed the wax portrait of the Bolognese Anna Maria Calegari Zucchini, who, like Chiarini, died in odour of sanctity, thus providing an effigy that would be ready for her cult.

Sometimes modelled from death masks, wax portraits were characterized by an attention to minute physical details and the use of original clothing and personal effects that had belonged to the sitter.[146] In some cases, the wax portraits of individuals who died in odour of sanctity contained relics such as hair and fingernails. The result was a highly personalized setting, where the marks of individuality were traced down to the minutest particularities and, like in a shrine, the presence of bodily relics and personal belongings enhanced the sense of authenticity associated with the portrait.

Like other Bolognese wax modellers, Anna Morandi made wax portraits of individuals who died in odour of sanctity, such as the Bolognese nobleman and clergyman Ercole Isolani. When Isolani died in November 1756, an impressive crowd gathered around the body that was exhibited for public worship. In line with the tradition that viewed the saintly body as a resource for holy and healing relics, a tooth was removed, Isolani's clothes were shredded, and scraps of fabric and strands of hair were taken away.[147] At the same time, Isolani's memory was also cherished

[142] Giovanni Ricci, 'Masks of Power. Funeral Effigies in Early Modern Europe', in Daninos (ed.), *Waxing Eloquent*, 61.

[143] Panzanelli, 'Compelling Presence', 21.

[144] On the creation of effigies that were aimed at promoting the cult of aspiring saints, see Ditchfield, 'Il mondo della Riforma e della Controriforma'.

[145] Tumidei, 'Terrecotte bolognesi', 36–7.

[146] On the history of wax portraiture, see Schlosser, 'History of Portraiture in Wax'; Daninos (ed.), *Waxing Eloquent*. According to Schlosser, the wax portrait replaced the defunct like a simulacrum that bridged life and the afterlife; its history overlaps with the history of death rituals. On death masks, see Marcia Pointon, 'Casts, Imprints and the Deathliness of Things: Artefacts at the Edge', *Art Bulletin*, 96 (2014), 170–95.

[147] Carlo Barbieri, *Memorie della vita e virtù del servo di Dio Ercole Maria Giuseppe Isolani, prete della Congregazione dell'Oratorio di Bologna* (Venice: Simone Occhi, 1761), 36. See also ASB, Archivio Isolani-Lupari, Istrumenti, G 2, 1–45, Filza 1734–77, n. 23, 28 November 1756. See also Fantuzzi, *Notizie degli scrittori bolognesi*, vol. 4, 368.

through death masks and wax portraits made by local artificers including Morandi. Morandi also made a wax-portrait of Laura Pepoli Malvezzi, another member of the Bolognese aristocracy who died in odour of sanctity.[148] Laura's confessor, Domenico Savorini, was also portrayed in wax. In line with the custom of including relics of the sitter in the wax portrait, part of Laura's heart was embalmed, preserved in oil of turpentine, and stored in the drawer of the portrait's case along with a lock of her hair. When, in 1770, Laura's daughter found that the relic manifested signs of decay, she asked the anatomist Carlo Mondini to treat it to ensure its preservation.[149]

Morandi's own anatomical self-portrait did not contain relics, but it did enclose tokens of her relationship with Bolognese religious charities and congregations. For instance, the interior of the portrait contained an invoice for her *Unione di Sant'Anna* membership in the amount of 24 bajocchi due in July 1760 (Figure 4.2). As we have seen, the *Unione* was a congregation created within the church of the

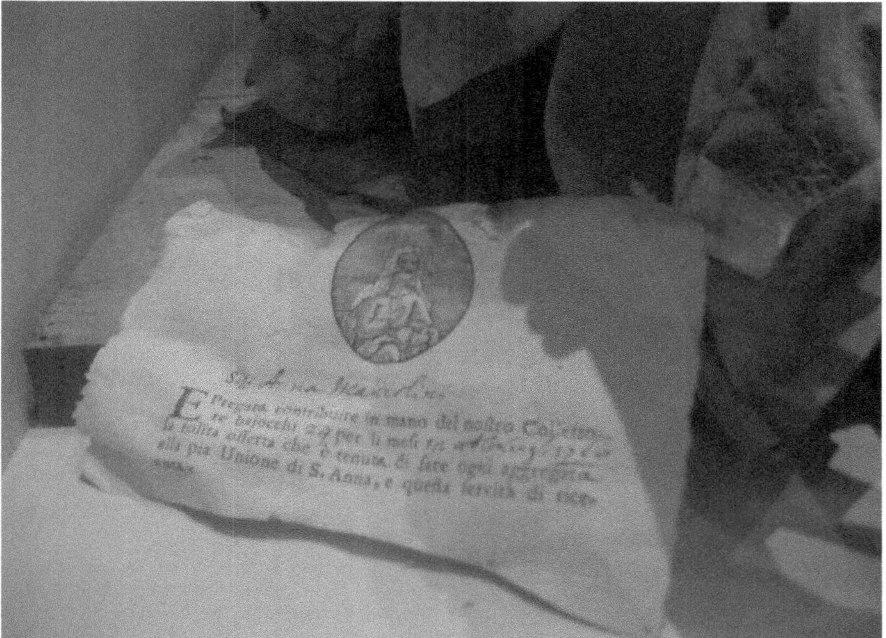

E' Pregata contribuire in mano del nostro Collettore bajocchi 24 per li mesi

la solita offerta che è tenuta di fare ogni aggregata

alla pia Unione di S. Anna, e questa servirà di

Figure 4.2 Membership invoice of the *Unione di Sant'Anna*, a congregation created within the church of the hospital of Santa Maria della Morte with the purpose of engaging in charitable activities. The note invites Morandi to contribute her fees for 1760, and is supposed to serve as a receipt of payment. The document was found inside Morandi's self-portrait and was apparently used along with other similar notes to support the portrait's internal parts.

[148] Carolina Isolani, *Donne di virtù nella baraonda bolognese del Settecento* (Bologna: Zanichelli, 1915), 156.

[149] ASB, Archivio Malvezzi Lupari, busta 29, notes of 30 July 1770 and 15 December 1770.

hospital of Santa Maria della Morte. The invoice found inside Morandi's portrait is apparently one among many similar notes used to support the portrait's internal parts. It is not, strictly speaking, a relic. And yet, one may wonder whether, by incorporating evidence of her commitment to local charities into the self-portrait, Morandi was only driven by practical considerations.

In his classic *The King's Two Bodies*, Ernst Kantorowicz described the tradition of displaying sovereigns' effigies in pre-modern royal funerals.[150] Well into the eighteenth century, wax portraits carried on this tradition and functioned as effigies in funerary celebrations of lay, as well as religious, individuals. When the famous Bolognese artist Elizabetta Sirani died in 1665, her wax portrait was exhibited on top of the grandiose catafalque erected in the church of San Domenico.[151] Again, in 1749 the wax bust of the Bolognese Reverend Alessandro Garofali was displayed at his funeral in the church of the hospital of Santa Maria della Morte—the same hospital that supplied cadavers to Morandi. Notably, Garofali taught how to provide spiritual support to prisoners awaiting execution in this hospital's *Scuola della Confortaria* (school of consolation).[152] In the mid-eighteenth century, the vogue of making wax portraits spread rapidly beyond religious and funerary settings. Over a few years, increasing numbers of Bolognese individuals, including aristocrats, artists, natural philosophers, and physicians joined the ranks of religious individuals who had their portrait made in wax. At a time when the city was elaborating new aspirations about its role on the transnational map of knowledge, many were involved in this collective effort of self-representation. Often displayed in the private-cum-public spaces of patrician houses, wax portraits came to showcase a reliable who's who of the city's noteworthy individuals, a kind of visual inventory of local celebrities. One of the heroines of the age, Laura Bassi, had her portrait made in wax.[153] So did the architect Carlo Francesco Dotti, who designed the sanctuary of the Madonna di San Luca, as well as the notable physician Giuseppe Azzoguidi, father of the anatomist Germano Azzoguidi, who was one of Morandi's supporters. Morandi was involved in the creation of this material inventory of contemporary celebrities. And when Jérôme Richard paid her a visit, he observed that she had realized a number of wax portraits of 'renowned' fellow citizens.[154]

[150] Kantorowicz's well-known work on 'the two bodies of the king' famously drew attention to how in medieval and early modern royal burials, the effigy of the defunct sovereign accompanied the royal funerary procession to symbolize the continuity of the political institution of the monarchy beyond the mortality and contingencies of its embodied representatives; see Ernst Kantorowicz, *The King's Two Bodies: A Study in Mediaeval Political Theology* (Princeton: Princeton University Press, 1957), esp. 419–37.

[151] Schlosser, 'History of Portraiture in Wax', 205.

[152] BUB, ms. 3718, capsula XXXIV, Giornale di Antonio Barilli dal 1746 al 9 dicembre 1750 di quanto è successo a Bologna, vol. 11, 1749, Bologna, 20 December 1749. On the *Scuola della Confortaria* at the hospital of Santa Maria della Morte, see Pellegrino Antonio Orlandi, *Notizie degli scrittori bolognesi e dell' opere loro stampate e manoscritte* (Bologna: Constantino Pisarri, 1714), 29–30. On early modern practices of the consolation of prisoners condemned to execution, see Nicholas Terpstra (ed.), *The Art of Executing Well: Rituals of Execution in Renaissance Italy* (Kirksville, MO: Truman State University Press, 2008).

[153] Bassi's wax portrait was realized by Nicola Toselli and was suitably displayed in Casa Bassi; see BCABo, ms. B 133, Marcello Oretti, *Notizie de' Professori del Dissegno*, vol. 11, 15.

[154] Richard, *Description historique*, vol. 2, 119.

Much as it drew attention to the exemplary character of renowned individuals, famous and infamous alike, wax portraiture constituted a privileged site for mediating moral messages related to the positive versus negative models offered by the lives of saints and criminals.[155] It also operated as a powerful marker of celebrity, and helped to shape new notions of renown that re-elaborated and expanded contemporary views of the exemplarity of the sitter.[156] While factors such as the spreading of new media informed novel ways of achieving renown, wax portraiture offered a particularly felicitous means of expression to the emerging culture of celebrity. Marie Grosholtz, the well-known Madame Tussaud (1761–1850), has traditionally been regarded as the prime interpreter of a new relationship between celebrity and wax portraiture.[157] However, the intense production of wax portraits of local celebrities in mid-eighteenth-century Bologna shows that the circumstances that linked this genre of wax modelling with the rise of celebrity culture may well be extended beyond Tussaud's collection.

As one of the main protagonists of eighteenth-century wax modelling, and a celebrity in her own right, Morandi included herself and her husband among the Bolognese personalities who participated in the city's collective aspiration to 'make an impression', and were appropriately depicted in wax.[158] Along with the wax portrait of Laura Bassi, her self-portrait constituted a powerful marker of celebrity status accomplished by the women who had received papal patronage. As is well known, Agnesi did not take up the lectureship in mathematics offered to her by the pope and instead dedicated herself to works of charity.[159] But Bassi and Morandi became icons of the Bolognese world of learning.[160] In doing so, they acted as chief interpreters of Lambertini's support for a new model of the female mind. As well as highlighting their status as local celebrities, their wax portraits also acted as testimonials of this new model of female accomplishment. In 1755, Giovanni Bianchi rejoiced to hear about the great success and popularity of Laura Bassi's lectures in experimental philosophy and concluded that philosophy was better learned 'by her than by any man'.[161] Notably, he did so in the same epistle in which he emphasized that anatomy was at the time better pursued by Bolognese artists such as Lelli, Manzolini, and Morandi than by physicians.[162]

[155] See, for instance, *Gabinetto di diecisette figure di cera di statura d'uomo rappresentanti i cinque capi ribelli della Transilvania, e Valacchia Imperiale unitamente ai più grandi malfattori della Francia spiegato in versi martegliani* (Alessadria: Ignazio Vimercati, 1785).

[156] Kornmeier, 'The Famous and the Infamous'.

[157] Ibid. On Tussaud and her waxworks, see Pamela Pilbeam, *Madame Tussaud and the History of Waxworks* (London: Hambledon & London, 2003).

[158] On the use of wax as a means of 'making an impression' in the classical period, see Verity Platt, 'Making an Impression: Replication and the Ontology of the Graeco-Roman Seal Stone', *Art History*, 29 (2006), 233–57.

[159] See, for instance, Mazzotti, *The World of Maria Gaetana Agnesi*.

[160] See, for instance, Antonio Meloni (ed.), *Raccolta ferrarese di opuscoli scientifici e letterari*, vol. 4 (Venice: Coleti, 1780), xxix.

[161] BUB, ms. 233, vol. 7, Lettere di Giovanni Bianchi (6 February 1751–29 December 1761), Letter of 22 November 1755 from Giovanni Bianchi to Ferdinando Bassi, fols. 111v–112r.

[162] This observation by Bianchi is discussed in Chapter 3.

As Bologna's accomplished women and wax modellers came to the fore of the city's aspirations, their wax portraits presented visitors with a powerful token of their status as transnational celebrities. Being the most famous woman philosopher in town, Bassi was entrusted with the task of welcoming the learned women who happened to visit Bologna. When, at the end of January 1750, a 'virtuous *dottoressa*' in medicine and law from Padua stopped in Bologna on her way to Rome, it fell on Laura Bassi to chaperon her to the university, take her to the public anatomy lesson, and show her 'the rarities that are to be seen' at the Institute of the Sciences.[163] Archival documentation is largely silent about the personal contacts and relationship between Bassi and Morandi, but travellers often ended up attending the demonstrations of these women in sequence. When, in 1769, the Holy Roman Emperor Joseph II visited Bologna, he attended both Morandi's and Bassi's demonstrations. In the same period, Count Maximilian Joseph von Lamberg, who served for a while as chamberlain to Joseph II, first admired Laura Bassi demonstrating 'many curious experiences' with an electrical machine, and was then taken by Giuseppe Veratti, Bassi's husband, to visit the '*Signora* Anna Morandi' who 'had for some time perfected the anatomies in wax displayed at the Institute of the Sciences'.[164]

News of the learned women of Bologna and their demonstrations spread rapidly. The section on '*hommes illustres*' in the second edition of Lalande's *Voyage en Italie* (1786), which followed one year after his *Astronomie des dames*, mentioned that women had 'distinguished themselves for their learning [*science*] in Bologna', and singled out Morandi and Bassi as recent examples of an honourable tradition that dated back to the fourteenth century.[165] Still others referred to Bassi and Morandi as examples of the city's engagement with knowledge and its commitment to women's learning.[166] To some, it looked like a world of promise. Having sojourned in Bologna in 1784, Hester Lynch Piozzi noticed that 'the University has been particularly civil to women' and 'many very learned ladies of France and Germany have been and are still members of it'.[167]

When, in the previous decades, Bassi and Morandi had acted as ambassadors of the new model of the female mind supported by Lambertini, travellers visiting Bologna felt they could not leave the city without paying them a visit. In 1765, the Scottish writer James Boswell, famous author of *The Life of Samuel Johnson* (1791), stopped in Bologna for two days and was hopeful that he could squeeze in a visit to Bassi. He addressed a note to her in Latin emphasizing that her fame had reached 'our Northern land' and entreating her to meet him despite the short notice.[168]

[163] BUB, ms. 3718, capsula XXXIV, 'Giornale di Antonio Barilli dal 1746 al 9 dicembre 1750 di quanto è successo a Bologna', vol. 11, 1750, entry for '31 January 1750'.

[164] Maximilian Joseph von Lamberg, *Mémorial d'un mondain*, 2nd edn., vol. 1 (London: n.p., 1776), 138–9.

[165] Lalande, *Voyage en Italie*, vol. 2, 352. On eighteenth-century celebrations of learned women in medieval Bologna, see Chapter 3, n. 4.

[166] See, for instance, Meloni (ed.), *Raccolta ferrarese di opuscoli scientifici e letterari*, vol. 4, xxix; Lady Morgan [Sydney Owenson], *Italy*, vol.1 (London: Henry Colburn and Co., 1821), 292.

[167] Piozzi, *Observations*, vol. 1, 260.

[168] Beinecke Rare Book and Manuscript Library, Yale University (New Haven), Boswell Collection, Letters, GEN 89, no. 1, box 1, folder 14, L 51.

Even after their deaths, the memory of Bassi and Morandi continued to feed both local narratives and travel accounts. During her visit to the Institute of the Sciences, Hester Piozzi saw Morandi's 'specimens of a human figure in wax', and noticed that they had been 'reckoned incomparable of their kind'.[169] She then reached the spot where Laura Bassi used to lecture and heard her guide sigh '*che brava donnetta che era!*' ('Ah, what a fine woman she was!'), while his eyes filled with tears.[170] Likewise, when the astronomer Jean Bernoulli arrived in Bologna shortly after Morandi's demise, he could barely conceal his disappointment in his laconic remark: 'the sublime artificer Anna Manzolini lives no more'.[171]

Thus, while at the local level keeping things separate was not easy, it was seemingly the gaze of viewers, and in particular that of Grand Tour travellers, that ultimately made the difference. And if the boundaries of natural and holy displays might have looked hazy to locals, many foreigners seemed to have no qualms about where to draw the line. For instance, while Caterina Vigri lay at the centre of the city's healing, devotional, and social practices and rituals, travellers found that despite the magnificent decorations, the jewels, the ornaments, the silver gown, and the diamond-studded golden crown, the sight of *La Santa*'s dried body was frightening and hideous.[172] Conversely, the accomplished women who had received papal patronage received travellers' unconditional appreciation. As their wax portraits came to mark their acquisition of status as representatives of Bolognese learning and papal patronage, they also ended up interpreting a novel model of female renown that could complement that of saintly women. On the other hand, even in the case of Bolognese wax portraiture, patterns of continuity and discontinuity could potentially affect the range of meanings and agencies associated with this popular genre of wax modelling.

In conclusion, it is worth taking another look at Morandi's self-portrait and her wax portrait of her husband to highlight how, even in the case of these anatomical wax portraits, wax modelling inscribed meanings and messages in complex ways (Plate 30). As we saw in Chapter 3, Morandi's wax portraits represented the couple engaged in anatomical dissections and articulated an assertion of anatomical authority. However, while Morandi portrayed herself as a woman whose capacity to engage in anatomical dissections spoke to her ability to keep her senses in check, she depicted her husband as a melancholic man in the act of touching an opened heart, in fact, almost offering it to the viewer (Plates 30 and 31). Completed after Giovanni's death, his portrait stood out as a tribute to the deceased modeller and a statement about Anna's own moral standing as a dutiful widow venerating the memory of her departed husband.[173] Here, Giovanni's hand holding the scalpel seemingly replicates the model of the hand that Morandi had completed for

[169] Piozzi, *Observations*, vol. 1, 260. [170] Ibid.

[171] Jean Bernoulli, *Zusätze zu den neuesten Reisebeschreibungen von Italien*, vol. 1 (Leipzig: Caspar Fritsch, 1777), 170.

[172] See Lalande, *Voyage d'un François en Italie*, vol. 2, 66; British Library, Add ms. 19739, M. Housset, *Observations sur les Voyage d'Italie* (1752), 122–3.

[173] On the visual culture of widowhood see Allison Levy (ed.), *Widowhood and Visual Culture in Early Modern Europe* (Aldershot: Ashgate, 2003).

the series on the senses, the one she presented as the depiction of a suffering and contracted hand. Likewise, his other hand sitting on the heart imitates the hand that, in the model, is resting serenely on a surface that is soft and tender, and enjoys a pleasant sensation (Plate 28). Thus, on the one hand, Giovanni's portrait situated him in the world of anatomical dissection and modelling. On the other hand, as a monument memorializing the man's sufferings, the portrait may also have been reminiscent of the rich devotional tradition, ranging from ex-votos to artefacts and specimens associated with the cult of saints, which informed wax modelling and representations of the heart. For instance, while linking the mysteries of the Eucharist with the portrayal of the heart as the physiological site of love, the cult of the Sacred Heart of Jesus had grown in the aftermath of Marguerite-Marie Alacoque's mystical visions, and gained status as an independent cult in 1765, namely, in the period following Morandi's completion of the portraits.[174] Thus, looking at Giovanni's melancholic eyes, his hands, and the opened heart sitting in front of him, we may wonder whether, in the eyes of his contemporaries, the borders between the devotional, anatomical, and artistic aspects of wax portraiture were sharply defined.

[174] In 1765, the Sacred Heart of Jesus also became a universally celebrated festivity. On its cult in the early modern period, see Stevens, 'Sacred Heart and Secular Brain'.

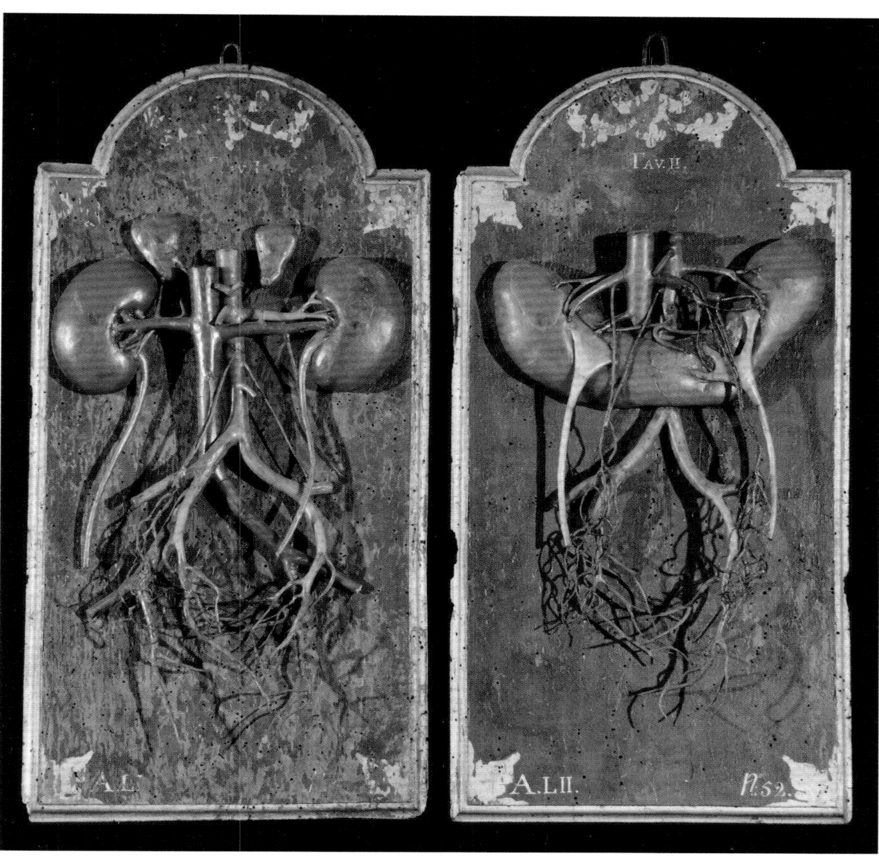

Plate 1. Two wax models of kidneys (one of which is 'horseshoe') made by Ercole Lelli in 1731 for the dissector Lorenzo Bonazzoli; wax and wood, table of the kidneys on the left hand side: 57 cm × 29 cm × 8 cm, table of the 'horseshoe' kidney on the right hand side: 60 cm × 29 cm × 8 cm.

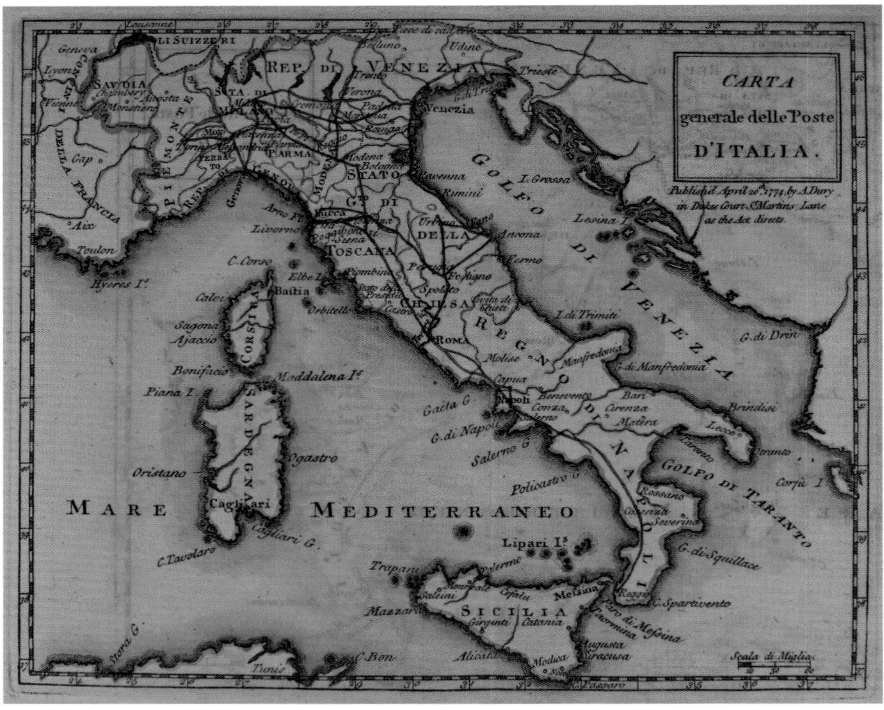

Plate 2. Map of the postal routes of the Italian peninsula for Grand Tour travellers, printed in both French and Italian, in *Le portefeuille nécessaire à tous les seigneurs qui font le tour d'Italie/Il Portafoglio necessario a tutti quelli che fanno il giro d'Italia*, London: A. Dury, 1774, 9; hand-coloured etching.

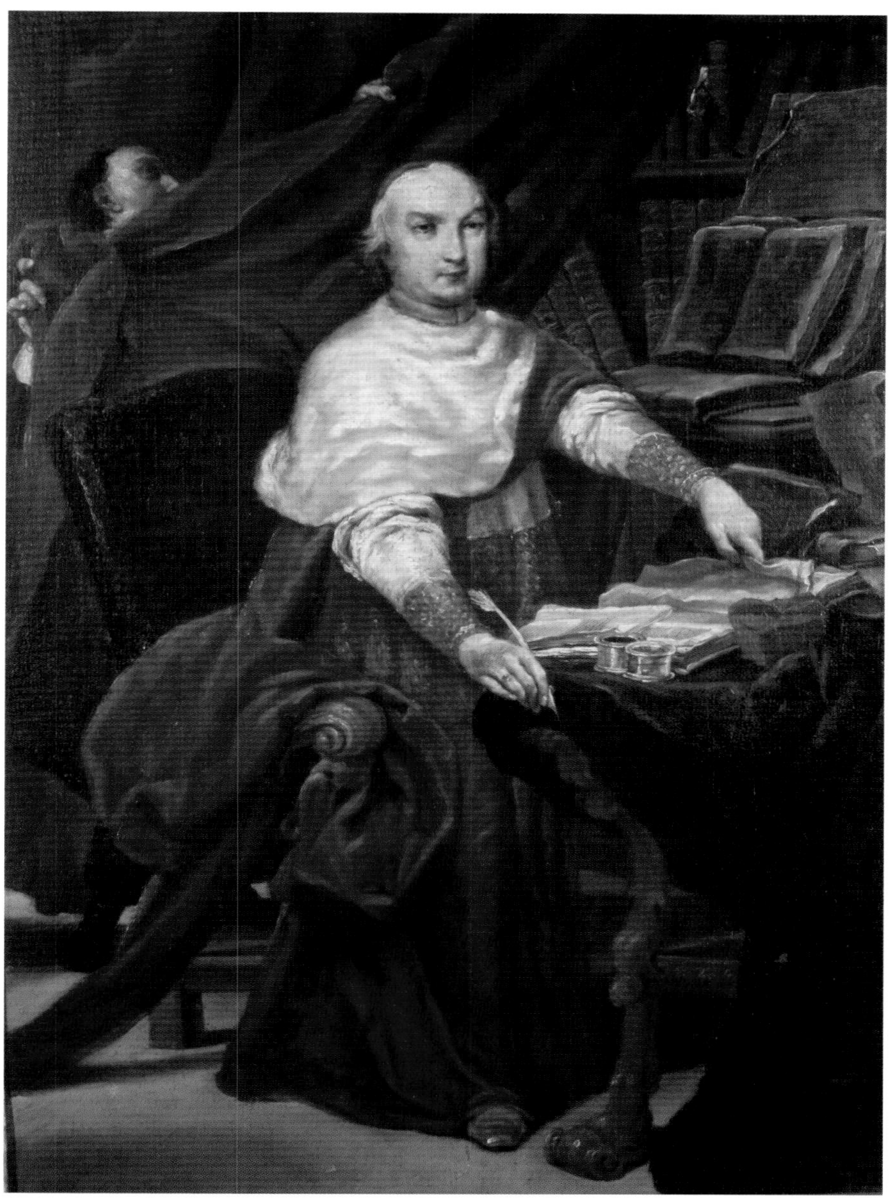

Plate 3. Giuseppe Maria Crespi, *Il cardinal Lambertini* (1739/40), realized shortly before Lambertini became pope; oil on canvas, 79 cm × 58 cm.

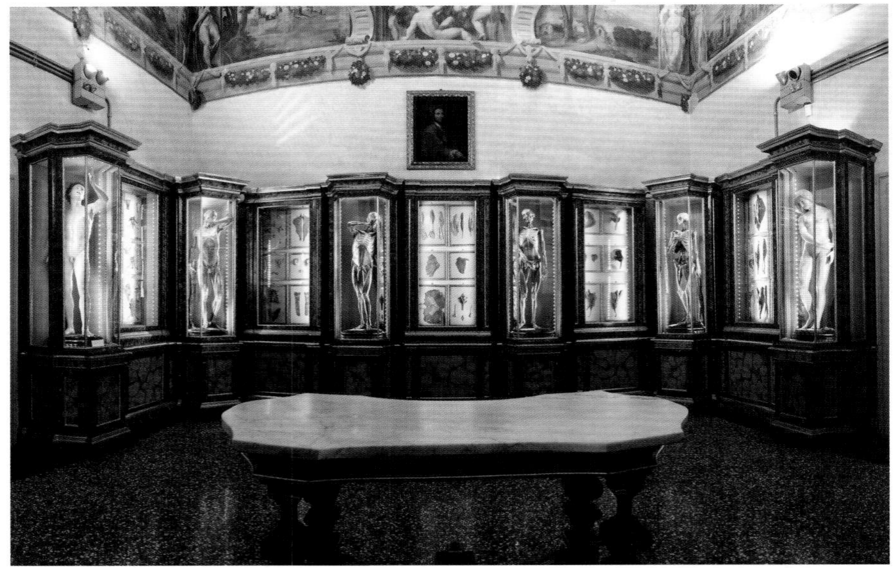

Plate 4. Anatomy room, the anatomical display sponsored by Pope Benedict XIV at the Institute of the Sciences.

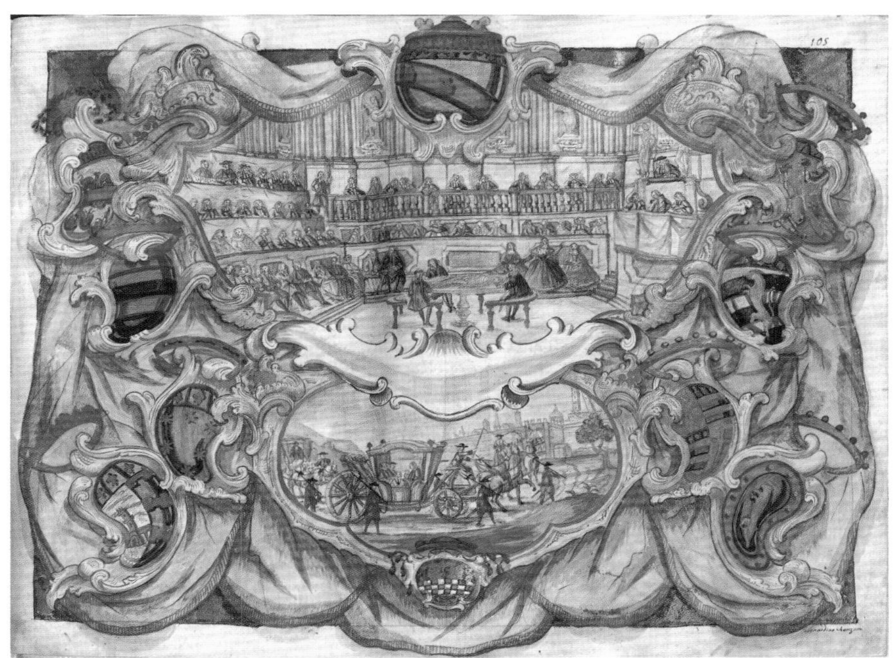

Plate 5. Bernardino Sconzani, *Insignia degli Anziani* depicting a public anatomy lesson during the carnival period where Laura Bassi is engaged in anatomical argumentation with the anatomist in cathedra. Lambertini is sitting in the left upper gallery dressed in the characteristic red cardinal's attire (1st bimester of 1734), in Archivio di Stato di Bologna, Anziani Consoli, Insignia, vol. 13, c. 105a.

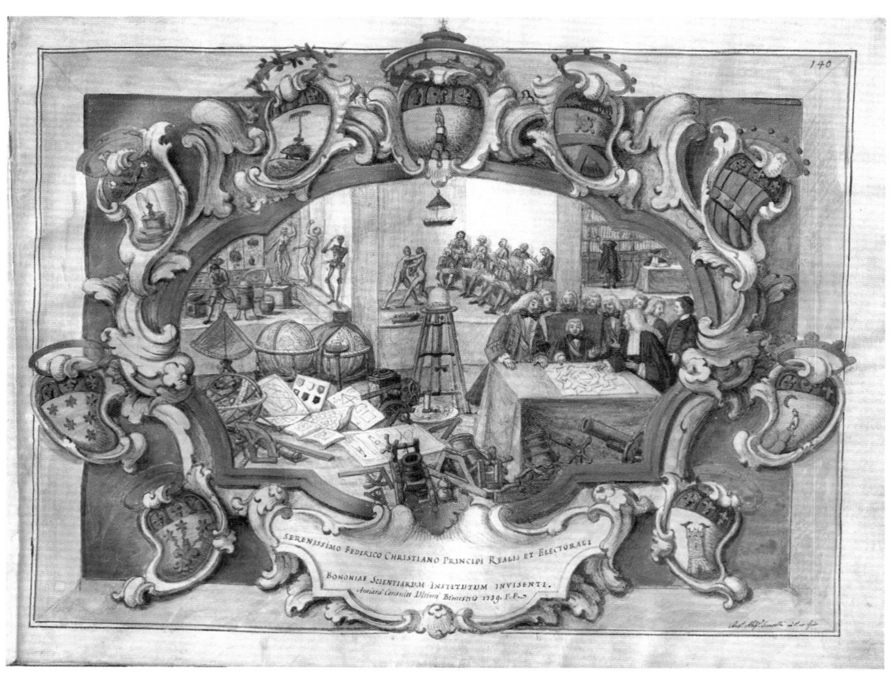
140
SERENISSIMO FEDERICO CHRISTIANO PRINCIPI REALIS ET ELECTORALI
BONONIAE SCIENTIARUM INSTITUTUM INVISENTI.
Anziani Consules Ultimi Bimestris 1739. P.P.

Plate 6. Antonio Alessandro Scarselli, *Insignia degli Anziani* commemorating the visit of the Prince Frederick Christian to the Institute of the Sciences (6th bimester of 1739), in Archivio di Stato di Bologna, Anziani Consoli, Insignia, vol. 13, c. 140a.

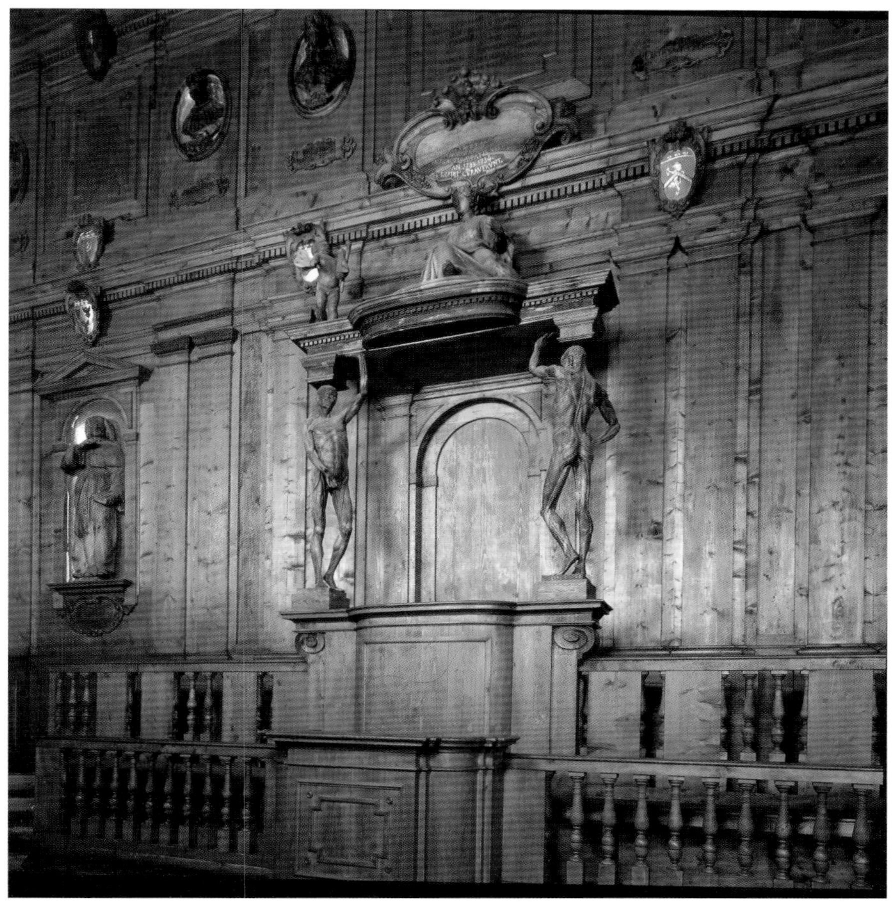

Plate 7. Silvestro Giannotti and Ercole Lelli, two wooden écorché caryatids supporting the roof of the professor's cathedra in Bologna's anatomical theatre; wood.

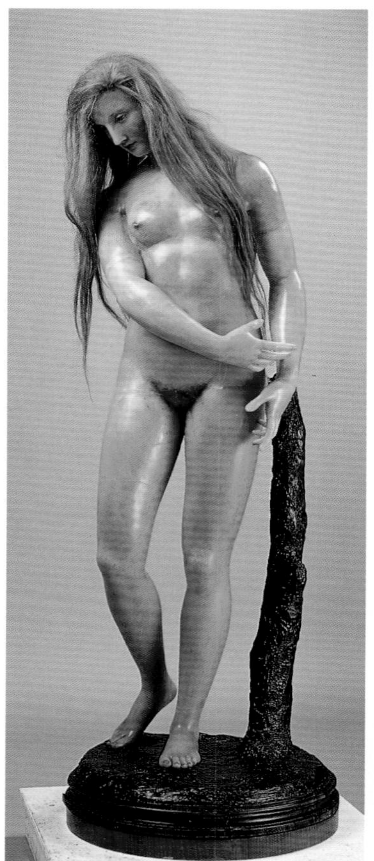

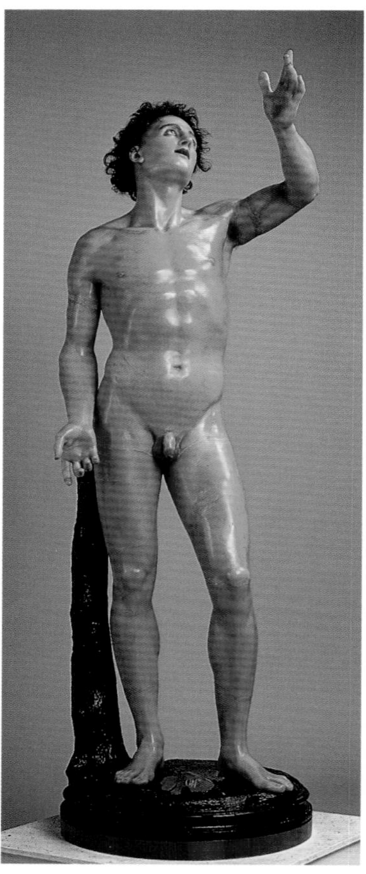

Plates 8 and 9. Ercole Lelli, wax figures of a woman and man, dubbed Eve and Adam, in the anatomy room of the Institute of the Sciences; wax and wood.

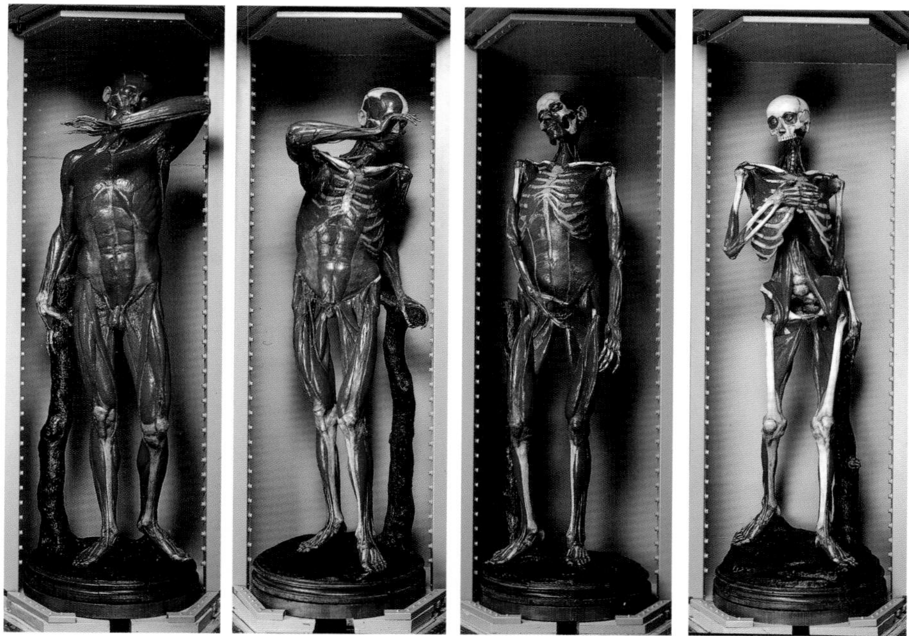

Plates 10–13. Ercole Lelli, series of four écorchés built on natural skeletons to reveal the different muscular layers of the male body in the anatomy room of the Institute of the Sciences; bone, wax, and wood.

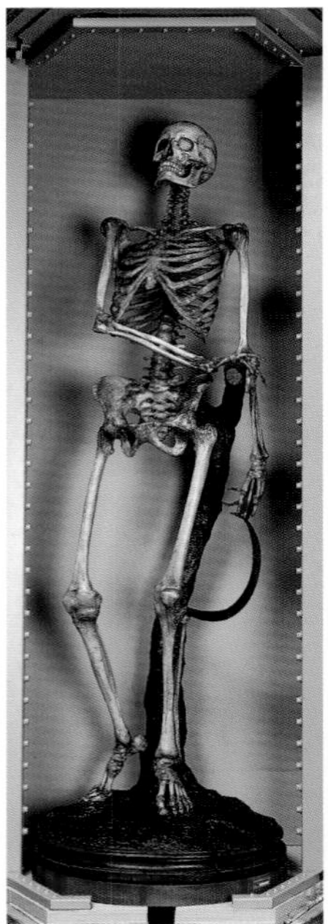

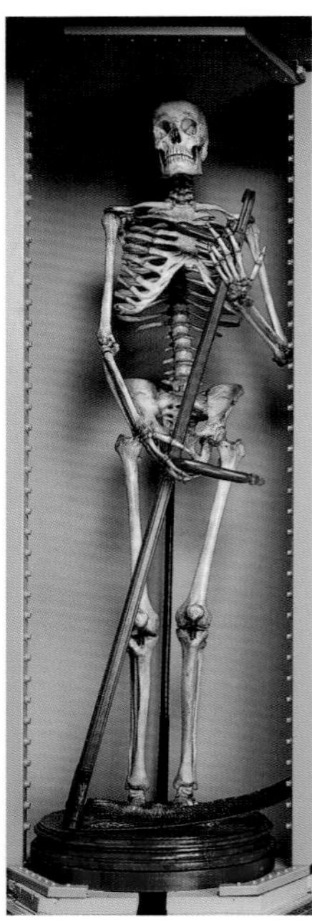

Plates 14 and 15. Ercole Lelli, female (left) and male (right) skeletons in the anatomy room of the Institute of the Sciences; bone, wax, and wood.

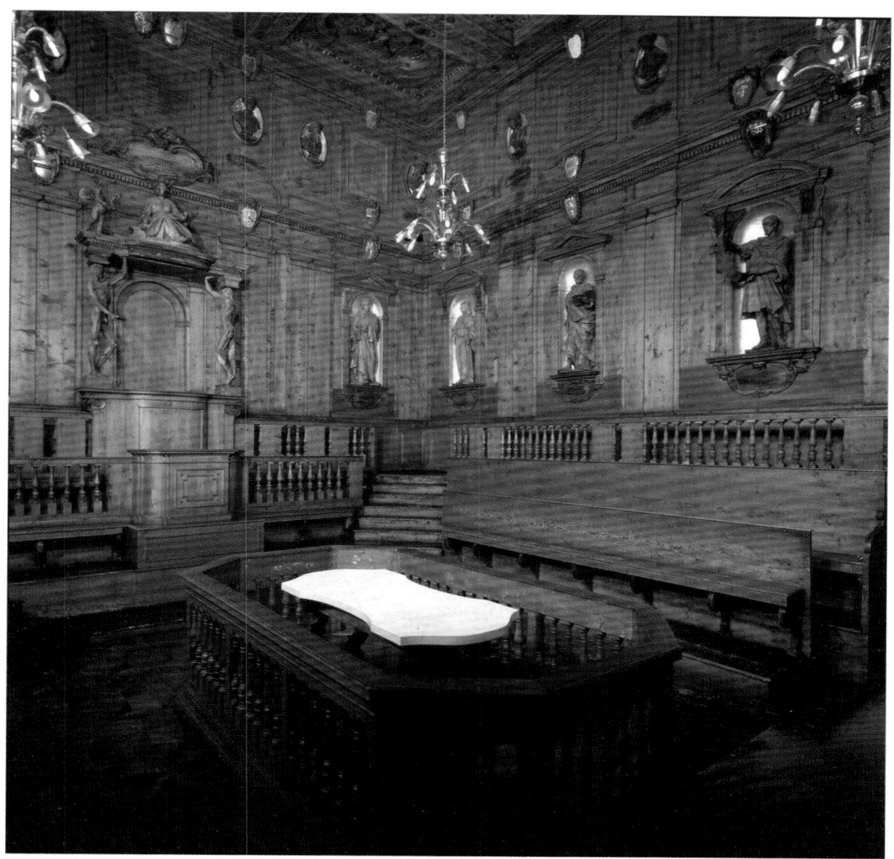

Plate 16. The anatomical theatre of Bologna.

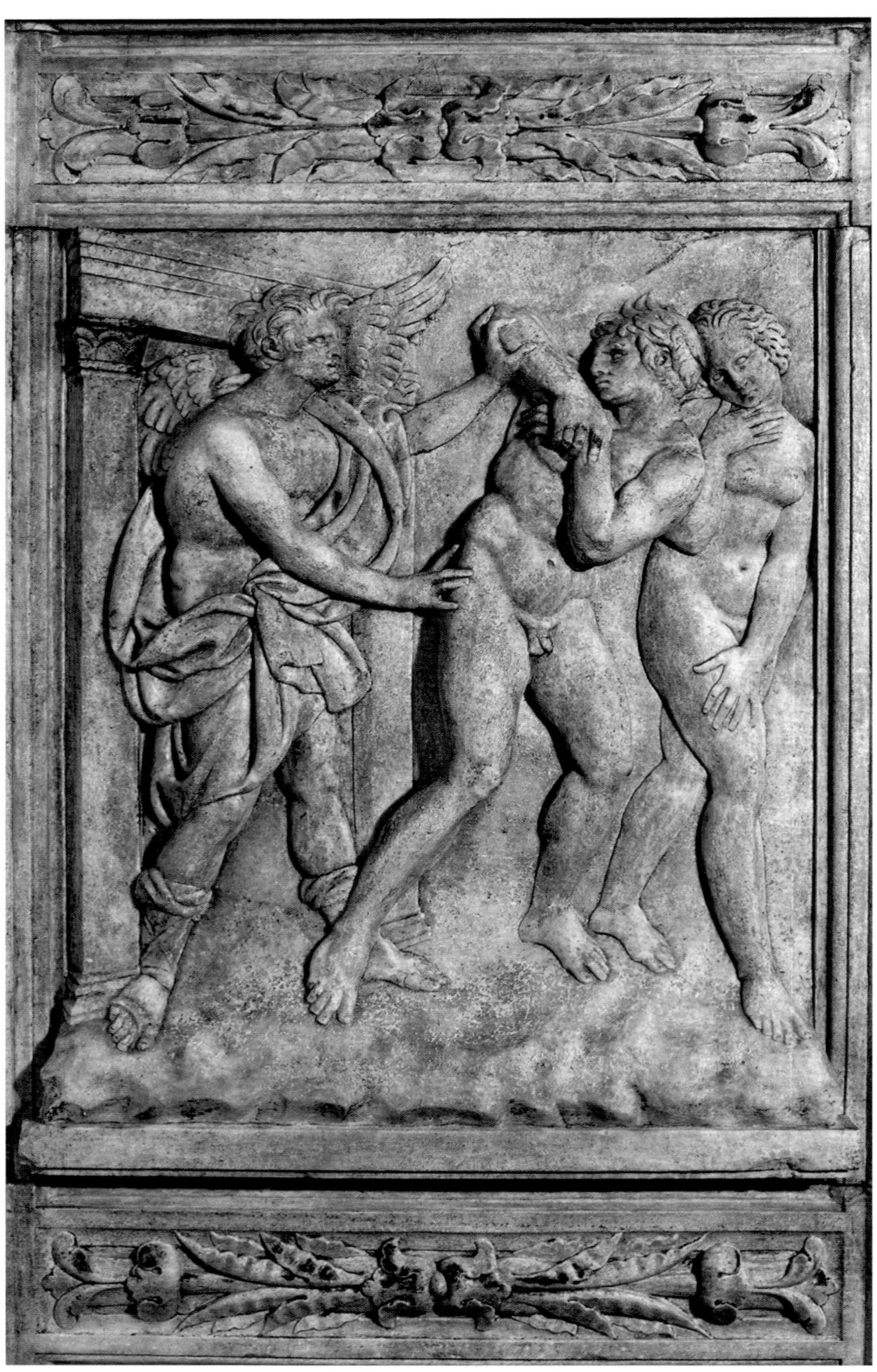

Plate 17. Jacopo della Quercia, Expulsion of Adam and Eve from the Garden of Eden, highlighting the figures' anatomical and muscular features, relief panel, main portal of the Basilica of San Petronio, Bologna, first half of the XV century.

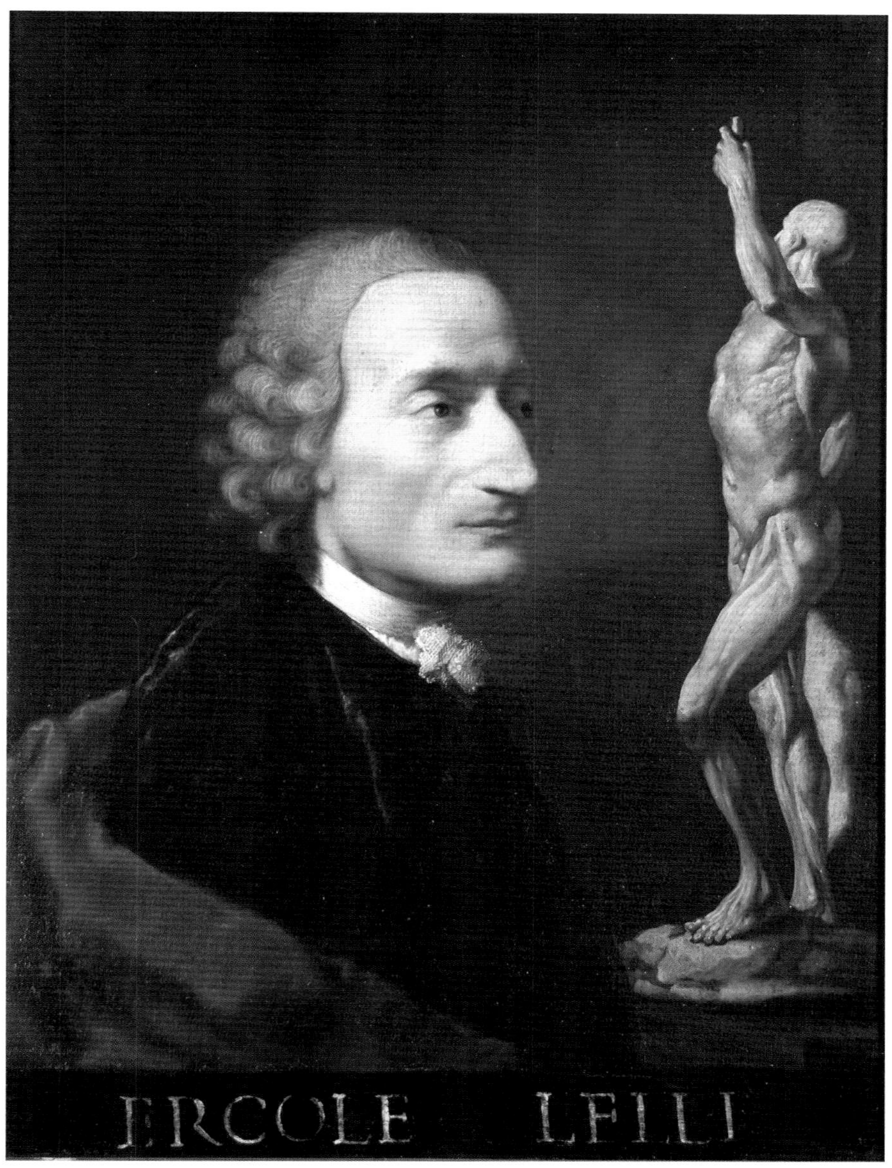

Plate 18. Ercole Lelli, self-portrait, where the author depicts himself contemplating his anatomical statuette; oil on canvas, 77 cm × 57 cm.

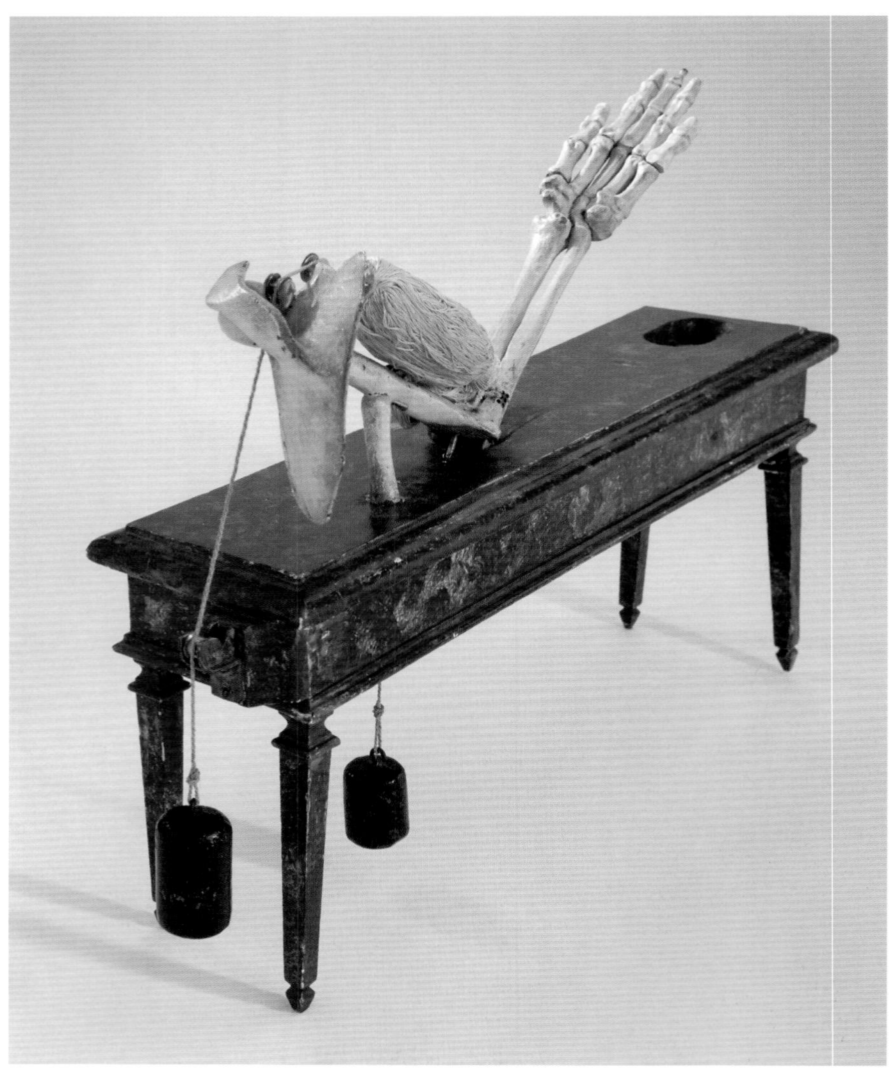

Plate 19. Model depicting the human arm as a third-class lever, where a skein of silk is used to portray the muscle, second half of the XVIII century; wood, lead, silk, brass, 72.5 cm × 18 cm × 51 cm, Inv. fot. 23858.

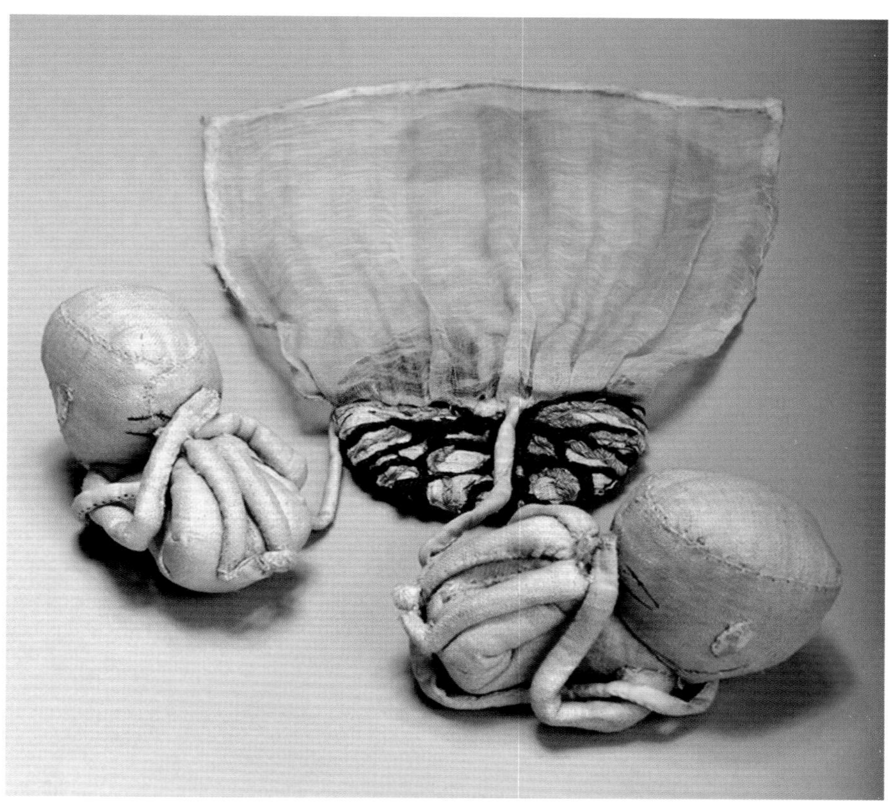

Plate 20. Angélique-Marguerite Le Boursier du Coudray, model of twins made out of fabric, XVIII century.

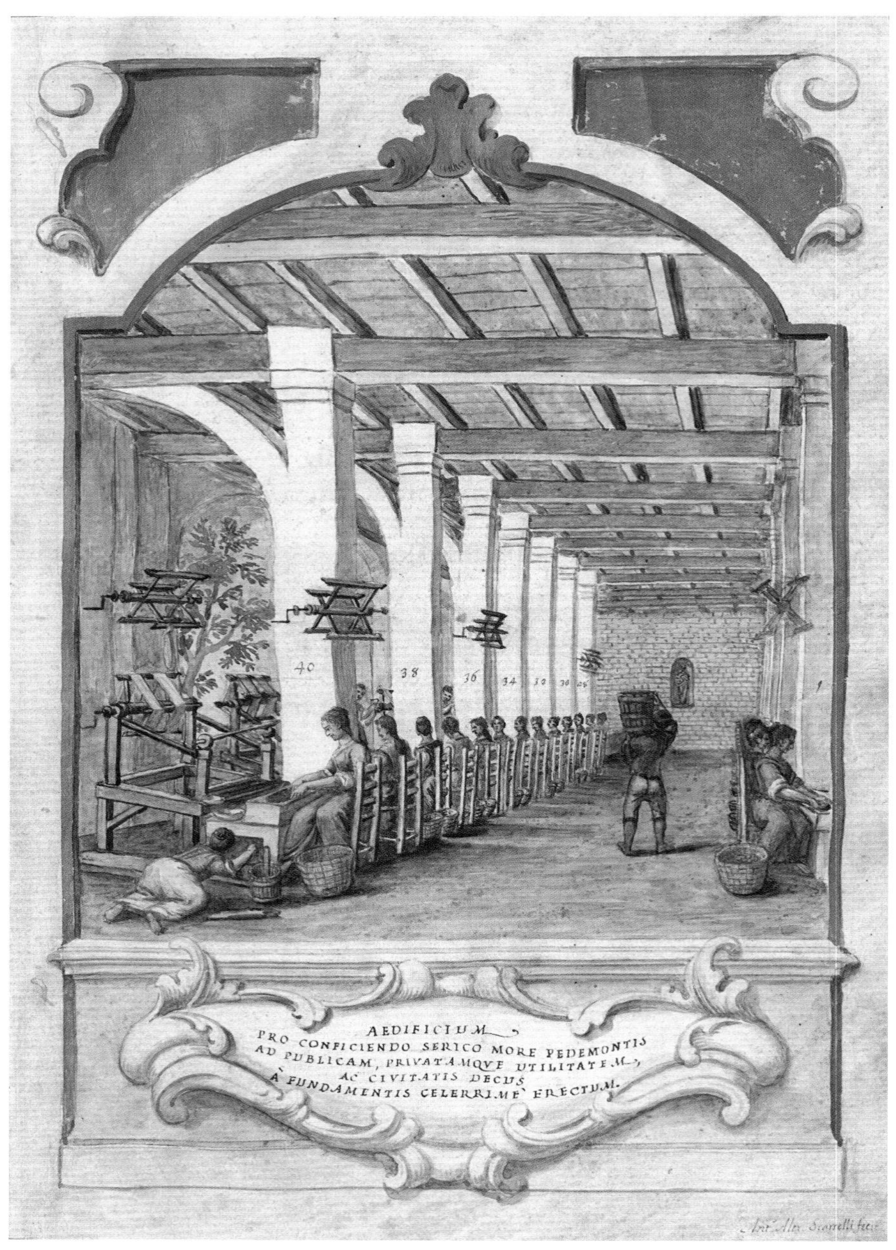
AEDIFICIUM
PRO CONFICIENDO SERICO MORE PEDEMONTIS
AD PUBLICAM, PRIVATAMQUE UTILITATEM,
AC CIVITATIS DECUS
À FUNDAMENTIS CELERRIMÈ ERECTUM.

Plate 21. Antonio Alessandro Scarselli, *Insignia degli Anziani* depicting women working in a silk factory constructed 'for both public and private utility' (3rd bimester of 1750), in Archivio di Stato di Bologna, Anziani Consoli, Insignia, vol. 14, c. 052a.

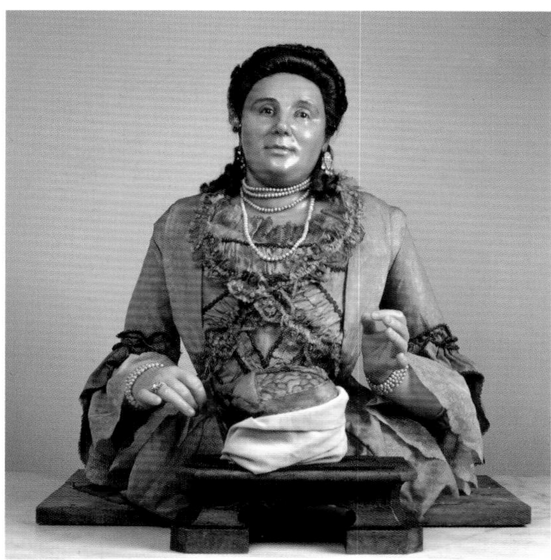

Plate 22. Anna Morandi, self-portrait where the modeller depicts herself dissecting a brain; wax, wood, metal, silk, hair, 90 cm × 82 cm × 68 cm.

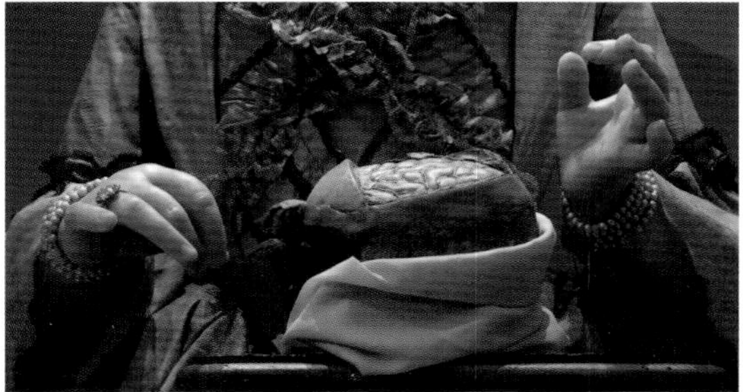

Plate 23. Anna Morandi, self-portrait: detail of Morandi's hands.

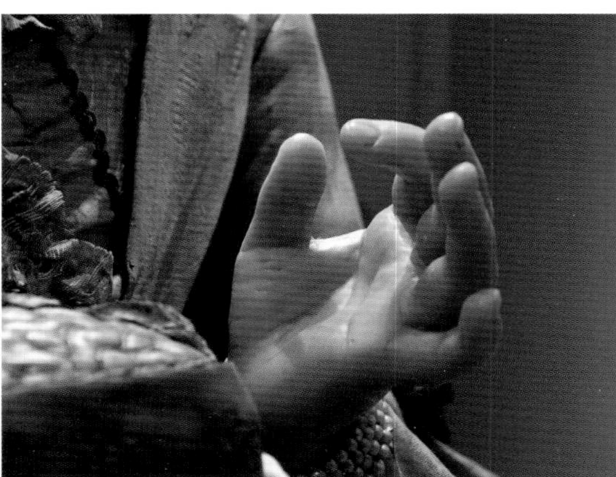

Plate 24. Anna Morandi, self-portrait: detail of Morandi's hand performing a gesture that seemingly superimposes the realm of needlework over that of anatomical practice.

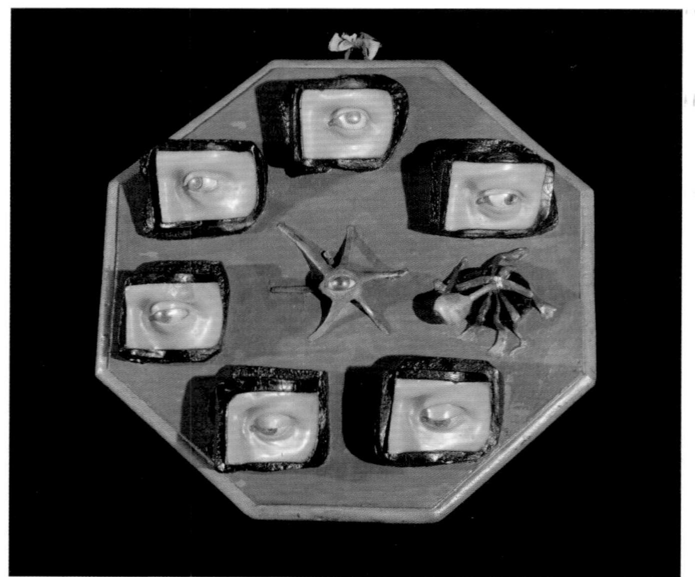

Plate 25. Anna Morandi, table of the eye; wax and wood, 35 cm × 35 cm × 7 cm.

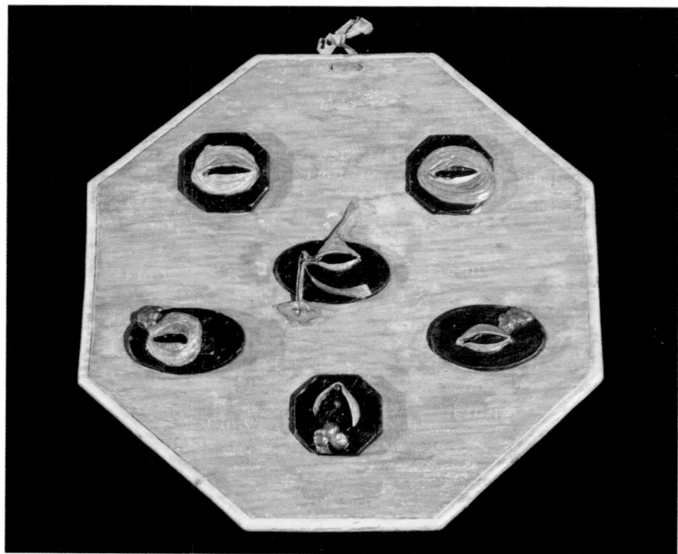

Plate 26. Anna Morandi, table of the eye; wax and wood, 35 cm × 35 cm × 4 cm.

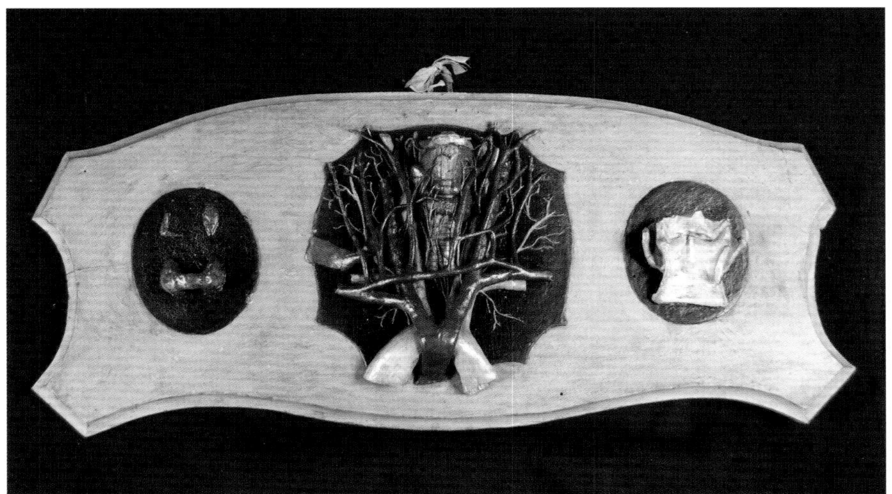

Plate 27. Anna Morandi, table of the larynx; wax and wood, 57 cm × 28 cm × 5.5 cm.

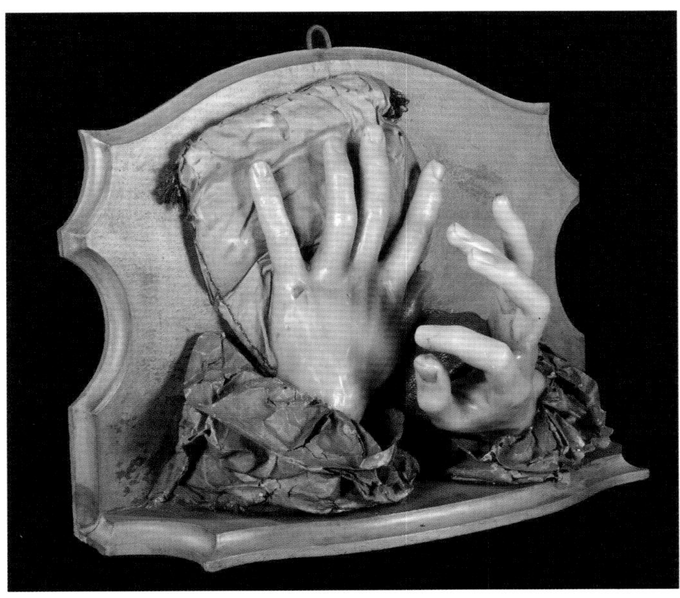

Plate 28. Anna Morandi, model of the hands; wax, wood, and fabric, 41 cm × 41 cm × 8 cm.

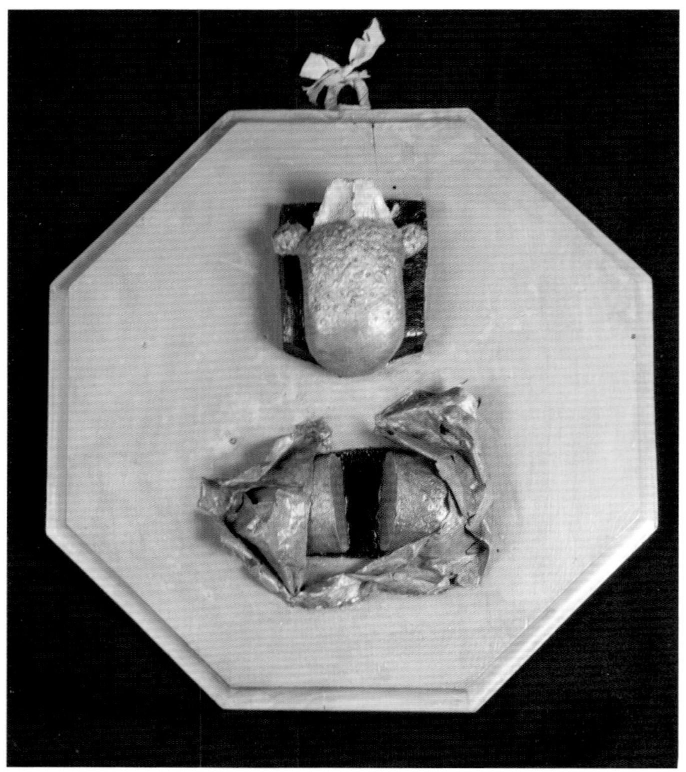

Plate 29. Anna Morandi, table of the tongue displaying enlarged anatomical details; wax, wood and fabric, 35 cm × 35 cm × 5.5 cm.

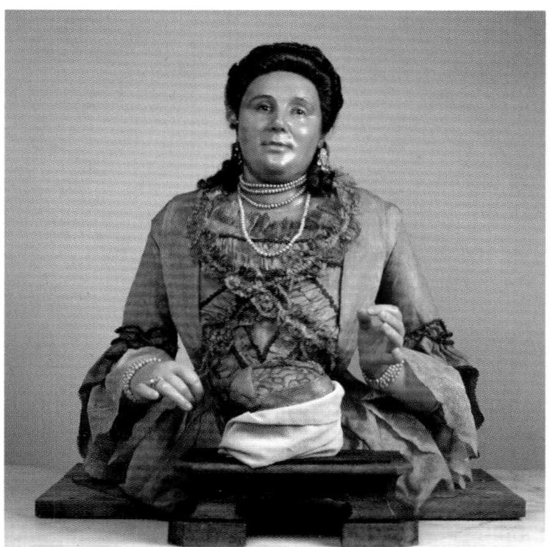

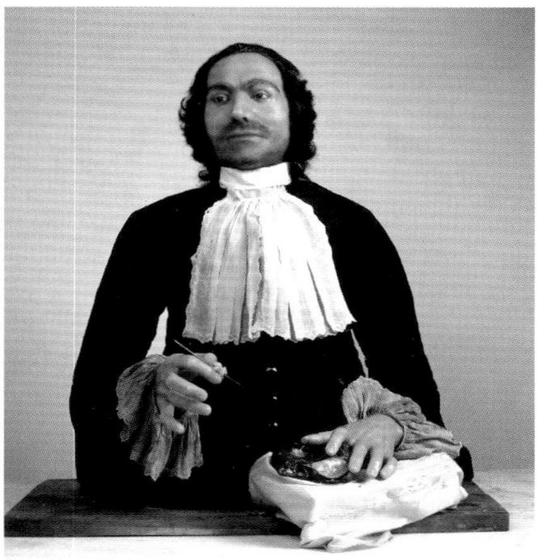

Plate 30. Anna Morandi, self-portrait and portrait of her husband Giovanni Manzolini depicted in the act of dissecting, respectively, a brain and a heart; wax, wood, metal, silk, hair, self-portrait: 90 cm × 82 cm × 68 cm, portrait of Manzolini: 90 cm × 82 cm × 68 cm.

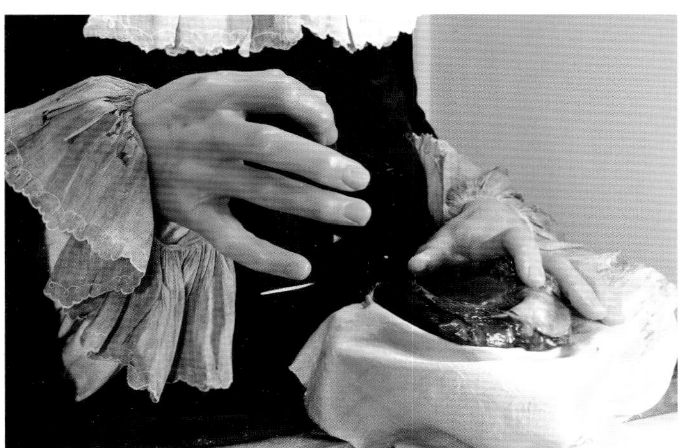

Plate 31. Anna Morandi, portrait of Giovanni Manzolini: detail of Manzolini's hands.

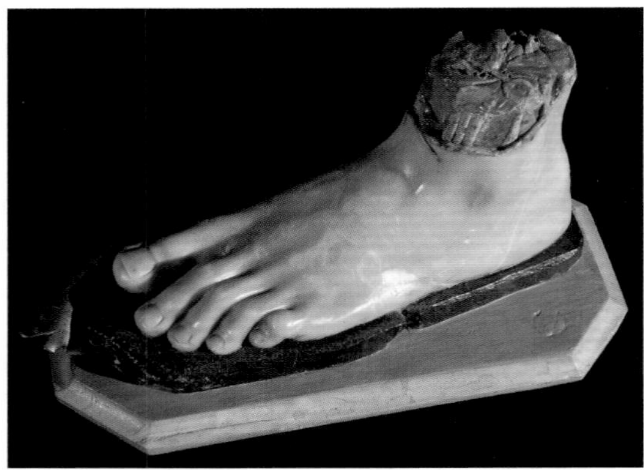

Plate 32. Giovanni Manzolini and Anna Morandi, model of the foot; wax and wood, 30 cm × 14 cm × 18 cm.

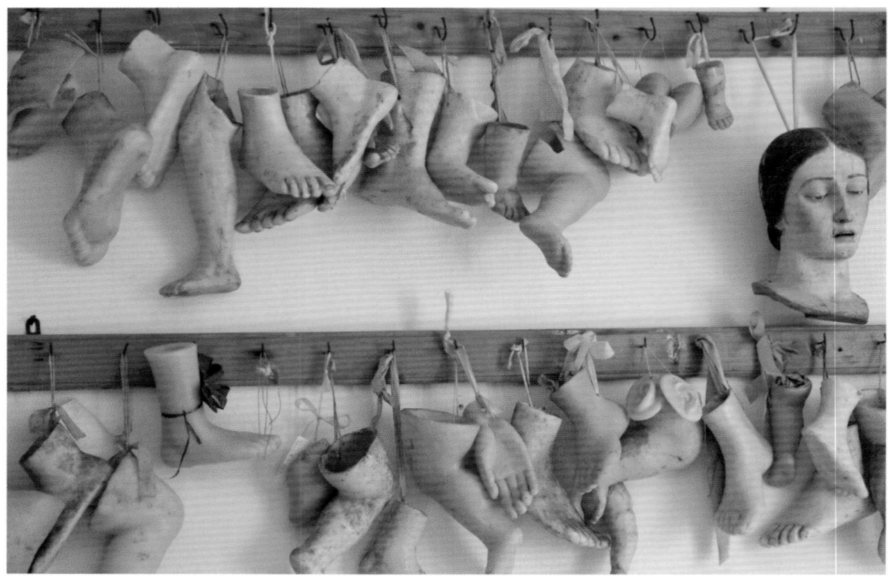

Plate 33. Ex-votos in wax from the Museum of Ex-votos in Altavilla Milicia, Sicily.

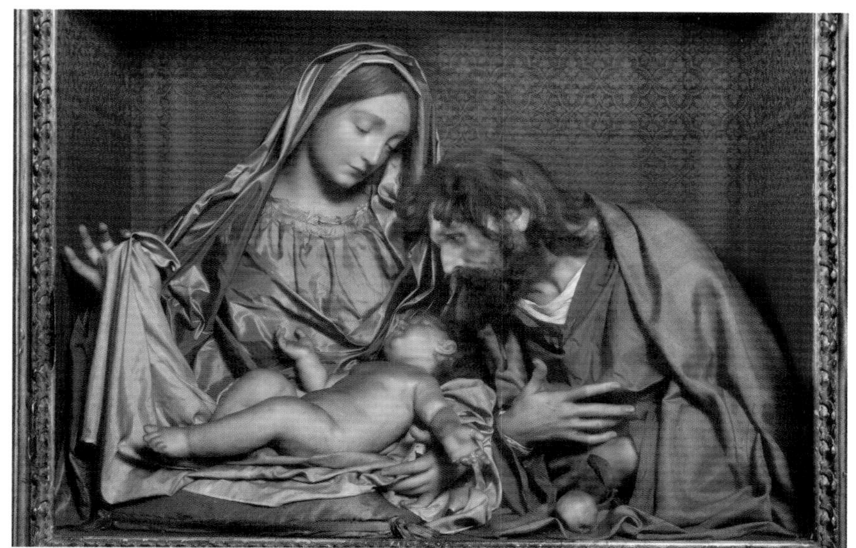

Plate 34. Angelo Piò, Sacra Famiglia (Holy Family), in Church of Santi Vitale e Agricola, Bologna, Italy, mid-XVIII century; wax and silk, 61.3 cm (height) × 96 cm (breadth).

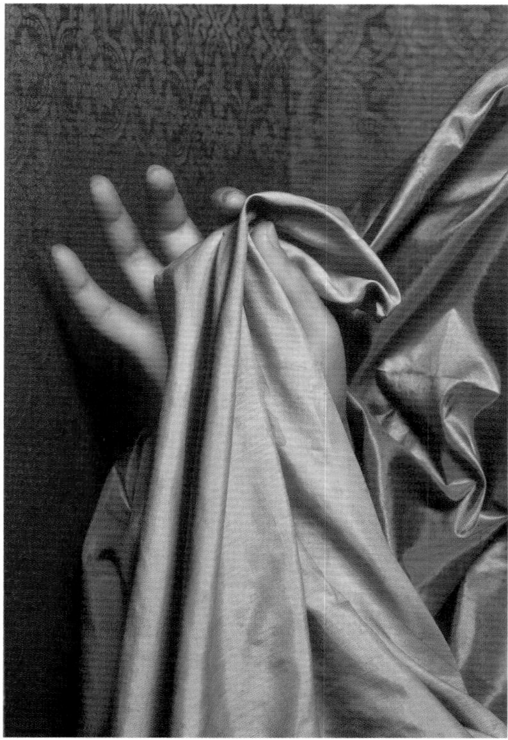

Plate 35. Angelo Piò, Sacra Famiglia (Holy Family): detail of the hand of Mary.

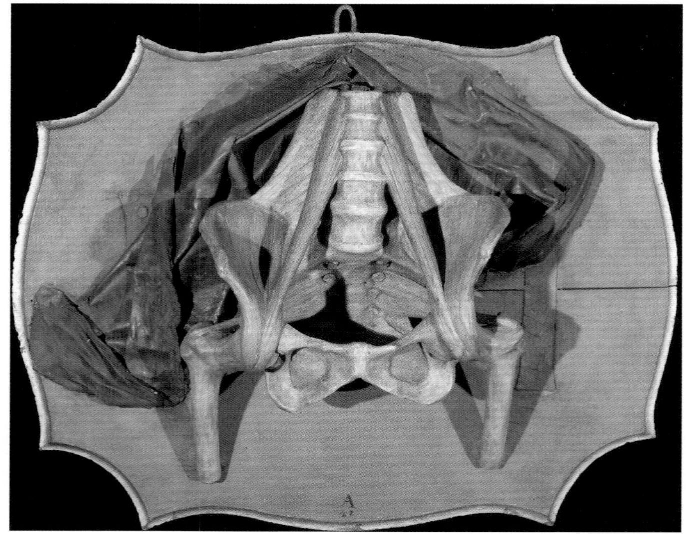

Plate 36. Giovanni Manzolini and Anna Morandi, model of the pelvis displaying the internal muscles and ligaments; wax, wood, and cloth, 47 cm × 61 cm × 18 cm.

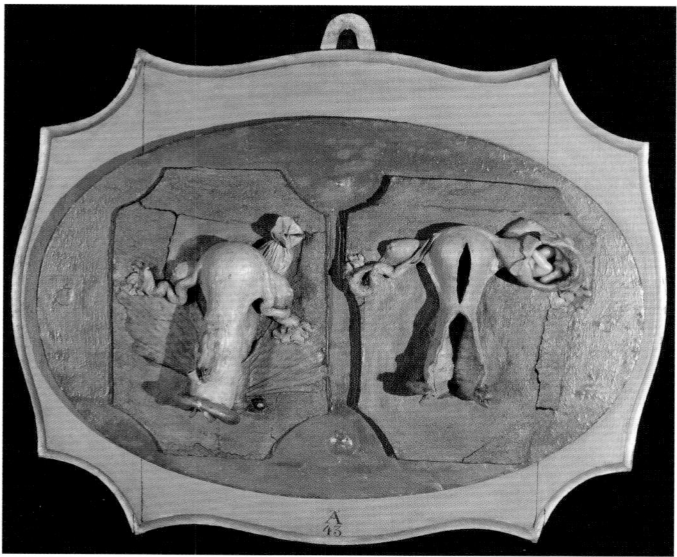

Plate 37. Giovanni Manzolini and Anna Morandi, table displaying two wax models of the womb, one showing a pregnancy in the womb's left tube; wax and wood, 50 cm × 63 cm × 11 cm.

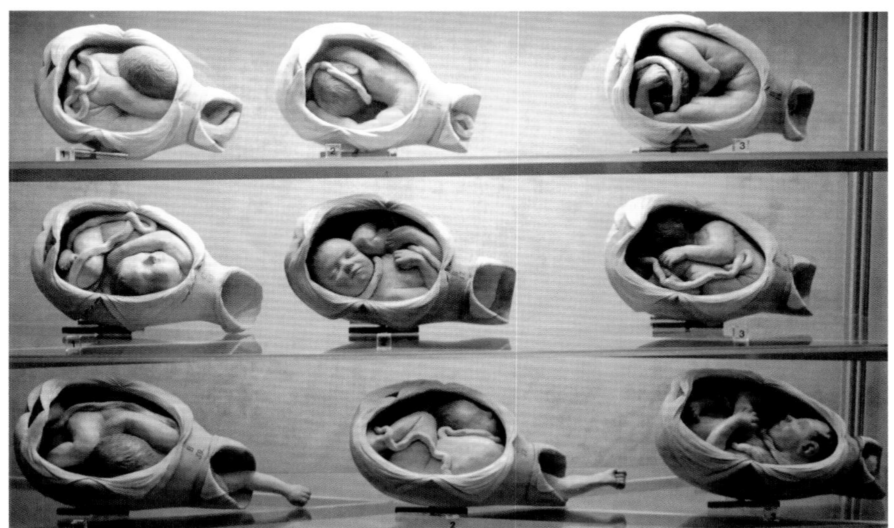

Plate 38. Sequence of clay models of the gravid uterus in Giovanni Antonio Galli's midwifery collection.

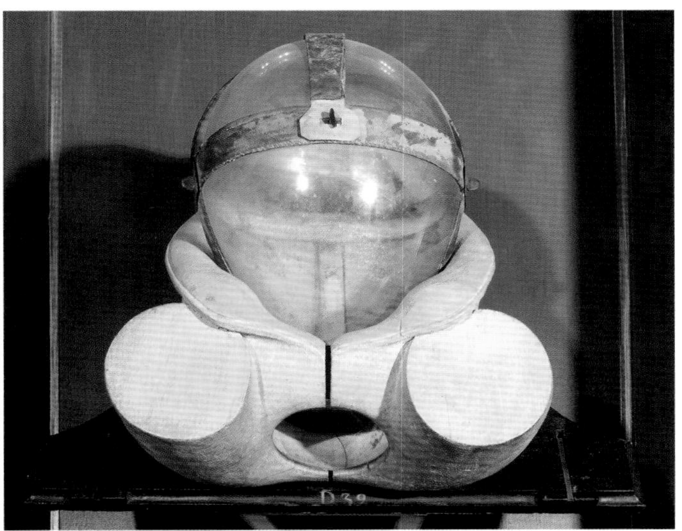

Plate 39. Antonio Cartolari, 'Abdomen and pelvis with crystal womb' (midwifery machine), where a puppet could be inserted and extracted during midwifery training; glass, wood, and metal, 64 cm × 50 cm × 40 cm.

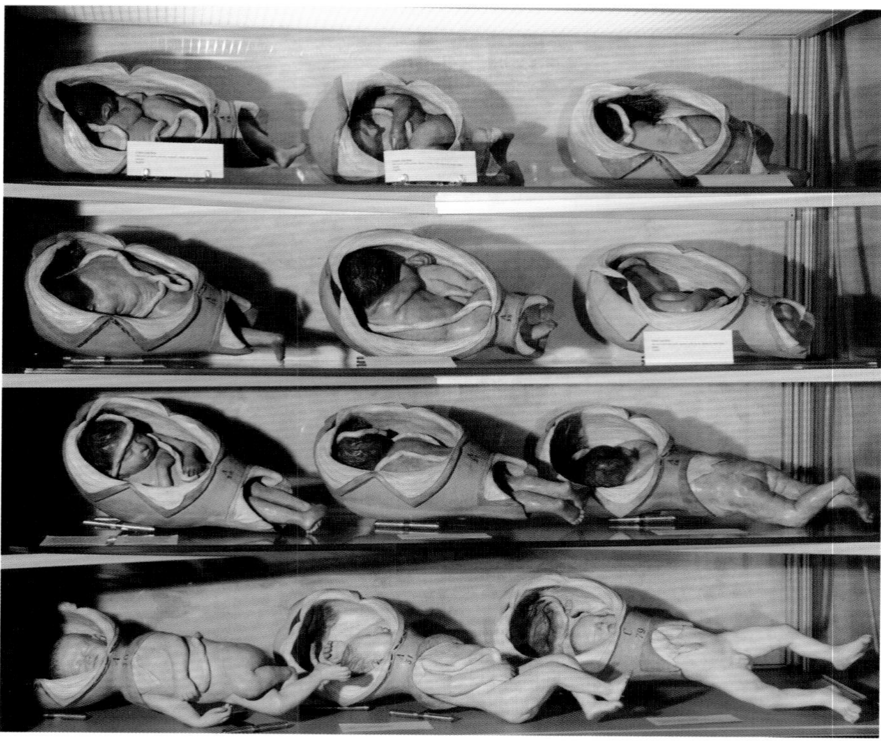

Plate 40. Series of clay wombs presenting unborn children in anomalous situations in Giovanni Antonio Galli's midwifery collection.

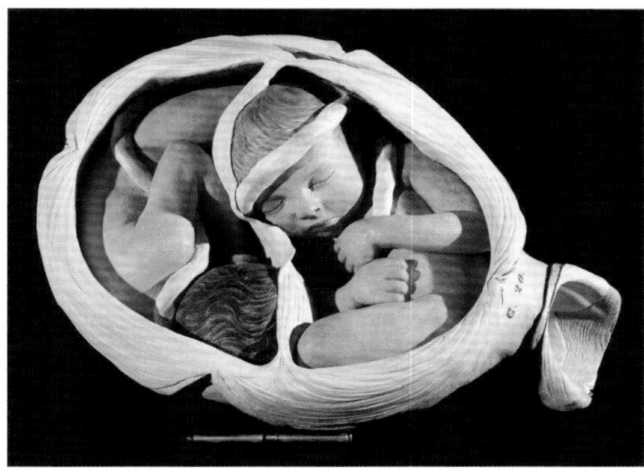

Plate 41. Model of the gravid uterus with nine-month-old unborn twins; clay, 40 cm × 28 cm × 17 cm.

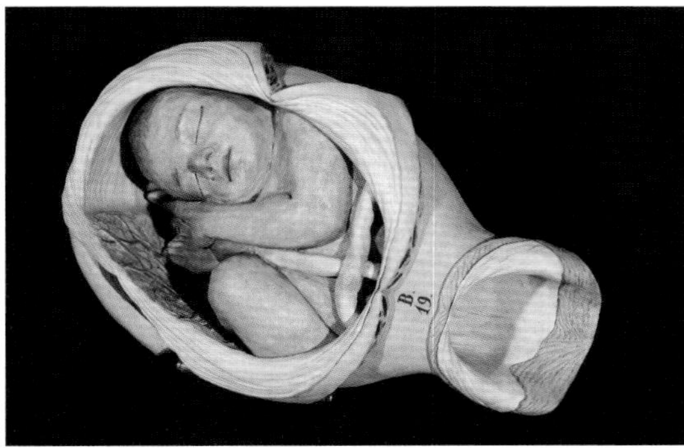

Plate 42. Model of the gravid uterus with unborn child; clay, 31 cm × 21cm × 13 cm.

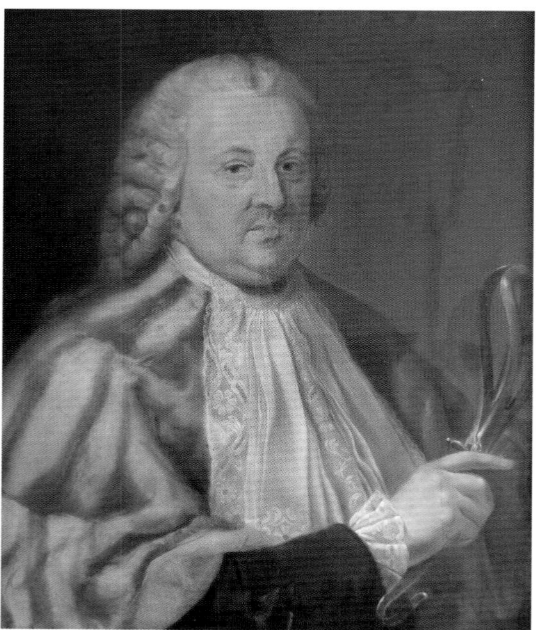

Plate 43. Angelo Crescimbeni, portrait of Giovanni Antonio Galli (1775); pastel on paper, 73 cm × 68 cm.

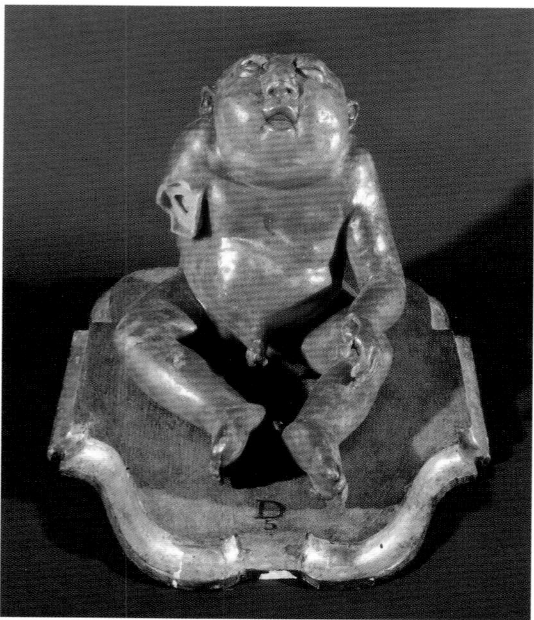

Plate 44. Wax model of a malformed child described by Galli in a presentation at the Academy of the Sciences on 10 May 1764; wax and wood, 18 cm × 22 cm× 30 cm.

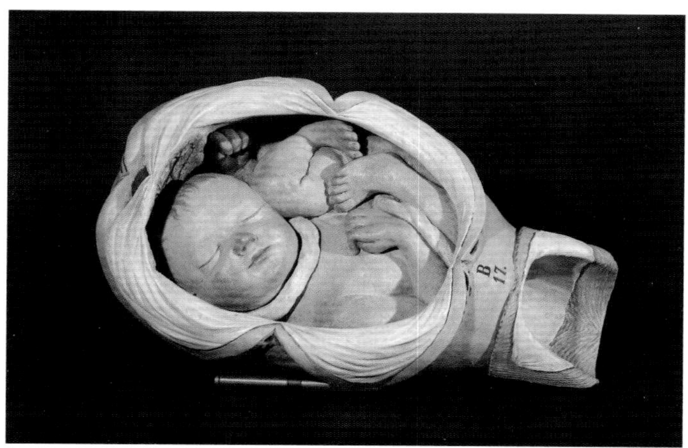

Plate 45. Model of the gravid uterus with unborn child in unordinary position displaying a calm and beatific expression; clay, 36 cm × 22cm × 14 cm.

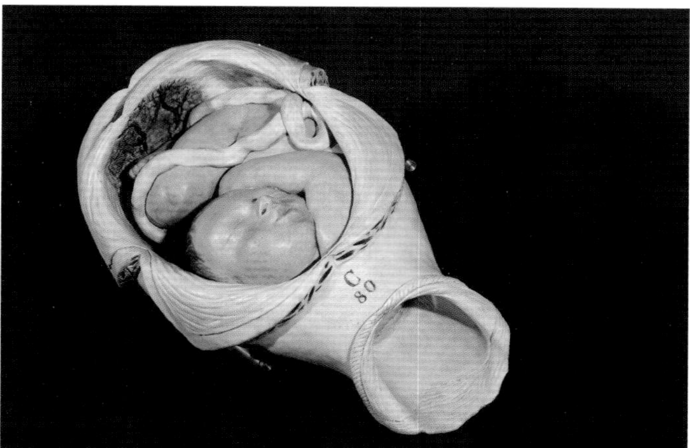

Plate 46. Model of the gravid uterus with unborn child in unordinary position displaying a serene and peaceful expression; clay, 36 cm × 22 cm × 15 cm.

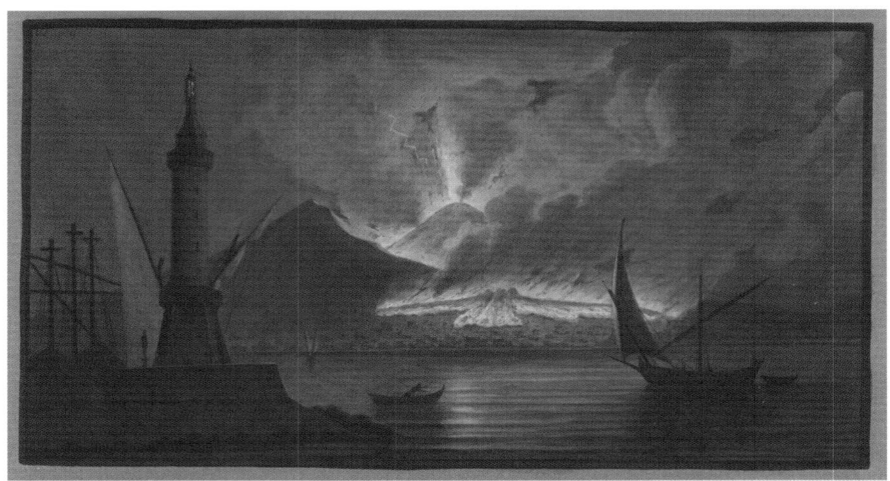

Plate 47. 'View of the great eruption of Vesuvius from the mole of Naples in the night of the 20th of October 1767', from William Hamilton, *Campi Phlegraei: Osservazioni sui vulcani delle Due Sicilie*, Naples: Pietro Fabris, 1776–9, Plate VI; hand-coloured etching by Pietro Fabris.

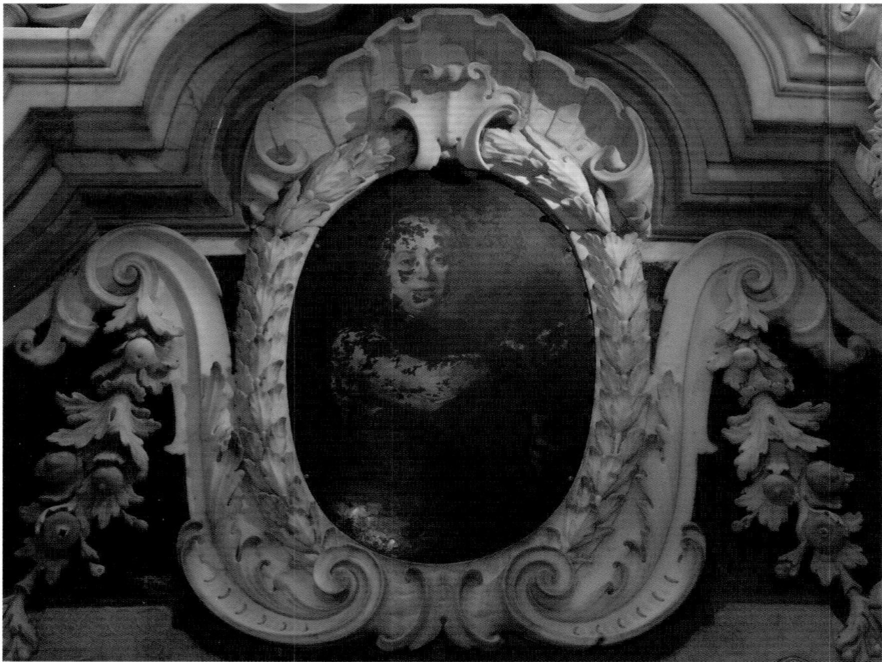

Plate 48. Carlo Amalfi, portrait of Raimondo di Sangro, c.1759 (?), in Museo Cappella di Sansevero, Naples; oil on copper.

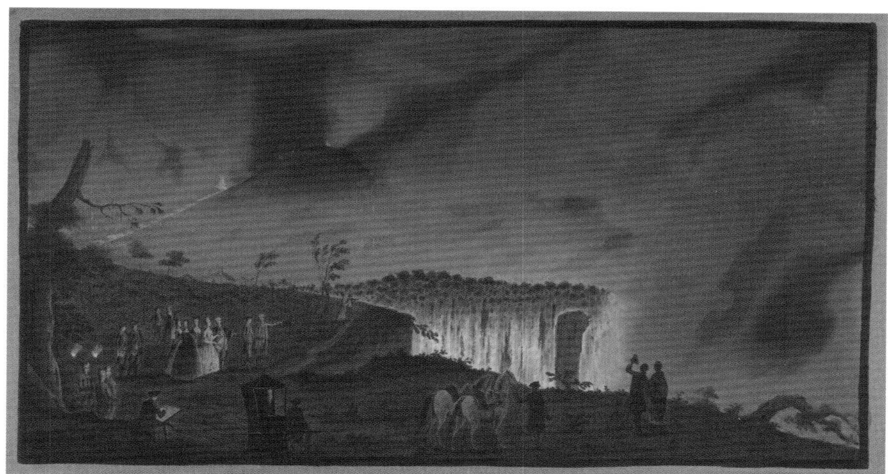

Plate 49. William Hamilton escorting the Neapolitan sovereigns to view the stream of lava running from Mount Vesuvius towards Resina on the night of 11 May 1771, from William Hamilton, *Campi Phlegraei: Osservazioni sui vulcani delle Due Sicilie*, Naples: Pietro Fabris, 1776–9, Plate XXXVIII; hand-coloured etching made by Pietro Fabris after his drawing.

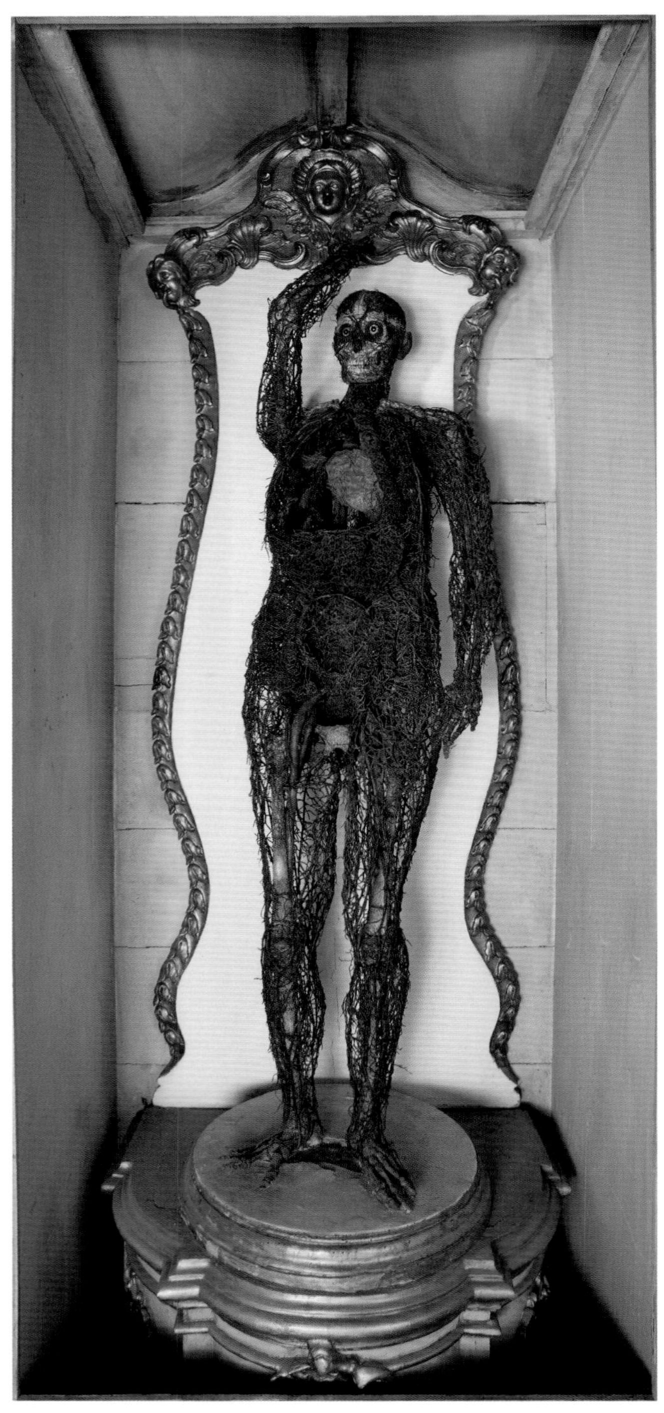

Plate 50. Giuseppe Salerno, 'Anatomical machine' displaying the complex web of blood vessels on a female skeleton.

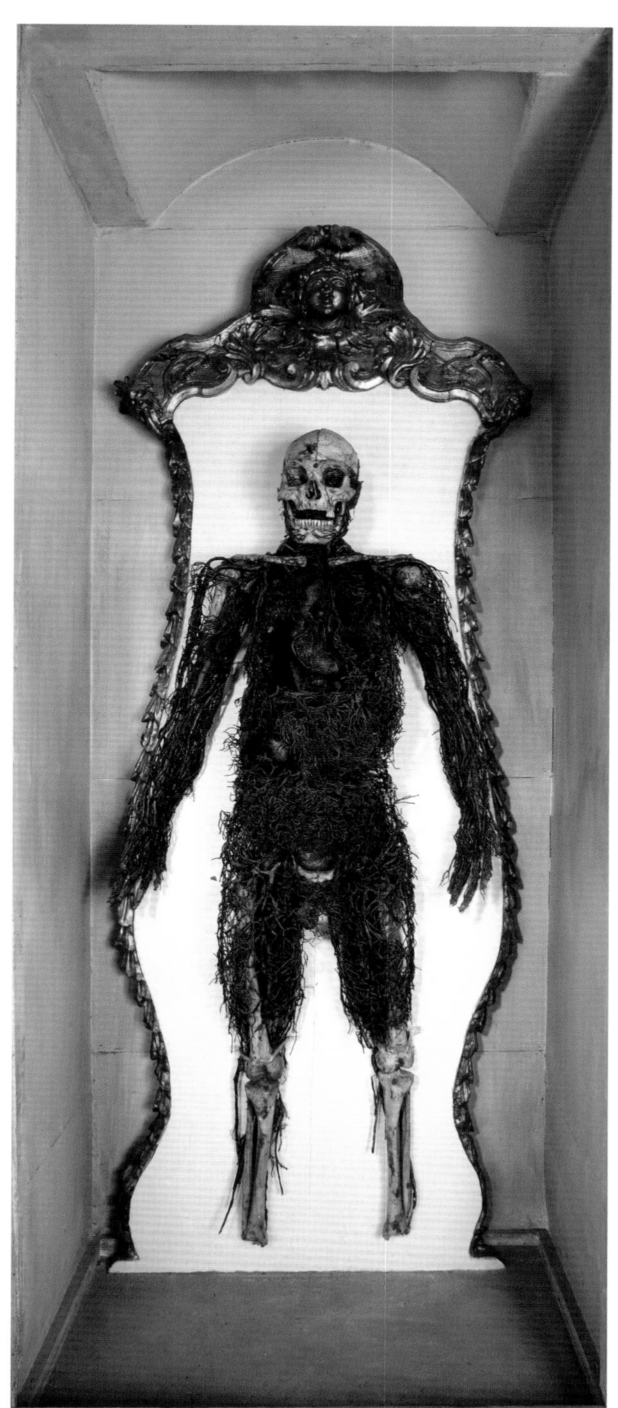

Plate 51. Giuseppe Salerno, 'Anatomical machine' displaying the complex web of blood vessels on a male skeleton.

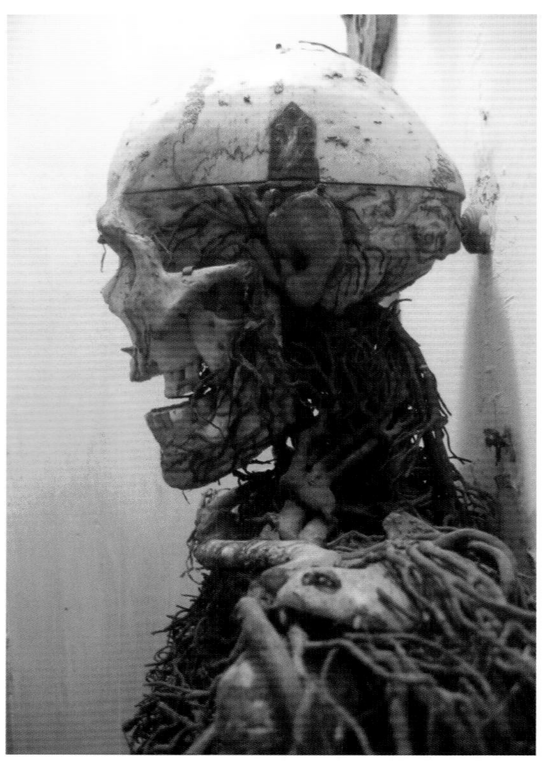

Plate 52. Giuseppe Salerno, 'Anatomical machine': detail of the upper body of the male skeleton.

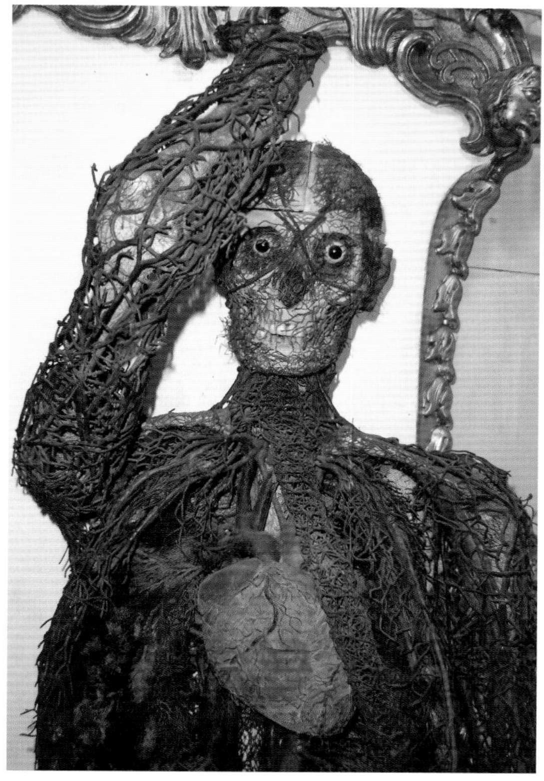

Plate 53. Giuseppe Salerno, 'Anatomical machine': detail of the upper body of the female skeleton.

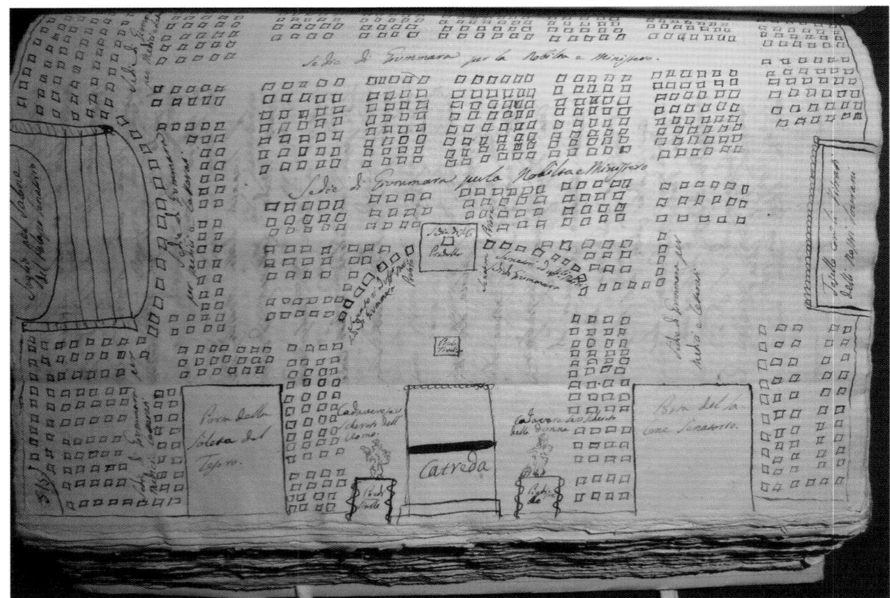

Plate 54. Seating plan for Giuseppe Salerno's anatomical demonstration of 1789 at the Palermitan Senate. The plan highlights the display of Salerno's two skeletons on the sides of the cathedra (at the bottom of the image), the central seat of the Viceroy, and the location of the physicians, aristocrats, and literati around the hall, in Archivio Storico del Comune di Palermo, ms. Cerimoniali (1789), vol. 38, 515.

5

Blindfolding the Midwives

ANATOMY AND MIDWIFERY

To all those concerned in Bologna, the end of 1751 was the harbinger of good news. At long last, the anatomy room of the Bolognese Institute of the Sciences was completed, the wax modellers Giovanni Manzolini and Anna Morandi were working on their own collection of anatomical models, and the rumour that the surgeon Giovanni Antonio Galli had gathered yet another anatomical collection had started to spread both in town and beyond the city's walls.[1] In early November 1751, the physician Jacopo Bartolomeo Beccari visited the residence of the '*buon Dottor* Galli' to check his midwifery collection and remained deeply impressed. As he encountered a 'very beautiful and numerous' series of anatomical and midwifery models, he could barely contain his enthusiasm: 'I assure you', he wrote the next day to his cousin and friend Flaminio Scarselli, secretary of Bologna's embassy in Rome, 'the thing is amazing':

> when I saw it, I felt dazzled to the point of confusion, partly for the marvel, and partly due to a compelling feeling of approval for something that will be of such great distinction and decorum for our poor country, which has citizens capable of ideas that could please a sovereign.[2]

What Beccari saw was a breathtaking sequence of some 200 midwifery models, which showed all the situations that could occur in childbirth and 'filled a big room'.[3] The collection included tables of the pelvis (Plate 36), waxworks that showed the anatomical details of the parts of generation and pregnancy (Plate 37), dozens of models in clay of the gravid uterus (Plate 38), specimens of foetuses

[1] On Galli's collection, see Marco Bortolotti, 'Insegnamento, ricerca e professione nel museo ostetrico di Giovanni Antonio Galli', in *I materiali dell'Istituto delle Scienze*, 239–47; Marco Bortolotti et al., *Ars obstetricia bononiensis: Catalogo ed inventario del Museo Ostetrico Giovan Antonio Galli* (Bologna: Clueb, 1988); Olimpia Sanlorenzo, *L'insegnamento di ostetricia nell'Università di Bologna* (Bologna: Alma Mater Studiorum Saecularia Nona, 1988), 27–37; Ambre Murard, *La collection du médicin-chirurgien Giovan Antonio Galli à Bologne* (Mémoire de maîtrise en Langue et Civilisation italiennes, Université de Paris III, 1997); Ambre Murard, 'La rappresentazione del corpo femminile nell'ostetricia settecentesca', in Claudia Pancino (ed.), *Corpi: Storia, metafore, rappresentazioni fra Medioevo ed età contemporanea* (Venice: Marsilio, 2000), 41–54; Pancino, 'Questioni di genere'; Claudia Pancino, 'Malati, medici, mammane, saltimbanchi: Malattia e cura nella Bologna d'età moderna', in Prosperi (ed.), *Storia di Bologna*, vol. 3/II, 720–4.

[2] BUB, ms. 243, Lettere di Jacopo Bartolomeo Beccari a Flaminio Scarselli, Letter of 6 November 1751 from Jacopo Bartolomeo Beccari in Bologna to Flaminio Scarselli.

[3] Ibid.

preserved in 'spirit of wine', and several midwifery machines that mimicked the circumstances of childbirth. Placing three-dimensional anatomical visualization at the centre of midwifery training, Galli's collection relied on sequences of anatomical models that were intended to instruct practitioners and promised to shed light on the mysterious and opaque domains of generation and pregnancy.[4] In doing so, the collection fashioned Galli's residence as both a training venue and a site of wonder and amazement. Like Beccari, others marvelled at the sight of a display that pledged to expose pregnancy's secrets at a glance. Beccari felt dazzled and confused. Galli was ready to cash in.

To be sure, Galli was neither the first nor the only mid-eighteenth-century practitioner to employ models in the training of midwives.[5] In the British Isles, man-midwives such as Richard Manningham (1690–1759) and William Smellie (1697–1763) also used midwifery models and machines in their training practices. In France, Madame du Coudray crafted mannequins and models that were meant to speak directly to the eyes and hands of training midwives (Plate 20).[6] However, Galli's collection was special because of its unprecedented size. When Beccari saw it in 1751, one of the things that struck him was precisely its magnitude. The 'immense' number of models continued to impress viewers for years to come.[7] Featuring models that were made in a variety of materials, such as clay, crystal, soft fabric, and wood, as well as wax, Galli's collection partly differed from the other Bolognese anatomical displays in that it was a hands-on, working collection, allowing users to handle some of the models, as well as inspect them visually.[8] Seeking to provide a comprehensive overview of the world of generation, it staged a visual and material archive of pregnancy and childbirth where the models' orderly arrangement promised to turn the complex and mysterious domain of childbearing into a distinctively accessible site of learning. A crystal model of the womb marked one of the high points of the display by presenting the womb as an allegedly transparent object of knowledge (Plate 39).[9]

Well into the eighteenth century, pregnancy conjured up a complex, elusive, and ambiguous state of affairs of the body, a corporeal condition characterized by confusing and variable signs that changed in unforeseeable and potentially deceitful ways.[10] As is well known, the attempt to unveil and clarify the 'hidden truths

[4] ASB, Assunteria di Studio, Requisiti dei Lettori, busta 40, cartella 17, 'Relazione alle SS.rie VV. Ill:me ed Ecc.se degli Assunti di Studio'.

[5] See Nina Rattern Gelbart, *The King's Midwife: A History and Mystery of Madame du Coudray* (Berkeley: University of California Press, 1998); Helen King, *Midwifery, Obstetrics and the Rise of Gynaecology: The Uses of a Sixteenth-Century Compendium* (Aldershot: Ashgate, 2007), 79 and 134; Pam Lieske, '"Made in Imitation of Real Women and Children": Obstetrical Machines in Eighteenth-Century Britain', in Andrew Mangham and Greta Depledge (eds.), *The Female Body in Medicine and Literature* (Liverpool: Liverpool University Press, 2011), 69–88.

[6] Gelbart, *The King's Midwife*, 61.

[7] Lalande, *Voyage d'un François en Italie*, vol. 2, 35.

[8] On the use of touch in anatomical collections, see Knoeff, 'Touching Anatomy'.

[9] Notably, Morandi herself had made glass models of the womb.

[10] See Duden, *The Woman Beneath the Skin*; Barbara Duden, 'The Fetus on the "Farther Shore": Toward a History of the Unborn', in Lynn M. Morgan and Meredith W. Michaels (eds.), *Fetal Subjects, Feminist Positions* (Philadelphia: University of Pennsylvania Press, 1999), 14; Cathy McClive, 'The Hidden Truths of the Belly: The Uncertainties of Pregnancy in Early Modern Europe', *Social History*

of the belly', as Cathy McClive has put it, has historically provided a privileged locus of negotiation and contention for different medical practitioners. While generation and pregnancy long remained the epitome of 'corporeal uncertainty', claims related to the unveiling of their workings offered a privileged avenue to anatomical and medical prestige.[11] A canonical narrative of the history of seventeenth- and eighteenth-century midwifery tells the story of the emergence of man-midwives as a story of conflict and competition between female practitioners and medical men who sought to take over the realm of childbirth on the basis of claims of medical and anatomical expertise.[12] In its most traditional formulation, this narrative largely focuses on the British Isles and ends badly—with a finale that closes with the displacement of midwives from their long-lasting centrality at the scene of childbirth. This account has been nuanced in a number of ways. It has been rearticulated as a story of collaboration as well as competition, and the very issue of the disappearance of midwives has been, at least in part, reappraised.[13] This chapter revisits traditional narratives of the eighteenth-century world of midwifery in light of the specificities related to the conspicuous material culture of pregnancy and childbirth in the Italian peninsula.[14] While attention has been drawn to the

of Medicine, 15:2 (2002), 209–27; Park, *Secrets of Women*; Maria Conforti, '"Affirmare quid intus sit divinare est": mole, mostri e vermi in un caso di falsa gravidanza di fine Seicento', in Federica Favino (ed.), 'Oggetti di scienza', special issue, *Quaderni storici* 130:1 (2009), 125–51; John Christopoulos, *Abortion in Counter-Reformation Italy* (PhD Thesis, University of Toronto, December 2012); John Christopoulos, 'Abortion and the Confessional in Counter-Reformation Italy', *Renaissance Quarterly*, 65:2 (2012), 443–84.

[11] See McClive, 'The Hidden Truths of the Belly'; Cathy McClive, 'Blood and Expertise: The Trials of the Female Medical Expert in the Ancien-Régime Courtroom', *Bulletin of the History of Medicine*, 82:1 (2008), 86–108, esp. 93. On the rise of medical men who fashioned themselves as the best candidates to seize the complexity of the female body and expose its secrets, see Mary Fissell, *Vernacular Bodies: The Politics of Reproduction in Early Modern England* (Oxford: Oxford University Press, 2004); Monica Green, *Making Women's Medicine Masculine: The Rise of Male Authority in Pre-Modern Gynaecology* (Oxford: Oxford University Press, 2008); Park, *Secrets of Women*; Silvia De Renzi, 'The Risks of Childbirth: Physicians, Finance, and Women's Deaths in the Law Courts of Seventeenth-Century Rome', *Bulletin of the History of Medicine*, 84:4 (2011), 549–77.

[12] See, for instance, Adrian Wilson, *The Making of the Man-Midwifery: Childbirth in England, 1660–1770* (London: UCL Press, 1995).

[13] See Eve Keller, 'The Subject of Touch: Medical Authority in Early Modern Midwifery', in Elizabeth D. Harvey (ed.), *Sensible Flesh: On Touch in Early Modern Culture* (Philadelphia: University of Pennsylvania Press, 2003), 62–80; Lisa Cody, *Birthing the Nation: Sex, Science, and the Conception of Britons* (Oxford: Oxford University Press, 2005); King, *Midwifery*, esp. 73–6. See also Samuel S. Thomas, 'Early Modern Midwifery: Splitting the Profession, Connecting the History', *Journal of Social History*, 43:1 (2009), 115–38.

[14] As Claudia Pancino has suggested, in the Italian peninsula the emergence of man-midwives did not necessarily amount to the marginalization of midwives. Rather, as mid-eighteenth-century midwifery schools sought to create a class of midwives that were conversant with the language of anatomy, they generated internal divisions between the midwives who were trained in such schools and those who were not; see Claudia Pancino, *Il bambino e l'acqua sporca: Storia dell'assistenza al parto dalle mammane alle ostetriche (secoli XVI–XIX)* (Milan: Franco Angeli, 1984); Claudia Pancino, 'L'ostetricia del Settecento e la scuola bolognese di Giovanni Antonio Galli', in Bortolotti et al., *Ars obstetricia*, 24–31. On midwifery in pre-modern Italy, see also Pomata, 'Barbieri e comari'; Nadia Maria Filippini, 'Levatrici e ostetricanti a Venezia tra Sette e Ottocento', *Quaderni storici*, 58 (1985), 149–80; Nadia Maria Filippini, 'The Church, the State and Childbirth: The Midwife in Italy during the Eighteenth Century', in Hilary Marland (ed.), *The Art of Midwifery: Early Modern Midwives in Europe* (London: Routledge, 1993), 152–75; Nadia Maria Filippini, *La nascita straordinaria: Tra madre e figlio la*

role of instruments—notably forceps—in the surge of man-midwives, with a few exceptions little is still known about the historical significance and the specific contexts of the making and use of eighteenth-century midwifery models and machines.[15]

Created at a time of booming mania for anatomical displays, Galli's collection tackled the uncertainties of pregnancy and childbirth through series of anatomical models that concentrated on the parts of generation and the womb at the expense of the whole body. In doing so, it participated in the process that made female anatomy publicly available through the display of dismembered bodily parts. The collection also focused on the position of the child in the gravid uterus as the key to a successful delivery. A large number of clay wombs serialized the atypical by presenting unborn children in anomalous situations (Plates 38 and 40).[16] These models participated in the delineation of boundaries between natural (or ordinary) and preternatural (or unordinary, also called by Galli 'non-natural') childbirth, which identified those cases where delivery was particularly difficult, laborious, and dangerous.[17] In what follows, I suggest that while conjuring up these boundaries for both lay viewers and midwifery trainees, the collection drew some of its affective power from cultural as well as medical repertoires that gave visual and material expression to the realm of maternity.

Jacqueline Marie Musacchio has remarked that in early modern Italy artefacts played a central part in the culture of childbirth: 'childbirth was encouraged, celebrated and commemorated with a variety of objects', including dolls and figures of infants as well as wooden trays decorated with childbirth scenes, ceramic wares, and majolica bowls.[18] In many ways, these objects mediated between different domains of childbearing. As Christiane Klapisch-Zuber has suggested, in early modern Italy 'the borderline between devotional practices and play activities' related to maternity was a narrow one.[19] This chapter explores how the boundaries between these arenas and the medical culture of maternity were equally fluid.

rivoluzione del taglio cesareo, sec. XVII–XIX (Milan: Franco Angeli, 1995); Alessandro Pastore, *Il medico in tribunale: La perizia medica nella procedura penale d'antico regime (secoli XVI–XVIII)*, 2nd edn. (Bellinzona: Edizioni Casagrande, 2004), 129–48 and 230–6; Pancino, 'Malati, medici, mammane', 719–24.

[15] On eighteenth-century models, mannequins, and machines in midwifery schools, see Gelbart, *The King's Midwife*; King, *Midwifery*, 133–4; Lieske, '"Made in Imitation of Real Women and Children"'; Claudia Pancino and Jean d'Yvoire, *Formato nel segreto: Nascituri e feti fra immagini e immaginario dal XVI al XXI secolo* (Rome: Carocci, 2006); Lyle Massey, 'On Waxes and Wombs', in Panzanelli (ed.), *Ephemeral Bodies*, 83–105; Margaret Eileen Carlyle, *Cultures of Anatomy in Enlightenment France (c.1700–c.1795)* (PhD Thesis, McGill University, August 2012), chapter 6.

[16] On seriality in the history of nineteenth-century science, see Nick Hopwood, Simon Schaffer, and Jim Secord (eds.), 'Seriality and Scientific Objects in the Nineteenth Century', special double issue, *History of Science*, 48 (2010).

[17] Francesco Antonio Zaccaria, *Storia letteraria d'Italia*, vol. 5 (Venice: Poletti, 1753), 726. As Silvia De Renzi has observed, in early modern Italy the distinction between natural and preternatural pregnancy and childbirth was a contentious matter and played a part in legal disputes; see De Renzi, 'The Risks of Childbirth'.

[18] Jacqueline Marie Musacchio, *The Art and Ritual of Childbirth in Renaissance Italy* (New Haven: Yale University Press, 1999).

[19] See Christiane Klapisch-Zuber, *Women, Family and Ritual in Renaissance Italy*, trans. Lydia G. Cochrane (Chicago: University of Chicago Press, 1985), 310.

When Francesco Maria Zanotti presented Galli's midwifery collection in the *Commentarii*, he remarked that, in the residence of the Bolognese surgeon, childbirth was presented like a most beautiful game.[20]

Well into the eighteenth century, the use of dolls, models, and statuettes of infants made in clay, wax, wood, and soft fabric similarly bridged medical, devotional, and ludic domains.[21] As we saw in Chapter 4, at the time in which Galli commissioned a number of models from Anna Morandi, nuns like Laura Chiarini were involved in making wax figures of holy babies. Dolls and models of infants were equally employed in domains that crossed borders between the quotidian and the medical, such as the practices that were inspired by medical views on 'callipaedia', the art of generating a healthy and handsome progeny.[22] Galli's collection similarly inscribed practices and representations of pregnancy and childbirth that took place outside as well as inside the medical realm. Building on some of the representational features and conventions that characterized these domains, it brought some of their culture's affective power to bear on the world of midwifery (Plates 41 and 42). This chapter examines how Galli's midwifery models tackled the uncertainties and mysteries that were proverbially associated with generation and pregnancy through a visual and material language that addressed users' senses and affects. I argue that, while doing so, the models translated midwives' tacit and gestural knowledge into a demonstrative regime of learning that was still nonverbal and yet could be publicly communicated. As Galli's collection acquired increasing importance in the Bolognese world of licensing regulations, it came to enact a special relationship between training and licensing. As the collection participated in the creation of new forms of transfer and control of midwifery knowledge, it also redefined the relationship between skill, knowledge, and expertise.

'TIRELESS STUDIES, AFFABLE MANNERS'

Galli's pursuit of a surgical career made him a very busy man. Teaching at home and in the 'public schools', offering medical services for free in Bolognese hospitals, attending difficult births and instructing midwives and medical students, Galli was always on the move. He also made presentations at the Academy of the Sciences, cultivated a clientele of affluent patients, and engaged in correspondence with medical colleagues and friends. Even before gathering his midwifery collection, Galli had started to make a name for himself as a man-midwife. After his collection became a celebrated site of midwifery learning, he became a renowned medical practitioner. Yet, in the early years of his surgical career, obtaining

[20] Zanotti, 'De re obstetricia', 88.

[21] As Pancino and d'Yvoire have suggested, statues of the Virgin Mary whose opening belly revealed the unborn Jesus, and wax figures of baby Jesus and baby Mary mediated the worlds of maternity and childbearing to believers; see Pancino and d'Yvoire, *Formato nel segreto*, 52–3. See also Niccoli, *La vita religiosa*, 178.

[22] See Jean Louis Fischer, *L'art de faire de beaux enfants: Histoire de la callipèdie* (Paris: Albin Michel, 2009).

recognition for his efforts had not been easy. Galli had started to study medicine under the guidance of the physician Gian Antonio Stancari and the surgeon Antonio Sebastiano Trombelli.[23] In 1727, he became an assistant at the hospital of Santa Maria della Morte at a time when the high concentration of pilgrims and foreigners kept him 'extremely busy'.[24] He attended the University of Bologna while working in hospitals and dissecting cadavers. Having studied rhetoric and philosophy as well as anatomy, medicine, and surgery, in December 1731 Galli graduated both in philosophy and medicine.[25] To mark the occasion, his friends published a book of rhymes highlighting 'his tireless studies, affable manners' and the three years he had spent as assistant at Santa Maria della Morte.[26] In the following years, Galli continued to work in the hospital, and taught suturing techniques, surgical operations, and anatomy in private sessions where he noted that students lacked anatomical knowledge.[27]

In many ways, then, Galli's early career did not differ substantially from that of many other surgeons. However, things changed after he decided to devote himself to the investigation of childbirth, maintaining that this study was 'more than any other useful and necessary', though it had been overlooked.[28] In 1734, he defended 'a thesis' on 'women's deliveries', in which he presented his successful extractions of both dead and living foetuses in preternatural situations.[29] On 25 January of the following year, Galli reported at the Bolognese Academy of the Sciences on the dissection of a woman who had died in the eighth month of pregnancy.[30] The decision to study the realms of generation and childbirth seemingly paid off. In 1736, Galli became a lecturer in philosophy at the University of Bologna and subsequently taught surgery both publicly and at home.[31] Two years later, he was elected as an honorary member of the Academy of the Sciences. In 1739, he felt ready for an increase in salary. He diligently penned a list of his medical services and teaching activities, and submitted it to the Senate, but his request was turned down.[32] In 1744, he presented a new request, this time successfully, having taught surgery

[23] On Galli, see Michele Medici, 'Elogio di Gian Antonio Galli', in *Memorie della Accademia delle Scienze dell'Istituto di Bologna*, vol. 8 (Bologna: San Tommaso d'Aquino, 1857), 423–50.

[24] ASB, Assunteria di Studio, Requisiti dei Lettori, busta 40, cartella 17, 'Giovanni Antonio Galli, 1736–1782'; 'Agl'Illmi ed Eccsi SSig.ri Il Sig. Gonfaloniere, e Senatori del Reggimento di Bologna per il Dottore Gio. Antonio Andrea Galli'.

[25] Sanlorenzo, *L'insegnamento di ostetricia*, 27.

[26] *Rime in occasione di conferirsi la laurea dottorale in Filosofia, e Medicina al molt' illustre signore Gian-Antonio Galli, cittadino Bolognese, ed assistente nell'insigne Arciospedale di Santa Maria della Morte di Bologna* (Bologna: Insegna della Rosa, 1731), 3.

[27] ASB, Assunteria di Studio, Requisiti dei Lettori, busta 40, cartella 17, 'Giovanni Antonio Galli, 1736–1782'.

[28] Ibid. On the place of physicians in the pre-modern worlds of pregnancy and childbirth, see Pastore, *Il medico in tribunale*, 88–90; Park, *Secrets of Women*; Green, *Making Women's Medicine Masculine*; King, *Midwifery*; De Renzi, 'The Risks of Childbirth'.

[29] ASB, Assunteria di Studio, Requisiti dei Lettori, busta 40, cartella 17, 'Giovanni Antonio Galli, 1736–1782'.

[30] Medici, 'Elogio di Gian Antonio Galli', 436; Sanlorenzo, *L'insegnamento di ostetricia*, 27, 33, and 35.

[31] Fantuzzi, *Notizie degli scrittori bolognesi*, vol. 4 (1784), 31.

[32] ASB, Assunteria di Studio, Requisiti dei Lettori, busta 40, cartella 17, 'Giovanni Antonio Galli, 1736–1782'.

for six years to many students, including numerous foreigners, both publicly and 'privately in his house'.[33] By then, Galli had also started to offer training to midwives and assistance with difficult births. In the following years, he gathered 'at his own expense' a large collection of midwifery models that displayed all that was 'necessary to know in the art of midwifery'.[34] In 1751, when Galli submitted another request for an increase in salary, he could rely on this new, compelling credential.

The visit that dazzled Jacopo Bartolomeo Beccari 'to the point of confusion' was precisely aimed at assessing the merits of this new accomplishment.[35] Having served as *protomedico*, and having supervised medical licensing, Beccari was well positioned to assess the promise and value of Galli's collection for midwifery practice.[36] A few weeks later, on 22 November, a report to the *Assunti di Studio* illustrated the advantages of Galli's collection and concluded that it 'was bound to increase the credit of the University' and 'lure foreigners' to move to Bologna 'to practice in a matter that was of so much importance for humankind'.[37] By then, Galli had already started using the collection to teach 'young students and midwives' from the city and beyond, who gathered in his residence 'in no small number', and received instruction in the autumn and the spring in different time slots.[38]

By the time the collection was completed, calls for integrating anatomical knowledge into the world of midwifery had grown increasingly loud. Midwifery manuals, such as Sebastiano Melli's popular *La comare levatrice* (1721), encouraged midwives to attend demonstrations of the anatomy of the womb and 'the genital parts of the woman', and accordingly obtain certification from an anatomical sector.[39] The need to extend anatomy to the world of midwifery also became part of wider discussions on the 'public good'. In his *Della pubblica felicità* (1749), Ludovico Antonio Muratori emphasized that the employment of public midwives

[33] Ibid., 'Gio. Antonio Galli Lettore pubblico di Chirurgia avendo compiuto altro triennio coll'aver sempre letto a buon numero di scolari, supplica perciò riverentemente le Signorie loro Illustrissime ed Eccelsi per l'aumento del suo onorario' (25 August 1744).

[34] ASB, Assunteria di Studio, Requisiti dei Lettori, busta 40, cartella 17, 'Giovanni Antonio Galli, 1736–1782'; ASB, Assunteria di Studio, Requisiti dei Lettori, busta 40, cartella 17, 'Relazione alle SS.rie VV. Ill:me ed Ecc.se degli Assunti di Studio'. Fantuzzi reports that Galli had in his residence an inscription dating the collection to 1750; see Fantuzzi, *Notizie degli scrittori bolognesi*, vol. 4, 31.

[35] See n. 2 above. As we saw in Chapter 4, in 1756, Jacopo Bartolomeo Beccari would be entrusted with the task of assessing Anna Morandi's credentials before she was offered a position as an anatomical demonstrator at the university.

[36] See, for instance, ASB, Studio, busta 233, 'Notificazione ad ogni, e qualunque persona, che esercita l'Arte di Commare, o sia Allevatrice nel Contado di Bologna' of 20 December 1746.

[37] See ASB, Assunteria di Studio, Requisiti dei Lettori, busta 40, cartella 17, 'Relazione alle SS.rie VV. Ill:me ed Ecc.se degli Assunti di Studio'. Notably, the 'Relazione' reported almost verbatim what Beccari had already written to Scarselli; see BUB, ms. 243, Lettere di Jacopo Bartolomeo Beccari a Flaminio Scarselli, Letter of 6 November 1751 from Jacopo Bartolomeo Beccari in Bologna to Flaminio Scarselli.

[38] ASB, Assunteria di Studio, Requisiti dei Lettori, busta 40, cartella 17, 'Gio: Antonio Galli Dottore di Filosofia e Medicina Pubblico Lettore di Chirurgia umiliss.mo Oratore delle Signorie Loro Ill.me, ed Eccelse riverentem.e le supplica a graziarlo dell'aumento della lettura. [. . .] Li 30 del 1750'. See also Zaccaria, *Storia letteraria d'Italia*, vol. 5, 725–7. The training of both women and men in the practice of midwifery was not uncommon in the eighteenth century; see King, *Midwifery*, 74.

[39] Melli, *La comare levatrice*, 152.

contributed to the welfare of societies. Accordingly, he urged 'the cities, or the prince' to hire a physician or a person with expertise in anatomy to instruct women who had been chosen for this task.[40] In the same period, the process of integrating anatomy into midwifery found expression in the rich material culture of childbirth that filled the cabinets of newly founded midwifery schools, ranging from models and specimens to instruments, mannequins, dolls, and midwifery machines or 'phantoms'.

In Bologna, the idea of using artefacts and specimens to integrate anatomy into midwifery practice found a particularly fertile ground. As anatomical modelling was blossoming in the city, the development of Galli's collection intersected with that of the other Bolognese anatomical displays. As we have seen, in 1749 Giovanni Manzolini made a clay cast of the womb of a woman who had died after giving birth for the surgeon Pier Paolo Molinelli, Galli's teacher. Morandi subsequently made a copy of this model in wax.[41] Galli also commissioned some twenty wax models from Manzolini (and probably Morandi) in order to use them for the midwifery lessons that he offered in his residence. Being satisfied with the result, he decided to expand the collection. Since wax models were costly and time-consuming, the collection ended up including a large number of clay models as well as models in wax and other materials. Moreover, it resulted from the work of different artificers, including Giovanni Battista Sandri, Antonio Cartolari, and the brothers Ottavio and Nicola Toselli as well as Anna Morandi and Giovanni Manzolini.[42] By and large, however, Manzolini and especially Morandi ended up being credited as the collection's main artificers. In the *Commentarii* of 1755 Francesco Maria Zanotti, secretary of the Institute of the Sciences, praised them as the main modellers of Galli's collection.[43] Others, such as Johann Jacob Volkmann and Jérôme de Lalande, mentioned only 'Anna Manzolini' among the artificers of the collection.[44] Likewise, while reporting his visit to Galli's collection, the famous musician and music historian Charles Burney annotated in his manuscript 'Travel Diary' that 'Anna Manzolini' had made some preparations for Galli that were meant 'to show in what manner the foetus receives nourishment in the womb', a matter that, as we have seen, engaged and divided eighteenth-century anatomists.[45] Some travellers ended up associating Anna Morandi Manzolini so closely with Galli's collection that they presented her as a midwife.[46]

[40] Ludovico Antonio Muratori, *Della pubblica felicità, oggetto de buoni principi* (Lucca: n. p., 1749), 142. See also Pancino, *Il bambino e l'acqua sporca*, 85.

[41] Crespi, *Felsina pittrice*, vol. 3, 307 and 329; Medici, 'Elogio di Giovanni, e di Anna Morandi coniugi Manzolini', 6.

[42] See Marco Bortolotti, 'Il maestro alla lavagna. Il museo Galli dall'inventario al catalogo', in Bortolotti et al, *Ars obstetricia*, 21–2.

[43] Zanotti, 'De re obstetricia', 87–9.

[44] See Lalande, *Voyage d'un François en Italie*, vol. 2, 34; Volkmann, *Historisch-kritische Nachrichten von Italien*, vol. 1, 391.

[45] The Beinecke Rare Book & Manuscript Library, Yale University, New Haven, Osborn ms. c. 194, Charles Burney, 'Travel Diary', vol. 2, 9. See also Chapter 3 n. 138.

[46] See, for instance, Ekaterina Bariatinskaia's observation, in Elena Gretchanaia and Catherine Viollet (eds.), *Si tu lis jamais ce journal: Diaristes russes francophones, 1780–1854* (Paris: CNRS Éditions, 2008), 55.

SENSING CHILDBIRTH

Part of the lure of Galli's collection was that it conveyed knowledge 'visually' rather than through words. In doing so, it created a special site of non-verbal learning. As the Jesuit theologian Francesco Antonio Zaccaria (1714–1795), who succeeded Ludovico Antonio Muratori as the archivist and librarian of the duke of Modena, put it, the collection made it possible to apprehend 'materially and visually' what one 'needs to know in order to practice proficiently as a midwife'.[47] The biographer Giovanni Fantuzzi, similarly observed that Galli's models enacted a visual mode of learning.[48] Fantuzzi also noticed that the collection represented the main source of Galli's accomplishments and rewards as a medical practitioner. In fact, Galli 'did not become illustrious through a multiplicity of works published in print' but managed nonetheless to obtain renown 'through a new method no less useful for the advancement of the sciences and more advantageous to humanity'.[49] Still, printed works did play a part in the collection.

In order to make sure 'that nothing was missing', Galli's collection included 'a choice of the best books' that one could find in the art.[50] In the history of a manually based practice like midwifery, books did not feature as core training tools.[51] Yet, in Galli's collection books allowed the transfer of some of the prestige of print culture to the display. In some cases, the collection's models took inspiration from the illustrations of anatomical and midwifery treatises, and this could in turn support claims to accurate and truthful knowledge.[52] The very act of writing could provide a useful resource to redeploy the labour of the hand from the realm of manual work to that of learning.[53] A number of eighteenth-century man-midwives took up the pen and wrote midwifery manuals for courses that were offered in their newly opened midwifery schools.[54] Galli himself engaged in writing a midwifery manual in the form of dialogue, which he intended to use in his midwifery school, though he never published it. Midwifery manuals frequently encouraged midwives to learn how to read and write. However, Galli remarked that his training did not require any writing: he did not dictate to students, nor in fact did he ask them to write at all.[55] Rather, he tested their progress on the basis

47 Zaccaria, *Storia letteraria d'Italia*, vol. 5, 725–7. Here Galli's collection was discussed in the section that covered the period from September 1751 to March 1752.

48 Fantuzzi, *Notizie degli scrittori bolognesi*, vol. 4, 31.

49 Ibid., 30.

50 BUB, ms. 243, Lettere di Jacopo Bartolomeo Beccari a Flaminio Scarselli, Letter of 6 November 1751 from Jacopo Bartolomeo Beccari in Bologna to Flaminio Scarselli.

51 King, *Midwifery*, 67–8. According Mary Fissell, printing played a role in disseminating man-midwives' views; see Fissell, *Vernacular Bodies*. See also Thomas, 'Early Modern Midwifery', 126–7.

52 See Viviana Lanzarini, 'Un museo per la didattica e la sanità ostetrica', in Bortolotti et al., *Ars obstetricia*, 38.

53 See Lianne McTavish, *Childbirth and the Display of Authority in Early Modern France* (Aldershot: Ashgate, 2005), 137.

54 See, for instance, Giuseppe Vespa, *Dell'arte ostetricia* (Florence: Andrea Bonducci, 1761). See also Keller, 'The Subject of Touch', 67–8.

55 See ASM, Luoghi pii, p.a., cartella 382, '1765. Osservazioni per le scuole di Chirurgia ed Ostetricia nell'Ospital Maggiore di Milano', 'Informazione del Dottore Galli di Bologna'. On calls for midwives' need to learn to read, see, for instance, Melli, *La comare levatrice*, 152.

of 'private exercises in which he looked for the knowledge that he had publicly communicated to them'.[56]

In fact, if Galli's collection made it possible to 'apprehend visually', it was also because its models' orderly arrangement was such that it 'could be instructive by itself'.[57] A putatively self-explanatory *crescendo* was supposed to guide viewers through the sequences of models by taking them from the anatomy of the pelvis to the parts of generation, and from the study of pregnancy to the mimicking of the delivery through midwifery machines. Likewise, multiple sets of comparisons were supposed to direct the process of acquisition of midwifery knowledge. In line with the view that the study of anatomy had to start from the skeleton, the structure of the pelvis inaugurated the collection (Plate 36). Just as in the anatomy room of the Institute of the Sciences, where the skeleton was taken to reveal sexual specificity, the pelvis of a woman was placed next to that of a man 'to show the differences'.[58] The pelvis of a woman who had delivered many children was then displayed next to that of a woman who had never given birth. Galli also intended to include the model of the pelvis of a tall woman next to that of a shorter woman, but did not find a specimen that could appropriately illustrate the case. The principle of comparison similarly guided trainees' acquaintance with the bodily changes that occurred during the months of pregnancy. Accordingly, the collection showed pregnancy's temporal growth and development through differently sized models of the gravid uterus.[59]

Just like Beccari, viewers were thrilled and bewildered. Some celebrated the novelty of Galli's mode of training.[60] Yet, the techniques inscribed into Galli's collection, and notably the use of comparison, were hardly new to the world of midwifery. In fact, well before Galli gathered his collection, early modern midwives had already devised practices that relied on similar forms of visual and tactual comparison to recognize and appraise the variability of the female body. As Alessandro Pastore has noted, when, in early modern Rovio, a village in the region of Ticino, the midwife Elisabetta Prestini had to assess the case of Caterina's alleged pregnancy, she simultaneously checked and compared both visually and tactually the breasts and parts of generation of both Caterina and Giovannina, a woman of similar age who was not pregnant.[61] The method raised the eyebrows of the clergy. Yet, it was recorded as part of the midwife's expert legal report.[62] Galli's own midwifery collection drew on similar techniques of comparison to account for bodily variability: it paired bodies, compared them, and organized them in

[56] ASM, Luoghi pii, p.a., cartella 382, '1765. Osservazioni per le scuole di Chirurgia ed Ostetricia nell'Ospital Maggiore di Milano', 'Informazione del Dottore Galli di Bologna'.

[57] BUB, ms. 243, Lettere di Jacopo Bartolomeo Beccari a Flaminio Scarselli, Letter of 6 November 1751 from Jacopo Bartolomeo Beccari in Bologna to Flaminio Scarselli.

[58] ASB, Assunteria d'Istituto, Diversorum, busta 11, n. 10, 'Inventario di quanto si trova nelle due camere dell'Instituto destinate ad istruzione dell'Arte Ostetricia'. See also Lanzarini, 'Un museo per la didattica', 32–47; Murard, *La collection du médicin-chirurgien Giovan Antonio Galli*, chapter 2.

[59] ASB, Assunteria d'Istituto, Diversorum, busta 11, n. 10, 'Inventario di quanto si trova nelle due camere dell'Instituto destinate ad istruzione dell'Arte Ostetricia'.

[60] Fantuzzi, *Notizie degli scrittori bolognesi*, vol. 4, 31.

[61] Pastore, *Il medico in tribunale*, 231–3. [62] Ibid., 232.

sequences that were meant to unveil pregnancy's circumstances, clarify its ambiguities, and predict its course.[63] In many ways, then, Galli's models inscribed forms of knowledge that had long been available to midwives and spelled them out in a communicable form through the material and visual medium of the model. Turning these long-established midwifery techniques into anatomical visualizations, the collection offered Galli the opportunity to deploy this knowledge, take control over it, and advance claims of authority.

It is worth noting that Galli's models implicated the senses of users and viewers in different ways. As we have seen in the case of visitors like Beccari, models addressed the eyes and generated a sense of wonder at the sight of a display that pledged to unveil the proverbially opaque worlds of pregnancy and generation. However, in the case of training midwives, different types of models engaged users' senses in different ways. Although midwifery was typically associated with manual dexterity, midwives' long-established practices of inspection of the female body relied on the employment of both touch and sight. Galli's wax and clay models similarly introduced trainees to the anatomies of pregnancy and childbirth by engaging both the eyes and the hands. Notably, they did so in different, sometimes complementary, ways. When, in 1765, Galli wrote a memoir concerning the origins of his collection for the hospital Maggiore in Milan, which had contacted him about the prospect of creating a midwifery collection there, he noted that the high cost of wax models had weighed in favour of realizing the majority of models in clay instead.[64] However, the choice of materials was not merely driven by economic considerations. Thanks to their capacity to capture anatomical details with particular effectiveness, wax models informed the eyes about the state of affairs of the body, but were too fragile to be handled manually. Clay models offered the opportunity to highlight critical anatomical features such as figure, position, structure, and size as well as the connection between the parts, and could be examined visually or manually.[65] For instance, a number of clay models of the gravid uterus showed 'the vagina open' in order to visualize changes in the mouth of the womb during the later stages of pregnancy.[66] In another clay model, however, the vagina was closed and only an external orifice was left open to allow manual examination of the mouth of the womb.

Along with wax and clay models, the collection also included a number of 'machines'. In one of these machines, which has not survived to this day, a 'folding' puppet could be fitted in a variety of different positions in the opening and closing belly and womb of a life-size model of a woman.[67] Galli had planned to add

[63] ASB, Assunteria d'Istituto, Diversorum, busta 11, n. 10, 'Inventario di quanto si trova nelle due camere dell'Instituto destinate ad istruzione dell'Arte Ostetricia'.

[64] ASM, Luoghi pii, p.a. cartella 382, '1765. Osservazioni per le scuole di Chirurgia ed Ostetricia nell'Ospital Maggiore di Milano', 'Informazione del Dottore Galli di Bologna'.

[65] See Zaccaria, *Storia letteraria d'Italia*, vol. 5, 725–7; ASB, Assunteria d'Istituto, Diversorum, busta 11, n.10, 'Inventario di quanto si trova nelle due camere dell'Instituto destinate ad istruzione dell'Arte Ostetricia'.

[66] ASB, Assunteria d'Istituto, Diversorum, busta 11, n.10, 'Inventario di quanto si trova nelle due camere dell'Instituto destinate ad istruzione dell'Arte Ostetricia'.

[67] Ibid.

another machine with a contracting womb to give trainees the opportunity to familiarize themselves with 'the pressure and distress' of labour. However, he did not find a satisfactory mechanical device that could serve the purpose, and in the end this machine was not realized.[68] A further machine consisted of a wooden base and an opening crystal ball in lieu of the womb where a folding puppet could be fitted in a variety of different positions (Plate 39).[69] Attributed to Antonio Cartolari, a Bolognese wood carver, designer, and mechanic, this machine depicts full term pregnancy by presenting a life-size section of a mutilated female body that has been truncated from the abdomen to the cross-sectioned thighs. The model is characterized by schematic anatomical features and lacks detail. Likewise, the external genitals are replaced by a foregrounded circular cavity through which trainees were supposed to extract the folding puppet.

While clay models displayed the wide range of situations that could be encountered during pregnancy, midwifery machines were meant to test how knowledge obtained through the models translated into manual dexterity. In the case of the crystal womb, Galli inserted the puppet in the model when the students were not around. The trainees then came in blindfolded and extracted the puppet with their eyes covered. Meanwhile, Galli visually scrutinized their hands through the glass and admonished them when they did not perform the right manoeuvres.[70] The scene represented one of the pivotal moments of Galli's training. It was a spectacular act, one which combined training and surveillance with a striking performance. By blindfolding the midwives, Galli could downplay their visual skills and, at the same time, subordinate their tactual expertise to his own visual control. In doing so, he could literally and symbolically blind the midwives and use visual inspection to exercise power over their manual skills. In his *Description historique et critique de l'Italie*, Jérôme Richard further reported on midwives working blindfolded on one of Galli's midwifery machines. He noted that, while extracting the puppet from the machine, midwives had to account for their actions. They thus articulated gestural knowledge into speech. Only after they had offered enough proof of 'their intelligence and dexterity', Richard observed, was Galli willing 'to let them exercise their talents'.[71]

BLINDING KNOWLEDGE

Peculiar as it may have looked, Galli's employment of blindfolded practice in midwifery training was not carried out in isolation. And if Galli turned the act of blindfolding into an assertion of authority over midwives' visual skills, images of blindness had, in turn, been used by man-midwives to assert their own credentials

[68] Ibid.

[69] Ibid. See also ASB, Assunteria di Studio, Requisiti dei Lettori, busta 40, cartella 17, 'Relazione alle SS.rie VV. Ill: me ed Ecc.se degli Assunti di Studio'.

[70] Zanotti, 'De re obstetricia', 88.

[71] Richard, *Description historique*, vol. 2, 120–1. See also De La Porte, *Le voyageur françois*, vol. 26, 41–2.

in the world of midwifery. Since their viewing of the body of a parturient woman was restricted, early modern man-midwives sought to present their limited access to the female body as an advantage rather than a limitation.[72] A number of midwifery surgeons emphasized the benefits of relying exclusively on touch, and used their status as 'blindfolded practitioners' to construct their claims to authority on the assumption that the act of touching was more fundamental than the act of looking. As Lianne McTavish has suggested, early modern French midwifery surgeons 'claimed that obstetrical emergencies were the most demanding type of surgical procedure precisely because practitioners could see neither their clients nor what their own hands were doing inside the opaque womb'.[73]

Eighteenth-century debates on the interaction and reciprocity of the senses developed in the shadow of the so-called 'problem of Molyneux'. Suppose a man blind from birth suddenly recovers his sight—would he be able to distinguish a sphere from a cube? The question had originally been formulated in 1688 by the natural philosopher and political writer William Molyneux (1656–1698) in a letter to John Locke. The letter was then published by Locke in the second edition of his *Essay Concerning Human Understanding* (1694), and garnered much attention.[74] Raising questions about the status and reciprocity of the senses, images of blind savants permeated experimental culture. As 'the problem of Molyneux' became a much beloved topic for debate among literati and savants, it triggered numerous discussions, salon conversations, and epistolary exchanges. Denis Diderot's *Lettres sur les Aveugles* (1749) tapped into the discussion by considering the accomplishments of the blind mathematician Nicholas Saunderson.[75] In 1744, the Roman periodical *Giornale de' Letterati* presented the problem of Molyneux to Italian readers along with the review of the *Traité des sens* by the French surgeon Claude-Nicolas le Cat (1700–1768), chief-surgeon at the Hôtel-Dieu in Rouen, who had himself operated on patients suffering from cataracts.[76] Le Cat presented the case of a blind organist who could distinguish money by touch, was familiar with colours, learnt how to play cards and ended up being regarded as a dangerous adversary who could recognize the cards' figures just by shuffling them.[77] The *Giornale de' Letterati* similarly concluded that size, direction, and distance (which, as we have seen, constituted important anatomical features) belonged to the domain of touch rather than of sight and, in fact, even the sense of sight ultimately relied on it.[78]

72 McTavish, *Childbirth and the Display of Authority*, 186.

73 Ibid. On man-midwives's reliance on touch, see also King, *Midwifery*; Keller, 'The Subject of Touch'.

74 On the problem of Molyneux see, for instance, Jessica Riskin, *Science in the Age of Sensibility: The Sentimental Empiricists of the French Enlightenment* (Chicago: University of Chicago Press, 2002), chapter 2.

75 Denis Diderot, *Lettres sur les aveugles, à l'usage de ceux qui voient* (London [i.e. Paris?]: n.p., 1749).

76 See 'Riflessioni sopra i sensi Umani', *Giornale de' Letterati per l'anno MDCCXLIV pubblicato col titolo di Novelle letterarie oltramontane* (Rome: Fratelli Pagliarini, 1744), 263–70. On touching colours in the early modern period, see Schaffer, 'Regeneration', 90–2.

77 Claude-Nicolas Le Cat, *Traité des sens* (Rouen: n.p., 1740).

78 'Riflessioni sopra i sensi Umani', 270.

As touch was given primacy over sight, practices involving tactile experience promised to acquire ever more significance in the domain of knowledge. Surgeons and man-midwives seized the opportunity to turn midwifery into an arena where touch could be redeployed as a privileged attribute of learning.[79] Much as Diderot's blind mathematician could solve geometrical problems, 'blind' man-midwives characterized childbirth in terms of geometry and mechanics. The French physician Jean Astruc famously boasted of having never seen a delivery, and characterized childbirth as a mechanical problem.[80] André Levret (1703–1780) similarly maintained that childbirth was a mechanical operation that was susceptible to geometrical demonstration and, on this basis, redesigned the forceps.[81] After studying obstetrics in Paris with Levret, the surgeon Giuseppe Vespa (1727–1804), who opened a midwifery school at the Florentine hospital of Santa Maria Nuova and used anatomical and midwifery models to teach students, similarly emphasized that exact knowledge of the mechanical laws of childbirth was necessary for practising obstetrics.[82]

Signposting the transformation of midwives' manual dexterity into a realm of instrument-led precision and controlled gesturality, midwifery instruments like the forceps became the material correlate of calls for the transformation of childbirth into a geometrically defined mechanical phenomenon based on the primacy of touch. As is well known, not everybody surrendered to the forceps' lure and eighteenth-century satires and caricatures warned about its risks.[83] Even some famous man-midwives, such as William Hunter (1718–1783), had misgivings about its use.[84] Yet, the forceps ended up being fashioned as an emblem of the accomplished man-midwife, and entered the world of portraiture. Realized by the Bolognese artist Angelo Crescimbeni, Galli's own portrait drew on this repertoire. Completed in 1775, the portrait presented Galli at the height of his career, sporting a large wig and an ermine while brandishing the Levret forceps acquired when Benedict XIV purchased his collection (Plate 43).[85] Taking a closer look at the image, however, one may wonder whether Galli's somewhat faltering grasp of the forceps raises questions about his attitude towards it. Upon visiting the collection, Beccari noticed that Galli had gathered as many instruments as possible 'for the extraction

[79] Keller, 'The Subject of Touch', 70.

[80] Jean Astruc, *L'art d'accoucher réduit à ses principes, où l'on expose les pratiques les plus sûres & les plus usitées dans les différentes espèces d'accouchements* (Paris: Cavelier, 1771).

[81] André Levret, *L'art des accouchemens, démontré par des principes de physique et de mécanique*, 3rd edn. (Paris: Didot Le Jeune, 1766).

[82] Vespa, *Dell'arte ostetricia.*

[83] See, for instance, Laurence Sterne, *The Life and Opinions of Tristram Shandy, Gentleman* (London: J. Dosdley, 1761), 70ff. See also Keller, 'The Subject of Touch'.

[84] Wilson, *The Making of Man-Midwifery*, part 2. As Lianne McTavish has remarked, in late seventeenth-/early eighteenth-century France the use of instruments remained controversial, and man-midwives insisted 'that their hands were specialised tools capable of managing any delivery'; see McTavish, *Childbirth and the Display of Authority*, 13.

[85] On the acquisition of the Levret forceps, see ASB, Assunteria d'Istituto, Diversorum, busta 11, n. 10, 'Nota di spese fatta dal Dottore Gio. Ant.o Galli intorno la suppellettile ostetricia, dopocche fù acquistata da Papa Benedetto XIV'. See also Lanzarini, 'Un museo per la didattica', 40–1.

of the foetus'.[86] Likewise, when Galli presented the midwifery machines in the inventory of the collection, he mentioned that the extraction of the foetus would take place 'with the help of the hand or of the instruments'.[87] Yet, a close look at the records of Galli's collection, practice, and training seems to suggest that he might have favoured manual dexterity over the use of instruments. Galli's own views of generation, and in particular his endorsement of the role of the maternal imagination, were seemingly at odds with the use of invasive tools.

MODELLING MATERNITY

Views of the maternal imagination postulated that the body of the unborn child was soft and malleable and thus had to be handled with particular care. Such views maintained that the imagination of the expectant mother had the power to model the soft physical matter of the unborn. In particular, striking sights, unruly thoughts and passions, and unfulfilled cravings experienced by mothers at the time of conception and during pregnancy were taken to affect the shape of the child.[88] While attributing special powers to the relationship between the mothers' sights and desires and the soft fabric of the child, the notion of material imagination ascribed an almost tangible quality to visual perception. Dating back to the ancient period, accounts of maternal imagination sat well with views of generation that drew on the language of impression.[89] They portrayed women's bodies as soft and malleable, and generation as the result of the impression of soft matter.[90] By the mid-eighteenth century, generation had become contested terrain.[91] Supporters of epigenesis who conceptualized generation as a process were set against preformationists who maintained that the preformed child was provided by one parent and grew

[86] BUB, ms. 243, Lettere di Jacopo Bartolomeo Beccari a Flaminio Scarselli, Letter of 6 November 1751 from Jacopo Bartolomeo Beccari in Bologna to Flaminio Scarselli.

[87] ASB, Assunteria d'Istituto, Diversorum, busta 11, n.10, 'Inventario di quanto si trova nelle due camere dell'Instituto destinate ad istruzione dell'Arte Ostetricia'.

[88] See Herman W. Roodenburg, 'The Maternal Imagination: The Fears of Pregnant Women in Seventeenth-Century Holland', *Journal of Social History*, 21:4 (1988), 701–16; Massimo Angelini, 'Il potere plastico dell'immaginazione nelle gestanti tra XVI e XVIII secolo: La fortuna di un'idea', *Intersezioni*, 14:1 (1994), 53–69; Claudia Pancino, *Voglie materne: Storia di una credenza* (Bologna: CLUEB, 1996); De Renzi, 'Resemblance, Paternity and Imagination', 61–83; Mary Terrall, 'Material Impressions: Conception, Sensibility, and Inheritance', in Helen Deutsch and Mary Terrall (eds.) *Vital Matters: Eighteenth-Century Ideas about Conception, Life and Death* (Toronto: University of Toronto Press, 2012), 109–29.

[89] See Jane Fair Bestor, 'Ideas about Procreation and Their Influence on Ancient and Medieval Views of Kinship', in David I. Kertzer and Richard P. Saller (eds.), *The Family in Italy from Antiquity to the Present* (New Haven: Yale University Press, 1991), 150–67, esp. 152–9; Katharine Park, 'Impressed Images: Reproducing Wonders', in Peter Galison and Caroline A. Jones (eds.), *Picturing Science, Producing Art* (New York: Routledge, 1998), 254–71, esp. 257–9.

[90] Margreta de Grazia, 'Imprints: Shakespeare, Gutenberg and Descartes', in Terence Hawkes (ed.), *Alternative Shakespeares* (London: Routledge, 1996), vol. 2, 63–94.

[91] See Clara Pinto-Correia, *The Ovary of Eve: Egg and Sperm and Preformation* (Chicago: University of Chicago Press, 1997); Ivano dal Prete, 'Cultures and Politics of Preformationism in Eighteenth-Century Italy', in Raymond Stephanson and Darren N. Wagner (eds.), *The Secrets of Generation: Reproduction in the Long Eighteenth Century* (Toronto: University of Toronto Press, 2015), 59–78.

only in dimension. Over the course of the eighteenth century, preformationism remained largely dominant and was in turn divided into ovists and animalculists, depending on whether, respectively, the mother or the father was taken to supply the preformed child.

Controversies over the nature of generation had implications for the doctrine of maternal imagination.[92] Some preformationists raised doubts about the likelihood that maternal imagination might affect a body whose shape was already determined. Still, support for maternal imagination continued to have wide currency, and numerous naturalists and medical practitioners endorsed it even when they declared that they were unable to account for it. In 1721, for instance, Antonio Vallisneri, a defender of ovist preformationism, observed that portraits of ancestors played a part in granting family resemblance over time because they affected the imagination of the mother and thus contributed to shape the appearance of the child along the lines of family resemblance.[93] Yet, he admitted that he was uncertain about the workings of the maternal imagination.[94] In the following decades, others, such as the anatomist Giambattista Morgagni, were not quite sure what to think.[95] Ludovico Antonio Muratori similarly expressed perplexity. But he also maintained that if animal spirits impressed the brain with the ideas of figures, colours, smells, sounds, and tastes, nothing in principle prevented them from imprinting the 'very soft' bodies of unborn children with particular marks and shapes.[96] Muratori thus associated the maternal imagination with the imprinting of ideas of the senses on the soft matter of the brain. As we noticed in Chapter 4, wax offered a particularly well-suited material to express such patterns of impression. In Galli's collection, one of the wax models visually recorded the case of a malformed child whose mother had skinned frogs for the bakery where she had worked while pregnant (Plate 44). Galli had presented the case on 10 May 1764 at the Bolognese Academy of the Sciences.[97]

Much has been written on the role of the maternal imagination in early modern accounts of 'monstrous births'.[98] But precisely because views of the influence of

[92] See Philip K. Wilson, '"Out of Sight, Out of Mind?": The Daniel Turner-James Blondel Dispute Over the Power of the Maternal Imagination', *Annals of Science*, 49:1 (1992), 63–85.

[93] Antonio Vallisneri, *Istoria della generazione dell' uomo e degli animali; se sia da'vermicelli spermatici, o dalle uova* (Venice: Gio. Gabbriel Hertz, 1721), 240–1. On resemblance and maternal imagination in early modern Italy, see De Renzi, 'Resemblance, Paternity and Imagination'.

[94] Vallisneri, *Istoria della generazione*, 59–60.

[95] Alfonso Corradi, *Dell'ostetricia in Italia dalla metà dello scorso secolo fino al presente* (Bologna: Gamberini e Parmeggiani, 1874), 355.

[96] Muratori, *Della forza della fantasia umana*, 104–6 (citation p. 106).

[97] Archivio dell'Antica Accademia delle Scienze, Bologna, Reg. Atti, Giovanni Antonio Galli, 'Sopra alcuni mostri', 10 May 1764. See also Medici, 'Elogio di Gian Antonio Galli', 444–5; Pancino, *Voglie materne*, 141; Valeria P. Babini, 'Anatomica, medica, chirurgica', in Walter Tega (ed.), *Anatomie Accademiche*, vol. 2 (Bologna: Il Mulino, 1987), 71 and n. 20; Lanzarini, 'Un museo per la didattica', 42; Marco Bortolotti and Viviana Lanzarini, 'Catalogo ed inventario', in Bortolotti et al., *Ars obstetricia*, 100.

[98] See, for instance, Marie-Hélène Huet, *Monstrous Imagination* (Cambridge, MA: Harvard University Press, 1993); Valeria Finucci, 'Maternal Imagination and Monstrous Birth: Tasso's *Gerusalemme Liberata*', in Valeria Finucci and Kevin Brownlee (eds.), *Generation and Degeneration: Tropes of Reproduction in Literature and History from Antiquity through Early Modern Europe* (Durham: Duke University Press, 2001), 41–77; Mary E. Fissell, 'Hairy Women and Naked Truths: Gender and

maternal imagination were centred on the relationship between seeing, craving, and imagining, a whole apparatus of images, portraits, paintings, and sculptures also accompanied early modern domains of conception and pregnancy with the purpose of enhancing the generation of beautiful and healthy progeny. Elaborating on artistic ideals of beauty, nuptial dolls made in wax, sugar, and plaster similarly circulated among pregnant women in order to propitiate the making of beautiful children.[99] In his popular poem *Callipaedia, seu de pulchrae prolis habendae ratione* (1655), the seventeenth-century physician Claude Quillet invited mothers who wanted to give birth to beautiful daughters to look at images of the 'Paphian Goddess' (Venus), such as the one painted by Titian, and those wishing to generate good-looking sons to gaze upon pictures of the statue of Apollo.[100] As well as attributing special powers to the mother's thoughts and cravings, accounts of maternal imagination also presupposed that the body of the child was soft and impressionable. In the sixteenth century, the French surgeon Ambroise Paré (1510–1590) characterized the unborn child as consisting of soft matter that was like wax, and was therefore ready to receive forms and shapes from the imagination of the mother.[101] Unborn children's tender and malleable bodies put them at risk of being disfigured during delivery.[102] Midwives were then encouraged to take particular care in order not to compromise the children's appearance. Quillet, for instance, urged midwives 'not to spoil the Figure of the coming Boy / Nor with

the Politics of Knowledge in *Aristotle's Masterpiece*', *The William and Mary Quarterly*, 60:1 (2003), 43–74; Fissell, *Vernacular Bodies*, esp. 207ff. See also Ottavia Niccoli, '"Menstruum Quasi Monstruum": Monstrous Births and Menstrual Taboo in the Sixteenth Century', trans. Mary M. Gallucci, in Edward Muir and Guido Ruggiero (eds.), *Sex and Gender in Historical Perspective* (Baltimore: Johns Hopkins University Press, 1990), 1–25.

99 See Klapisch-Zuber, *Women, Family, and Ritual*, 317–18. Leon Battista Alberti famously suggested decorating the places of conception with 'portraits of men of dignity, and handsome appearance' because they could influence 'the fertility of the mother and the appearance of future offspring'. In the mid-sixteenth century, Giovan Battista della Porta similarly observed that women who wanted to generate beautiful children had to adorn their bedroom with beautiful figures, either in sculpture or painting; see Leon Battista Alberti, *On the Art of Building in Ten Books*, trans. J. Rykwert et al. (Cambridge, MA: MIT Press, 1988 [1452]), 299; Giovan Battista Della Porta, *De i miracoli et marauigliosi effetti dalla natura prodotti, Libri IIII* (Venice: Marc'Antonio Zaltieri, 1584 [1560]), 91–2. See also Park, 'Impressed Images'; Finucci, 'Maternal Imagination', 54 and 59; Geraldine A. Johnson, 'Beautiful Brides and Model Mothers: The Devotional and Talismanic Functions of Early Modern Marian Reliefs', in McClanan and Rosoff Encarnación (eds.), *The Material Culture of Sex*, 135–61.

100 Claude Quillet, *Callipaedia: or, the Art of getting Beautiful Children; a Poem, in Four Books, Written in Latin by Claudius*, trans. N. Rowe (London: W. Feales, 1733), 74. Quillet's book underwent numerous editions and was translated into different languages well into the eighteenth century. On the art of making beautiful children, see Fischer, *L'art de faire de beaux enfants*.

101 Ambroise Paré, *On Monsters and Marvels*, trans. Janis L. Pallister (Chicago: University of Chicago Press, 1983), 54.

102 The idea that the bodies of unborn children were soft and pliable was reflected in eighteenth-century anatomical displays. In his project for an anatomy room at the Institute of the Sciences, for instance, Ercole Lelli remarked that 'the skeleton of a foetus' was displayed to show that 'the bones of foetuses are for the most part cartilaginous and membranous', see ASB, Assunteria d'Istituto, Diversorum, busta 10, n. 2.

distorted Limbs the beauteous Work destroy' for in fact the 'little Joints' were 'pliant to command / Tender, and waxen to the moulding Hand'.[103]

Well into the eighteenth century, views of maternal imagination continued to draw attention to the tender nature of the unborn child, warning about the risk that an improperly handled childbirth could end up affecting its bodily integrity.[104] Portraying handsomely formed babies as angelic and cute *putti*, Galli's models evoked the visual world that populated the art of making beautiful children (Plates 41 and 42). Made in malleable materials such as clay and wax, they reminded viewers of the soft corporeal nature of the child. Presenting the unborn in a multiplicity of situations, the clay models also recalled how the mishandling of childbirth could end in disaster. Lianne McTavish has drawn attention to early modern images of unborn children portrayed in situations of impending risk while showing 'blissful expressions on their faces'.[105] She has argued that such images instantiated sites of negotiation for midwifery authority because they created a space for the intervention of the surgeon to guarantee the safety and integrity of the newborn.[106] In the case of Galli's collection, the models of handsome children caught in situations of imminent danger evoked the risks and uncertainties related to childbirth. In doing so, they called for the need to acquire appropriate manual and anatomical skills. The models presented in Plates 45 and 46, for instance, seemingly warned trainees and viewers about the challenges of a situation in which unborn children, who showed the most serene and beatific expressions, were presented in unordinary situations and trapped in a tangle of twisted and contorted limbs.

A *PORTELLA* AT THE INSTITUTE OF THE SCIENCES

Just like the other anatomical displays of Bologna, Galli's midwifery collection promised to take the city to the forefront of the anatomical world and attracted the interest of Grand Tour travellers. Its models came to define a multifunctional space of touristic curiosity and training practice as well as anatomical knowledge and bodily spectacle, a site for defining human nature and celebrating the promises of anatomy in tackling bodily mysteries even in as elusive and uncertain an arena as that of generation and pregnancy. Like Beccari, many remained deeply impressed, being amazed by the display's marvel and excited by its practical promise. As Beccari noticed in 1751, a 'Swedish physician', who had seen Galli's collection, had commented that the art of midwifery would not be better learnt in Paris than in Bologna.[107] Two years later, Zaccaria similarly observed that

[103] Quillet, *Callipaedia*, 87. According to McTavish, the appearance in early modern France of perfectly formed, intact, and undamaged infants in the portraits of man-midwives pointed to the latter's claims of expertise in preserving the integrity of the newborn; see McTavish, *Childbirth and the Display of Authority*, 128–9.

[104] Corradi, *Dell'ostetricia*, 354–5.

[105] McTavish, *Childbirth and the Display of Authority*, 173.

[106] Ibid., chapter 6.

[107] BUB, ms. 243, Lettere di Jacopo Bartolomeo Beccari a Flaminio Scarselli, Letter of 6 November 1751 from Jacopo Bartolomeo Beccari in Bologna to Flaminio Scarselli.

French and English visitors had been dazzled by its '*maraviglia*'.[108] Just like Bologna's other anatomical displays, the collection was celebrated in travellers' reports as well as in the local press. Jérôme de Lalande famously referred to it as 'one of the most singular things in Europe for the study of anatomy'.[109] Charles Burney similarly raved about the 'wonderful collection of preparation or models of all parts of the uterus and matrix in every state and of the foetus in all situations, for the use of young students in midwifery and anatomy'.[110]

While generating widespread satisfaction, foreigners' enthusiasm also raised some concerns. In 1751, Galli had assured the Senate that he had no intention of selling the collection.[111] However, two years later Zaccaria warned that foreign buyers could become interested in acquiring it and transferring it abroad.[112] Meanwhile, news about the midwifery models continued to spread. In 1755, when Francesco Maria Zanotti presented the collection in the Institute's *Commentarii*, he increased its visibility among learned readers and literati.[113] The following year, Cardinal Giovanni Giacomo Millo, prefect of the Congregation of the Council and prodatary, tried to convince Pope Benedict XIV to acquire Galli's *supellettile* for the benefit of the Institute of the Sciences. In the summer of 1757, Flaminio Scarselli informed Galli that the pope had expressed interest in the proposal. Galli was pleased, but remained cautious.[114] As he mentioned to Scarselli, he was aware that the collection had triggered jealousy and hostility as much as it had generated appreciation. For one thing, the Marquis Sigismondo Malvezzi, the Institute's representative who had been designated as the broker of the affair, had not even bothered to visit it, in spite of repeated invitations. According to Galli, Malvezzi did not do anything in the Institute without the advice and guidance of Ercole Lelli. But Lelli had kept his distance from the midwifery models because of their association with Morandi and Manzolini. Moreover, in Galli's view, Lelli had also adopted a hostile stance because, compared to the midwifery collection, the models he had made for the anatomy room showed signs of deterioration and cracking.[115] Even Galli's friend and colleague Pier Paolo Molinelli had not had anything good to say about the midwifery collection. Quite the opposite: possibly because he had not been involved in its making and use, Molinelli had bad-mouthed the collection, discouraging some people from going to see it, and praising and employing midwifery practitioners who had not trained with Galli.[116]

Still, things moved forward quickly. By the end of August, Marco Antonio Laurenti offered Galli 1000 scudi (*c.*5,000 Bolognese lire) for the collection.[117]

[108] Zaccaria, *Storia letteraria d'Italia*, vol. 5, 727.

[109] Lalande, *Voyage d'un François en Italie*, vol. 2, 34.

[110] The Beinecke Rare Book & Manuscript Library, Yale University, New Haven, Osborn ms. c. 194, Charles Burney, 'Travel Diary', vol. 2, 9.

[111] ASB, Assunteria di Studio, Requisiti dei Lettori, busta 40, cartella 17, 'Relazione alle SS.rie VV. Ill: me ed Ecc.se degli Assunti di Studio'.

[112] Zaccaria, *Storia letteraria d'Italia*, vol. 5, 727.

[113] Zanotti, 'De re obstetricia', 87–9.

[114] BUB, ms. 72, Corrispondenza Letteraria dell'abate Flaminio Scarselli, vol. 1, Letter of 20 August 1757 from Giovanni Antonio Galli in Bologna to Flaminio Scarselli, fols. 100v–101r.

[115] Ibid., fol. 100r.

[116] Ibid., fols. 100v–101r.

[117] Ibid., vol. 1, Letter of 29 August 1757 from Giovanni Antonio Galli in Bologna to Flaminio Scarselli, fols. 102r–103v.

Cardinal Millo was called in to mediate the affair and the Marquis Malvezzi was in charge of finalizing the agreement. The contract was signed on 14 November 1757.[118] Two days later, Millo's untimely demise did not interfere with the plan. On 19 November, a letter addressed to the ambassador in Rome celebrated the purchase of the midwifery collection as the highlight of an already very fruitful year of papal patronage at the Institute of the Sciences.[119] Two rooms were then allocated to the midwifery collection on the ground floor of the Institute: one for the models, and the other for training on the machines.[120] Galli was keen to make sure that the order and layout of the collection at the Institute remained the same as in his residence.[121] Fearing that the ever-hostile Lelli might be charged with the task of supervising the display, and could therefore be in a position to boycott it, he asked and obtained permission to maintain control over the arrangement of the collection.[122]

The transferral of the collection to the Institute of the Sciences marked a rare entrée of midwives and midwifery practice into the world of eighteenth-century academies. However, finding a suitable space for midwifery learning within academic premises was not an easy task. Issues concerning the display of artefacts and specimens occupied the thoughts and energies of the *Assunti* of the Institute of the Sciences, generating recurrent discussions and negotiations about the location, dislocation, and arrangement of things. More importantly, locating midwifery practice within the Bolognese temple of natural inquiry and experimental culture was no straightforward matter. Along with Galli's models, midwives entered the academic world. But their admission did not take place without reservations. Part of the fame of the Institute of the Sciences was associated with the activities of the very famous natural philosopher Laura Bassi who, along with the mathematician Maria Gaetana Agnesi and the anatomical modeller Anna Morandi, had benefited from papal patronage.[123] Yet, accommodating less famous and lower-status women such as midwives within academic premises was quite another thing. Upon donating the collection to the Institute of the Sciences, Pope Benedict XIV explicitly requested that a small door (*portella* or *portino*) be opened on the side of the building to prevent midwives from entering the Institute through the main door.[124] The room adjoined to the *portella* was assigned to 'the women'.[125] The fireplace was then dismantled, and benches were provided for the midwives to sit on when they assembled before accessing the collection.[126]

[118] ASB, Ufficio del Registro, Libro delle Copie, n. 674, fol. 191v.

[119] ASB, Assunteria d'Istituto, Lettere dell'Istituto, n. 4 (1756–65), Letter of 19 November 1757 from the Institute to the ambassador.

[120] Richard, *Description historique*, vol. 2, 120–1; De La Porte, *Le voyageur françois*, vol. 26, 41–2. See also Fantuzzi, *Notizie degli scrittori bolognesi*, vol. 4, 32.

[121] ASB, Assunteria di Studio, Requisiti dei Lettori, busta 40, cartella 17, 'Relazione alle SS.rie VV. Ill:me ed Ecc.se degli Assunti di Studio'.

[122] BUB, ms. 72, Corrispondenza Letteraria dell'abate Flaminio Scarselli, vol. 1, Letter of 20 August 1757 from Giovanni Antonio Galli in Bologna to Flaminio Scarselli, fol. 101r.

[123] See Chapter 4.

[124] ASB, Ufficio del Registro, Libro delle Copie, n. 674, fol. 191v.

[125] ASB, Assunteria d'Istituto, Atti, n. 5 (1754–60), 5 April 1759.

[126] See ASB, Assunteria d'Istituto, Atti, n.5 (1754–60), 4 November 1757 and 20 April 1759; ASB, Assunteria d'Istituto, Diversorum, busta 11, n. 10, Letter of 7 November 1757 from Cardinal Millo.

The opening of a side entrance for midwives pointed to a difference in status. It also revealed a concern about the possibility that midwives could wander around the Institute and mingle with other visitors. Galli's own teaching sessions were supposed to be scheduled in the days 'in which the other Professors' were 'not busy in their exercises', namely, when nobody else was around.[127] However, as we have seen, some visitors did report on Galli's training practices. Notably, while the arrival of midwives brought about a spatial segregation within the Institute's premises, the need to keep spaces that were representative of the public image of the Institute under control was of more general concern. Now and again, apprehensions were expressed about the levels of decorum of the area surrounding the Institute's entrance and 'under the arcades'. On 5 April 1759, moreover, the Institute's *Assunti* decided that medical students who attended Galli's lessons had to gather in the 'room of the Painters' or 'the rooms of the Assunteria' so as to avoid hanging out in front of the Institute's entrance before their classes.[128]

Upon selling the collection, Galli had hoped to receive some personal reward, and to continue to teach and make demonstrations based on the models.[129] On 3 December 1757, his wishes were fulfilled as the Institute's *Assunti* read the papal letter that recommended appointing him as 'professor of obstetrics' to carry out midwifery teaching at the Institute. He would then receive an annual emolument of 200 lire as a complement to his salary as a university professor.[130] When, in October 1758, the time came to publish the list of the Institute's professors, it was decided to include Galli's name, though 'after the name of Pier Paolo Molinelli'.[131] For Galli, the benefits of having his collection relocated to the Institute's premises were manifold. Along with periodicals' accounts and Grand Tourists' reports, the papal acquisition further fuelled Galli's medical fame. In the spring of 1758, while the models were still making their way from his residence to the Institute of the Sciences, Galli was called to the Principality of Monaco to become the *accoucheur* of the Princess Maria Caterina di Brignole-Sale, who was about to deliver her first child. Galli arrived in Monaco along with a student and a servant on 13 April 1758, and spent the following days studying while waiting for the delivery. When he was drawn into courtly betting on the sex of the unborn, he argued against Père Serafin's prediction that the child would be a boy, proving himself wrong.[132] But overall the trip was a success. After the birth of Prince Honoré IV on 17 May, Galli returned to Bologna where he cultivated a clientele of affluent patients among prominent Bolognese families.[133]

[127] ASB, Assunteria d'Istituto, Atti, n. 5 (1754–60), 26 October 1758.

[128] Ibid., 5 April 1759.

[129] BUB, ms. 72, Corrispondenza Letteraria dell'abate Flaminio Scarselli, vol. 1, Letter of 24 August 1757 from Giovanni Antonio Galli in Bologna to Flaminio Scarselli, fols. 102r–v.

[130] ASB, Assunteria d'Istituto, Atti, n. 5 (1754–60), 3 December 1757; ASB, Assunteria d'Istituto, Diversorum, busta 15, n. 34; ASB, Senato, Partiti, n. 39 (1756–61), 17 December 1757, fols. 63r–64r.

[131] ASB, Assunteria d'Istituto, Atti, n. 5 (1754–60), 26 October 1758.

[132] Archives du Palais Princier (Principality of Monaco), ms. B 28, Letter of 14 April 1758.

[133] For instance, as soon as he came back from Monaco, Galli attended the pregnancy and childbirth of the Countess Marsigli; see BUB, ms. 72, Corrispondenza Letteraria dell'abate Flaminio Scarselli, vol. 1, Letter of 1 May 1758.

Back at the Institute, Galli started to offer midwifery courses consisting of fifty-five to sixty lessons taking place in the springtime.[134] In 1760, he was assigned an assistant to help with the demonstrations.[135] Over time, training on Galli's collection was integrated with anatomical teaching carried out in the Institute's anatomy room. Due to Lelli's negative attitude towards Galli's collection, in the years following its arrival at the Institute of the Sciences coordinating the teaching activities on the two collections was not easy. However, as we observed in Chapter 2, after Lelli died in March 1766, and Luigi Galvani replaced him as the demonstrator of the anatomy room, it was decided that teaching in the two rooms would be synchronized so that Galvani would perform demonstrations from Lent to May or June, or at the time in which '*Dottor* Galli teaches the art of obstetrics'.[136] The teaching schedule accordingly had to avoid conflicts between Galli's and Galvani's lessons, thus giving students the opportunity to attend both.[137] By the early 1770s, training on both collections turned into a significant qualification for applicants to the position of assistant surgeon at the hospital of Santa Maria della Morte.[138] Over time, Galli's models also acquired increasing significance in the licensing system that sought to regulate and scrutinize midwifery practice.[139]

MODELS, TRAINING, AND LICENSING

One of the purposes of Galli's training activities was to prepare midwives for their licensing exams at the Protomedicato. Originally established in Bologna in 1517 as part of the College of Physicians, the Protomedicato was in charge of monitoring healers and practitioners, and issuing licences to those who passed the examination successfully.[140] In 1686 it extended its control to midwives, who had formerly relied on the bishopric for their licensing.[141] Along with other practitioners such as barber-surgeons and apothecaries, midwives were regularly required to take licensing exams. Well into the eighteenth century, public notices such as *bandi*, *editti*, and *notificazioni* urged practitioners to present their licences to the medical authorities as a condition for inclusion in the new register (*catalogo*) of *speziali*,

[134] ASB, Assunteria d'Istituto, Atti, n. 5 (1754–60), 26 October 1758. See also ASB, Assunteria di Studio, Requisiti dei Lettori, busta 40, cartella 17, 'Relazione alle SS.rie VV. Ill:me ed Ecc.se degli Assunti di Studio'. Over time, the lectures ended up being reduced to thirty.

[135] See ASB, Assunteria d'Istituto, Diversorum, busta 15, n. 34; ASB, Assunteria d'Istituto, Atti, n.5 (1754–60), 3 December 1757 and 26 October 1758.

[136] ASB, Assunteria Instituto, Atti, n. 6 (1761–75), fol. 76v.

[137] Ibid., fol. 78v. On Galvani's midwifery teaching, see Leonardo Giardina (ed.), *Lezioni inedite di ostetricia di Luigi Galvani* (Bologna: CLUEB, 1965).

[138] See Chapter 2 n. 144.

[139] ASM, Luoghi pii, p.a., cartella 382, '1765. Osservazioni per le scuole di Chirurgia ed Ostetricia nell'Ospital Maggiore di Milano', 'Informazione del Dottore Galli di Bologna'.

[140] On the history of the Protomedicato and its impact on healing practice, see, for instance, Gentilcore, *Healers and Healing*, esp. chapter 2; Gentilcore, *Medical Charlatanism*; Pomata, *Contracting a Cure*.

[141] Pomata, *Contracting a Cure*, 64.

surgeons, and midwives.[142] Notices also reminded midwives of the constraints of their practice, such as the prohibition on prescribing internal remedies and carrying out bloodletting without a request from a physician, as well as on teaching how to perform abortions or prescribing abortifacients.[143] As Gianna Pomata has observed, in early modern Bologna healers were not so much punished 'for being unskilled' as 'simply for not having a license'.[144] The renewal of their licence was accordingly given priority over other requirements. The frequency with which the Protomedicato issued *bandi* 'on the abuses introduced in Bologna concerning the Profession of Medicine', and called on barbers, midwives, and apothecaries to renew their licences, may be a sign that, recurrent and insistent as they might have been, attempts to monitor practitioners were only partially successful. A large number of these *bandi* were undersigned by Bolognese physicians and surgeons whom we have encountered in the course of this work, such as Germano Azzoguidi, Jacopo Bartolomeo Beccari, Lorenzo Antonio Bonazzoli, Marco Antonio Laurenti and, indeed, Giovanni Antonio Galli, who participated in the activities of the Protomedicato and its attempt to regulate and monitor medical and midwifery practice in the city.[145] Galli's own collection promised to expand the scope of institutional control over midwives and became increasingly associated with the circumstances of licensing regulations. It is worth noting that not long before visiting and assessing Galli's collection, Jacopo Bartolomeo Beccari had served as a *protomedico*, and in this capacity he undersigned *notificazioni* and *bandi* that addressed midwives, surgeons, and apothecaries.[146] Galli himself occupied influential positions within the Bolognese licensing board and served both as prior of the College of Physicians and *protomedico*.[147] Moreover, he participated in the system of control set out by the Protomedicato by preparing midwives for the licensing exams. In a note of 27 April 1746, for instance, he certified that he had

[142] See, for instance, ASB, Assunteria di Studio, busta 233, 'Bandi, Editti, e Notificazioni del Protomedicato e provviggioni spettanti alla Citta' di Bologna dal 1571 a tutto il 1769': 'Notificazioni alli Barbieri, e Comari' of 21 August 1710 and 'Notificazioni alli Barbieri, e Comari' of 5 May 1711, and 'Notificazione alli Speziali, Chirurghi, e Comari' of 8 April 1772. Practitioners residing in the city were normally given 'fifteen days' to report to the Protomedicato, though allowances of up to thirty days were granted to those living in the countryside.

[143] See ASB, Studio, busta 233, 'Bandi, Editti, e Notificazioni del Protomedicato e provviggioni spettanti alla Citta' di Bologna dal 1571 a tutto il 1769', 'Editto per li Speciali, Barbiari, Comari, & altri' of 26 August 1683'.

[144] Pomata, *Contracting a Cure*, 83–4 (citation p. 84).

[145] 'Bandi, Editti, e Notificazioni del Protomedicato e provviggioni spettanti alla Citta' di Bologna dal 1571 a tutto il 1769'.

[146] Ibid., 'Notificazione ad ogni, e qualunque persona, che esercita l'Arte di Commare, o sia Allevatrice nel Contado di Bologna' of 20 December 1746; 'Notificazione alli chirurghi di primo grado' of 13 October 1749; 'Notificazione' of 27 July 1763'.

[147] For example, Giovanni Antonio Galli was prior of the College of Physicians and of the Protomedicato at the time of the publication of the 'Notificazione sopra l'osservanza della Tariffa dei Medicinali Semplici, Composti, e Spagirici' of 31 January 1765, and *protomedico* at the time of the publication of the 'Bando, e Provisione. Sopra gli abusi introdotti a Bologna, intorno la Professione della Medicina' on 25 November 1768; see ASB, Assunteria di Studio, busta 233, 'Bandi, Editti, e Notificazioni del Protomedicato e provviggioni spettanti alla Citta' di Bologna dal 1571 a tutto il 1769'.

trained Maria Flaminia Mellini, who was then ready to take the exams and was fit for 'the art of obstetrics'.[148] Two days later, Mellini was approved for practise.[149]

After Galli started to base his training on the collection, he continued to certify midwives who took their licensing exams. Although training under Galli and obtaining his certification was not a necessary requirement for licensing, his collection acquired increasing significance as a licensing as well as a training tool. When, in 1765, Galli discussed the origins of his collection for the benefit of the hospital Maggiore in Milan, he explained that at the time no law obliged midwives to train on the collection. Even if they received training elsewhere, they could still be approved so long as they passed the exam. However, Galli added, the *Assunteria di Studio* and the College of Physicians were about to deliberate on the proposal that every woman who wanted to exercise the art of obstetrics should be required to attend his midwifery course. In any case, a certification from the 'professor of obstetrics' at the Institute of the Sciences was undoubtedly advantageous to 'those women who wanted to take the exam at the College of Physicians' and be licensed.[150] And indeed the registers of the Protomedicato indicated when midwives had trained with Galli.[151] In the 1760s, Jérôme Richard similarly noticed a close connection between licensing and training on Galli's collection. He wrote that midwives were allowed to practise 'only after having done a course of study at the Institute'.[152]

RELIGIOUS LICENSING

As Galli's collection became the object of papal patronage, it also intersected with the system of religious licensing that the pope himself had addressed as part of his intense legislative activity as the city's archbishop. In fact, the pope's intervention in Bolognese midwifery practice dated back at least to September 1732, when, shortly after returning to Bologna, Lambertini had discussed the issue of midwifery licensing in one of his notifications.[153] After becoming pope, in a *Breve* of 10 May 1741, Lambertini extended the right to practice 'hic, et ubique terrarum' ('here and everywhere on earth'), which had been formerly granted only to physicians who graduated from the University of Bologna, to licensed surgeons, apothecaries, and midwives.[154] As we saw in

[148] BUB, ms. 4737, Autografi, IX, 5.

[149] ASB, Studio, busta 322, Registro degli Atti del Protomedicato, Seconda Serie (27 January 1744–2 August 1746), fol. 35v.

[150] ASM, Luoghi pii, p.a., cartella 382, '1765. Osservazioni per le scuole di Chirurgia ed Ostetricia nell'Ospital Maggiore di Milano', 'Informazione del Dottore Galli di Bologna'.

[151] See, for instance, ASB, Assunteria di Studio, busta 326, 28 January 1764, fol. 20v; ASB, Assunteria di Studio, busta 327, 21 January 1769, fol. 18v.

[152] Richard, *Description historique*, vol. 2, 120.

[153] Prospero Lambertini, 'Delle Ostetrici, o Mammane, o sieno Comari da Putti [...]', in *Raccolta di alcune notificazioni, editti, ed istruzioni pubblicate dall'Eminentissimo, e Reverendissimo Signor Cardinale Prospero Lambertini, Arcivescovo di Bologna, e Principe del S.R.I. pel buon governo della sua Diocesi*, vol. 1 (Bologna: Longhi, 1733), 78–85.

[154] See Serafino Mazzetti, *Memorie storiche sopra l'università e l'istituto delle scienze di Bologna* (Bologna: San Tommaso d'Aquino, 1840), 56–7.

previous chapters, Lambertini's involvement in the Bolognese anatomical world set new parameters of ecclesiastical control over anatomical practice. In his notification 'Delle Ostetrici, o Mammane, o sieno Comari da Putti' (1732), Lambertini similarly emphasized the need to subject midwives to religious licensing. Moreover, he spelled out the procedures that midwives had to follow in administering emergency baptism, which was aimed at saving the child's soul in cases of difficult deliveries.[155]

Baptism was a critically important rite of passage that was carried out through a highly symbolic ceremony.[156] Along with the cult of saints, it represented one of the cornerstones of Counter-Reformation identity. Since baptism marked a child's entrance into the religious community, it became the object of endless discussions about the circumstances of its administration. As a performative ritual that ran the risk of being invalidated if carried out incorrectly, it raised special concerns: was baptism *in utero* legitimate? What if the baptismal water did not reach enough of the unborn's body or the right bodily parts? What if the midwife did not perform the ritual or pronounce the baptismal formula correctly?[157] After becoming pope, Lambertini intervened on such matters in his *De Synodo diocesana* (1748), where he discussed the circumstances of baptism *in utero*.[158] In ensuing years, baptismal syringes ended up becoming part of midwives' toolkits. In 1771, Galli himself weighed in on the issue of emergency baptism in a report on caesarean sections, where he concluded that it was licit to operate immediately after the body of the mother showed signs of death, as long as the dimensions of the surgical cut were not larger than what was needed to baptize the child.[159] In November 1745, Galli had presented an account of a caesarean section he had carried out in a case of extrauterine pregnancy at the Bolognese Academy of the Sciences.[160] In the same year, the Sicilian clergyman Francesco Emanuele Cangiamila advocated caesarean sections as the most suitable procedure to employ in the baptism of unborn children in cases of emergency, thus giving priority to the spiritual being of the unborn over the life of the mother.[161]

[155] Lambertini, 'Delle Ostetrici, o Mammane'.

[156] See Adriano Prosperi, 'Scienza e immaginazione teologica nel Seicento: Il battesimo e le origini dell'individuo', *Quaderni storici*, 100:1 (1999), 173–98; Adriano Prosperi, 'Battesimo e identità tra Medio evo e prima età moderna', in Peter von Moos (ed.), *Unverwechselbarkeit: Persönliche Identität und Identifikation in der vormodernen Gesellschaft* (Cologne: Böhlau, 2004), 325–54.

[157] Prosperi, 'Battesimo e identità', 325–53.

[158] Prospero Lambertini, *De Synodo diocesana, libri octo* (Rome: Komarek, 1748), 197–201.

[159] Medici, 'Elogio di Gian Antonio Galli', 442. Galli's 'De tempore sectionis mulierum, quae gravidae moriuntur, ut foetus posit vivus baptizari, extrahi per abdomen' was delivered at the Academy of the Sciences on 28 November 1771.

[160] Giovan Antonio Galli, 'De nominestri foetu extra utero aucto, et mortuo per abdomen vivae matris extracto', in *De Bononiensi Scientiarum et Artium Instituto atque Academia Commentarii*, vol. 2/III (Bologna: Lelio dalla Volpe, 1747), 251–61. See also Sanlorenzo, *L'insegnamento di ostetricia*, 35.

[161] Francesco Emanuele Cangiamila, *Embriologia sacra: ovvero dell'uffizio de' sacerdoti, medici, e superiori, circa l'eterna salute dei bambini racchiusi nell'utero* (Palermo: Francesco Valenza, 1745). On the history of caesarian section in the eighteenth and nineteenth centuries, see, for instance, Filippini, *La nascita straordinaria*; Nadia Maria Filippini, '"Sanctuaire de la nature ou prison du fœtus": nature et corps féminin sous le combat sur la césarienne en France au XVIIIe siècle', in Daston and Pomata (eds.), *The Faces of Nature*, 259–82; Pancino, *Il bambino e l'acqua sporca*, 143–5.

The theological centrality of baptism also affected midwifery and licensing practices. Because of their position of centrality in the worlds of sexuality, generation, and childbirth, midwives were subjected to tight religious surveillance.[162] Due to their role in emergency baptism, they had to receive the approval of the parish priest and were 'often chosen by him'.[163] The very ritual of baptism provided a valuable opportunity for priests to keep in touch with midwives, and thus gather information about the sexual life of fellow parishioners.[164] Midwives' role as performers of emergency baptism equally exposed them to a pressing need for religious certification.[165] Diocesan synods accordingly prescribed that midwives had to learn the baptismal formula and be regularly checked to ensure that they were up to the goal of administering such an important sacrament.

Even before the Protomedicato became the institution in charge of issuing midwifery licences, references to the requirement for submitting evidence of religious certification had appeared in its notifications and *editti*.[166] After Lambertini issued the notification on midwives, medical and religious powers in Bologna joined forces to increase control over midwifery practices. Quite inevitably, the establishment of a dual system of religious and medical licensing also increased the chances of confusion. In his notification on midwifery, Lambertini structured the religious licensing of midwives in a way that was symmetrical to their medical licensing.[167] The very format of the licensing certificates ran the risk of creating some misunderstanding as it gave permission to practise without referring to the need for obtaining medical licensing as well.[168] And confusion indeed there was. In the mid-eighteenth century, public notices of the Bolognese Protomedicato addressed those midwives who, having received religious approval, had not obtained medical licensing.[169] Nor were midwives alone in being the subject of misunderstanding. In 1769, the members of the Protomedicato were displeased to hear that a number of midwives who served at the hospital of the Esposti had received only religious licensing, and urged the hospital's board to fire those who had not received medical

[162] Filippini, 'The Church, the State and Childbirth', 157–61 (citation p. 159).

[163] Ibid., 158.

[164] Ibid., 159; Pastore, *Il medico in tribunale*, 136; Pancino, 'Malati, medici, mammane', 719–24.

[165] Filippini, 'The Church, the State and Childbirth', 158–9; For a comparison with midwives' ecclesiastical licensing in early modern Britain and France, see Doreen A. Evendeen, *The Midwives of Seventeenth-Century London* (Cambridge: Cambridge University Press, 2000); Tiffany D. Vann Sprecher and Ruth Mazo Karras, 'The Midwife and the Church: Ecclesiastical Regulation of Midwives in Brie, 1499–1504', *Bulletin of the History of Medicine*, 85:2 (2011), 171–92.

[166] In 1682, for instance, an 'Editto per speciali, barbieri, comari & altri' issued by the Protomedicato, required midwives to bring to the prior or the *protomedici* a certificate 'de vita, & moribus' ('of good life and morals') provided by their parish curate; see ASB, Studio, busta 233, 'Bandi, Editti, e Notificazioni del Protomedicato e provviggioni spettanti alla Citta' di Bologna dal 1571 a tutto il 1769'.

[167] For instance, just as in the case of the medical exam, religious licences required that midwives be tested by three examiners; see Lambertini, 'Delle Ostetrici, o Mammane', 80–1.

[168] AAB, cart. 6, fasc. 6, 'Certificati di Levatrici approvate dal 1742 al 1817'.

[169] ASB, Studio, busta 233, 'Bandi, Editti, e Notificazioni del Protomedicato e provviggioni spettanti alla Citta' di Bologna dal 1571 a tutto il 1769', 'Notificazione ad ogni, e qualunque persona, che esercita l'Arte di Commare, o sia Allevatrice nel Contado di Bologna' of 20 December 1746.

approval as well.[170] When, in 1757, some twenty-five years after the publication of his notification on midwifery, Lambertini purchased Galli's collection to donate it to the Institute of the Sciences, he created particularly favourable conditions for implementing religious as well as medical control.[171] Once transferred to the Institute, Galli's collection provided a site for defining what kind of practices, gestures, and tools midwifery relied on; what knowledge it generated, displayed, and mediated; and what type of expertise it created. In short, as the collection gained increasing significance within the world of training and licensing, it participated in defining what the practice of midwifery was all about. Meanwhile, calls for the need of training on Galli's collection continued to grow. When, in the mid-1770s, a number of deliveries that were attended by surgeons ended in disaster, the Bolognese Senate turned to Galli as the ultimate saviour.

TRANSLATING GESTURAL KNOWLEDGE

In early 1776, an anonymous letter reached the Bolognese Senate asking for the public funding of a surgeon who would help poor women in the city in cases of difficult and laborious births.[172] One year later, a new anonymous letter resubmitted the proposal, lamenting the disastrous childbirth incidents that had taken place at the hands of unskilled surgeons. Galli was appalled: how could something like that happen in a city where midwifery had been taught for many years on the basis of his collection and where the surgeon in charge—namely himself—had successfully engaged in so many diverse midwifery operations?[173] The discussion dragged on.[174] In March 1778, the proposal was relaunched along with the suggestion to sponsor the position by reassigning funds allocated to the lectureship of the late Laura Bassi.[175] Galli offered advice on pay, certification, lodgings, and monitoring while recommending that the appointed surgeons ought neither to 'argue or quarrel with the midwives' nor to show themselves 'partial to any'. Rather, they should 'gain the esteem of all those approved by the College of Physicians'.[176] Galli also suggested instructing more countryside midwives as an alternative to the plan of training and hiring surgeons. Since the worst incidents usually took place in the countryside, and the city of Bologna could already count on well-trained 'midwives and skilled practitioners', he instead proposed spending the allocated sum

[170] ASB, Studio, busta 261, 'Mammane: Istruzioni per abusi ed abilitazioni', fols. 182r–v. In the summer of 1769, the names of the midwives who practised at the Hospital but did not have a medical licence were recorded. A note including the names of some midwives also recalled that they needed the certification *de vita et moribus* from the parish priest and the certification of a physician 'concerning women's practice', ibid., fols. 180–1.

[171] ASB, Assunteria d'Istituto, Lettere dell'Istituto, n. 4 (1756–65), Letter of 19 November 1757 from the Institute to the ambassador.

[172] ASB, Assunteria di Studio, Diversorum, Servizi Pubblici, Sec. XVI–XVIII, busta 98, fasc. n. 3: 'Recapiti diversi riguardanti il Progetto di stabilire alcuni Chirurghi in Città, e Levatrici in Campagna per l'assistenza de' Parti a spese pubbliche'.

[173] Ibid. [174] Ibid. [175] Ibid., note of 14 March 1778.

[176] ASB, Assunteria di Studio, Diversorum, Servizi Pubblici, Sec. XVI–XVIII, busta 98, fasc. n. 3, 'Recapiti diversi'.

on instructing four countryside midwives each year. These midwives would move to Bologna in May and June to attend the midwifery lectures held at the Institute, and would accordingly be trained in 'non-natural and laborious' as well as 'in easy and natural' deliveries.[177]

As the foregoing story shows, in Bologna midwives remained central to the world of midwifery. The surge of man-midwives like Galli did not amount to their displacement. In fact, as contemporaries noted, the collection purportedly expanded midwives' domain of action in that it introduced them to a realm of training that included difficult and unordinary as well as ordinary and unproblematic deliveries.[178] For a period, midwives also played a role in the training of medical students. In May 1783, for example, Margherita Sandri, a public midwife (*comare pubblica*) in Bologna, certified that the *Dottor* Agostino Fantini had long trained in the art of midwifery with her, and had made 'various laborious operations' which she had personally witnessed.[179] Highlighting a situation in which a midwife trained and certified an aspiring man-midwife, Sandri's note points to the continuing role of female practitioners in midwifery training, including the training of the new class of surgeons looking for occupation in the realm of hands-on practices.[180] Still, the claims of authoritative knowledge that ended up being associated with Galli's collection, its integration into eighteenth-century academic culture, and its growing importance within the licensing realm, placed its models at the centre of the process of reorganization of the midwifery world. For one thing, as much as Galli's models focused on spelling out and casting light on the world of pregnancy and childbirth, they contributed to the reframing of midwives' realm of expertise. In doing so, they participated in the process that redesigned it from the more broadly defined domains of female sexuality and generation to those of pregnancy and childbirth.[181] For another thing, while seeking to tackle the proverbial aura of ambiguity and uncertainty characterizing the realms of generation and pregnancy, models translated and articulated in anatomical form the practices that had long characterized midwives' skills and techniques.

In fact, by the time Galli established a midwifery school based on anatomical models, midwives had long been devising bodily techniques and had elaborated complex traditions of manual dexterity on the basis of the same principles of sight-cum-touch expertise that also ended up being inscribed into Galli's models, such as the use of comparison in the assessment of bodily variability.[182] At a time when calls for midwives to learn anatomy were becoming ever more insistent, some midwives refused to comply with the request to attend anatomical demonstrations on the grounds that there was nothing new for them to learn.[183] Furthermore, the

[177] Ibid. [178] Zaccaria, *Storia letteraria d'Italia*, vol. 5, 725–6.

[179] ASB, Assunteria d'Istituto, Diversorum, busta 15, Note of 30 May 1783.

[180] Pomata, 'Barbieri e comari', especially 179ff.

[181] On midwives' expertise on women's sexuality in early modern Italy, see, for instance, ibid., 175–6; Pomata, *Contracting a Cure*, 77–8; Pastore, *Il medico in tribunale*, 129–48 and 230–6.

[182] See, for instance, the case of Bortola Marchesini, who was training in Venice as described by Filippini in 'The Church, the State and Childbirth', 156.

[183] Ibid., 173 n. 47.

anatomical expertise of early modern midwives is extensively recorded in judicial records, where midwives served as expert witnesses in cases of sexual offence. In early modern Bologna, two midwives were appointed by the court (*Tribunale del Torrone*) to inspect the bodies of the victims of sexual crimes and to produce expert legal reports, a practice that continued even after the establishment of Galli's midwifery school.[184] But just as in the case of other early modern hands-on practitioners, midwives' practice relied on tacit skills and embodied knowledge that was transmitted through gestural techniques and was largely incommunicable. Midwifery models such as Galli's promised to articulate this knowledge in the visual language of anatomy, make it publicly communicable, and transfer it to the hands or, as in the case of the crystal womb, to the eyes of the man-midwife.

The history of the making and early employment and viewing of Galli's collection of midwifery models may then be regarded as an instance of the wider history of the processes of translation of tacit knowledge, gestural performance, and embodied skill into forms of natural or, in this case, anatomical knowledge.[185] Well into the eighteenth century, such processes accompanied and marked the many points of encounter, conflict, and negotiation between hands-on practitioners and physicians or natural philosophers in artisanal and academic settings. As Galli's models translated and redeployed midwifery techniques such as bodily comparison in the form of anatomical sequences, they entered the premises of eighteenth-century academies. The story of the *portella* created on the side of the Institute of the Sciences illustrates the implications of this process for midwifery practice. Midwives continued to practise midwifery, but they ended up accessing skill via the side door.

[184] The archival record concerning such cases is vast. For a selection of cases in the mid- to late eighteenth century, see ASB, Torrone, Processi (1671), 6953, fasc. 62; Torrone, Processi (1731–2), 7952/2, fasc. 5; Torrone, Processi (1749–50), 8122/3, fasc. 72 and 78; Torrone, Processi (1749–50), 8127/2, fasc. 19; Torrone, Processi (1774–6), 8321/2, fasc. 21 and 39; Torrone, Processi (1781–2): 8355/3, fasc. 101; Torrone, Processi (1784–5), 8368/3, fasc. 83. My thanks to Cesarina Casanova for sharing with me her knowledge of this archival corpus. See also Pastore, *Il medico in tribunale*, 129–48; Pancino, 'Malati, medici, mammane', 719; Giancarlo Angelozzi and Cesarina Casanova, *La giustizia criminale in una città di antico regime: Il tribunale del Torrone di Bologna (secc. XVI–XVII)* (Bologna: CLUEB, 2009).

[185] On embodied, incommunicable knowledge and its translation see, for instance, Heinz Otto Sibum, 'Reworking the Mechanical Value of Heat: Instruments of Precision and Gestures of Accuracy in Early Victorian England', *Studies in History and Philosophy of Science*, 26:1 (1995), 73–106, esp. 96; Schaffer, 'Experimenters' Techniques'.

6

Transferring Value

VALUABLE MATTERS

On 11 July 1774, the funeral rites of the wax modeller Anna Morandi Manzolini were celebrated with 'the solemn pomp that was appropriate to the singular merits of such an excellent woman'.[1] As the chronicler Petronio Cavallazzi reported in his *Memorie storiche* and the gazzette *Bologna* observed on the next day, a requiem mass was held in the church of San Procolo and a special composition by the abbot Valerio Tesei, a member of the Accademia Filarmonica, was sung before interment.[2] Morandi's sons paid for the funeral and everyone mourned the loss of such a 'rare and renowned woman' who, thanks to 'her famous operations' often commissioned by foreign princes, 'increased the prestige and decorum of our city'.[3] The news was then reported in the Venetian *Giornale Enciclopedico* of July 1774, where it was emphasized that Morandi's death constituted a great loss for the city of Bologna.[4] Other tributes were to follow.[5] Reactions to Morandi's demise point to the extent to which her work was appreciated. Notably, in previous years, Morandi had both lost the ownership of her collection and achieved the height of her celebrity while joining the pantheon of local heroines. This chapter shifts attention from Galli's midwifery collection back to Morandi's practice. It focuses on how anatomical displays participated in commercial as well as medical and cultural networks, and generated value for viewers, makers, and collectors alike. In order to do so, it examines the developments of Bolognese anatomical modelling during the last part of Morandi's life, and explores the period when, having received papal patronage, she consolidated her role as a transnational celebrity. I suggest that following the fate of Morandi and her collection in this later period provides a felicitous point of entry into the processes of valorization that implicated models at a time when appreciation of anatomical collections had reached a high point.

Issues related to the creation and distribution of value are, of course, complex and in many ways intractable. Any attempt to address them would have to take into account that value is variable and volatile, socially and culturally embedded, and contingent on specific circumstances and particularities related to time and

[1] *Bologna*, 28, 12 July 1774.

[2] Ibid.; BCABo, Gozz. 351, 'Memorie storiche bolognesi dall'anno 1760 all'anno 1796 raccolte da Petronio Cavallazzi', n.p. (11 July 1774).

[3] *Bologna*, 28, 12 July 1774.

[4] 'Aneddoti', *Giornale enciclopedico,* Luglio 1774, vol. 7 (Venice: Stamperia Fenziana, 1774), 92.

[5] See, for instance, *Münchner Zeitung*, 123, 4 August 1774, 'Bononien, den 19. Juli'.

place.[6] With regard to the early modern period, historians have highlighted the role of collections as social and cultural assets that generated value and blurred the boundaries between knowledge value and commercial value.[7] Attention has also been drawn to the part played by precious specimens and rarities in increasing the worth and prestige of collections. Anatomical models similarly had the capacity to generate value. Fashioned as veritable tools of knowledge and sites of evidence about the state of affairs of the body, they acted as cultural currencies that had the capacity to accumulate and transfer value across medical, cultural, and commercial domains. Recent literature on early modern anatomical displays in the Netherlands and the British Isles has shed light on how specimens embodied economic and cultural values that extended beyond their functions as tools of teaching and investigation.[8] Focusing on the processes of valorization related to anatomical displays realized in the Italian peninsula in the mid-eighteenth century, this chapter and Chapter 7 consider how in Bologna and Naples anatomical models acted as both tools of knowledge and luxury goods, and came to be regarded as cultural currencies that had the capacity to transfer value. Both chapters also investigate the transformative power of value, and look at anatomical models as capable of extending their worth not only to other items within the same collection, but also to the broader context of their collectors' pursuits. This chapter, in particular, explores the process of valorization involved with Morandi's collection by drawing attention to the events related to the sale of her anatomical models to the Bolognese senator Girolamo Ranuzzi. More specifically, I examine how Ranuzzi's acquisition of the collection took place at a time when the Bolognese senator was busy trying to relaunch the family's spa. In a related manner, I reconstruct how the transferral of the modeller and her collection to the Ranuzzi Palace offered the opportunity to impart a broader scope to Ranuzzi's own ambitions and commercial pursuits. I argue that not only did anatomical models act as powerful vehicles for transforming their makers into celebrities, they also became precious collectibles that could

[6] See, for instance, Appadurai (ed.), *The Social Life of Things*; Thomas, *Entangled Objects*; Fred R. Myers (ed.), *The Empire of Things: Regimes of Value and Material Culture* (Santa Fe, NM: School of American Research Press, 2001); Paula Findlen (ed.), *Early Modern Things: Objects and their Histories, 1500–1800* (New York: Routledge, 2013).

[7] See Findlen, *Possessing Nature*; Cook, *Matters of Exchange*; Smith and Findlen (eds.), *Merchants and Marvels*; Anne Goldgar, *Tulipmania: Money, Honor, and Knowledge in the Dutch Golden Age* (Chicago: University of Chicago Press, 2007); Daniela Bleichmar and Peter C. Mancall (eds.), *Collecting Across Cultures: Material Exchanges in the Early Modern Atlantic* (Philadelphia: University of Pennsylvania Press, 2011).

[8] Harold Cook has examined how, in seventeenth-century Netherlands, anatomical preparations' capacity to defy decay turned them into vehicles for the accumulation of value. Similarly focusing on early modern Dutch anatomists, Dániel Margócsy has explored the circumstances that made it possible to fashion anatomical preparations as 'consumer goods that circulate commercially'. Shifting attention to eighteenth-century Britain, Simon Chaplin has further observed that the specimens displayed in John Hunter's anatomical museum in London played an important part as cultural capitals 'which not only embodied the values of a community of practitioners, but served to project these values to a wider audience'; see Cook, 'Time's Bodies'; Cook, *Matters of Exchange*, chapter 2; Margócsy, 'Advertising Cadavers'; Margócsy, 'A Museum of Wonders' (citation p. 213); Margócsy, *Commercial Visions*; Chaplin, 'Nature Dissected', 137; Chaplin, 'John Hunter'. On the concept of cultural capital, see Pierre Bourdieu's classic 'The Forms of Capital', in John G. Richardson (ed.) *Handbook of Theory and Research for the Sociology of Education* (New York: Greenwood, 1986), 241–58.

act as testimonials of their collectors' involvement in natural inquiries and medical enterprises while, at the same time, adding value and prestige to them.

ENTERING THE BOOKISH WORLD OF ANATOMY

As was to be expected, the years following Benedict XIV's response to Morandi's plea for help brought about a dramatic series of events, leading to new commissions, additional tributes, and enhanced celebrity status. As early as 3 December 1755, shortly after the pope intervened on her behalf, Morandi was elected honorary member of the Accademia Clementina and 'was acclaimed by the whole Academy' in a session where her long-term adversary Ercole Lelli was among the presentees.[9] In the same period, Morandi was busy working on commissions. As Giovanni Bianchi recalled in the *Novelle letterarie*, in September 1754 she was working on anatomical specimens commissioned by a number of sovereigns and illustrious buyers.[10] Writing in December 1756 to the mathematician Eraclito Manfredi, who mediated the payment for Morandi's models for the king of Sardinia, the physician Ignazio Somis was glad to hear that 'the anatomical box' was on its way to Turin.[11] In March 1758, Somis was in charge of paying Anna Morandi 'for the other four boxes' containing the preparations of the organs of hearing, smelling, taste, and touch.[12] Morandi also made new models for Giovanni Antonio Galli's midwifery collection, which Pope Benedict XIV had purchased and donated to the Institute of the Sciences in 1757. This meant that even those viewers who did not personally visit Morandi's cabinet could become acquainted with her work there.[13] When, months after the death of Benedict XIV, Morandi donated to the Senate an anatomical statue made by Giovanni Manzolini, which would then be exhibited at the Institute, she may have hoped to mend her relationship with an institution that already displayed some of her and her husband's work, in spite of Lelli's ongoing reservations.[14]

The demise of Morandi's patron on 3 May 1758 did not amount to the end of her growing celebrity and public recognition. When, in 1759, the *Diario bolognese* started chronicling the most important news and events concerning Bologna's

[9] AABAB, Atti dell'Accademia Clementina, vol. 1, 189–90. Miriam Focaccia has noticed that although Luigi Crespi and Giovanni Fantuzzi mentioned that Morandi was aggregated to the Academy of the Sciences in the Institute, this does not appear to be confirmed by the records; see Focaccia, 'Anna Morandi Manzolini', 7.

[10] Bianchi, 'Lettera del Signor Dottor Giovanni Bianchi', 711.

[11] BCABo, Fondo Speciale *Collezione degli Autografi*, LXV, 17584–17754, Letter n. 17587, Letter of 15 December 1756 from Ignazio Somis in Turin to Eraclito Manfredi.

[12] Archivio Storico dell'Università di Torino, Spese, XII, c. 3, 'Registro mandati', vol. 8, fols. 17–18 (2 March 1758); BCABo, Fondo Speciale *Collezione degli Autografi*, LXV, 17584–17754, Letter n. 17710, Letter of 29 March 1758 from Ignazio Somis in Turin to Eraclito Manfredi; ibid., Letter n. 17712, Letter of 12 April 1758 from Ignazio Somis in Turin to Eraclito Manfredi.

[13] See, for instance, Lalande, *Voyage d'un François en Italie*, vol. 2, 34; Beinecke Rare Book and Manuscript Library, Yale University (New Haven), Osborn ms. c. 194, Charles Burney, 'Travel Diary', vol. 2, 9.

[14] See ASB, Assunteria d'Istituto, Atti, n. 5 (1754–60), 4 January 1759.

'secular and ecclesiastical governments', including the university, the Institute of the Sciences, noble families, and charitable institutions, Morandi found a place among the 'professors nominated by the Senate and salaried with the revenues of the University' as a 'wax-modeller of the parts of the human body and demonstrator of anatomy to *studiosi* at home'.[15] The same wording continued to appear in the subsequent issues of the *Diario bolognese* until her death. In the same period, recognitions started to pour in. In 1761, Morandi was aggregated to Florence's Accademia del Disegno.[16] In 1762, her name appeared on the list of associates of the Respublica Literaria Umbrorum, which also included a number of learned women—not only Laura Bassi and Maria Gaetana Agnesi but also Anna Manfredi Costa, the daughter of the Bolognese mathematician Gabriele Manfredi, and many more.[17] The academy also counted among its members the anatomist Giovanni Bianchi and Raimondo di Sangro, the Neapolitan nobleman and savant who befriended Girolamo Ranuzzi, and whose display of anatomical models in Naples will be the subject matter of Chapter 7.[18] Contemporaries also noticed that Morandi received 'splendid' offers from London, Milan, and St Petersburg.[19] Meanwhile, ever more travellers reported and commented on her collection, anatomical abilities, new method of teaching, and anatomical demonstrations.

While travel reports and periodicals crucially contributed to making Morandi known to a wide audience, in the later part of her life she also entered the bookish canon of anatomy and her name started to appear in anatomical treatises and encyclopaedias. Notably, in his *Encyclopédie ou Dictionnaire universel raisonné des connoissances humaines* (1770–80), also known as the *Encyclopédie d'Yverdon*, which aimed at expanding Diderot and D'Alembert's *Encyclopédie*, Fortunato Bartolomeo De Felice (1723–1789) referred to the models made by Morandi for Galli's midwifery collection.[20] In the same period Germano Azzoguidi turned to Morandi's authority and referred to her anatomical proficiency in his *Observationes ad uteri constructionem pertinentes* (1773). Here Azzoguidi associated Morandi's name with those of prominent anatomical figures and noticed that she was known both 'among anatomists' and lay 'non-ordinary individuals' ('non vulgares homines').[21] When Azzoguidi's book was reviewed in the *Giornale de' Letterati* of 1773, readers of the periodical came across the name of the 'famous Anna Manzolina' along with that of Giambattista Morgagni and those of the famous 'anatomists of London'.[22] In the following decades, the news was reported in medical

[15] *Diario bolognese, ecclesiastico e civile, per l'anno MDCCLIX*, 1759, 126.

[16] Fantuzzi, *Notizie degli scrittori bolognesi*, vol. 6, 115.

[17] See 'Album sodalium Reip. Litterariae Umbrorum' in *Acta Reipublicae Litterariae Umbrorum* (Foligno: Excudebat Franciscus Fofus, 1762), ii and ix. According to Fantuzzi, Morandi was aggregated to Foligno's Literary Society in 1760; see Fantuzzi, *Notizie degli scrittori bolognesi*, vol. 6, 115.

[18] 'Album sodalium Reip. Litterariae Umbrorum', vi and xi.

[19] On the tributes conferred to Morandi, see for instance BCABo, ms. B 133, Marcello Oretti, *Notizie de' Professori del Dissegno*, vol. 11, 228; Crespi, *Felsina pittrice*, vol. 3, 311; Fantuzzi, *Notizie degli scrittori bolognesi*, vol. 5, 115; Giordani, *Articolo di biografia*, 10.

[20] Fortunato Bartolomeo De Felice, *Encyclopédie; ou, Dictionnaire universel raisonné des connoissances humaine*, vol. 24 (Yverdon: n.p., 1770–80), 656.

[21] Azzoguidi, *Observationes ad uteri constructionem pertinentes*, 36–7.

[22] Anon., Articolo III: 'Observationes ad uteri costructionem pertinentes', in *Giornale de' Letterati*, vol. 16 (Pisa: Fratelli Pizzorni, 1773), 85.

texts across the Alps. In 1785, the German translation of the first volume of Giovanni Battista Borsieri di Kanifeld's *Institutionum medicinae practicae* (1785) referred to Azzoguidi's reliance on the authority and experience of 'Anna Manzolina' as well as that of Morgagni and Pietro Moscati.[23] The English translation of Borsieri di Kanifeld's work similarly included a note highlighting that in his *Observationes* Azzoguidi referred both to 'the authority of Morgagni, which is of great weight, and that of Anna Manzolina, distinguished for her anatomical research, together with the observations of the celebrated Moscatus, professor of anatomy, a man of incredible skill'.[24]

IN A STATE OF EXTREME NEED

It is worth noting that while the realms of mothering and domesticity informed the making of Morandi's public persona, the dramatic sequence of rewards that followed Morandi's reception of papal patronage also found a counterpart in her family life. As Morandi obtained the patronage of the pope, became a university demonstrator, and consolidated her role as a living monument of the Grand Tour, her children were likely to benefit from their mother's new standing. Morandi's son Giuseppe had entered the orphanage of San Bartolomeo di Reno in October 1756, and in February 1758 he won a lottery that was organized to assign the inheritance and title of the nobleman Flaminio Solimei, who had died without male descendants.[25] Becoming rich and noble overnight, Giuseppe took the name of the Solimei family and moved to its patrician residence in the palace-lined Strada Maggiore.[26] The event generated much fanfare. It was reported in local chronicles and recorded in Grand Tour accounts, and entered the stories that shaped Morandi's public persona by drawing, once again, attention to her family life. It also offered the opportunity to celebrate the city's charity networks to transnational audiences. In his *Description historique et critique de l'Italie*, the abbé Jérôme Richard observed that Morandi would have encountered great difficulty in granting her children a proper education had it not been for the support offered by the city's charitable institutions and the habit of patrician families without male descendants to choose their heirs from among these institutions' well-educated children.[27]

Just as in the case of the criteria that regulated admission to the orphanage of San Bartolomeo, inclusion in the group of orphans who could participate in the lottery

[23] Giambattista Borsieri de Kanilfeld, *Anleitung zur Kenntnis und Heilung der Fiebe*, trans. Georg Conrad Hinderer (Giessen and Marburg: Krieger, 1785), 729.

[24] Giambattista Borsieri de Kanilfeld, *The Institutions of the Practice of Medicine [...] Translated from the Latin by William Cullen Brown*, vol. 2 (Edinburgh: Cadell and Davis et al., 1801), 186.

[25] ASB, Orfanotrofio di San Bartolomeo, Filze e Congregazioni, n. 9, fasc. 3 ('Libri degli Atti dei Governatori, 1720–61)', fols. 113v–114r; ASB, Orfanotrofio di San Bartolomeo: Documenti, n. 41, fasc. 45 (1 and 2) and 46. On patriliny in early modern Italy, see, for instance, Gianna Pomata, 'Family and Gender', in John A. Marino (ed.), *Early Modern Italy: 1550–1796* (Oxford: Oxford University Press, 2002), 69–86.

[26] BCABo, Gozz. 351, 'Memorie storiche Bolognesi di Petronio Cavallazzi', n.p. (11 July 1774).

[27] Richard, *Description historique*, vol. 2, 142–5.

required having 'parents of good life and reputation'.[28] Giuseppe's presence in the pool of selected children was likely to have benefited from Morandi's accomplishments and enhanced status as a recipient of papal patronage. For her part, despite her ever-increasing fame and her son's stroke of luck, Morandi continued with her usual modest lifestyle. When Richard visited her in the early 1760s, he found her living in a state of '*grande médiocrité*'.[29] In the following years, Morandi fell sick, was unable to work and had to leave her residence. In early September 1765, she pleaded with Marcello Oretti for help in a letter written in Bertalia, a neighbourhood located outside the city's walls where some Bolognese patrician families, including the famous castrato opera singer Carlo Broschi, known as Farinelli, owned large villas and mansions.[30] In all likelihood this was meant to be a temporary abode, and in fact Morandi's name was not included in the annual parish censuses (*stati delle anime*).[31] As Morandi explained in her missive, a 'serious and long infirmity' and 'other costly circumstances' had led her to a state of 'extreme need'.[32] Accordingly, she asked Oretti to plead with the Senate on her behalf for an increase of 200 lire in her salary. Amidst the papers addressed to Oretti, a note written by Morandi highlighted that she had not received 'the necessary help' by those who should do their duty.[33] It was the second time that Morandi turned to local institutions for help. But this time she could no longer count on the help of a mighty patron. Her plea to the Senate was turned down with a bureaucratic excuse that exploited the grey areas of the relationship between town and gown: it was remarked that, since Morandi was among university employees paid by the *Gabella Grossa*, she could not benefit from the limited resources made available by the death of 'public lecturers'. Her request was then deferred to future consideration in case resources became available after the demise of employees that belonged to her group.[34]

The reply could not have been more disappointing. Yet, while Morandi's request was turned down, her celebrity continued to grow. As she recovered from her illness, travellers recommenced their anatomical pilgrimages to her collection. Famous travelogues that were published in this period, such as Richard's, added further lustre to her name.[35] Growing interest in Morandi's anatomical cabinet also paved the way for new commercial prospects. As Morandi resumed her anatomical encounters and demonstrations, novel rumours about foreign

[28] ASB, Orfanotrofio di San Bartolomeo, Filze e Congregazioni, n. 9, fasc. 3 ('Libri degli Atti dei Governatori', 1720–61).

[29] Richard, *Description historique*, vol. 2, 142.

[30] See BCABo, ms. B 120, 'Lettere di diversi al S.r Oretti', fols. 182r–191r.

[31] Archivio Parrocchiale di San Martino di Bertalia (Bologna), Stati delle Anime (1765 and 1766).

[32] BCABo, ms. B 120, 'Lettere di diversi al S.r Oretti', fols. 182r–191r.

[33] Ibid., esp. fols. 182r and 183r.

[34] ASB, Atti dell'Assunteria di studio, n. 25 (1756–77), 27 November 1765. On the disparity of treatment between Morandi and Laura Bassi, who had received a higher salary than Morandi, and in 1759 requested and obtained an increase, Cavazza, 'Dottrici e lettrici'; Berti Logan, 'Women and the Practice'.

[35] Richard, *Description historique*, vol. 2, 118–19 and 142–5. In his *Voyage*, Lalande did not mention a direct encounter with Morandi, possibly because he visited Bologna when Morandi had temporarily moved to the neighbourhood of Bertalia. However, as we saw in Chapter 5, he did refer to the models that Morandi had completed for Galli's midwifery collection; see Lalande, *Voyage d'un François en Italie*, vol. 2, 34.

buyers' interest in the collection started to spread. In 1766, for instance, two British travellers visited 'the *signora Manzolini*' and penned in their diary that the hereditary Prince of Brunswick, who toured the Italian peninsula in the same year, had proposed purchasing the 'curious cabinet' of this 'famous anatomist'.[36] As we have seen, shortly after becoming a widow Morandi had become sufficiently renowned and valuable to the city to prompt the pope to respond favourably to her request for help, lest she accept offers to move abroad.[37] As she found herself anew in a situation of hardship, she may have used the offers of potential buyers as a bargaining chip to improve her financial situation.

When, in 1769, the Bolognese nobleman and senator Girolamo Ranuzzi stepped in to purchase Morandi's collection, he capitalized on the same rhetoric: in the opening lines of the sale contract he emphasized that his offer to Morandi was made at a time when the modeller was negotiating the sale of her collection to foreign buyers. His purchase of the collection would ensure that it remained in the city. Thus, by acquiring the collection, Ranuzzi fashioned himself as a saviour and a civic champion.[38] In fact, as Elio Vassena and others have remarked, even contemporaries such as Marcello Oretti observed that Ranuzzi 'took advantage' of the situation.[39] Of course, Ranuzzi could easily exploit the situation. Regardless of her celebrity, Morandi was still a widow who had lost her powerful patron. She could count on limited means and found herself in a situation of 'extreme need'. Although recent literature on Morandi has referred to Oretti's allegation, little is still known about the wider context of Ranuzzi's purchase.[40] Drawing attention to some of the circumstances that accompanied the senator's acquisition of Morandi's collection can help to shed light on the backdrop of Oretti's remark. Exploring the nature of the advantages that Ranuzzi could have gained from the purchase further affords the opportunity to reconstruct how, over time, Morandi's models acquired special status as cultural currencies that had the capacity to transfer value.

MEDICAL ENTERPRISES

Dated 6 May 1769 and signed six days later, the sale contract sanctioned Ranuzzi's purchase of Morandi's anatomical collection for 12,000 Bolognese lire. As part of the contract, Morandi's children were asked to put down in writing that they

[36] Bodleian Library (Oxford), ms. Add. A. 366, 'A Journal kept by Mr Tracy and Mr Dentand, during their Travels through France and Italy', entry for 26 November 1766, unpaginated. On the visit of the Prince of Brunswick to Bologna, see BCABo, ms. B 89, vol. 10, 'Diario e memorie varie dall'anno MDL all'anno MDCCLXXXXVI raccolte e scritte dal Domenico Maria D'Andrea Galeati', 137; BCABo, Gozz. 351, 'Memorie storiche bolognesi dall'anno 1760 all'anno 1796 raccolte da Petronio Cavallazzi', fol. 91r.

[37] As we saw in Chapter 5, the rumour that Giovanni Antonio Galli's midwifery collection might travel abroad had similarly generated concern; see Zaccaria, *Storia letteraria d'Italia*, vol. 5, 727.

[38] ASB, Archivio Ranuzzi, Scritture diverse spettanti alla Nobil Casa Ranuzzi (1769–73), Lib. 124, fasc. 6.

[39] BCABo, ms. B 133, Marcello Oretti, *Notizie de' Professori del Dissegno*, vol. 11, 228.

[40] See, for instance, Vassena, *La fortuna dei ceroplasti bolognesi*, section on 'Anna Morandi Manzolini'; Messbarger, *The Lady Anatomist*, 164; Focaccia, 'Anna Morandi Manzolini', 11.

renounced any claim to the collection. Ranuzzi granted Morandi a salary, victuals, and lodgings in the Ranuzzi Palace, where the modeller moved along with her younger son Carlo and her maid Lucia Grifoni.[41] Two years later, Ranuzzi also acquired the anatomical books and the set of surgical and anatomical instruments that Morandi had 'purchased with the fruit of her personal industry and effort' as well as her wax portrait of Ercole Isolani.[42] As Gabriella Berti Logan suggested, the offer for Morandi to move into the Ranuzzi Palace may have been intended to provide the famous modeller with a more prestigious venue where she could pursue her work and make anatomical demonstrations.[43] It also meant entrusting Morandi's celebrated collection to a well-established senatorial family. Throughout the early modern period, the Ranuzzi family had been at the centre of the city's political and cultural life, actively engaging in the patronage of the arts and natural knowledge.[44] By the eighteenth century, the family had lost some of its influence and a significant portion of its resources. Yet, it maintained a prominent role as one of the senatorial families that played a central part in the city's intellectual and academic life. In 1732, for instance, the Countess Maria Ranuzzi, Girolamo's mother, was in charge of accompanying Laura Bassi in her memorable graduation ceremony. Even before acquiring Morandi's collection, Girolamo Ranuzzi had himself acted as a patron of medical practitioners, such as the anatomist Petronio Ignazio Zecchini.

In the summer of 1763, Zecchini wrote to Girolamo Ranuzzi to express his gratitude for the senator's support and his wish for continued protection.[45] Notably, shortly after Ranuzzi purchased Morandi's collection, Zecchini became a staunch adversary of women's learning and famously triggered a debate on the topic through the anonymous publication of a venomous booklet titled *Dì geniali. Della Dialettica delle Donne ridotta al suo vero principio* ('Genial days. On women's dialectics reduced to its true principle').[46] Launched after the transferral of Morandi's collection to Ranuzzi's palace, Zecchini's attack on women's learning was brought out at the end of a period in which his relationship with the University of Bologna had been particularly tense. Between the end of 1768 and the beginning of 1769, Zecchini had been offered the onerous honour of lecturing in the 1770 public anatomy lesson.[47] But he was unavailable, and the anatomist Germano

[41] ASB, Archivio Ranuzzi, Scritture diverse spettanti alla Nobil Casa Ranuzzi (1769–73), Lib. 124, fasc. n. 6.

[42] Ibid., Lib. 124, fasc. n. 21.

[43] Berti Logan, 'Women and the Practice', 515.

[44] Annibale Ranuzzi (1625–1697) owned a famous library and his son, Vincenzo Ferdinando Antonio Ranuzzi (1658–1726), served at the Medici court.

[45] ASB, Ranuzzi, Carte di Famiglia, Lettere di casa (1763), Letters of 19 July and 6 August 1763 from Petronio Ignazio Zecchini. On Zecchini, see Fantuzzi, *Notizie degli scrittori bolognesi*, vol. 9, 201–2.

[46] See Paul Mengal (ed.), *Giacomo Casanova, Lana Caprina: Une controverse médicale sur l'utérus pensant à l'Université de Bologne en 1771–1772*, trans. Roberto Poma (Paris: Honoré Champion, 1999). See also Cavazza, 'Women's Dialectics'.

[47] ASB, Assunteria di studio, Atti, n. 25 (1756–77), 17 December 1768. In January 1768, Zecchini had also been involved in an argument concerning the public anatomy lesson with the students' prior; see ibid., 22 January 1768.

Azzoguidi took his place.[48] Zecchini then moved to Ferrara to teach medicine there. Before leaving, he made a deal with the University of Bologna: were he to return, he would be able to take on the first available lectureship. However, when, at the end of 1771, he intended to go back to Bologna, he grew unhappy with the terms of the agreement and requested that the university offer him a salaried lectureship without delay. The university did not yield to the pressure, and Zecchini flew into a rage.[49] In the same period, he anonymously published his *Dì geniali*, where he famously disparaged female participation in the world of learning by arguing that women's intellectual capacities were influenced by their womb.

According to Zecchini, as the womb lay at the origin of women's proverbial inconstancy and concupiscence, women's intellect was bound to be equally unstable and unreliable. Germano Azzoguidi replied with a defence of women and, as we saw in Chapter 3, referred to the two famous women of Bologna (Bassi and Morandi) who, with their demonstrations, impressed viewers and managed to convince even those who did not agree with them to change their minds.[50] The traveller and adventurer Giacomo Casanova, who was at the time sojourning in Bologna, joined the debate. Both Azzoguidi and Casanova defended women from Zecchini's accusations. They emphasized the importance of education and downplayed the role of nature in creating differences between the sexes. Casanova, for his part, did not spare Azzoguidi and criticized both university professors. The dispute enjoyed considerable notoriety. Foreign travellers touring the Italian peninsula reported on it, and within fifteen days from the appearance of his *Lana caprina*, Casanova claimed to have sold all his 500 copies, and was pleased with his gains.[51]

Zecchini's pamphlet has been regarded as a remarkable example of the 'misogynist' attitude of eighteenth-century medical practitioners who supported views of the animal economy of the female body.[52] However, we should read the booklet against the events that preceded and accompanied its publication, such as Zecchini's conflict with the University of Bologna and Ranuzzi's acquisition of Morandi's collection. Such a reading sheds light on how the complex dynamics of local academic politics, patronage networks, and personal acrimonies contextualize the season in which Bologna became renowned for its group of accomplished women who received papal patronage and acquired celebrity status. As Zecchini's ambition to return to the University of Bologna floundered, he may have resented Ranuzzi's purchase of Morandi's collection as the sign that his former patron was showing a preference for a woman over himself.

In fact, Girolamo Ranuzzi had good reasons for acquiring Morandi's famous anatomical collection. As well as pursuing the family's tradition of patronage of

[48] ASB, Atti dell'Assunteria di studio, n. 25 (1756–77), 12 and 19 April 1769, and 15 December 1770.

[49] See ASB, Assunteria di Studio, Lettere dell'Assunteria, n. 66 (1744–95), Letters of 4, 14, and 28 December 1771, and of 5 February 1772 to the ambassador.

[50] [Azzoguidi], *Lettres de Madame Cunégonde*, 122.

[51] Andrés, *Cartas familiares*, vol. 1, 18.

[52] See Paul Mengal, 'Introduction', in Mengal (ed.), *Giacomo Casanova*, 8; Messbarger, *The Lady Anatomist*, 144–5.

natural and medical knowledge, in the same period he actively engaged in promoting its commercial interests and reviving its name among European aristocratic circles. Ranuzzi's pursuits led to the creation of an impressive network of agents and brokers across Italian and European cities and ports. They also brought about a conspicuous movement of supplies, letters, specimens, luxury goods, and books in and out of the grand arcade of the Ranuzzi Palace. Embarking on trips across Europe and in the Italian peninsula further allowed Ranuzzi to create a rich and tightly interwoven web of acquaintances, which generated massive epistolary exchange. During his trip to Naples in 1762 Ranuzzi befriended Carlotta Gaetani dell'Aquila d'Aragona (1718–1779), the Princess of San Severo who, together with her spouse Raimondo di Sangro, the Prince of San Severo, were featured prominently in Ranuzzi's contact book, being listed among the family's 'correspondents and friends'.[53] As we shall see in Chapter 7, since the mid-1750s the Prince of San Severo had housed an impressive anatomical specimen in his palace in Naples. Here, Ranuzzi may have come across di Sangro's anatomical display and acquainted himself with the benefits of accommodating an anatomical collection under one's roof. Indeed, as models became highly appreciated tools of knowledge, they not only brought their makers fame and fortune but also promised to add value to their owners' collections and pursuits. Notably, Ranuzzi acquired anatomical models at a time when he was seeking legitimation for his initiatives related to the world of health. Just like Raimondo di Sangro, who invested in anatomical models when he was trying to enhance the reputation of his cabinet of curiosities and his own standing as a savant, Ranuzzi's purchase of Morandi's anatomical collection took place at the height of his efforts to boost the family's name and commercial aspirations by relaunching the family's spa.[54]

THE SALT OF THE LION

Ranuzzi's spa was located in Porretta, a town situated in the hilly region south of Bologna. It had belonged to the Ranuzzi family since the fifteenth century, when Girolamo Ranuzzi's homonymous and illustrious ancestor, the second Count of Porretta, had received it as a papal donation. The spa was inherited on the basis of the right of primogeniture, namely the right of the eldest child to be bequeathed the family estate. Being the first child, Girolamo became the twelfth Count of Porretta upon his father's death in 1735. Since he was only eleven then, his mother Maria remained in charge of the spa until 1748, when Girolamo made his first official visit. As Anna Rosa Bambi has observed, the Porretta spa was of 'great importance' in Ranuzzi's projects, absorbing much of his energy.[55]

[53] See ASB, Archivio Ranuzzi, Carte politiche, Indici relativi a Girolamo Ranuzzi, busta 1, 'Registro di tutti quelli a' quali per ragione di Commercio, di Civiltà, e Parentela giornalmente si scrive da S.E. il Sig: Senatore Girolamo Ranuzzi, Conte XII della Porretta', 2 and 72.

[54] Biblioteca Gambalunga (Rimini), Fondo Gambetti, Lettere autografe al Dott. Giovanni Bianchi, fasc. Ferdinando Bassi, Letter of 12 September 1759 from Ferdinando Bassi in Bologna to Giovanni Bianchi.

[55] Anna Rosa Bambi, 'Il conte Girolamo Ranuzzi, un eclettico bolognese del 700', *Il Carrobbio*, 24 (1998), 137–56 (citation p. 138).

Over the course of the eighteenth century, spa resorts gained ever more prominence as places of healing, leisure, and socialization.[56] They also offered ideal locations to spend a *villeggiatura* (leisurely time spent away from the city and urban commitments). In Britain, the spa city of Bath became a renowned place of leisure and cultural entertainment as well as a healing site attracting people interested in its mineral waters. Over a few decades Bath had turned from a provincial town into one of the most fashionable centres outside the capital, so much so that members of the elite who participated in the famous London season in the winter relocated to Bath during the summer months. As in Bath, in the Italian peninsula spa resorts frequently boasted ancient origins. As such, they were particularly well positioned to be included in the itineraries of travellers who toured Italy in search of fresh contact with the ancient world.

To Ranuzzi, the prospect of transforming the family spa into a Grand Tour destination was no doubt alluring. When he started to dedicate himself to revamping the site, the beneficial effects of spa waters were being discussed in a number of medical works written by prominent literati. In the 1750s, for instance, Antonio Cocchi and Giovanni Bianchi, the famous anatomists and antiquarians that we encountered in earlier parts of this work, published writings on the Bagni di Pisa.[57] Others celebrated the salubriousness of a variety of hot springs scattered throughout the Italian peninsula in locations such as Ischia and Montecatini.[58] In 1761, Ranuzzi followed the lead of spa enthusiasts and called on the naturalist Ferdinando Bassi to shed light on the nature of the new hot mineral water found at the Porretta spa, inquiring as to whether it could be identified as 'the salt of the lion'.[59] He then decided to commission a book on the spa waters and involve savants, such as Jacopo Bartolomeo Beccari, the prominent Bolognese physician and supporter of anatomical collections, as well as Bassi. Bassi agreed to complete the book under the condition of remaining anonymous.[60] Ranuzzi was eager to see the project completed, and started to put pressure on Bassi, urging him to finish the book as soon as possible so as to enhance the repute of the Porretta spa and attract foreign visitors.[61] Over time, Ranuzzi became ever more insistent. On 5 January 1765, for instance, he exhorted Bassi to end the book during that very winter so as to encourage visitors to head to Porretta in the coming spring.[62]

[56] On spas and their relationship with bathing practices in early modern Italy, see Cavallo and Storey, *Healthy Living*, 254.

[57] See Antonio Cocchi, *Dei Bagni di Pisa* (Florence: Stamperia Imperiale, 1750); Giovanni Bianchi, *Dei Bagni di Pisa posti a pie' del monte di San Giuliano* (Florence: a spese della Stamperia Paperiniana, 1757).

[58] Giovanni Andrea D'Aloisio, *L'infermo istruito nel vero salutevole uso dei rimedi minerali dell'isola d'Ischia* (Naples: G. di Domenico e V. Manfredi, 1757).

[59] BUB, ms. 233, vol. 8, Letter of 16 December 1761 from Girolamo Ranuzzi in Rome to Ferdinando Bassi, fol. 104r.

[60] Bambi, 'Il conte Girolamo Ranuzzi', 149–50. See also ASB, Archivio Ranuzzi, Feudo della Porretta, Miscellanea, Recapiti spettanti alle Terme Porrettane, busta 3, 'Notizie spettanti all'acque porrettane con documenti'.

[61] BUB, ms. 233, vol. 8, Letters of Girolamo Ranuzzi to Ferdinando Bassi, fols. 104r–129v.

[62] Ibid., fol. 125r (Letter of 5 January 1765).

In fact, the book was only one aspect of the vast operation that was intended to make the Porretta estate profitable. Keen to integrate the Porretta waters into the lucrative market of medical remedies, Ranuzzi gathered samples of the waters and sent them around Europe. Making extensive use of his network of acquaintances, throughout the 1760s he dispatched dozens of samples to locations as diverse as Alessandria (in Piedmont), Amsterdam, Ancona, Avignon, Bergamo, Ferrara, Florence, Lisbon, London, Marseille, Milan, Modena, Padua, Rome, Turin, Venice, Verona, Vienna, and many more. The main aim was to collect information about the waters' healing properties. Apparently, Ranuzzi also wished to check how the Porretta waters compared to the salt that had made Bath so famous.[63] In some cases, he sent the water samples directly to his medical acquaintances such as the physician Leopoldo Marco Antonio Caldani in Padua.[64] In other cases, he asked his correspondents to forward the samples to their physicians, surgeons, and apothecaries. He also reached out to hospitals and, notably, to the famous hospital of Santo Spirito in Rome, where he wrested the promise that all the 'chief physicians' ('*medici primari*') would use the 'water of the lion' and examine its effects.[65]

Gifts regularly accompanied the water samples to curry favour with the addressees. After the book on the Porretta waters was finally published in 1768, it was sent out to Ranuzzi's contacts along with the samples. Offering a means to advertise the waters' properties, the book added the prestige of a publication to the spa resort and its travelling samples. Elegant prints depicting the newly refurbished Ranuzzi Palace were also included in some of the shipments. Whilst the book on the waters of Porretta provided background information on the samples, the prints of the Ranuzzi Palace were intended as a precious gift for those in charge of negotiating with local practitioners. After Ranuzzi acquired Morandi's collection and the modeller moved to the Ranuzzi Palace, waxworks also started to travel alongside the water samples. In 1770, Ranuzzi sent a box containing figures in wax to some addressees in Marseille who in the same period also received a package containing the 'salt of the lion'.[66]

Focused as he was on his commercial agenda, Ranuzzi urged some correspondents to sell the water samples as well as to check out their properties and advertise them.[67] Not everybody, however, was willing to yield to the pressure. In September 1769, an irritated Domenico Controni, Ranuzzi's long-term Amsterdam broker,

[63] In November 1768, for instance, Gaspare Moretti reported to Ranuzzi about his trip to Bath; see ASB, Archivio Ranuzzi, Carte di Famiglia, Lettere di casa (1768), Letter of 22 November 1768 from Gaspare Moretti in London.

[64] ASB, Archivio Ranuzzi, Carte di Famiglia, Lettere di casa (1769), Letter of 24 March 1769 from Leopoldo Caldani in Padua.

[65] ASB, Archivio Ranuzzi, Carte di Famiglia, Lettere di casa (1767), Letter of 14 October 1767 from Orazio Orlandini in Rome.

[66] See ASB, Archivio Ranuzzi, Carte di Famiglia, Lettere di Casa (1770), Letters of 21 September and 19 October 1770 from Gio. G. Dufour in Livorno. On early modern cultures of gift, see, for instance, Natalie Zemon Davis's classic *The Gift in Sixteenth-Century France* (Oxford: Oxford University Press, 2000).

[67] In June 1767, for instance, Luigi Lolli from Rome acknowledged reception of the 'salt of the lion', promising that he would both check its effects and try to sell it; see ASB, Archivio Ranuzzi, Carte di Famiglia, Lettere di casa (1767), Letter of 13 June 1767 from Luigi Lolli in Rome.

informed Ranuzzi that, although he was willing to promote the salt, he had no intention of selling it, for 'we are bankers, not shop-keepers or sellers of remedies'.[68] However, when, some ten months later, the water samples arrived in Amsterdam, Controni talked with his physician, 'one of the most important ones', and with the hospital's apothecary, and when he wrote back to Ranuzzi he was able to offer sound advice: before seeking to commercialize the 'salt of the lion', Ranuzzi should first verify whether or not it was better and cheaper than 'the English one'.[69]

The late 1760s saw a flurry of correspondence on the 'salt of the lion'. In the same period, Ranuzzi purchased Morandi's collection. The timing could not have been better. By the late 1760s, Morandi's anatomical demonstrations had become one of Bologna's Grand Tour landmarks. Accommodating a famous collection and an anatomical celebrity like Morandi promised to augment the tourist traffic to the Ranuzzi Palace and to bolster the effort to increase the worth and repute of the senator's pursuits. Thanks to its Palladian façade, handsome staircase, noble hall, and gallery of paintings, the Ranuzzi Palace was by then already considered a tourist attraction.[70] However, it received mixed reviews. For instance, the British traveller Anna Riggs Miller noted in her popular *Letters from Italy* that the Ranuzzi Palace held 'the largest collection we have yet seen of bad pictures'.[71] The arrival of Morandi and her collection promised to transform the palace into a unique site of anatomical learning and spectacle that could easily reach those travellers whom Ranuzzi had hoped to attract to the Porretta spa. Upon visiting the palace, visitors could familiarize themselves with anatomical knowledge and become acquainted with what lay behind the cultivation of a healthy body. They could then travel to the Porretta spa as part of their engagement in the pursuit of health.

The plan seemed well thought out and in the beginning it appeared to pay off. Shortly after the purchase of Morandi's collection, Ranuzzi welcomed the Holy Roman Emperor Joseph II to his residence. The emperor had arrived in Bologna in March 1769 incognito, under his characteristic alias Count of Falkenstein, and resided at the Pellegrino, the inn that frequently offered hospitality to foreigners, before setting off for Rome.[72] Back in Bologna on May 9, he left again for Parma and returned to the city on 13 May.[73] As the emperor expressed the wish to visit Morandi's collection, the following morning, on the day of the Pentecost, he was escorted to the Ranuzzi Palace by a delegation of local authorities, including the Maresciallo Pallavicini, his son, the Count Giuseppe Pallavicini,

[68] ASB, Archivio Ranuzzi, Carte di Famiglia, Lettere di casa (1768), Letter of 14 November 1768 from Domenico Cotroni.

[69] ASB, Archivio Ranuzzi, Carte di Famiglia, Lettere di casa (1769), Letter of 14 July 1769 from Domenico Cotroni. See also Letters of 1 September and 24 November 1769.

[70] See Edward Wright, *Some Observations Made in Travelling Through France, Italy,* &c. *in the years 1720, 1721, and 1722*, vol. 2 (London: Tho. Ward and E. Wicksteed, 1730), 442.

[71] [Anna Riggs Miller], *Letters from Italy, Describing the Manners, Customs, Antiquities, Paintings, &c. of that Country, in the Years MDCCLXX and MDCCLXXI, to a Friend Residing in France, by an English Woman*, 2nd edn., vol. 1 (London: Edward and Charles Dilly, 1777), 336.

[72] BCABo, ms. B 89, 'Diario e memorie varie dall'anno MDL all'anno MDCCLXXXXVI raccolte e scritte dal Domenico Maria D'Andrea Galeati', vol. 10, 203 and 205–6.

[73] ASB, Assunteria d'Istituto, Diversorum, busta 18, n.16, 'Visita all'Istituto dell'Imperatore Giuseppe II'.

and the Count Marulli.[74] As eighteenth-century reports have it, the emperor spent about an hour and a half in conversation with Morandi, and gifted her both a golden box and a golden medal that bore his effigy.[75]

It is not easy to assess whether the fact that the contract between Morandi and Ranuzzi was signed on 6 May 1769, that is, only a few days before Joseph II's visit to her collection, was as a matter of mere coincidence.[76] One can only speculate about whether Ranuzzi had tried to finalize the agreement before Joseph II returned from Rome so as to ensure that everything was in order in case the emperor showed interest in purchasing the collection. As is well known, in the following years the emperor's brother Pietro Leopoldo, the Grand Duke of Tuscany, supported the large anatomical collection that opened in Florence in 1775.[77] In 1785, Joseph II himself would sponsor a copy of the Florentine anatomical collection of La Specola for the medico-surgical military academy of the Josephinum in Vienna.[78] Without question, Joseph II's visit marked a crucial moment in Morandi's career. News of the visit appeared in gazettes and periodicals and continued to be mentioned in travellers' diaries and local chronicles for years to come.[79] In 1777, the event was evoked, yet again, by Luigi Galvani as the ultimate evidence of Morandi's merits.[80]

Morandi tried to keep in contact with the illustrious visitor, with mixed results. Months after the imperial visit, in early January 1770 the Bolognese biographer and writer Vincenzo Camillo Alberti, a relative of the surgeon and man-midwife Giovanni Antonio Galli, interceded on Morandi's behalf and sent a letter to the emperor via his friend, the famous poet and librettist Pietro Metastasio who lived in Vienna. Metastasio was not sure whether proper etiquette allowed him to present a closed letter to the emperor and did not appreciate the request to act as a go-between. Still, he reluctantly delivered the missive to the cabinet secretary only to discover that in fact the emperor appreciated receiving the letter, and praised Morandi as 'a truly distinguished woman' who created 'marvellous works', which he had seen and admired.[81] Yet, when Morandi directly contacted Metastasio the following December to ask him to forward a Christmas card to the emperor, the

[74] See *Bologna*, 20, 17 May 1769.

[75] BCABo, ms. B 133, Marcello Oretti, *Notizie de' Professori del Dissegno*, vol. 11, 228.

[76] See ASB, Archivio Ranuzzi, Scritture diverse spettanti alla Nobil Casa Ranuzzi (1769–73), Lib. 124, fasc. n. 6.

[77] See, for instance, Maerker, *Model Experts*. [78] Ibid., part 3.

[79] See, for instance, BCABo, ms. B 1275, Lorenzo Tarozzi, 'Giornale delle funzioni dell'Illmo, ed Ecclso Magistrato de' Sri Anziani fatto da me D. Lorenzo Dottor Tarozzi moderno Cappellano Cerimoniere del suddetto Magistrato eletto li 11 Febbraio 1757', fols. 20–21; *Bologna*, 20, 17 May 1769; BCABo, B 89, 'Diario e memorie varie dall'anno MDL all'anno MDCCLXXXXVI raccolte e scritte dal Domenico Maria D'Andrea Galeati', vol. 10, 203 and 205–6; BCABo, ms. B 133, Marcello Oretti, *Notizie de' Professori del Dissegno*, vol. 11, 228; Jacob Jonas Björnståhl, *Lettere ne' suoi viaggj stranieri di Giacomo Giona Bjoernstaehl, professore di Filosofia in Upsala, scritte al Signor Gjörwell, bibliotecario regio in Istocolma, tradotte dallo svezzese in tedesco da Giusto Ernesto Groskurd e dal tedesco in italiano recate da Baldassar Domenico Zini di Val di Non*, vol. 3 (Poschiavo: Giuseppe Ambrosioni, 1782–7), 147.

[80] Galvani, *De Manzoliniana supellectili*, 53.

[81] Pietro Metastasio, *Lettere*, in *Tutte le opere di Pietro Metastasio*, ed. Bruno Brunelli, vol. 4 (Milan: Arnoldo Mondadori Editore, 1954), 787–8 (Letter 1829: Letter of 7 January 1770 from Pietro Metastasio in Vienna).

libretto writer refused to do so on account of his insignificant position at the Habsburg court.[82]

Metastasio's different responses to Morandi's requests are worth noting as they point, once again, to her position as a very famous practitioner who, despite her celebrity, enjoyed limited negotiating power and had to rely on men of higher social rank like Oretti and Alberti to intercede on her behalf. In general, in addition to marking a crucial moment in Morandi's career, Joseph II's visit also constituted a critical event for her patron, who could capitalize on the prestige and authority bestowed upon his estate by the royal visit. Benefiting from Morandi's presence in his palace, Ranuzzi adopted a protective attitude towards the collection. He exercised control over her work, and seemingly influenced and brokered her engagements and commissions. We see this, for example, in the case of Anna Sapieha Jablonowska, a Polish noblewoman who owned a cabinet of natural history, launched a programme of reforms concerning estate management (including her own), and acted as a patroness of hospitals and midwifery training. Having admired Morandi's tables of the senses in Turin, Jablonowska contacted Morandi to commission a copy of the series from her. However, Morandi died before completing the job, and Jablonowska risked disappointment after Ranuzzi initially refused to let her have the original models copied and finalized by someone else, on account that such a course of action would run the risk of lessening the models' value 'as unique things in Europe'.[83]

TRANSFERABLE SKILLS

Just when everything seemed perfect, a flood of letters reached the Ranuzzi Palace with disappointing news about the 'salt of the lion'. To be sure, some correspondents were satisfied with the salt and managed to convince local apothecaries to keep samples in their shops. In September 1769, for instance, a certain Filippo Chiesa from the town of Cento, near Ferrara, reported on three case histories of patients cured by the salt.[84] But many more correspondents reported bad news, and highlighted that their attempts to evaluate the effectiveness of the salt had been either incomplete or inconclusive.[85] While such letters started to pile up, Ranuzzi had to

[82] Ibid., vol. 5, 61 (Letter 1911: Letter of 17 December 1770 from Pietro Metastasio in Vienna to Anna Morandi Manzolini).

[83] ASB, Archivio Ranuzzi, Carte di Famiglia, Lettere di Casa (1770), Letter of 20 June 1770; ASB, Archivio Ranuzzi, Scritture diverse spettanti alla Nobil Casa Ranuzzi (1774–8), Lib. 125, 'Pro-memoria al Monsig. Illmo e Rmo Ranuzzi' and 'Risposta alla pro-memoria indirizzata a Mon. Ranuzzi, da Monsig. Lascaris'. See also Dacome, 'Women, Wax and Anatomy', 547; Messbarger, *The Lady Anatomist*, 165.

[84] ASB, Archivio Ranuzzi, Carte di Famiglia, Lettere di Casa (1769), Letter of 26 September 1769 from Filippo Chiesa in Cento. The physician Leopoldo Marco Antonio Caldani also sent encouraging words from Padua, declaring himself 'persuaded that the 'salt of the lion' had very good effects'; see ibid., Letter of 24 March 1769 from Leopoldo Caldani in Padua.

[85] See, for instance, ibid., Letter of 28 February 1769 from Orazio Orlandini; ibid., Letter of 4 September 1769 from Giosepantonio Badia in Turin; ASB, Archivio Ranuzzi, Carte di Famiglia, Lettere di Casa (1770), Letter of 22 July 1770 from Luigi Stampini in Ancona, and Letter of 6 February 1770 from Girolamo Ranuzzi to Gaspare Moretti in London.

reconsider his plan to transform Porretta into the new Bath. Morandi's role in Ranuzzi's ambitious programme of self-promotion was also likely to be affected. While, to start with, the presence of Morandi and her collection in the palace could support the senator's ambitions to join the profitable market of spa cures and remedies, the fading promise of the Porretta waters seemingly led Ranuzzi to employ the artificer in different ways. In particular, as Ranuzzi sought to expand his vast network of powerful acquaintances, he relied on Morandi's skills as a portrait artist as well as an anatomical modeller and a maker of wax figures. Morandi's portraits were accordingly integrated into Ranuzzi's elaborate rituals of gift exchange and joined the traffic of luxuries that transited in and out of the Ranuzzi Palace.

When in the summer of 1769, shortly after the purchase of Morandi's collection, Ranuzzi advertised the talents of 'a certain artificer' to the marquise Benedetta Hercolani Zagnoni, he was likely referring to Morandi. The marquise replied favourably to Ranuzzi's recommendation and mentioned that she was already acquainted with the 'ability and value of the artificer', who in fact had made a portrait for her niece.[86] Two years later, in 1771, the Institute of the Sciences started negotiations for the acquisition of Morandi's portrait of the late Jacopo Bartolomeo Beccari, though in the end the sale was not finalized.[87] At times, Morandi's creations could serve as currency for the payment of Ranuzzi's debts. In August 1771, Agnese Marchesini, a supplier based in Volterra from whom Ranuzzi had acquired a number of alabaster vases, asked not to be compensated with cash. Rather, she preferred to have the famous female wax sculptor make a portrait of a fellow citizen, the antiquarian and literatus Mario Guarnacci (1701–1785), as a way to pay back the debt she had contracted with him.[88]

Guarnacci was the author of famous antiquarian works such as the *Origini italiche o siano memorie istorico–etrusche sopra l'antichissimo regno d'Italia* (1767–72), where he somewhat controversially claimed the superiority of ancient Italian culture over that of Greece. Being in regular epistolary contact with Ranuzzi, Guarnacci exchanged with him books, artefacts, ideas, and considerations on the 'salt of the lion'. On 12 October 1769, for instance, he wrote to Ranuzzi to acknowledge the receipt of a text that elucidated the properties of the 'salt of the lion' as a solvent of iron, gold, and steel, as well as a medicinal substance. Guarnacci was willing to pass the news on to some friends and maintained that it could be publicized in 'some gazette, at least a literary one'.[89] Keeping in regular contact with Ranuzzi, Guarnacci likely knew about the presence of Morandi and her collection in the senator's palace. In December 1772, he was thrilled to hear that a

[86] ASB, Archivio Ranuzzi, Carte di Famiglia, Lettere di Casa (1769), Letter of 7 August 1769 written by proxy for the Marquise Benedetta Hercolani Zagnoni.

[87] ASB, Assunteria d'Istituto, Atti, n. 6 (1761–75), 17 May 1771, fols. 129v–130r.

[88] ASB, Archivio Ranuzzi, Carte di Famiglia, Lettere di Casa (1771), Letter of 17 August 1771 from Agnese Marchesini in Volterra.

[89] ASB, Archivio Ranuzzi, Carte di Famiglia, Lettere di Casa (1769), Letter of 12 October 1769 from Mario Guarnacci in Volterra. Emphasis on the salt's capacity to dissolve metals may have perhaps pointed to Ranuzzi's interest in alchemy. On Ranuzzi's alchemical and Masonic interests, see Gianna Paola Tomasina, *'All'uso di Francia': Dalla moda all'industria. Carte decorate, papier peint e tessile stampato nel sec. XVIII: la Bottega Bertinazzi, Bologna, 1760–1896* (Bologna: Pàtron, 2001).

portrait made by the '*brava Professora*' ('skilled female professor') was on its way to Volterra. He then wanted to send some expression of gratitude to the artificer, but Ranuzzi stopped him on the grounds that this had already been taken care of.[90] The story of Guarnacci's portrait sheds further light on the considerable level of control exercised by Ranuzzi over Morandi's activities. It also shows how Ranuzzi traded Morandi's portraits as gifts that could help him weave together a tight web of favours and obligations. Indeed, with the exception of Jablonowska's case, there is little evidence that, after selling the collection to Ranuzzi and moving to his palace, Morandi continued to entertain direct relations with the addressees and the beneficiaries of her work. Thus, while Morandi's growing popularity as an anatomical celebrity increased the value of her creations, Ranuzzi could capitalize on some of this added value to support his own pursuits. Not surprisingly, as Morandi's own effigy became itself the correlate of her celebrity, it ended up playing into Ranuzzi's networking strategies.

PORTRAYING CELEBRITY

When Jérôme Richard met Morandi in the early 1760s, he had words of praise for her anatomical collection and remarked that she 'made busts in wax that were as true as nature'.[91] However, he was not completely satisfied with her self-portrait and believed that in this case she 'had not perfectly succeeded with regard to likeness'.[92] Still, Morandi's self-portrait was a great success. Becoming a powerful token of Morandi's status as a celebrity, it was turned into a cherished memento that was imitated and replicated in its own right. In 1770, shortly after purchasing Morandi's collection, Ranuzzi asked the British sculptor Joseph Nollekens to realize a bust of Morandi. At the time, Nollekens was about to return to London, having lived for a number of years in Rome where he had sculpted the busts of British travellers and established a reputation as a portrait sculptor. His portrait of Morandi corroborated even further the modeller's status as a celebrity and an icon of the Grand Tour.

For his part, Ranuzzi capitalized on Morandi's effigy and used it as yet another tool of gift exchange. In the summer of 1771, just before starting his journey to Turin, he offered 'the well-known portrait of Manzolini' to the king of Sardinia. The king gladly accepted the offer and ordered the display of the portrait at the university where Morandi's models of the senses had already found a home.[93] In October 1771, Ranuzzi was in Turin, happily reporting that the portrait had

[90] ASB, Archivio Ranuzzi, Carte di Famiglia, Lettere di Casa (1772), Letters of 6 December and 28 December 1772 from Mario Guarnacci in Volterra. On the reception of the portrait, see also ASB, Archivio Ranuzzi, Carte di Famiglia, Lettere di Casa (1773), Letter of 5 January 1773 from Mario Guarnacci in Volterra. Apparently, the bust ended up being made in clay rather than wax; see ASB, Archivio Ranuzzi, Carte di Famiglia, Lettere di Casa (1772), Letter of 29 December 1772 from Luigi Spulcioni in Florence.

[91] Richard, *Description historique*, vol. 2, 119.

[92] Ibid.

[93] ASB, Archivio Ranuzzi, Carte di Famiglia, Lettere di Casa (1771), Letter of 21 August 1771 from Count Lascaris in Turin to Girolamo Ranuzzi.

arrived safely.[94] The timing was hardly accidental. In the same period Vincenzo Ranuzzi, Girolamo's brother, was seeking to advance his ecclesiastical career in Rome and was therefore in search of a powerful patron capable of supporting his ambitions. Notably, in 1750 the king of Sardinia had already interceded on behalf of Vincenzo with the papal court.[95] Some twenty years later, however, things had seemingly changed: Count Giuseppe Lascaris, the king's chamberlain and first secretary of foreign affairs, warned Girolamo Ranuzzi that the sovereign was reluctant to make recommendations to the pope. Yet, perhaps also thanks to the precious gift, the king changed his mind. In April 1772, he declared himself willing to support Vincenzo's aspirations in Rome.[96]

In the following years, Ranuzzi's engagement in gift exchange practices based on Morandi's effigy grew in parallel to the senator's ambitions. In 1773, Ranuzzi offered 'the bust of the famous Manzolini' together with the book of prints of the Ranuzzi Palace to Maximilian Friedrich von Königsegg-Rothenfels, the Archbishop-Elector of Cologne and Bishop of Münster, who, the following year, would act as godfather at the baptism of the senator's daughter.[97] Two years earlier, Ranuzzi had proposed sending a copy of the bust to the Russian Empress Catherine II. As Ranuzzi was likely to know, in the previous decades the Russian court had extensively engaged in acquiring anatomical models. Most famously, Peter the Great had purchased Frederik Ruysch's celebrated collection of anatomical preparations for a remarkable sum of money, making the famous Dutch anatomist a rich man.[98] An 'artificial anatomy' made by the French anatomical modeller Marie Marguerite Bihéron was furthermore included in the collection of surgical 'instruments, machines and models necessary for surgery' that the Empress Elizabeth, Peter's daughter, had commissioned from the French surgeon Sauveur-François Morand (1697–1773).[99] Catherine II also manifested a keen interest in both Morandi and Bihéron, and invited them to move to Russia along with their collections.[100] In July 1771, a box containing a 'bust or portrait sculpture' in plaster left the Ranuzzi Palace heading to the 'Empress of Moscovia'. It arrived first in the port city of Livorno, and from there travelled to Amsterdam, though it did not reach its destination.[101] In March 1774, the Baron de Staal wrote to Ranuzzi from St Petersburg to inform him

[94] Ibid., Letter of 8 October 1771 from Girolamo Ranuzzi in Turin.

[95] Bambi, 'Il conte Girolamo Ranuzzi', 143.

[96] ASTo, Materie politiche per rapporti all'interno, Lettere diverse Real Casa, Registri delle Lettere della Segreteria Esteri a particolari, n. 10 (1766–73), Letter of 1 April 1772 from Count Lascaris to Girolamo Ranuzzi.

[97] ASB, Archivio Ranuzzi, Carte politiche dei vari membri della famiglia, busta 78, Letter of 23 May 1773 from Maximilian Friedrich von Königsegg-Rothenfels, Elector of Cologne. On the bishop's participation in the baptism of the senator's daughter, see BCABo, Gozz. 351, 'Memorie storiche bolognesi dall'anno 1760 all'anno 1796 raccolte da Petronio Cavallazzi', n.p. (13 July 1774).

[98] See, for instance, Margócsy, 'Advertising Cadavers'; Margócsy, 'A Museum of Wonders?'; Margócsy, *Commercial Visions*; Knoeff, 'Touching Anatomy'.

[99] [G. de Simpré], *Voyage en France de M. le comte de Falckenstein*, vol. 1 (London [i.e. Paris]: Cailleau, 1778), 180.

[100] Messbarger, *The Lady Anatomist*, 167; Gargam, 'Marie-Marguerite Biheron'; Dacome, '"Une dentelle"'.

[101] On the portrait that left the Ranuzzi Palace to head towards Moscow, see ASB, Archivio Ranuzzi, Carte di Famiglia, Lettere di casa, 1771, Letters of 12 and 19 July, and 2 August 1771, from Gio. G. Dufour in Livorno to Girolamo Ranuzzi.

that he 'had not been able to find out what had happened to the bust of the famous Manzolini'.[102] In May 1776, Ranuzzi again offered Morandi's portrait to the empress. This time the gift arrived safely.[103] Writing to the diplomat and writer Friedrich Melchior, Baron von Grimm (1723–1807), in August 1776 Catherine mentioned having received the portrait: she had displayed it on her desk in Peterhof Palace and told those who inquired about the sitter's identity that the woman was her grandmother.[104] Turned into an object capable of both stimulating curiosity and generating conversation, the portrait helped to preserve and consolidate Morandi's fame and memory well after her death.

CELEBRITY AND MODESTY

Morandi's death had taken place before her effigy reached the Russian empress and started to prompt curious inquiries in Peterhof. By then, Morandi's collection had found a new home. Once the artificer was no longer around to demonstrate her models and make portraits for Ranuzzi's acquaintances, the collection was seemingly divested of its value as cultural capital capable of supporting the senator's own ambitions and pursuits. Indeed, shortly after the modeller died, Ranuzzi engaged in negotiations to sell her collection. In January 1775, Vincenzo Ranuzzi, who had by then become a cardinal in Rome, wrote to his brother Girolamo to let him know that a 'prince' was eager to buy the collection for the conspicuous sum of 7,000 scudi (about 35,000 Bolognese lire). Accordingly, he urged his brother to prepare a copy of the inventory and send it to Rome.[105] Vincenzo did not like the idea of selling, though he reckoned that the offer was very tempting. For his part, Girolamo did not waste any time. He turned to the Institute of the Sciences, flagged, once again, the risk of the collection falling into foreign hands, and offered to sell it to them for 6,000 scudi (about 30,000 Bolognese lire). The Institute's *Assunti* considered the request too onerous and, 'with great regret', turned it down.[106] Ranuzzi, however, had no intention of giving up and engaged in forceful negotiations.[107] The *Assunti* reconvened only to ascertain once more that the scarcity of resources prevented the Institute from accepting the offer. This time, however, they decided to send a plea to the new pope to check whether, given the examples of his predecessors, he might be willing to help.[108] Meanwhile, the negotiations continued.

[102] ASB, Archivio Ranuzzi, Carte politiche dei vari membri della famiglia, busta 78, Letter of 4/15 March 1774 from the Baron de Staal in St Petersburg.

[103] The portrait that Ranuzzi sent to the empress was apparently a plaster cast of the bust made by Nollekens; see Messbarger, *The Lady Anatomist*, 167–8.

[104] Catherine II, 'Lettres de l'impératrice Catherine II à Grimm (1774–1796), publiées avec les notes explicatives de Grote', in *Recueil de la Société Impériale russe d'histoire*, vol. 2 (St Petersburg: n.p., 1878), 52.

[105] ASB, Archivio Ranuzzi, Scritture diverse spettanti alla Nobil Casa Ranuzzi (1774–8), Lib. 125, Letter of 28 January 1775 from Vincenzo Ranuzzi to Girolamo Ranuzzi. As we have seen, Ranuzzi had purchased Morandi's collection in 1769 for 12,000 lire.

[106] ASB, Assunteria d'Istituto, Atti, n. 6 (1761–75), fol. 180r (6 April 1775).

[107] Ibid., fol. 178v (27 February 1775).

[108] Ibid., fols. 183r–v (6 April 1775).

The anatomist Luigi Galvani was charged with the task of checking the state of the models and eventually the Institute agreed to purchase the collection for a more reasonable 16,000 lire.[109]

The contract was finalized to general satisfaction, though the *Assunteria dei Magistrati* did receive an anonymous letter from a seemingly displeased 'citizen lover of the public good' inquiring whether the Institute had acquired the waxworks of the late Manzolini and asking 'with what faculty, what money, what contract and what economy' the purchase had taken place.[110] In fact, the news rapidly entered the public domain. In June 1777, Luigi Galvani famously delivered an *oratio* that celebrated the arrival of the collection at the Institute of the Sciences. The acquisition ensured, once again, that the collection would remain in Bologna and in fact, according to Galvani, it fulfilled Morandi's own wish to have her models displayed at the Institute of the Sciences.[111] In the *oratio*, Galvani also took the opportunity to take sides in the long-standing contention among the Bolognese modellers: he granted Morandi's models primacy over the other anatomical collections, and highlighted their utility as a complement to Lelli's models in the teaching of surgery. Delivered to general acclaim, Galvani's speech was published the following November, when the anatomy lessons at the Institute were just about to start, and contributed to Galvani's own career as well as to Morandi's consecration as a local heroine.[112]

Recent literature has taken Galvani's emphasis on Morandi's manual work, and his employment of the appellative 'artificer' to describe her occupation, as a sign that ultimately Morandi was not fully granted anatomical authority.[113] However, as the foregoing chapters have shown, mid-eighteenth-century Bolognese anatomical artificers like Lelli, Morandi, and Manzolini gained considerable anatomical standing and great renown precisely because of their extraordinary manual skills and their capacity to exemplify a special relationship between making and knowing; so much so that, as we have seen, they were praised by renowned anatomists such as Giovanni Bianchi as being capable of cultivating anatomy better than physicians.[114] It may be appealing to frame Morandi's life in terms of the story of an exceptionally talented woman whose accomplishments were only partially recognized by her fellow citizens. As is documented in the meagre paper trail that she has left behind, Morandi's capacity to capitalize on her achievements and celebrity did indeed remain limited. Yet, one may wonder whether these limitations ought

[109] ASB, Assunteria d'Istituto, Atti, n. 7 (1776–9), fols. 18v–19v; ASB: Assunteria d'Istituto, Lettere dell'Istituto, n. 5 (1766–82), Letter of 1 June 1776 from the Institute to the ambassador; Letter of 21 September 1776 from the Institute to the ambassador; Letter of 19 October 1776 from the Institute to the ambassador; ASB Lettere all'Istituto, n. 7, (1771–83), Letters of 8 June and 14 September 1776 from Filippo Gozzadini Parti Bonfiglioli in Rome.

[110] ASB, Assunteria dei Magistrati, Affari diversi, Istituto delle Scienze, busta 78, fasc. 8. The note is not dated.

[111] Galvani, *De Manzoliniana supellectili*.

[112] ASB, Assunteria d'Istituto, Lettere dell'Istituto, n. 5 (1766–82), Letter of 19 November 1777 from the Institute to the ambassador.

[113] Messbarger, *The Lady Anatomist*, 173.

[114] BUB, ms. 233, vol. 7, Lettere di Giovanni Bianchi (6 February 1751–29 December 1761), Letter of 22 November 1755 from Giovanni Bianchi in Rimini to Ferdinando Bassi, fols. 111v–112r.

to be looked at as the consequence of the lack of support of her fellow citizens rather than as the expression of how social as well as gender norms and constraints affected the lives of many eighteenth-century women, even when they ended up becoming widely appreciated public figures.

It may be worth drawing attention to how such factors equally played a part in the narratives that accompanied the making of Morandi's public persona. As Felicity Nussbaum and Laura Engel have remarked, over the course of the eighteenth century the emerging phenomenon of celebrity allowed some women, such as performers, to use the stage to challenge narratives of passive womanhood and accordingly find special spaces of agency. At the same time, public exposure also subjected these women to intense scrutiny, leading them sometimes to conceal their ambitions in the public domain and embrace narratives that complied with prescribed codes of female modesty.[115] Similarly, we have seen that, as Morandi's rise to celebrity developed alongside close observation of her personal life, her acquisition of public renown took place in conjunction with narratives of maternity and domesticity that framed her accomplishments and public presence within accepted codes of female conduct.[116]

In an essay on eighteenth-century accomplished women, such as Bassi and Agnesi, who dedicated themselves to natural knowledge and became particularly famous public figures, Marta Cavazza has observed that public exposure did not necessarily sit well with the many calls for modesty and moderation that were regularly addressed to them.[117] Some of these calls were articulated by famous 'enlightened' savants, such as Jean-Jacques Rousseau (1712–1778) and the Italian writer Pietro Verri (1728–1797), who took categories of modesty or moderation to be the ultimate foundation for female conduct, and the defining features of the social conventions with which women, including educated and learned women, had to comply. In his letter to Agnesi published by Caraccioli (which we encountered in Chapter 4), Lambertini similarly mentioned that he would be glad to find in libraries ('alongside our doctors') women who could be knowledgeable and still modest.[118] As Cavazza has suggested, modesty was a requirement placed on learned women because it 'offered reassurance that knowledge would not be used to demand a less subordinate role or even a public role'.[119] At the same time, such a request was at odds with the equally pressing requirement to perform in public and to make, as Eustachio Manfredi put it with regard to Laura Bassi, 'an almost continual spectacle of herself'.[120] As Morandi was becoming a prominent female

[115] Nussbaum, *Rival Queens*; Engel, *Fashioning Celebrity*. See also Waltraud Maierhofer, '"Angelicamad" – Then and Now', in Czennia (ed.), *Celebrity*, 107–30.

[116] On eighteenth-century learned women's strategies to safeguard their public reputation, see, for instance, Mary Terrall, 'The Uses of Anonymity in the Age of Reason', in Mario Biagioli and Peter Galison (eds.) *Scientific Authorship: Credit and Intellectual Property in Science* (New York: Routledge, 2003), 91–112; Paola Bertucci, 'The In/visible Woman: Mariangela Ardinghelli and the Circulation of Knowledge between Paris and Naples in the Eighteenth Century', *Isis*, 104:2 (2013), 226–49.

[117] Cavazza, 'Between Modesty and Spectacle', 289.

[118] Caraccioli, *La vie du pape Benoît XIV*, 104.

[119] Cavazza, 'Between Modesty and Spectacle', 289.

[120] Quoted in Cavazza, 'Between Modesty and Spectacle', 285.

anatomist who revealed the body's inner secrets in spectacular performances, and whose own body was subjected to public scrutiny, narratives of modesty and moderation accompanied her acquisition of celebrity status.[121] In the 1760s, the Scottish traveller William Patoun observed: 'there is a famous female Anatomist at Bologna whose works in wax are extremely Curious. She is a very ingenious Modest Woman.'[122] In a letter dated 19 August 1772, the Turinese architect Giuseppe Pazienza further remarked that Morandi deserved 'much praise for her moderation'.[123] Other famous contemporary women, such as Laura Bassi and Marie Marguerite Bihéron, who regularly engaged in theatrical demonstrations, were equally commended as exemplars of modesty and moderation.[124]

By the end of her life Morandi had become a champion of civic and moral standing and had received the honours and tributes that were due to a local heroine. Despite the conflict with Lelli, which exposed her to long-term contention, Morandi's contemporaries continued to sing her praises well after her death. In one of the ten poems on 'illustrious women' published not long after she died, the poet and abbot Francesco Clodoveo Maria Pentolini concluded his tribute to Morandi in a spirit of reconciliation: he emphasized that 'as much as a drop of water is similar to the other, so the kind and polite (*gentile*) Anna is equal to Ercole'.[125] When, on 31 July 1786, the Bolognese Accademia dei Gelati decided that the eulogy of 'an illustrious Bolognese man' had to be read at every gathering, its members included Morandi's name among those who deserved 'the honour'.[126] The fact that the Institute of the Sciences decided to acquire Morandi's collection in spite of the shortage of resources further points to the level of appreciation that Morandi had acquired in the city. When, a few years after the acquisition of the collection, the marquis Angelelli updated Bolletti's *Dell'origine e de' progressi dell'Instituto delle Scienze*, he gave ample space to the description of Morandi's collection, which was newly displayed at the Institute, and wondered whether Morandi was to be considered 'an excellent sculptor or a learned anatomist', concluding that she had excelled in both arts.[127] Angelelli's words point to how, thanks to her modelling activities, Morandi had acquired status as an authoritative creator of anatomical knowledge. If this had been possible, it was also because in the previous decades she had become a chief interpreter of the intimate relationship between making and knowing, and her sculpting skills had been regarded as

[121] It is worth noting that complex dynamics of modesty and spectacle also characterized the representation of female bodies in early modern anatomy; see Park, *Secrets of Women*; Massey, 'On Waxes and Wombs', 85.

[122] Patoun, 'Advice on Travel', xliv.

[123] Giuseppe Piacenza, 'Letter of 19 August 1772 from Turin', in Michelangelo Gualandi, *Memorie originali, italiane riguardanti le belle arti*, vol. 1 (Bologna: Marsigli, 1840), 105–6.

[124] See, for instance, Andrés, *Cartas familiares*, vol. 1, 20; Aubin-Louis Millin, *Magasin encyclopédique, ou Journal des sciences, des lettres et des arts*, vol. 4 (Paris: Imprimerie du Magasin Encyclopédique, 1796), 415.

[125] Francesco Clodoveo Maria Pentolini, *Donne illustri: Canti dieci*, vol. 2 (Livorno: Vincenzo Falorni, 1776–7), 14.

[126] *Regolamenti per gli Esercizi Letterari dell'Accademia de' Gelati, restituiti nella sessione del 31 luglio 1786*, n. 11, 5.

[127] Angelelli, *Notizie dell'origine*, 117.

constitutive of anatomical knowledge.[128] It is true that, as the foregoing story shows, Morandi only partially enjoyed the advantages brought about by the added value generated by her models. Yet, one may argue that her children did in fact end up benefiting from her accomplishments. Giuseppe became rich and noble overnight as the recipient of the Solimei inheritance. Morandi's other son, Carlo, became professor of theology at the University of Bologna and had a successful career in the Bolognese ecclesiastical world.[129] In short, much as Morandi's public persona ended up being elaborated through an emphasis on her family life and the relationship between mothering and the creation of anatomical knowledge, her children became the ultimate beneficiaries of her fame.

[128] Galvani, *De Manzoliniana supellectili*.
[129] ASB, Assunteria di Studio, Requisiti dei Lettori, busta 45, fasc. 36, 'D. Carlo Manzolini'.

7

Injecting Knowledge

GIUSEPPE GOES TO NAPLES

The fame of the Bolognese anatomical collections spread rapidly across Europe. After accounts of the anatomical models made by Lelli, Manzolini, and Morandi appeared in periodicals, travellers' reports, and local chronicles, Bologna started to look like an attractive hub for anatomical modellers in search of fortune. In 1756, when the Palermitan anatomist and priest Giuseppe Salerno (1728–1792) packed his anatomical specimen ('skeleton') and headed towards Bologna, he may have hoped to replicate the successes of these celebrated Bolognese modellers. Yet, when he stopped in Naples to make a public anatomical demonstration, he did not have to go any farther to find his luck.[1] This chapter travels down the Italian peninsula to follow the practice of anatomical modelling along the routes of the Grand Tour. Shifting attention from the Papal States to the colonial kingdoms of Naples and Sicily under Bourbonic rule, and from papal patronage to patrician collecting, it sets off to reconstruct the story of Salerno's anatomical specimen that did not arrive at its intended destination.

Created in Palermo and envisioned as a potential addition to the Bolognese anatomical displays, Salerno's skeleton ended up being purchased by the aristocrat Raimondo di Sangro, the seventh Prince of San Severo, to be displayed in his palace in Naples. Following the Palermitan anatomist on his journey, and exploring the setting in which his specimen ended up being displayed and viewed, this chapter considers another domain of the early history of anatomical displays that has received limited historical attention. While doing so, it offers an opportunity to expand the scope of our investigation of the early stages of anatomical modelling and provide a more comprehensive picture of the diversified world of mid-eighteenth-century anatomical displays. Like the anatomical models of Bologna, Salerno's anatomical specimens became renowned before the large Florentine anatomical collection of La Specola would define new modes of realization and display that would be endorsed and pursued by others. The story of Salerno's skeleton travelling north with its maker brings into focus the transformative power of

[1] Giuseppe De Gregorio e Russo, 'Ad Augustinum Giuffrida Ex Archiatris Catanensibus, Epistola, De notatu dignis Regalis Panh. Medicorum Academiae', in *Opuscoli di autori siciliani*, vol. 7 (Palermo: Stamperia de' Ss. Apostoli in Piazza Vigliena per Pietro Bentivegna, 1762), esp. 246–9; Francesco Buoncuore, 'Lettera di Francesco Buoncuore medico del nostro re Carlo Borbone indirizzata a S. E. sig. marchese Fogliani vicerè, e capitan generale di Sicilia' (Naples, 27 May 1757), in Francisco Maria Vesco, *De eloquentia apud siculos, orta, aucta, et absoluta [...]* (Palermo: Solli, 1797), 126–8.

movement in shaping the meaning and value of anatomical specimens as they journeyed across spaces, geographies, and cultural settings. It also sheds further light on the fluidity and malleability of the meanings of mid-eighteenth-century anatomical displays.

What follows expands on Chapter 6's exploration of anatomical models as cultural currencies that had the capacity to transfer value. As we have seen, in Bologna Ranuzzi purchased Morandi's anatomical collection at the same time that he was trying to promote the family's commercial prospects and market the city of Porretta and its spa waters to foreign travellers. In Naples, di Sangro's acquisition of anatomical specimens similarly promised to increase the value of his cabinet and consolidate his role and reputation as a savant. Just as in the case of Ranuzzi's acquisition of Morandi's collection, di Sangro's purchase of Salerno's anatomical work took place when the Prince of San Severo was transforming his palace into a Grand Tour destination. Thus, the history of Salerno's anatomical work further speaks to the significance of Grand Tour culture and spectatorship in the development of mid-eighteenth-century anatomical displays. Since Salerno's anatomical specimens were presented as the result of anatomical injections, theirs is also a story about how different techniques created distinctive forms of visualization of the inner body and informed different knowledge claims.

Although in recent years anatomical models have begun to receive scholarly attention, many aspects of the history of anatomical injections remain largely unexplored. This is possibly because injected specimens have suffered more than their fair share of damage, and only a limited number of them has survived to this day.[2] Quite understandably, recent literature has focused on the seminal season of engagement with the practice that took place in the Netherlands during the late seventeenth and early eighteenth centuries.[3] Yet, well into the eighteenth century, anatomical injections gathered the interest and aspirations of many practitioners and audiences across different regions. Promising a high degree of accuracy, anatomical preparations based on injections were considered capable of accounting for the state of affairs of the body like never before. As such, they were likened to the microscope and regarded as the vehicles of a new era of anatomical discovery and visualization. The expectation that the injection of materials, such as wax, resins, and oil of turpentine would make it possible to visualize anatomical parts that would otherwise remain unseen swept the anatomical world.

The use of injecting techniques to visualize blood vessels generated particular enthusiasm. Although by the mid-eighteenth century blood circulation was widely endorsed, issues related to the nature of blood, the ramification of blood vessels,

[2] On early modern anatomical injections, see Francis J. Cole, 'The History of Anatomical Injections', in Charles Joseph Singer (ed.), *Studies in the History and Method of Science*, vol. 2 (Oxford: Clarendon Press, 1921), 285–343.

[3] See, for instance, Cook, 'Time's Bodies'; Cook, *Matters of Exchange*, esp. chapter 7; Harold J. Cook, 'The Preservation of Specimens and the Takeoff in Anatomical Knowledge in the Early Modern Period', in Smith, Meyers, and Cook (eds.), *Ways of Making and Knowing*, 302–29; Margócsy, 'Advertising Cadavers'; Margócsy, 'A Museum of Wonders'; Margócsy, *Commercial Visions*; Knoeff, 'Touching Anatomy'. See also Marieke M.A. Hendriksen, *Elegant Anatomy: The Eighteenth-Century Leiden Anatomical Collections* (Leiden: Brill, 2015).

and their implications for medical practice, continued to raise questions and generate puzzlement. Mapping the complex web of blood vessels with the help of anatomical injections promised to shed light on these ongoing perplexities. Just as in the case of anatomical modelling, anatomical injections pledged to translate this promise into social and cultural as well as medical assets that could benefit makers, patrons, and collectors alike. This chapter examines the factors that both nourished and constrained the capacity of Salerno's anatomical specimens to act as instruments of credit.[4] It reconstructs how their biographical trajectories ended up being entangled in the contingencies related to di Sangro's own pursuits and vicissitudes.

A SKELETON AT THE NEAPOLITAN COURT

Unlike the famous anatomical modellers of Bologna, the Palermitan priest and anatomist Giuseppe Salerno had a degree in medicine. Much like the Bolognese artificers, however, he gained his anatomical reputation thanks to his hands-on work on anatomical specimens. In fact, Salerno was not the first Sicilian practitioner who travelled north in search of fortune. As he headed in the direction of Bologna with his skeleton, he may have been trying to walk in the footsteps of the Sicilian abbot Gaetano Giulio Zumbo, who found his way to success as a wax modeller while travelling to Naples, Florence, Bologna, Genoa, and Paris.[5] By the time Salerno left Palermo, the city had become a centre of anatomical modelling in its own right.[6] In 1738, the Palermitan Senate set up a committee to select a physician to send to Paris in order to receive surgical training. Among the candidates, Giuseppe Mastiani (1715–1756) impressed the committee with a model of the head, which generated 'no less delight than admiration'.[7] On 30 April 1738, Mastiani set off to Paris, where he studied with famous surgeons and anatomists such as Jacques-Bénigne Winslow (1669–1760), Sauveur-François Morand, and Georges de la Faye (1699–1781), who appreciated his 'anatomical manufactures'.[8] Mastiani's contemporaries observed that he had greater talent for modelling than for writing, and therefore his anatomical models constituted the bulk of his medical legacy.[9] In Paris, his skills as a maker of anatomical models helped him secure a place in prestigious medical circles. In 1743, at the French Academy of the Sciences Mastiani

[4] On the role of artefacts, instruments, and techniques in early modern strategies of credit in the Italian peninsula, see Mario Biagioli, *Galileo's Instruments of Credit: Telescopes, Images, Secrecy* (Chicago: University of Chicago Press, 2006).

[5] On Zumbo, see Chapter 2, note 86.

[6] A long-standing tradition of cadaver preservation found expression in the city's Capuchin Crypt, where the environmental circumstances seemed to preserve cadavers from decaying, and where the upper classes and the clergy buried their dead.

[7] [Domenico Schiavo], *Memorie per servire alla storia letteraria di Sicilia*, vol. 2 (Palermo: Stamperia de' SS. Apostoli per Pietro Bentivenga, 1756), 100–2 (citation p. 101).

[8] Ibid., 100–3.

[9] As we saw in Chapter 5, Galli's biographers similarly noticed that the Bolognese surgeon had become renowned thanks to his deployment of models in midwifery teaching rather than by authoring books.

demonstrated a set of wooden models of the ear and the eye, realized 'in conformity to Winslow's anatomical presentation'.[10] Some of Mastiani's models ended up in the Cabinet du Roi, and in 1749 the naturalist Louis-Jean-Marie Daubenton described them in Georges Louis Leclerc de Buffon's monumental *Histoire naturelle, générale et particulière* alongside the other anatomical specimens and models gathered in the royal cabinet (Figure 7.1).[11]

In 1744, Mastiani was back in Palermo where Charles de Bourbon had reformed the Royal Academy of Physicians so as to include anatomy in the medical curriculum. Mastiani was then appointed professor of anatomy and surgery and chief surgeon in the city's hospital. When he died of consumption shortly before turning forty-one in April 1756, Palermo could count on a sizeable group of anatomists who engaged in the making of anatomical models and preparations. In 1753, the surgeon Paolo Graffeo built 'a human skeleton in wax' showing the blood vessels of a male body, to which he added a similar 'female skeleton in wax' in 1758.[12] Giuseppe Salerno likewise made an anatomical specimen that displayed the complex web of blood vessels over a natural skeleton. In May 1756, he gave a demonstration of the specimen in front of the vice-royalty at the Royal Academy of Physicians in Palermo. The demonstration focused on the anatomy of blood vessels and bones, and was a great success.[13] A few months later, Salerno packed up his specimen and left the city.

Heading north, Salerno intended to take his skeleton to Bologna.[14] As he stopped in Naples to demonstrate this 'very elaborate product of his hands', he introduced viewers to the 'fabric' ('*tessitura*') of the human body and left his audience agape.[15] Among others, Francesco Buoncuore, physician to the king of Naples and *protomedico*, remained deeply impressed. In a letter to the Sicilian viceroy Giovanni Fogliano, who had asked him to introduce Salerno's work to Neapolitan society, he highly praised Salerno's anatomical specimen. He remarked that if the king of Denmark could boast that the artificial skeleton in his cabinet was 'a miracle of anatomy', Salerno's skeleton equally deserved to be placed in one of 'the most sumptuous' galleries of Europe.[16] In all likelihood this was Salerno's own aspiration when he set off to Bologna. Instead, his skeleton ended up travelling down Naples' streets and narrow alleys to the patrician residence of the nobleman Raimondo di Sangro. As the story has it, the day following the

[10] See 'Diverse ouvrages et diverses observations d'anatomie', in *Histoire de l'Académie Royale des Sciences, Année 1743* (Paris: Imprimerie Royale, 1746), 85.

[11] See Georges-Louis Leclerc, Comte de Buffon, and Louis-Jean-Marie Daubenton, *Histoire naturelle, générale et particulière, avec la description du cabinet du Roi*, vol. 3 (Paris: Imprimerie Royale, 1749), 238–42.

[12] See Luigi Del Pozzo, *Cronaca civile e militare delle Due Sicilie sotto la dinastia Borbonica dall'anno 1734 in poi* (Naples: Stamperia Reale, 1857), 64 and 70; Domenico Scinà, *Prospetto della storia letteraria di Sicilia nel secolo decimottavo*, vol. 1 (Palermo: Lo Bianco, 1859), 277; Luigi Sampolo, *La R. Accademia degli Studi di Palermo* (Palermo: Tipografia dello Statuto, 1888), 61.

[13] De Gregorio e Russo, 'Ad Augustinum Giuffrida', 246–7; Buoncuore, 'Lettera di Francesco Buoncuore', 126–8.

[14] De Gregorio e Russo, 'Ad Augustinum Giuffrida', 248; Buoncuore, 'Lettera di Francesco Buoncuore', 127.

[15] Buoncuore, 'Lettera di Francesco Buoncuore', 127.

[16] Ibid.

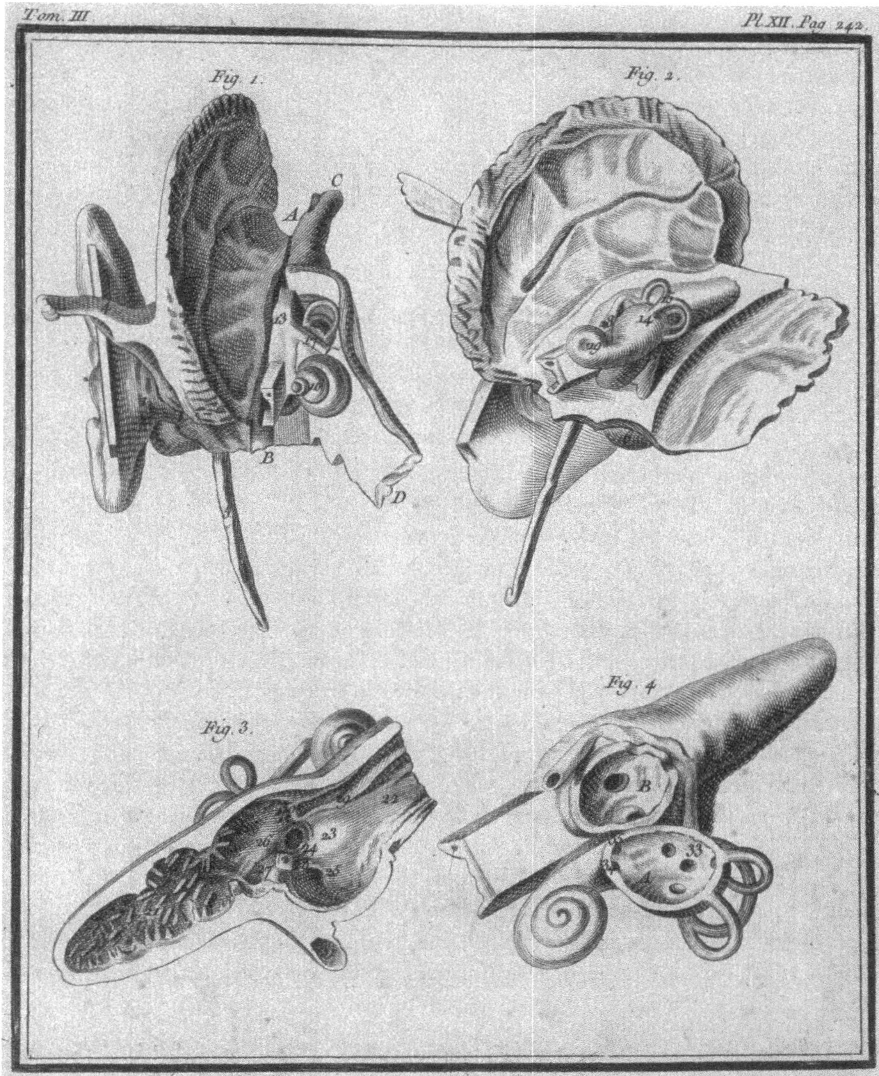

Figure 7.1 Picture of the models of the ear made by the Palerminan anatomist Giuseppe Mastiani, who used them in a demonstration of the organ of hearing at the Parisian Academy of the Sciences. The models became part of the Cabinet du Roi in Paris; in Georges-Louis Leclerc, Comte de Buffon, and Louis-Jean-Marie Daubenton, *Histoire naturelle, générale et particulière, avec la description du cabinet du Roi*, vol. 3 (Paris: Imprimerie Royale, 1749), pl. XII, 242.

demonstration, Salerno was ready to continue his journey to Bologna. But di Sangro, who had attended Salerno's anatomical demonstration, decided to buy his anatomical specimen and made him a 'splendid offer' that he could not refuse.[17] Faced with the prospect of a lifetime pension, Salerno changed his plans and travelled no more.[18] In doing so, he linked the destiny of his skeleton with di Sangro's pursuits and, more broadly, with the context of production and consumption of marvels in Naples, a city that was at the time negotiating its complex identity as a colonial capital and a major site of both antiquarian and natural wonder.

THE LURE OF THE VOLCANO

When Salerno landed in Naples with his anatomical specimen, the city was the capital of the colonial kingdom of Naples, one of the largest cities in Europe, and a very special place.[19] In 1734 the kingdoms of Naples and Sicily had returned to Spanish sovereignty under Charles de Bourbon. In the following years, excavations of the ancient cities of Herculaneum (in 1738), and Pompeii (in 1748), both of which had been buried in Mount Vesuvius' eruption of 79 CE, triggered widespread enthusiasm. Naples could now be compared with, and to some extent even surpass, Rome as a crucial destination for those who were in search of fresh contact with the classical world. The whole region became a major focus of antiquarian interest and a favourite Grand Tour destination. Upon his visit to Naples, the Holy Emperor Joseph II remarked that thanks to the discovery of Herculaneum and Pompeii, Mount Vesuvius would be an 'abundant goldmine' for the city.[20] Travellers were lured by the opportunity to be in close proximity to the newly unearthed specimens of the past. Some raved at the prospect of experiencing 'antiquity in the flesh'.[21] The arrival in Naples of the abbot Antonio Piaggio (1713–1796), a Scolopian priest from the Vatican Library, with an enticing machine that pledged to unroll the papyri found at Herculaneum, further nourished the hope of fresh access to ancient texts.

In their history as Spanish colonies, the Southern Italian territories fulfilled a specific function as sources of cultural prestige.[22] The vastly expanding Spanish

[17] De Gregorio e Russo, 'Ad Augustinum Giuffrida', 248.

[18] As we shall see in the Epilogue, Salerno then returned to Palermo where he continued to pursue his medical career.

[19] On eighteenth-century Naples see, for instance, Anna Maria Rao, *Il Regno di Napoli nel Settecento* (Naples: Guida, 1983); Girolamo Imbruglia (ed.), *Naples in the Eighteenth-Century: The Birth and Death of a Nation State* (Cambridge: Cambridge University Press, 2000); Elvira Chiosi, 'Academicians and Academies in Eighteenth-Century Naples', trans. Mark Weir, *Journal of the History of Collections*, 19:2 (2007), 177–90; Melissa Calaresu and Helen Hills (eds.), *New Approaches to Naples c.1500–c.1800: The Power of Place* (Farnham: Ashgate, 2013).

[20] Chiosi, 'Academicians and Academies', 183.

[21] Alain Schnapp, 'Introduction: Neapolitan Effervescence', trans. Mark Weir, *Journal of the History of Collections*, 19:2 (2007), 161.

[22] Anthony Pagden, *Spanish Imperialism and the Political Imagination: Studies in European and Spanish-American Social and Political Theory 1513–1830*, 2nd edn. (New Haven: Yale University Press, 1998).

empire projected its aspiration to establish a line of continuity with the vestiges of ancient empires onto the lands of the classical Magna Graecia. No other places promised to fulfil such a function better than Herculaneum and Pompeii, and the court was ready to capitalize on their discovery. Excavations were carried out under the aegis of the sovereign, and in 1755 the Reale Accademia Ercolanese was established under royal auspices.[23] Likewise, an ambitious plan of publication, resulting in the volumes of the *Antichità di Ercolano*, was meant to publicize the findings by presenting images of specimens that had been dug out, thus creating a virtual museum, which partly replicated on paper, and accordingly advertised, the antiquities displayed at the Royal Museum of Portici.[24] Nor were the antiquities of Herculaneum and Pompeii the only reason why travellers were being drawn to Naples.

As the clergyman Giovanni Vincenzo Antonio Ganganelli (1705–1774), the future pope Clement XIV, put it in a letter of 1750 to his friend Raimondo di Sangro, Naples was 'the most proper town in the world to exercise the genius of the learned' because it presented 'on all hands phenomena of every kind' that engaged their attention.[25] Some thirty years later the Marquis Dauvet similarly noticed that nature seemed to have chosen the region of Naples as its laboratory.[26] Indeed, thanks to its monuments, caverns, stones, waters, and especially the fire with which it was 'penetrated', as Ganganelli put it, Naples attracted fresh attention to its natural and historical sites.[27] Natural inquirers, dilettanti, connoisseurs, and antiquaries accordingly ended up working side by side in order to unearth both its historical and its natural past.[28] In the mid-eighteenth century, Mount Vesuvius underwent a season of great activity. Many flocked to see the grand spectacle of the volcano. The king entrusted the physician Francesco Serao with the task of writing a book on the 1737 eruption.[29] Others, such as the natural philosopher and Somascan father Giovanni Maria della Torre, who was in charge of the Royal Library and Museum, and, later on, the famous British envoy William Hamilton,

[23] Elvira Chiosi, 'Intellectuals and Academies', in Imbruglia (ed.), *Naples in the Eighteenth-Century*, 122; Chiosi, 'Academicians and Academies', esp. 183ff; Maria Toscano, 'The Figure of the Naturalist-Antiquary in the Kingdom of Naples: Giuseppe Giovene (1753–1837) and His Contemporaries', trans. Mark Weir, *Journal of the History of Collections*, 19:2 (2007), 226.

[24] Chiosi, 'Academicians and Academies', 185. The crown closely controlled the circulation of the volumes of the *Antichità di Ercolano* and sought to limit its dissemination to selected circles. Many requests beseeching the prime minister for a copy were denied. This generated frustration and complaints.

[25] Giovanni Vincenzo Antonio Ganganelli, *Interesting Letters of the Pope Clement XIV (Ganganelli): To Which Are Prefixed, Anedcotes of his Life*, trans. Lottin Le Jeune, 3rd edn., vol. 1 (London: for T. Becket, 1777), 106.

[26] BNF, ms. Fr. 7966, Marquis de Dauvet, 'Journal de Voyage. Voyage en Italie, et Lettres Écrites d'Italie', Letter of 12 May 1781 from the Marquis de Dauvet in Naples to his father, fol. 183v.

[27] Ganganelli, *Interesting Letters*, vol. 1 (1777), 106. See also Chiosi, 'Academicians and Academies', 183–4.

[28] Chiosi, 'Academicians and Academies', 183–4. On early modern views of Vesuvius, see Sean Cocco, *Watching Vesuvius: A History of Science and Culture in Early Modern Italy* (Chicago: University of Chicago Press, 2013).

[29] Francesco Serao, *Istoria dell'incendio del Vesuvio accaduto nel mese di maggio 1737* (Naples: Novello de Bonis, 1738).

regularly climbed up the volcano, guiding visitors who were eager to experience the thrill.[30] Many took notes, gathered information, made observations, and published accounts of the '*spaventoso spavento*' (frightening fright) generated by the volcano.[31] Artists equally captured the magic of the volcano that at times spewed smoke and, at other times, dramatically erupted and spat fire in spectacular day and night views (Plate 47). Fashioning Mount Vesuvius as Naples' most characteristic landmark, such scenes were filled with promise. As the city became a major centre of both antiquarian and natural interest, the court was keen to maintain its grip over the phenomena that generated an unprecedented influx of visitors.

In the course of the eighteenth century, the Bourbonic crown exploited natural knowledge as a viable tool of colonial and imperial power. After succeeding to the Spanish throne and moving to Madrid, in the 1760s Charles supported a series of botanical expeditions to the Americas, which aimed to rediscover the empire's natural resources.[32] But even during his time as the king of Naples and Sicily, Charles found natural knowledge to be a felicitous arena for shaping the image of the Southern Italian colonial territories. As well as offering support to the universities, he engaged in a number of activities including the creation of a new map of the kingdom, the completion of a museum of antiquities from Herculaneum and Pompeii, and the plan of a marine museum that would gather natural specimens from the area's sea and shores, such as corals, marine plants, and shells, which increasingly drew the interest of naturalists.[33] Giovanni Bianchi was involved in consultations about such a museum.[34] As we saw in Chapter 3, in 1754 he reported in the *Novelle letterarie* that the king of Naples had commissioned some anatomical specimens from Anna Morandi.[35] By then, Naples had developed its own tradition of wax modelling and anatomical displays.

Throughout the early modern period the city had enjoyed a reputation as a centre of wax modelling, which found expression in the large production of wax nativities, and saw the emergence of famous wax modellers such as Caterina de Julianis. In the late seventeenth century, the Sicilian wax modeller Gaetano Giulio Zumbo, who became renowned for both his devotional and his anatomical waxworks sojourned in Naples.[36] Furthermore, the surgeon and anatomist Marco Aurelio

[30] Chiosi, 'Academicians and Academies', 183.

[31] Ibid., 182–3 and 189 n. 29. The expression was used by Ferdinando Galiani in his satirical *Spaventosissima descrizione dello spaventoso spavento che ci spaventò tutti coll'eruzione del Vesuvio la sera degli otto d'agosto* (Naples: Gio. Battista Seguin, 1779).

[32] On these expeditions, see Bleichmar, *Visible Empire*. See also Juan Pimentel, 'The Iberian Vision: Science and Empire in the Framework of a Universal Monarchy, 1500–1800', in Roy MacLeod (ed.), *Nature and Empire: Science and the Colonial Enterprise*, *Osiris*, 15 (2000), 17–30; Antonio Lafuente, 'Enlightenment in an Imperial Context: Local Science in the Late-Eighteenth-Century Hispanic World', ibid., 155–73; Paula de Vos, 'Natural History and the Pursuit of Empire in Eighteenth-Century Spain', *Eighteenth-Century Studies*, 40:2 (2007), 209–39.

[33] On the circulation of marine specimens, see, for instance, ASN, Segreteria di Stato di Casa Reale, Affari Diversi, busta n. 855, Letter of 20 April 1757 from the Prince Fustenberg in Prague.

[34] On Bianchi's correspondence with the Neapolitan court about the creation of a museum of natural history, see ASN, Segreteria di Stato di Casa Reale, Affari Diversi, busta n. 870.

[35] Bianchi, 'Lettera del Signor Dottor Giovanni Bianchi', 711.

[36] See, for instance, Lemire, *Artistes et mortels*, 28; De Ceglia, 'Rotten Corpses', 420 and 424.

Severino (1580–1656) gathered a collection of anatomical wax models in the Neapolitan hospital of San Giacomo Apostolo. Not surprisingly, at a time of growing interest in anatomical displays, Naples continued to act as a centre of production and viewing of anatomical specimens.

In the mid-eighteenth century, the surgeon Anthonius Mayer realized and showed in Naples a cabinet of anatomical wax models. Having arrived in the city as part of a Swiss regiment, for which he served as its chief surgeon, Mayer displayed the models in his home and made anatomical demonstrations 'for public admiration'.[37] In 1766, he donated a large number of anatomical models to the Grand Master of Malta and in return was bestowed half a cross of the Order of Knights of Malta.[38] Just like the other anatomical displays we have encountered in this work, Mayer's anatomical collection was visited by Grand Tour travellers. When the Swedish traveller Jacob Jonas Björnståhl (1731–1779), Carl Linnaeus' correspondent, visited Morandi's cabinet in Bologna in 1772, he recalled having seen Mayer's anatomical models in Naples, as well as the anatomical collection of Marie Marguerite Bihéron in Paris and that of Felice Fontana in Florence, concluding that 'this Signora *Mansolini*' seemed to be 'the most accomplished of all'.[39]

In the second half of the eighteenth century, the anatomist Domenico Cotugno, who had visited the Institute's anatomy room in Bologna and discussed its models with Lelli, assembled an anatomical collection at the Neapolitan hospital of the Incurabili.[40] Even before purchasing Salerno's anatomical specimen, in 1750 Raimondo di Sangro had entrusted the artist Francesco Queirolo with the task of acquiring a skeleton in Rome for him.[41] This incident provides an early record of di Sangro's interest in anatomical specimens. In the following years, such interest would lead him to purchase Salerno's costly anatomical creations regardless of his family's growing debts.[42] In fact, in addition to acquiring the skeleton that Salerno had taken to Naples in 1756, in 1763 di Sangro commissioned from the Palermitan anatomist a new anatomical specimen for the conspicuous sum of 2000 *ducati*.[43]

[37] On Mayer and his anatomical cabinet, see Georges-Louis Leclerc, Comte de Buffon and Louis-Jean-Marie Daubenton, *Storia naturale generale, e particolare, con la descrizione del gabinetto del Re*, trans. from French, vol. 5 (Naples: Fratelli Raimondi, 1772), 334–5. On Mayer's donation of anatomical models to Malta, see NLM, AOM 637, fols. 109r–v. On the bestowing of half a cross of the Order of Knights of Malta upon him, see ibid., AOM 570 (Registri delle Bolle di Cancelleria, Liber Bullarum, 1766), fol. 175r. Some sources refer to a Franz or Francesco Mayer as the chief surgeon of the Swiss Guard in Naples who was a freemason and physician to Charles de Bourbon's son Philip. I have not been able to verify whether this is the same surgeon who also made anatomical models; see Carlo Francovich, *Storia della Massoneria in Italia: Dalle origini alla Rivoluzione francese* (Florence: La Nuova Italia, 1974), 204; Ruggiero Di Castiglione, *La Massoneria nelle Due Sicilie e i 'fratelli' meridionali del '700*, vol. 2 (Rome: Gangemi Editore, 2014), 428 n. 7.

[38] NLM, AOM 637, fols. 109r–v; ibid., AOM 570, fol. 175r.

[39] Björnståhl, *Lettere ne' suoi viaggj* [...], vol. 3, 147 (original spelling and emphasis).

[40] Cotugno's meeting with Lelli is discussed in Chapters 2 and 3.

[41] Bruno Crimaldi (ed.), *Chartulae desangriane: Il principe committente* (Naples: Alòs, 2006), 79.

[42] For an overview of di Sangro's economic problems, see Oderisio de Sangro, *Raimondo de Sangro e la Cappella Sansevero* (Rome: Bulzoni, 1991), 79–80.

[43] See ibid., 237–9; Eduardo Nappi, 'La famiglia, il palazzo e la cappella dei principi di Sansevero', *Revue Internationale d'Histoire de la Banque*, vol. 11 (Geneva: Droz, 1975), 142–3 and 145; Archivio Storico del Banco di Napoli, Banco di San Giacomo (1763), 1st semester, 14 May, Giornale Copiapolizze, Matricola 1562, 517. The payment for the poplar case that accommodated 'the skeleton' was finalized in April 1765.

ONE OF THE MOST PERFECT PHILOSOPHERS

It is not easy to build a clear image of Raimondo di Sangro, the seventh Prince of San Severo. Descendant of an old aristocratic family, gentleman of chamber to the king of Naples, Grand Master of the local Masonic lodge, natural inquirer, ingenious manufacturer, alchemist, healer, skilled mechanic, courtier, author of a dictionary of military terms, member of the Accademia della Crusca, and owner of a cabinet of curious objects largely made by himself, di Sangro resists any straightforward biographical characterization.[44] In the mid-eighteenth century, the philosopher Antonio Genovesi portrayed him as a 'gentleman of short height', large head, handsome and jovial, a philosopher in spirit, 'very devoted to the mechanical arts', of very charming and pleasant manners, 'studious and reserved', and a 'lover of conversation with men of letters' (Plate 48).[45] In fact, according to Genovesi, had di Sangro not been carried away by his powerful imagination, which sometimes brought him to believe things that were unlikely, 'he could have passed for one of the most perfect philosophers'.[46] In a letter to di Sangro of 1757, Ganganelli similarly praised his 'new discoveries' but expressed concern that his chemical experiments could harm his health. In the same letter, Ganganelli also highlighted the risks related to the excesses of the imagination.[47]

From an early age, di Sangro had enjoyed plenty of opportunities to cultivate his imagination and his dedication to the mechanical arts. Like many other aristocrats, he received a Jesuit education. At the Roman College, he would have come across the legacy of the Jesuit polymath Athanasius Kircher (1602–1680), who in the mid-seventeenth century had founded the college's museum and transformed it into one of Rome's most famous sites of wonder.[48] While in Rome, di Sangro actively participated in the college's tradition of mechanical and theatrical engineering by designing a folding stage for its yard.[49] Upon completing his studies, he headed back to Naples to face the demands of his rank and, like many fellow noblemen, undertook a career in the military. After becoming one of the heroes of the battle of Velletri, which consolidated Bourbonic rule over Southern Italy, di Sangro took his first steps into the world of authorship. In 1747, he published a book that described the military

[44] On di Sangro's life and pursuits see, for instance, Giovanni Giuseppe Origlia Paolino, *Istoria dello Studio di Napoli; in cui si comprendono gli avvenimenti di esso più notabili da' primi suoi principi fino a' tempi presenti, con buona parte della Storia Letteraria del Regno*, vol. 2 (Naples: Giovanni di Simone 1754), 320–89; Domenico Martuscelli, *Biografia degli uomini illustri del Regno di Napoli, ornata de loro rispettivi ritratti*, vol. 6 (Naples: Nicola Gervasi, 1813), entry on 'Raimondo di Sangro, Principe di San Severo', unpaginated; Fabio Colonna di Stigliano, 'La Cappella Sansevero e don Raimondo di Sangro', *Napoli nobilissima*, 4 (1894), 33–6, 52–8, 72–5, 90–4, 116–21, 138–42, and 152–5.

[45] Antonio Genovesi, *Autobiografia, lettere e altri scritti*, ed. Gennaro Savarese (Milan: Feltrinelli, 1962), 36.

[46] Ibid.

[47] Giovanni Vincenzo Antonio Ganganelli, *Interesting Letters of Pope Clement XIV (Ganganelli): To Which are Prefixed, Anecdotes of His Life*, trans. Lottin Le Jeune, 5th edn., vol. 2 (London: for T. Becket, 1781), 97–9.

[48] On Kircher, see, for instance, Paula Findlen (ed.), *Athanasius Kircher: The Last Man Who Knew Everything* (New York: Routledge, 2004).

[49] De Sangro, *Raimondo de Sangro*, 28–9; Martuscelli, *Biografia degli uomini illustri*, vol. 6, entry on 'Raimondo di Sangro, Principe di San Severo'.

exercises that he had first carried out on the battlefield.[50] He then spectacularly demonstrated these exercises at the Neapolitan court. Relying again on his military experience, di Sangro started working on a dictionary of military terms and, on that account, asked to be affiliated with the Accademia della Crusca, the academy overseeing the purity of the Italian language. The request drew mixed feelings. It left the generally 'scrupulous' academicians perplexed, compelling them to write to the famous diplomat, philosopher, and abbot Ferdinando Galiani (1728–1787) in order to gather information about di Sangro with the greatest 'secrecy and sincerity'.[51] Although di Sangro was 'not a man that could pass for a literato', the academy was inclined to admit him. However, it wanted to make sure that he was not a person 'so preposterous' as to make the whole academy look ridiculous.[52] In the end, di Sangro did obtain affiliation. However, this was not the end of his troubles: his chosen academic nickname was turned down, and di Sangro had to struggle to find one that could satisfy the academicians and be approved.[53]

Di Sangro's subsequent attempts to enter the world of learning were hardly received with any more enthusiasm. For instance, the publication of a series of letters in the *Novelle letterarie*, where di Sangro claimed to have recovered the ancient secret of inextinguishable lamps, generated mixed reactions.[54] Ferdinando Galiani was again involved in gossip about di Sangro when the literato Lorenzo Mehus mockingly wrote to him that the notoriously parsimonious people of Florence would no doubt appreciate di Sangro's discovery of imperishable lamps on account that it would allow them to save quite a bit on the consumption of oil.[55] And in a later letter to Mehus, Galiani suggested that the long entry praising di Sangro in the second volume of Giovanni Giuseppe Origlia Paolino's *Istoria dello Studio di Napoli* (1754) had been requested by di Sangro himself, who had supported its publication.[56] While the peninsula's literati were in two minds about di Sangro's claims, in the beginning his aspirations to gain intellectual reputation seemingly found better reception at the Neapolitan court.

THE MAKING OF A COURTIER SAVANT

A significant strand in the history of the sciences has drawn attention to the process of cross-fertilization between courtly culture and natural inquiry that led to the

[50] Raimondo di Sangro, *Pratica più agevole, e più utile di esercizj militari per l'infanteria* (Naples: Giovanni di Simone, 1747). See also De Sangro, *Raimondo de Sangro*, 34–6.

[51] Biblioteca della Società Napoletana di Storia Patria (Naples), ms. XXXI, B 1, 55–6.

[52] Ibid.

[53] See di Sangro's correspondence with the Accademia della Crusca in Archivio dell'Accademia della Crusca (Florence), ms. Carte Alamanni, Pezzi 107 and 108.

[54] Raimondo di Sangro, *Lettere del signore D. Raimondo di Sangro Principe di Sansevero di Napoli sopra alcune scoperte chimiche indirizzate al signor cavaliere Giovanni Giraldi Fiorentino e riportate ancora nelle Novelle Letterarie di Firenze del 1753* (Naples: n.p., after 1753).

[55] Giuseppe Nicoletti (ed.), *Ferdinando Galiani-Lorenzo Mehus: Carteggio (1753–1786)* (Naples: Bibliopolis, 2002), 61.

[56] According to Mehus, the incident had affected Origlia's legal career; see ibid., 117–18.

fashioning of early modern natural inquirers as courtiers.[57] Less attention has been devoted to those courtiers who pursued natural inquiries and, in some cases, relied on such engagements to define their identity and role within the court. Raimondo di Sangro was himself a courtier who gained a place of prominence within the Bourbonic court also as a result of his natural and mechanical pursuits. In fact, as natural knowledge helped to shape the identity and the public image of the new Spanish monarchy, it also became an integral part of the life of the courtiers.[58] The famous picture of William Hamilton escorting the Neapolitan sovereigns and part of the court to spectate an impressive lava flow on 11 May 1771, visually captured ongoing attempts to promote courtly engagements with nature (Plate 49). When di Sangro rushed to buy Salerno's anatomical specimen, he was working on his image as a courtier savant.[59] As the court actively engaged in the production and consumption of natural knowledge, curiosities were regularly presented to its members for their delight and edification.[60] From exotic animals to enticing machines and the optical marvels of the Royal Theatre of San Carlo (where di Sangro had a box and whose mirror-filled interior allowed the sovereign to watch over the courtiers), curiosity and wonder became part and parcel of courtly life. In 1742, the arrival of an elephant, allegedly donated by the Ottoman Sultan Mahmud I to the king of Naples, marked one of the highlights of the characterization of the city as a site of wonder.[61] The elephant was paraded around town, anatomically described, showcased in an opera at the San Carlo theatre, and eventually transformed into a natural specimen. Not surprisingly, when Salerno landed with his skeleton on the Neapolitan shores, he found an environment that was appreciative of marvel. In fact, demonstrations like the one made by Salerno were part of a routine of theatrical introductions of courtiers to natural wonder. Notably, on a summer evening of 1768 even Ercole Lelli's 'new, rare and never seen before

[57] See, for instance, Mario Biagioli, *Galileo, Courtier: The Practice of Science in the Culture of Absolutism* (Chicago: University of Chicago Press, 1993); Findlen, *Possessing Nature*.

[58] As Giovanni Montroni has suggested, the arrival of Charles de Bourbon in Naples brought about the reorganization of the state along the lines of the Spanish model, subjecting the local aristocracy to the new Spanish monarchic order. As a result, the court, its splendour, and its internal hierarchy became 'fundamental elements in the representation of the power of sovereignty'. The aristocracy equally played a key role in the construction of loyalty to the new Spanish crown and in the making of a new image of the monarchy; see Giovanni Montroni, 'The Court: Power Relations and Forms of Social Life', in Imbruglia (ed.), *Naples in the Eighteenth Century*, 22–43 (citation pp. 22–3).

[59] Ibid., 23–4 and 34.

[60] In the grand circulation of things, the attempt to give to the Neapolitan court a place of prominence on the Italian map of natural inquiry could sometimes generate confusion. When, in 1757, Francesco Maria Zanotti, secretary of the Bolognese Institute of the Sciences, mistakenly received Benjamin Gottfried Reyher's request of affiliation to the Neapolitan Royal Academy, he forwarded the parcel to Naples along with a note explaining that the Institute did not know about the court's customs and thus could not rule on it; see ASN, Segreteria di Stato di Casa Reale, Affari Diversi, busta n. 855, Letter of 26 March 1757 from Francesco Maria Zanotti in Bologna.

[61] Francesco Serao, *Descrizione dell'elefante pervenuto in dono dal Gran Sultano alla Regal Corte di Napoli* (Naples: Francesco e Cristoforo Ricciardi, 1742). In fact, the elephant had apparently been acquired by the king himself, and was 'presented as an important and valuable gift' and 'used to celebrate the power and prestige of the ruling monarchy'; see Rosita D'Amora, 'The Diplomatic Relations between Naples and the Ottoman Empire in Mid-Eighteenth Century: Cultural Perceptions', *Oriente Moderno*, 22:3 (2003), 715–27 (citation p. 725).

optical pictorial theatre', which we encountered in Chapter 2, was presented at the Neapolitan court.[62]

On the other hand, efforts to make the court conversant with the world of natural knowledge seemed to clash with a cliché that portrayed the Southern Italian aristocracy as lacking interest in the world of learning. When Lalande observed in his *Voyage d'un François en Italie* that as a legacy of 'the barbaric ignorance of the middle ages' in Naples 'learning and science' were still 'disdained by the nobility', his unflattering remark did not go down particularly well.[63] The city's literati engaged in vindicating local traditions of aristocratic learning. At a time when accomplished women were taken to provide a measure of Italy's engagement with natural knowledge, a number of the noblewomen who devoted themselves to natural pursuits in Naples, such as Faustina Pignatelli, Isabella Pignone del Carretto, Aurora Sanseverino, and Giuseppa Eleonora Barbapiccola, were also evoked in defence of the reputation of the Neapolitan aristocracy in the world of learning.[64] The name of Raimondo di Sangro was equally invoked as a remarkable example of dedication to learning and natural knowledge along with that of other Neapolitan aristocrats including Giovanni Caraffa, Paolo Mattia Doria, Francesco Maria Spinelli, Trojano Spinelli, and Niccolò Gaetano dell' Aquila d'Aragona.[65]

From the outset, di Sangro's creations and pursuits played a part in his attempts to fashion himself as a courtier savant. His military writing *Pratica più agevole* was dedicated to Charles de Bourbon who, in turn, donated a copy to an appreciative Frederick the Great.[66] Furthermore, di Sangro participated in the making of courtly spectacles, and in 1738 he claimed to have devised the rare colour green in fireworks for one such occasion.[67] When, in the following years, he produced garments for the king as the result of his own natural investigations, he brought his natural inquiries to bear on courtly patronage and royal splendour. Having contrived a special waterproof material, di Sangro used it to make a royal mantle that was meant to protect the king's body from bad weather during his hunting expeditions.[68]

[62] *Foglio ordinario*, n. 31, 2 August 1768.

[63] Lalande, *Voyage d'un François en Italie*, vol. 6, 364.

[64] Pietro Napoli Signorelli, *Vicende della coltura nelle Due Sicilie, o sia storia ragionata della loro legislazione e polizia, delle lettere, del commercio, delle arti, e degli spettacoli dalle colonie straniere insino a noi*, vol. 4 (Naples: Vincenzo Flauto, 1785), 496–7. In addition to these noblewomen, Mariangela Ardinghelli was in this period one of the most famous women who dedicated themselves to natural inquiry in Naples and the Italian peninsula as a whole; see, for instance, Paula Findlen, 'Translating the New Science: Women and the Circulation of Knowledge in Enlightenment Italy', *Configurations*, 3 (1995), 167–206; Bertucci,'The In/visible Woman'.

[65] See Björnståhl, *Lettere ne' suoi viaggj*, vol. 2, 149ff; Napoli Signorelli, *Vicende*, vol. 4, 495–6. On noblemen's involvement in the creation of centres of learning in the city, see also Paola Bertucci, 'The Architecture of Knowledge: Science, Collecting and Display in Eighteenth-Century Naples', in Calaresu and Hills (eds.), *New Approaches to Naples*, 149–74.

[66] Napoli Signorelli, *Vicende*, vol. 4, 487–8.

[67] See Raimondo di Sangro, *Lettera apologetica dell'Esercitato accademico della Crusca contenente la difesa del libro intitolato Lettere d' una Peruana per rispetto alla supposizione de' Quipu scritta dalla Duchessa di S**** e dalla medesima fatta pubblicare*, ed. Leen Spruit (Naples: Alòs, 2002 [1750]). On the colour green in eighteenth-century fireworks, see Werrett, *Fireworks*, 161.

[68] Lalande, *Voyage d'un François en Italie*, vol. 6, 248–9; Björnståhl, *Lettere ne' suoi viaggj*, vol. 2, 150–1. See also De Sangro, *Raimondo de Sangro*, 64.

He also made a dress for the king by using a special vegetable silk extracted from a local plant. Charles-Marie de La Condamine, who had travelled extensively in South America, found the material to be similar to the fabric obtained from the South American plant called *Apocynum*.[69] Bringing together the kingdom's natural resources with the outcome of his experimental pursuits, di Sangro dressed the body of the future Catholic king with the empire's natural products. In doing so, he placed the monarch's embodiment of natural knowledge at the centre of Naples' choreographies of power. Under Charles' rule, the degree of proximity to the king's body gave expression to a strictly regulated courtly hierarchy and was a measure of a courtier's status.[70] Rituals such as the kissing of the monarch's hand were accessible only to a handful of courtiers and were thus reflective of the court's hierarchies and ranks. Di Sangro was among the few who could enjoy such privileges. In 1740 he had been invested as a knight of the order of Saint Januarius, which gathered 'the most distinguished subjects of the monarchy' around the crown as a way to secure their loyalty.[71] His creation of royal garments similarly signalled his high standing at the court.

To be sure, not everybody was convinced by di Sangro's claim that the royal dress was, strictly speaking, made out of vegetable silk. Ferdinando Galiani found himself again drawn into gossip after he received a letter where the Marquis Alessandro Rinuccini reported that the dress was beautiful but remarked that di Sangro's 'vegetable silk' was a bit like cats' and dogs' fur: one could not really weave it without a substantial addition of regular fabric.[72] Charles did not seem to mind. By 1750, di Sangro's friendship with the sovereign seemed to be stronger than ever. In a letter to di Sangro of January 1750, his friend Ganganelli wrote that he was not surprised to hear about the king's favour for di Sangro, for 'every Monarch, who knows his own glory, is aware of how much the credit of the learned is reflected back upon him, when he protects them'.[73] However, troubles loomed ahead. Later that year, the publication of di Sangro's *Lettera apologetica* pushed things to the brink of disaster. The book took off from where the French writer and *salonnière* Françoise de Graffigny had left in her *Lettres d'une Péruvienne* (1747), and reconstructed the story of the *Quipu*, the Inca language based on the arrangements of knots along strings. In the footnotes, di Sangro took the opportunity to describe his activities and inquiries.[74] Yet, as the *Lettera apologetica* fell into the hands of detractors, such as the Jesuit Innocenzo Molinari, and the book was accused of

[69] La Condamine, 'Extrait d'un journal de voyage en Italie', 48; Björnståhl, *Lettere ne' suoi viaggj*, vol. 2, 150.

[70] Montroni, 'The Court', 30.

[71] Ibid., 30–1. See also, Richard, *Description historique*, vol. 4 (1770), 84–5.

[72] Biblioteca della Società Napoletana di Storia Patria (Naples), ms. XXXI, B18, 61 and 66.

[73] Ganganelli, *Interesting Letters*, vol. 1 (1777), 107.

[74] Di Sangro, *Lettera apologetica*. See also Leen Spruit, 'Introduzione', in di Sangro, *Lettera apologetica*; Patrizia Castelli, 'La rigenerazione ermetico-massonica del Principe Raimondo di Sansevero', in Paolo A. Rossi and Ida Li Vigni (eds.), *I veli di pietra: Il principe Raimondo di Sangro di San Severo (1710–1771)* (Genoa: Nova Scripta Edizioni, 2011), 77–116. The book was reviewed in periodicals such as the *Novelle letterarie* (in November 1751) and *Journal des Trévoux* (in February 1752), thus promising to give to di Sangro's work the exposure for which he had hoped.

reflecting cabbalistic principles and heretical views, things reached a critical stage.[75] Likewise, the situation came to a boiling point when di Sangro was exposed as the Grand Master of the Neapolitan lodge of Freemasons.

The episode followed Charles de Bourbon's decision to comply with Pope Benedict XIV's bull against Freemasonry by issuing an edict that banned it from the kingdoms of Naples and Siciliy.[76] As di Sangro ran the risk of being excommunicated, he addressed the pope in a letter of apology in Latin where he admitted to having joined the society of Freemasons in 1750, not long before being exposed as its Grand Master.[77] He furthermore portrayed the lodge as characterized by harmless engagements, and explained that it had interested him because it allowed individuals from any social background to converse amicably and promise reciprocal support in case of need, something that could be used to the city's advantage.[78] Di Sangro received the solidarity of savants and literati. Among them, Giovanni Lami, editor of the *Novelle letterarie*, himself a Freemason, published di Sangro's letters on the discovery of a perpetual, ever-burning lamp. According to Antonio Genovesi, the events surrounding the publication of the *Lettera apologetica* and di Sangro's participation in the Masonic lodge turned him into a target of the clergy and ran the risk of spoiling his friendship with the king.[79] However, thanks to the mediation of the Duke of Miranda, who was a close friend of the king, and who recovered from malignant fever thanks to di Sangro's treatment, he eventually got out of trouble.[80]

In the following years, di Sangro regained a prominent place within the court and was again at the service of the king. As a sign of reconciliation, he gave the king a press that he had devised, which could print different colours simultaneously. Having been formerly used by di Sangro to publish his controversial *Lettera*

[75] See Colonna di Stigliano, 'La Cappella Sansevero', 75; De Sangro, *Raimondo de Sangro*, 46–7. Di Sangro wrote a book-length *Supplica* to Pope Benedict XIV where he asked for forgiveness, and to have the *Lettera apologetica* taken out of the Index of Prohibited Books; see Raimondo di Sangro, *Supplica a Benedetto XIV*, ed. Leen Spruit (Naples: Alòs, 2006 [1753]); Biblioteca della Società Napoletana di Storia Patria (Naples), ms. XXXI, B 18, 66, Letter of Marchese Alessandro Rinuccini to Ferdinando Galiani from Naples of 27 December 1751. See also Leen Spruit, 'Introduzione', in di Sangro, *Supplica*, 11; Spruit, 'Introduzione', in di Sangro, *Lettera apologetica*, 53ff.

[76] On the Church's condemnation of Freemasonry, see José Antonio Ferrer Benimeli, 'Origini, motivazioni ed effetti della condanna vaticana', in Gian Mario Cazzaniga (ed.), *Storia d'Italia, Annali 21: La massoneria* (Turin: Einaudi, 2006), 143–65.

[77] In fact, a text published in the second volume of *L'étoile flamboyante* seemingly dates di Sangro's participation in the masonic lodge to an earlier period; see 'Discours prononcé à la réception de plusieurs Apprentifs, à la loge du Prince de S.S. à Naples, en 1745', in [Théodore Henri de Tschudy], *L'étoile flamboyante, ou la société des Francs-Maçons, considérée sous tous les aspects*, vol. 2 (Paris: À L'orient chez Le Silence, 1780), 31–4. *L'étoile flamboyante* was attributed to Théodore Henri de Tschudy, a friend of di Sangro, and served as a catechism of Freemasonic philosophy.

[78] Origlia Paolino, *Istoria*, vol. 2, 350–64. See also Harold Acton, *The Bourbons of Naples, 1734–1825*, 2nd edn. (London: Methuen, 1974 [1956]), 151.

[79] Genovesi, *Autobiografia*, 36–7.

[80] Ibid., 37; Bernardo Tanucci, *Epistolario III: 1752–1756*, ed. Anna Vittoria Migliorini (Rome: Edizioni di Storia e Letteratura, 1982), 22 (Letter of 1 August 1752 from Bernardo Tanucci in Naples to the Marquis of Narvaez in Florence). Here Tanucci observed that di Sangro was celebrated for having healed the Prince of Bisignano.

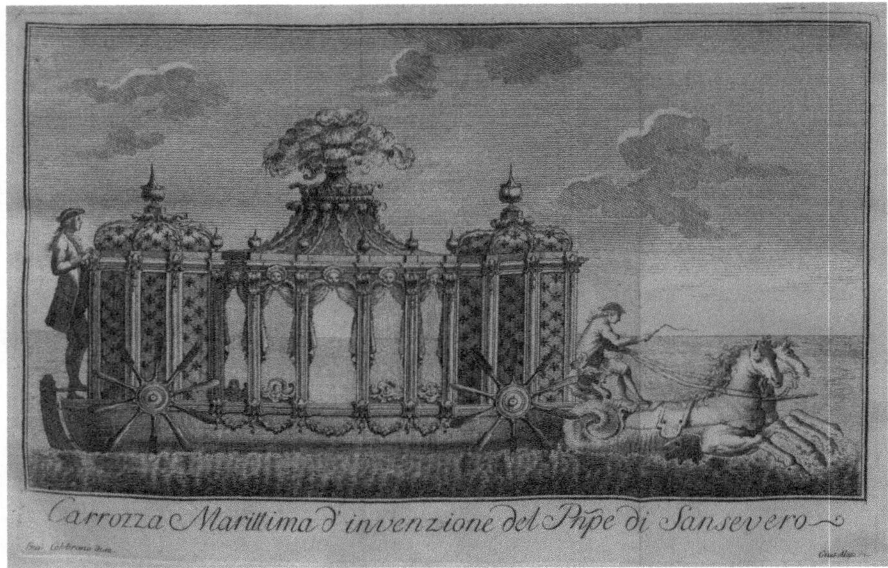

Figure 7.2 Francesco Celebrano, 'Maritime Carriage invented by the Prince of Sansevero' ('Carrozza Marittima d'invenzione del Principe di Sansevero'), in Pietro D'Onofri, *Elogio estemporaneo per la gloriosa memoria di Carlo III...*, Naples: Pietro Perger, n.d. [1789]; etching.

apologetica, di Sangro's press was now turned into the royal press.[81] In 1754, di Sangro was busy importing 'very curious' birds from the New World for 'the Emperor'.[82] Later in his life, he designed a maritime carriage that was originally supposed to be stationed in the artificial lake of the Royal Palace of Caserta for the use of the sovereigns (Figure 7.2). Bringing together mechanical spectacle and courtly sociability, di Sangro's maritime carriage was similar to a regular carriage, but was supposed to navigate merely by the propulsive action of water on its four wheels, without the help of either sails or oars. In July 1770, di Sangro tested the carriage near the shores of Posillipo, in the northern part of the Gulf of Naples.[83] And when the king saw it cruising in the sea, he found it delightfully surprising.[84]

In the previous years, di Sangro had continued to circulate his writings in courtly circles. When he sent his *Dissertation sur une lampe antique* to the Duke of Savoy in Turin in September 1756, the Chevalier Ossorio, minister of the king of Sardinia, welcomed the work on account of di Sangro's 'distinguished reputation among the

[81] Acton, *The Bourbons of Naples*, 100–1.
[82] Ganganelli, *Interesting Letters*, vol. 2 (1781), 29.
[83] *Diario ordinario*, n. 8181, 27 July 1770 (Rome: Stamperia del Chracas, 1770), 2–3. According to the *Diario ordinario*, in the end di Sangro decided to keep the maritime carriage for himself; see ibid., 2. See also De Sangro, *Raimondo de Sangro*, 73–5.
[84] Björnståhl, *Lettere ne' suoi viaggj*, vol. 2, 151.

savants'.[85] At the same time, di Sangro had also begun to look for new audiences. At a time in which Naples was attracting ever-increasing numbers of Grand Tour visitors, he capitalized on the potential benefits of extending his network of acquaintances to the transalpine world of travelling savants.[86] In order to do so, he transformed the San Severo Palace and Chapel into a Grand Tour destination, a curious corner within the city of wonders, a site of marvel where striking objects like Salerno's anatomical specimens could find a suitable home.

'A SECOND WORLD FROM THE FIRST'

In 1740, when Johann Georg Keyssler published a thorough report of his visit to Naples, he dedicated but a few lines to the San Severo premises.[87] However, by the time Jacob Jonas Björnståhl visited Naples in the early 1770s, he thought there was no need to describe at length all of di Sangro's 'useful and beautiful discoveries', simply because they had been mentioned in all travellers' accounts.[88] In the intervening years, di Sangro had opened the doors of the San Severo Palace and Chapel to the foreigners and travellers who visited Naples. Notably, in 1749 he had welcomed the abbé Jean-Antoine Nollet (1700–1770), the prominent French savant and member of the Parisian Academy of the Sciences.[89] While travelling in Italy on the Grand Tour, Nollet dined at the San Severo Palace and in his diary penned words of praise for di Sangro's work on the art of war and his knowledge of 'physics and mechanics'.[90] However, when di Sangro tested his guest's willingness to intercede on his behalf at the Academy of the Sciences, Nollet hesitated and discouraged his host. In the following years, when di Sangro published his *Lettres écrites par Monsieur le Prince de S. Sevère de Naples à Monsr. l'Abbé Nollet* and dedicated to Nollet his *Dissertation sur une lampe antique*, he may have hoped to convince his former guest to change his mind.[91] In fact, di Sangro never became a member of

[85] ASTo, Materie politiche per rapporti all'interno, Lettere diverse Real Casa, Registri delle Lettere della Segreteria Esteri a particolari (1754–8), n. 8, Letter of 1 September 1756 from 'Mr. Le Ch. Ossorio' to 'M. Le Prince de S.Severo'.

[86] On the relationship between Freemasonry and the Grand Tour, see Pierre-Yves Beaurepaire, '"Grand Tour", République des Lettres e reti massoniche: Una cultura della mobilità nell'Europe dei Lumi', in Cazzaniga (ed.), *Storia d'Italia*, 32–49.

[87] Keyssler, *Travels*, vol. 2, 416.

[88] Björnståhl, *Lettere ne' suoi viaggj*, vol. 2, 151. Grand Tourists who described di Sangro's pursuits and cabinet in their writings include La Condamine, 'Extrait d'un journal de voyage en Italie'; Lalande, *Voyage d'un François en Italie*, vol. 6, 240ff., 398ff., and 435; [Grosley], *New Observations*, vol. 2, 231–2.

[89] Officially, Nollet travelled around Italy in order to gather information on medical electricity but, unofficially, he was on an espionage mission that aimed at capturing the secrets of Italian silk-making; see Paola Bertucci, *Viaggio nel paese delle meraviglie: Scienza e curiosità nell'Italia del Settecento* (Turin: Bollati Boringhieri, 2007); Bertucci, 'Enlightened Secrets', 820–52.

[90] Jean Antoine Nollet, 'Journal du voyage de Piémont et d'Italie en 1749', Soisson, Bibliothèque Municipale de Soisson, ms. 150. I wish to thank Paola Bertucci for sharing this document with me.

[91] See Raimondo di Sangro, *Lettres écrites par Monsieur le Prince de S. Sevère de Naples à Mons.r l'Abbé Nollet l'Académie des Sciences à Paris, contenant la rélation d'une découverte qu'il a faite par le moyen de quelques expériences chimiques et l'explication physique de ses circonstances* (Naples: Joseph Raimondi, 1753); Raimondo di Sangro, *Dissertation sur une lampe antique trouvée à Munich en l'année*

the French Academy of the Sciences. Yet, news of his pursuits may have reached its members when, a few years later, La Condamine presented at the academy his 'Extrait d'un journal de voyage en Italie', which included a report of his encounter with di Sangro.[92] Over time the San Severo Palace and Chapel gained ever more visibility on the map of the Grand Tour. While di Sangro's early steps into the world of learning were largely taken within the Neapolitan court, the flocking of visitors to the Gulf of Naples created particularly favourable circumstances for the creation of new audiences for his pursuits. Di Sangro's own residence was being prepared to welcome literati and travelling savants.

When di Sangro married Carlotta Gaetani dell'Aquila d'Aragona, the famous philosopher Giambattista Vico wrote a sonnet in their honour.[93] Both Carlotta and Raimondo were part of a network of aristocrats who cultivated an interest in learning and natural and medical pursuits. Among them was Ranuzzi, the Bolognese count and senator we encountered in Chapter 6, who in 1769 purchased Morandi's anatomical collection. Having befriended the Princess and the Prince of San Severo, he was among the first to be informed when di Sangro died on the night of 21 March 1771.[94] Carlotta's and Raimondo's exquisite manners, hospitality, and pleasant conversation captivated many, transforming the Palace of San Severo into a site of sociable as well as curious learning that left visitors delighted, sated, and impressed. Convivial gatherings at the San Severo Palace became memorable. In 1751, the Marquis Alessandro Rinuccini remarked that he never dined out but gladly lunched at di Sangro's place.[95]

Over the course of the eighteenth century, the ability to comply with proper codes of sociability provided an important resource for natural inquirers. The fame of di Sangro's own polite sociability extended to his demonstrations of the curiosities on display in his palace. Visitors reported that di Sangro 'explained with great Politeness' the 'great many curiosities of Art that he himself hath performed'.[96] Among them, Jérôme Richard found di Sangro to be a 'sweet, honest and affable man' who received foreigners 'with the greatest politeness'.[97] Just as in the case of

1753, écrite par M. le Prince de St-Sévère, pour servir de suite à la première partie de ses lettres à M. l'Abbé Nollet, à Paris, sur une découverte qu'il a faite dans la Chimie (Naples: Morelli, 1756). The *Lettres* was largely a translation of the letters that had appeared in the *Novelle letterarie*, and his *Dissertation* expanded and complemented them.

[92] La Condamine, 'Extrait d'un journal de voyage en Italie', 382.

[93] Giambattista Vico, *Opere di Giambattista Vico*, vol. 4 (Naples: Giuseppe Jovene, 1840), 380.

[94] See ASB, Archivio Ranuzzi, Carte politiche dei vari membri della famiglia, Registro n. 1, 'Registro di tutti quelli a' quali per ragione di commercio, di civiltà e parentela giornalmente si scrive da S.E. il Sig: Senatore Girolamo Ranuzzi, Conte XII della Porretta A.D. MDCCLIV', 72; ASB, Archivio Ranuzzi, Carte di Famiglia, Lettere di Casa, 1771, 23 March 1771.

[95] Biblioteca della Società Napoletana di Storia Patria (Naples), ms. XXXI, B18, 66. With di Sangro's involvement in the secretive world of Freemasonry, the social and convivial gatherings that took place at his palace may have required the sheltering of sensitive information. Accordingly, di Sangro seemingly addressed the need of confidentiality by claiming to have devised a dinner-serving automaton that was aimed at protecting conversations from indiscreet ears; see De Sangro, *Raimondo de Sangro*, 72–3.

[96] Bodleian Library (Oxford), ms. Add. A. 366, 'A Journal kept by Mr Tracy and Mr Dent and during their Travel through France and Italy', unpaginated.

[97] Richard, *Description historique*, vol. 4, 212.

the Bolognese anatomical collections, the arrival in Naples of tourists who authored famous travelogues contributed to shaping di Sangro's reputation as a savant and consecrated his role as an icon of the Grand Tour. Devoting some ten pages to the Prince of San Severo, his palace, and his chapel, Lalande's *Voyage d'un François en Italie* provided a *summa* of di Sangro's creations and cabinet.

As well as personally guiding travellers through his cabinet and activities, in the mid-1760s di Sangro likely authored the booklet *Breve nota di quel che si vede in casa del Principe di Sansevero* ('A short note of what one can see in the house of the Prince of Sansevero'), which presented the curiosities displayed in his residence.[98] Introducing readers to the rich display of artefacts, specimens, artworks, materials, and mechanical devices housed in the San Severo Palace and Chapel, the booklet was handed out by di Sangro to visitors.[99] In addition to Salerno's anatomical specimens, the display included coloured marbles, vegetable wax, vegetable silk, waterproof fabric, paintings carried out by means of both encaustic and eloidric techniques, a special kind of porcelain, coloured glass, perfectly counterfeited gemstones such as inexpensive lapis lazuli, gemstones that changed colour, pieces of wood and carbon that did not burn, and much more.[100] Highlighting the transformation of the San Severo Palace into a Grand Tour destination, the *Breve nota* served both as a guide and as an inventory that organized for readers the visit to this large ensemble of 'all the curious effects of his [di Sangro's] Art'.[101] With the notable exception of Salerno's anatomical specimens, many of the curiosities were the results of di Sangro's 'own manufacture'.[102] They staged, as Ganganelli put it, 'a second world from the first', a newly invented world which duplicated the original one.[103]

In fact, the process of transforming the San Severo premises into a Grand Tour destination was not particularly smooth. And while the *Breve nota* introduced readers to what appeared to be a relatively well-organized site, the Palace itself was plagued by never ending works in progress. In the early 1760s, Jérôme Richard found it in a state of grand disarray.[104] In the mid-1770s, the Marquis de Sade, who travelled with Richard's *Description* in hand, complained that the palace was still in the same bad shape in which viewers had found it for some twenty years.[105] The task of fulfilling the expectation that a cabinet should be reasonably ordered fell on the *Breve nota*, which put everything into place and took readers through an ostensibly coherent itinerary. The booklet started with a description of di Sangro's

[98] *Breve nota di quel che si vede in casa del Principe di Sansevero D. Raimondo di Sangro nella città di Napoli* ([Naples]: n.p., 1766).

[99] See Bodleian Library (Oxford), ms. Add. A. 366, 'A Journal kept by Mr Tracy and Mr Dent and during their Travel through France and Italy', unpaginated; Lamberg, *Mémorial d'un mondain*, vol. 1, 167 (Letter of 10 April 1772 from Paul-Joseph Vallet in Grenoble). On the frontispiece of the 1766 copy of the *Breve nota* held in the British Library one can read in Italian: 'gift of the author, the Prince of Sansevero'.

[100] *Breve nota*, 19ff; Lalande, *Voyage d'un François en Italie*, vol. 6, 243–9.

[101] Bodleian Library (Oxford), ms. Add. A. 366, 'A Journal kept by Mr Tracy and Mr Dent and during their Travel through France and Italy', unpaginated.

[102] Beinecke Rare Book & Manuscript Library, Yale University (New Haven), Osborn ms. c. 200 (1754–5), 111.

[103] Ganganelli, *Interesting Letters*, vol. 2 (1781), 96.

[104] Richard, *Description historique*, vol. 4, 207.

[105] Sade, *Voyage d'Italie*, vol. 16, 429–30.

much cherished family chapel annexed to the palace, which di Sangro had been busy refurbishing in an ambitious project that had involved well-known artists such as Antonio Corradini, Francesco Queirolo, and Giuseppe Sammartino.[106] It then took readers to the Apartment of the Patriarch, which presented visitors with the family genealogy, and continued with the still unfinished Apartment of the Phoenix, where Giuseppe Salerno's two anatomical specimens were displayed amidst works in progress.

Enjoying a position of prominence in the virtual tour laid out by the *Breve nota*, Salerno's anatomical specimens became one of the highlights of the San Severo Palace. When a French translation of the *Breve nota* appeared in 1768 in *Le Journal encyclopédique*, a footnote highlighted that 'the English tourists, who have travelled most, consider these two anatomical pieces to be masterpieces'.[107] Here as well as in the *Breve nota*, Salerno's anatomical specimens were also called 'anatomical machines'. As we have seen, in the mid-eighteenth century calling anatomical models 'machines' was not unusual. It evoked, of course, contemporary accounts of the animal economy representing the body as a mechanical device composed of solid matter and fluids. By the time Salerno's anatomical specimens joined di Sangro's cabinet, reference to the body as a machine had become so common that it had entered the epistolary lexicon of letter writers who talked about the state of their 'machine' to refer to their health.[108] Automata, the ultimate bodily machines, were themselves called by the French maker Jacques de Vaucanson 'moving anatomies'.[109] As we saw in Chapter 5, the term 'machine' was also used to refer to instruments and tools like Galli's 'midwifery machines'. In early modern Italy, the Latin term 'machina' could equally refer to artifice and ingenious devices.[110] And, indeed, the anatomical machines were certainly artful and ingenious.

Characterized in the *Breve nota* as 'unique things in Europe' on account that they showed whole bodies and were made with the utmost diligence, the anatomical machines were presented as the result of anatomical injections and displayed a thick and intricate net of twisted red and blue blood vessels of various sizes that developed over the skeletons of a woman and a man (Plates 50 and 51). On the head of the skeletons, the skull and the mouth had opening devices to

[106] See, for instance, Colonna di Stigliano, 'La Cappella Sansevero'; Rosanna Cioffi, *La Cappella Sansevero: Arte barocca e ideologia massonica* (Salerno: Edizioni 10/17, 1987).

[107] The footnote may have been added by the editor; see 'Remarques sur quelques unes de curiosités observées en 1766, à Naples, dans le Palais du San-Severo, Seigneur Raimond de Sangro, Prince de San-Sévero', *Journal encyclopédique*, vol. 8 (15 November 1768), 108–15 (citation p. 114). See also 'Suites des remarques sur quelques unes de curiosités observes en 1766, à Naples, &c', ibid. (1 December 1768), 117–27. *Le Journal encyclopédique* was founded by Pierre Rousseau in 1756 to promote the ideas of Diderot and D'Alembert's *Encyclopédie*.

[108] See, for instance, the epistolary exchanges of Bernardo Tanucci who, in the mid-eighteenth century, served as prime minister in Naples and, in particular, Bernardo Tanucci, *Epistolario I: 1723–1746*, ed. Romano Paolo Coppini et al. (Rome: Edizioni di Storia e Letteratura, 1980), 221 and 260.

[109] See, for instance, Landes, 'Wax Fibers', 58. On eighteenth-century automata, see, for instance, Adelheid Voskuhl, *Androids in the Enlightenment: Mechanics, Artisans, and Cultures of the Self* (Chicago: University of Chicago Press, 2013).

[110] See *Vocabolario degli Accademici della Crusca* (Venice: Alberti, 1612), entries for 'Artificio', 'Ingegno', and 'Ordigno'.

show the vessels of the brain and the tongue (Plate 52).[111] The female skeleton was displayed along with the specimen of a foetus, which was worked with admirable 'delicacy', and whose skull also opened to display blood vessels.[112] Around the pubic bone of the female skeleton, the vessels thinned to reveal an anomalous pelvic structure that would have likely caused obstructed childbirth. As mentioned in Chapter 5, in his *Embriologia sacra* (1745) the Palermitan clergyman Francesco Emanuele Cangiamila, Salerno's fellow citizen, had advocated caesarean sections to facilitate the baptism of unborn children in cases of emergency. By drawing attention to the anomalies of the pelvis, Salerno's female skeleton visualized an anatomical situation that echoed contemporary debates on caesarian intervention.

It is worth noting that the anatomical machines presented some analogies with the anatomical displays of Bologna, where Salerno was originally headed. Like the models of the anatomy room at the Institute of the Sciences, they displayed anatomical parts over standing skeletons and, accordingly, offered demonstrations of the anatomy of bones as well as of soft anatomical parts. Moreover, just like the Bolognese écorchés, the female skeleton stood on a pedestal, which could be rotated around and shown to viewers from different sides. The anatomical machines also shared with Lelli's models a common anatomical iconography of postures and gestures that largely drew from classical sculpture and the visual repertoire of early modern anatomical works. Notably, in the female skeleton, the lifted arm evoked a canonic anatomical posture that took inspiration from classical statues and was usually associated with the display of male muscles in action. Here, however, the gesture was presented in the context of the demonstration of blood vessels in the arm of a female body (Plate 53). In general, by visualizing the complex web of blood vessels that unfolded over the skeleton, Salerno's specimens mapped the inner body in a way that complemented the focus on muscles characterizing the écorchés of the Bolognese anatomy room.[113] Unlike the Bolognese anatomical models, the anatomical machines were presented as the result of anatomical injections.

THICKENING BLOOD

By the time the anatomical machines appeared in the cabinet of curiosities of the Prince of San Severo, anatomical preparations based on injection had come to be regarded as a particularly effective means for investigating the inner body. Relying on elaborate techniques of anatomical preservation, they caused the hardening of bodily parts through the injection of materials such as wax, oil of turpentine, quicksilver, and resins, and through the employment of special instruments such as siphons and pneumatic machines. Thanks to the solidification of the injected

111 *Breve nota*, 20. 112 Ibid., 20–1.

113 Paolo A. Rossi, 'O' principe "haravec": le machine anatomiche e il sangue di San Gennaro', in Rossi and Li Vigni (eds.), *I veli di pietra*, 40–1.

materials and the corrosion of the soft parts around them, injections offered an impressive tool of visualization of the inner body. Revealing otherwise invisible and inaccessible corporeal recesses, they promised to chart the inner body with greater precision than any other anatomical technique could possibly do.

The eighteenth-century Bolognese collections included anatomical preparations that relied on actual bodily parts, as well as wax models. For instance, dry anatomical preparations were found in both Valsalva's collection and the cabinet of Morandi and Manzolini. Moreover, Galli's midwifery collection included a number of 'natural foetuses' preserved in spirit of wine.[114] None of these techniques however, were considered capable of achieving the same level of accuracy in unveiling the inner body as injections. Nor were injections absent from eighteenth-century Bolognese anatomy. In January 1705, the mathematician and physician Domenico Guglielmini noticed that an attempt to carry out wax injections in Bologna had not been particularly satisfactory.[115] However, as we saw in Chapter 2, in the 1750s the Bolognese anatomist Tommaso Laghi engaged in experimenting with injecting techniques. He recruited Ercole Lelli for this purpose and reported his pursuits in the *Commentarii* of the Institute of the Sciences.[116] Although these experiments did not lead to the addition of injected specimens to the Institute's anatomy room, Lelli injected the head of a man for the hospital of Santa Maria della Morte.[117] Anatomical injections also featured in the creation of mythical narratives of Bologna as a historical centre of anatomical knowledge. And when Alessandro Macchiavelli fabricated the story of Alessandra Giliani as the legendary medieval female anatomist and assistant of Mondino, he narrated that she cleaned the veins of cadavers and filled them with coloured liquids that solidified immediately and made them visible.[118] Regardless of its authenticity, the story points both to the role of injections in the pantheon of prominent anatomical techniques and to the place of women in eighteenth-century celebrations of Bolognese anatomy.

Indeed, anatomical injections were not new to the eighteenth century. In the course of the sixteenth century, the anatomist Jacopo Berengario da Carpi (*c.*1460–*c.*1530), who taught at the University of Bologna, recorded in his *Commentaria* (1521) the practice of injecting the veins of the kidney with warm water.[119] Other early modern medical practitioners, including the physician Amatus Lusitanus (1511–1568), the physician Franciscus Sylvius (1614–1672), and the anatomist Thomas Bartholin (1616–1680), made preparations of vessels and bodily parts by injecting liquids that cooled and solidified in the vessels.[120] In the following

[114] ASB, Assunteria d'Istituto, Diversorum, busta 11, n. 10, 'Inventario di quanto si trova nelle due camere dell'Instituto destinate ad istruzione dell'Arte Ostetricia'.

[115] Guillaume Desnoües, *Lettres de G. Desnoües, Professeur d'Anatomie, & de Chirurgie, de l'Académie de Bologne; et de Mr Guglielmini, Professeur de Medecine & de Mathematiques à Padoüe, de L'Académie Royale des Sciences; et d'autres Sâvans sur differentes nouvelles découvertes* (Rome: Antoine Rossi, 1706), 23.

[116] Laghi, 'De perficienda injectionum anatomicarum methodo'.

[117] See Medici, 'Elogio d'Ercole Lelli', 164.

[118] See Macchiavelli, *Effemeridi*, 40–1.

[119] Jacopo Berengario da Carpi, *Carpi Commentaria cum amplissimis additionibus super anatomia Mundini* (Bologna: H. de Benedictis, 1521).

[120] See Cole, 'The History of Anatomical Injections', 290.

period, a wave of enthusiasm for anatomical injections swept the world of anatomy.[121] Requiring much hands-on expertise as well as materials such as resins, wax, oil of turpentine, mercury, and spirit of wine, and instruments such as siphons and air pumps, anatomical injections became the object of an intense season of experimentation.[122] Marcello Malpighi, for instance, famously explored the structure of the kidneys by means of injections based on ink, mercury, urine, and spirit of wine.[123]

In the eyes of eighteenth-century practitioners, injections had entered a golden age of perfection largely due to the work of Dutch anatomists like Reinier de Graaf (1641–1673), Jan Swammerdam (1637–1680), and, most famously, Frederik Ruysch (1638–1731).[124] When eighteenth-century anatomists talked about instruments, they referred to de Graaf's copper and silver siphons and syringes.[125] When they discussed wax injections that solidified inner bodily parts, they mentioned Swammerdam. But when they celebrated the achievements of anatomical injections in visualizing the complexity of the circulatory system, they invoked the name of Ruysch who had contrived a way of injecting vessels all the way down to the minutest ramifications of the human body.[126] Unveiling what lay out of sight and revealing the smallest and most imperceptible bodily parts and ducts, anatomical injections ended up being regarded as the latest finding in a new age of visualization that equalled the promises of the microscope.[127]

In his 'Éloge de M. Ruysch', Bernard le Bovier de Fontenelle noticed that Ruysch's injections visualized even those vessels that were so minute that they could only be seen with the help of a microscope.[128] In the mid-eighteenth century, Alexander Monro *primus* (1697–1767), who taught anatomy at the University of Edinburgh, further remarked that through the assistance of 'injections and microscopes, wonderful plexuses of blood-vessels are discovered'.[129] Charles Bonnet equally observed that 'the scalpel, the microscope, and injections' had significantly contributed to the knowledge of animal anatomy (though not as much to the investigation of plants).[130] Others revisited the analogy in terms of the famous 'querelle des Anciens et des Modernes', which continued to engage and divide savants on the role and authority of ancient knowledge. Some argued that since anatomical injections and microscopes constituted genuine modern accomplishments, they showed the moderns' capacity to outdo the ancients. The British

[121] See [Pierre Tarin], *Anthropotomie; ou l' art de dissequer les muscles, les ligamens, les nerfs, & les vaisseaux sanguins du corps humain*, vol. 2 (Paris: Briasson, 1750), 103.

[122] Cook, *Matters of Exchange*, chapter 7; Cook, 'The Preservation of Specimens'.

[123] Cole, 'The History of Anatomical Injections', 288–90 and 294.

[124] Ibid.; Cook, 'Time's Bodies'.

[125] Cole, 'The History of Anatomical Injections', 297–9.

[126] See, for instance, Fontenelle, 'Éloge de M. Ruysch', esp. 102–3.

[127] On microscopes and their cultures in the eighteenth century, see Chapter 3, n. 116.

[128] Fontenelle, 'Éloge de M. Ruysch', 103.

[129] Alexander Monro, *The Anatomy of the Human Bones and Nerves* (Edinburgh: for G. Hamilton and J. Balfour and London by Innys et al., 1750), 343. On Monro, see Anita Guerrini, 'Alexander Monro Primus and the Moral Theatre of Anatomy', *The Eighteenth Century*, 47:1 (2006), 1–18.

[130] Charles Bonnet, *Contemplation de La Nature*, in *Oeuvres d'histoire naturelle et de philosophie de Charles Bonnet*, vol. 4/II (Neuchatel: Samuel Fauche, 1781), 112.

historian Edward Gibbon (1737–1794) observed that as far as anatomical knowledge was concerned 'the more solid and visible parts were known in the time of Galen', but 'the finer scrutiny of the human frame was reserved for the microscope and the injections of modern artists'.[131] Promising to offer better insights into the complexity of the body than any dissection could possibly do, injections became a privileged site for claims of discovery. As they seemed capable of providing a formidable means for mapping the inner body, they pledged to put an end to all anatomical disputes.[132]

As is well known, Ruysch had initially kept his recipes for anatomical injections secret. Only upon selling his collection to Peter the Great in 1717 did he reveal his injecting techniques for an additional 5000 guilders.[133] Even so, only few had access to it. When, following Ruysch's death, the text was finally disclosed to the wider learned world, it famously seemed to conceal as much as it revealed, turning out not to be very helpful. Still, Ruysch's work triggered much interest. In the 1740s the entry for 'injectio' in Robert James' *Medicinal Dictionary* reported Ruysch's 'method of injecting and preparing Bodies for anatomical purposes, from his own Manuscript'.[134] Notably, Ruysch's anatomical injections also provided an authoritative frame of reference for highlighting the importance of Salerno's own anatomical specimens. In May 1762, the Palermitan physician Giuseppe di Gregorio e Russo (1703–1771) referred to it in order to underscore the significance of Giuseppe Salerno's own anatomical work, which similarly unveiled the complex web of bodily vessels.[135] Situating Salerno's anatomical specimens within a distinguished anatomical tradition, di Gregorio e Russo also mentioned the anatomical work of Guillaume Desnoües, who had carried out anatomical injections and revealed his techniques to Domenico Guglielmini.[136]

Published in 1706 in Rome, the correspondence between Desnoües and Guglielmini described the painstaking complexity of the injecting process. Here Desnoües recalled the details of how, in order to preserve the cadavers of a mother and her unborn child, he had worked overnight for a whole month on the two bodies, in an area 'exposed to the Northern wind', first preparing the cadavers and then injecting them. He first opened and cleaned the cadavers, injected them with water through a hydraulic machine, and blew air into their vessels with the help of a pneumatic machine. He subsequently bathed the bodies in warm water before

[131] See Edward Gibbon, *The History of the Decline and Fall of the Roman Empire*, vol. 5 (London: A. Strahan and T. Cadell, 1788), 429.

[132] At the same time, as much as they were taken to provide the ultimate evidence of what lay underneath the skin, anatomical injections also stirred up controversy. For instance, having come to believe that bodies were made out of a web of vessels, as expressed in the famous adage 'totum corpus ex vasculis', Ruysch debated with Malpighi over the nature of glands; see Cole, 'The History of Anatomical Injections', 306. See also Guglielmini's defence of Malpighi in Desnoües, *Lettres de G. Desnoües*.

[133] See Margócsy, 'Advertising Cadavers', 306; Margócsy, *Commercial Visions*, 131.

[134] See Robert James, *A Medicinal Dictionary: Including Physic, Surgery, Anatomy, Chemistry, and Botany*, vol. 2 (London: T. Osborne, 1745), unpaginated, entry for 'Injectio'.

[135] De Gregorio e Russo, 'Ad Augustinum Giuffrida', 247–8. Although the author is known as 'di Gregorio e Russo', I have maintained the original spelling of the name when I refer to the source.

[136] Ibid.

injecting them first with coloured spirit of wine and then wax.[137] Ultimately, however, his efforts were to no avail. Much to his dismay, his elaborate anatomical preparation, which had required so much work and care, started gradually, if imperceptibly, to deteriorate. Desnoües then decided to make 'an anatomized artificial body', namely, a model in wax that portrayed the specimen of the injected woman. To begin with, he encountered 'many difficulties'. Yet, after he met the skilled Sicilian wax modeller Gaetano Giulio Zumbo, he created with him a collection of anatomical waxworks.[138]

Indeed, injecting vessels was not easy.[139] Something could go wrong at every step of the process. In order to solidify properly and maintain the vessels' natural features, the wax used in the injections needed to be neither too hot nor too cold, neither too hard nor too soft. Colouring, especially of small vessels, required particular care. Likewise, siphons had to be handled properly, for at any moment the presence of air in the emptied vessels ran the risk of wasting all efforts.[140] Another concern was that the pressure exercised on the vessels forced the injected material to areas where normally there was no blood. The possibility that injections could overly enlarge capillaries and lead to extravasation also ran the risk of affecting their capacity to map the inner body accurately. Finally, the presence of blockages in the vessels could equally frustrate efforts because the pressure exercised during injection could break the obstructed vessels. Still, arduous and laborious as the procedure may have been, the result was amazing. At the end of the process, Desnoües could not take his eyes away from the 'vast and marvellous forest' of vessels and 'the countless number of prepared parts' that had unfolded as the result of his injections.[141] In fact, according to Desnoües the outcome exceeded the imagination so much that it would take 'whole volumes' to describe it.[142]

While the details of injecting procedures had initially enjoyed limited circulation, Desnoües' description was followed by other reports discussing different injecting techniques. Wilhelm Homberg (1652–1715), for instance, a member of the Parisian Academy of the Sciences, who devoted himself to chemical inquiries, and whose work was known to di Sangro, presented the advantages of injecting a liquid made of wax, mercury, and oil of turpentine in cadavers in which the soft parts were removed by maceration.[143] For his part, Pierre Simon Rouhault, first surgeon to the king of Sardinia and professor of surgery at the University of Turin, expressed his preference for gland or fish glue dissolved in water.[144] In 1732,

[137] Desnoües, *Lettres de G. Desnoües*, 31–43. See also Taddia, 'Corpi', 172–3.

[138] Desnoües, *Lettres de G. Desnoües*, 82–3 (citations p. 82).

[139] In 1735 the anatomist Antonio Cocchi described the injection of the corpse of an infant where he highlighted the difficulties involved in the process; see Giorgio Weber, *Aspetti poco noti della storia dell'anatomia patologica tra '600 e '700: William Harvey, Marcello Malpighi, Antonio Cocchi, Giovanni Maria Lancisi; verso Morgagni* (Florence: Leo S. Olschki, 1997), 126 (Appendix II). See also Buffon and Daubenton, *Histoire naturelle*, vol. 3, 134ff.

[140] Desnoües, *Lettres de G. Desnoües*, 35–40. [141] Ibid., 41. [142] Ibid.

[143] On Homberg, see Bernard Le Bovier de Fontenelle, 'Éloge de Monsieur Homberg', in *Oeuvres de Monsieur de Fontenelle: Éloges des académiciens de l'Académie*, vol. 2 (London: Valade for H. M. Cazin, 1785), 110–30.

[144] Pierre Simon Rouhault, 'Sur les injections anatomiques', in *Histoire et Memoires de l'Académie des Sciences, Année 1718* (Paris: Imprimerie Royale, 1721), 219–21.

Alexander Monro published an account of the injecting techniques that he had employed hoping that it 'may save the young unexperienced [*sic*] anatomist the trouble of fruitless trials'.[145] Others followed suit. In Bologna, Tommaso Laghi engaged in perfecting Monro's injecting techniques.[146] Looking back at the developments that had taken place in the world of anatomical injections, in the mid-eighteenth century Louis-Jean-Marie Daubenton could conclude that after many attempts and mixed results, the art of anatomical injections had at last reached a high degree of perfection. This was also because chemists had come to the assistance of the anatomists and together they had contrived ingenious procedures.[147]

Thus, by the time Salerno's anatomical specimens joined the San Severo Palace, anatomical injections had come to be regarded as sites of truthful bodily knowledge. Although not all injections were aimed at showing blood vessels, their capacity to do so turned them into a much sought-after technique. By creating a thorough map of blood vessels, anatomical injections promised to address questions about the nature of blood and its circulation, and tackle ongoing frustrations. As François Quesnay, physician to Louis XV and author of the famous *Tableau économique*, put it in the mid-eighteenth century, circulation had proven a powerful tool of medical understanding, shedding light on the 'physics of the animal economy'. However, it had had little impact on medical practice, generating perplexity among practitioners and turning medicine into a more uncertain and dangerous activity.[148] Anatomical injections promised to tackle such perplexities while bringing knowledge of blood vessels to bear directly on the eye. In 1774, the British anatomist and man-midwife William Hunter famously celebrated anatomical injections as a fitting tribute to Harvey:

> Were the great Harvey to rise from his grave, to examine what has been done since his time, I imagine that nothing would give him more pleasure, than to view with attention, the cabinets of some of the Anatomists of the present times. He, and the Anatomists of former ages, had no other knowledge of the blood-vessels, than what they were able to collect from laborious dissections, and from examining the smaller branches of them, upon some lucky occasion, when they were found more than commonly loaded with red blood. But filling the vascular system with a bright coloured wax, enables us to trace the large vessels with great ease, renders the smaller much more conspicuous, and makes thousands of the very minute ones visible, which from their delicacy, and the transparency of their natural contents, are otherwise imperceptible.[149]

[145] Alexander Monro, 'An Essay on the Art of Injecting the Vessels of Animals', *Medical Essays and Observations, Revised and Published by a Society in Edinburgh*, 2nd edn., vol. 1 (Edinburgh: printed by T. and W. Ruddimans for W. Monro and W. Drummond et al., 1737), 94–111 (citation p. 95).

[146] Laghi, 'De perficienda injectionum anatomicarum methodo'.

[147] Buffon and Daubenton, *Histoire naturelle*, vol. 3, 135.

[148] François Quesnay, *Essai physique sur l'oeconomie animale, par M. Quesnay*, 2nd edn., vol. 3 (Paris: Guillame Cavelier, 1747), 418–19.

[149] William Hunter, *Two Introductory Lectures: Delivered by Dr. William Hunter, to his Last Course of Anatomical Lectures, at his Theatre in Windmill-Street: As They Were Left Corrected for the Press by Himself* (London: J. Johnson, 1784), 55–6.

Arguably, when the anatomical machines were put on display in the San Severo Palace, they pledged to transfer the complex ensemble of values related to skilled handcraft, discovery, amazement, and revelation, which had come to be associated with anatomical injections, to di Sangro's own cabinet and investigations. Being presented early on in the itinerary set out by the *Breve nota*, they were well positioned to contribute to the effort to persuade visitors and travellers about the value of di Sangro's own pursuits. Their characterization as injected specimens, the result of a happy cross-fertilization between anatomy and chemistry, further promised to reflect well on di Sangro's own chemical inquiries, especially his experiments with blood. As part of these pursuits, di Sangro claimed to have recreated blood by placing different kinds of well-chewed food in a jar, covering it with manure, and occasionally adding acid or lemon.[150] Unveiling the complex web of blood vessels, the anatomical machines expanded and complemented such investigations. In doing so, they participated in di Sangro's attempt to carve a special place for his cabinet and his pursuits among the wonders of 'the city of bloods'.

'THE CITY OF BLOODS'

When the French traveller Jean-Jacques Bouchard sojourned in Naples for eight months in 1632, he found plenty of opportunities to fill his diary with his impressions of what looked like an amazing place. However, nothing could quite parallel the some 3,000 relics that were scattered across town. Some of the blood relics miraculously liquefied on a periodic basis. Bouchard dubbed Naples '*urbs sanguinum*', the city of bloods.[151] The most famous instance of miraculous liquefaction encountered by Bouchard was, of course, that of Saint Januarius: on designated dates Saint Januarius' solidified blood miraculously liquefied in the city's *Duomo*. Dating back to the fourteenth century, the miraculous liquefaction lay at the centre of a ritual where the bust believed to contain the saint's head was presented with the reliquary where two ampoules were taken to preserve his solidified blood. The reliquary was then shaken in front of the bust and the miracle took place as the blood liquefied in front of the beholders. As Jean-Michel Sallmann has suggested, in Naples Saint Januarius was the saint of saints.[152] The liquefaction of Saint Januarius' blood similarly staged the miracle of miracles. The ceremony was also taken to test

[150] See Origlia Paolino, *Istoria*, vol. 2, 379–80; Napoli Signorelli, *Vicende*, vol. 4, 491.

[151] Jean-Jacques Bouchard, *Journal, II, Voyage dans le royaume de Naples, Voyage dans la campagne de Rome*, ed. Emanuele Kanceff (Turin: Giappichelli, 1977). On Naples as the 'city of bloods' characterized by miraculous liquefactions, see Marino Niola, *Il corpo mirabile: Miracolo, sangue, estasi nella Napoli barocca* (Rome: Meltemi, 1997), 84; Lucia Malafronte and Carmine Maturo, *Urbs Sanguinum: Itinerario alla ricerca dei prodigi di sangue a Napoli* (Naples: Intra Moenia, 2000); Francesco Paolo de Ceglia, 'Thinking with the Saint: The Miracle of Saint Januarius of Naples and Science in Early Modern Europe', *Early Science and Medicine*, 19:2 (2014), 133–73, esp. 138–9. On the miracle of Saint Januarius, see also Helen Hills, 'Through a Glass Darkly: Material Holiness and the Treasury Chapel of San Gennaro in Naples', in Calaresu and Hills (eds.), *New Approaches to Naples*, 31–62.

[152] Sallmann, *Naples et ses saints*.

the saint's protection over the city, which entailed sparing it from the volcano's eruptions as well as 'from war, pestilence, famine, and earthquakes', the assumption being that if the blood failed to liquefy, things were likely to take a turn for the worse.[153] In 1707 and in 1767, the successful liquefaction was taken to signal the saint's intercession to end catastrophic eruptions of Mount Vesuvius.

Early modern public and religious rituals provided a particularly felicitous arena for the exercise of power. In a colonial setting like the kingdoms of Naples and Sicily, religious rituals helped foreign sovereigns increase their grip over local subjects. As Giovanni Montroni has observed, 'through the cult of San Gennaro' the king 'was able to unite himself with the people of Naples more effectively than by the many attempts at political propaganda intended to conciliate various elements in society'.[154] Indeed, linking loyalty to the Church with the triumphal celebration of the Spanish crown, the miracle of Saint Januarius marked important moments in the establishment and consolidation of the new Spanish monarchy. Shortly after the victory over the Habsburg troops, in 1734 Charles de Bourbon triumphantly entered Naples as the new sovereign on the very day of the miracle, thus conveying the message that the Spanish dynasty received divine blessing and would rule by supernatural consent. A few years later, in 1738, the miracle also marked the wedding of Charles with Maria Amalia of Saxony. The occasion offered the opportunity to inaugurate the order of Saint Januarius, which counted Raimondo di Sangro among its ranks. The ritual of the liquefaction of Saint Januarius' blood also offered an arena for establishing patterns of continuity with long-standing local forms of devotion that sought the protection of the most important local saint and the welfare of the city. Not surprisingly, it became a key political event that manifested the joint control of crown and church over the public display of blood.

The miracles' political implications did not escape the Neapolitan literati. Savants like Antonio Genovesi and Paolo Mattia Doria deplored that the Spanish government had put much emphasis on 'elaborate public religious ceremonies', and encouraged forms of 'obsessive veneration' like that of Saint Januarius to distract 'the people from the correct understanding of their civic responsibilities'.[155] For their part, some travellers regarded the event as the ultimate manifestation of popish trickery. The editor of *The Spectator*, Joseph Addison, famously described the miraculous liquefaction as the most bungling trick he had ever seen.[156] In his *Lettres familières*, Charles de Brosses portrayed it as a very nice instance of chemistry.[157] Others noticed the charged atmosphere and the collective weeping

[153] Keyssler, *Travels*, vol. 2, 360–2; Vivant Denon, *Viaggio nel Regno di Napoli, 1777–1778*, trans. Teresa Leone (Naples: Paparo, 2001), 41.

[154] Montroni, 'The Court', 34.

[155] See Pagden, *Spanish Imperialism*, 80. On ritual and identity in early modern Naples, see John A. Marino, *Becoming Neapolitan: Citizen Culture in Baroque Naples* (Baltimore: Johns Hopkins University Press, 2011).

[156] Joseph Addison, *Remarks on Several Parts of Italy, &c in the Years 1701, 1702, 1703*, 2nd edn. (London: Tonson, 1718), 149.

[157] De Brosses, *Lettres familières*, vol. 1, 374.

and cheering that took place during the ceremony.[158] Some wrote that Protestants and, in general, non-Roman Catholic visitors were taken to be responsible for delays in the liquefaction of the relic. They were then asked to leave the cathedral because in their presence the relic could develop a bad mood and refuse to liquefy.[159] Still, regardless of the reservations, the ceremony did titillate the imagination of many who were keen to attend the event. Some travellers planned their journey so as to be in Naples at the time of the ceremony.[160] Having missed the celebration of the ritual during his first stay, the artist Richard de Saint-Non planned a second trip to Naples to attend it.[161]

In a setting in which the liquefaction of the blood relic drew so much attention, the news that di Sangro had replicated the miracle by natural means was unlikely to pass unnoticed. On 18 May 1751, Monsignor Gualtieri, the papal nuncio in Naples, passed the following news to Cardinal Valenti in Rome:

> I was told, in the greatest secret, that the Prince of San Severo has composed a material similar to the blood contained in the ampoule of Saint Januarius and, depending on the conditions of the air, seems to have the same effects, though this is kept in great secret.[162]

The timing could not have been worse. That year Saint Januarius' blood did not liquefy. The recently exposed Neapolitan lodge of Freemasonry was blamed for the failed liquefaction.[163] Being the Grand Master of the lodge, di Sangro was held directly responsible and had to relinquish his membership to the order of Saint Januarius. As the story has it, in his replica of the miracle, di Sangro commissioned 'an ostensory or reliquary', similar to Saint Januarius', which included 'a phial or ampoule of the same shape, and filled with a mixture of gold and mercury amalgamated with cinnabar, which imitated the colour of coagulated blood'. In order to liquefy this mixture, he then added more mercury in the empty neck of the phials, and added a valve that allowed the mercury to enter the phial when the reliquary was turned upside down.[164]

Di Sangro was not alone in engaging in such experiments. Having left Naples without being able to attend the ceremony, La Condamine found some consolation when he visited the Margravine of Bayreuth and participated in a collective experimental performance that conjured up di Sangro's own replica of the miraculous liquefaction. The Margravine of Bayreuth was the sister of Frederick the Great, one of the famous eighteenth-century learned princesses, and a friend of di Sangro

[158] Björnståhl, *Lettere ne' suoi viaggj*, vol. 2, 171–2; Saint-Non, *Panopticon italiano*; Denon, *Viaggio nel Regno di Napoli*.

[159] De Brosses, *Lettres familières*, vol. 1, 374.

[160] La Condamine, 'Extrait d'un journal de voyage en Italie', 383–4.

[161] Saint-Non, *Panopticon italiano*, 124–8.

[162] ASV, Napoli, vol. 234, fol. 98, quoted in Mario Buonoconto, *Viaggio fantastico alla luce del lume eterno: Le straordinarie invenzioni del principe di Sansevero* (Naples: Alòs, 2005), 65.

[163] Montroni, 'The Court', 39.

[164] Lalande, *Voyage d'un François en Italie*, vol. 6, 283–4. According to Harold Acton, di Sangro 'used to entertain his guests with such conjuring tricks'; see Acton, *The Bourbons of Naples*, 100. On early modern natural inquirers' interest in the miracle of Saint Januarius, see de Ceglia, 'Thinking with the Saint'.

who corresponded with him about recipes and 'secrets'.[165] Upon visiting her, La Condamine joined a group where a phial that 'appeared to be half filled with a gray-coloured fixed mass or paste', and 'had its sides tarnished with dust', was passed around the circle of participants with the result that

> on inclining it alternatively several ways, and shaking it for about half a minute, more or less, the paste became liquid, and melted; sometimes only partially; at other times it grew fixed again, and on shaking it anew it was either a shorter or a longer time in liquefying.[166]

La Condamine emphasized that he had witnessed this performance on several occasions, not only 'in the presence of their highnesses', but also 'more particularly, and in broad day, at the keeper's of the machine', where he 'had all the necessary time to examine it'.[167] A note added in the English translation of La Condamine's work remarked that the author's account clarified what Addison meant when he referred to the miracle as 'one of the most bungling tricks he ever saw'.[168]

Over the years, di Sangro's replica of the miracle ceased to be a whispered secret. In 1769, Lalande described it in his *Voyage d'un François en Italie*, though he only revealed di Sangro's name as the author of the replica in the second edition of the work, which was published in 1786, well after di Sangro's death.[169] In March 1771, Anna Riggs Miller reported to her 'friend residing in France' about her visit to Naples' *Duomo* and noticed that 'the ridiculous pretended miracle' of the liquefaction of St Januarius' blood on certain days had grown 'almost universally contemptible at Naples, even in the eyes of the vulgar'.[170] In particular, she had heard from 'the poor man who sweeps the church' that 'the Prince *Sansevero* had made a chymical preparation which exactly resembles St. Gennaro's blood, and caused it to liquefy in the same manner, by the warmth proceeding from his handling the phial, and turning it up and down'.[171]

It seems possible to situate di Sangro's replica of the blood miracle in the context of his various engagements with the study of blood including his production of artificial blood and his acquisition of anatomical specimens displaying blood vessels. In fact, both in the case of the replica of Saint Januarius' miracle and in that of the anatomical machines, blood lay at the centre of processes of material transformation related to solidification and liquefaction. Notably, from Mount Vesuvius' flowing lava that had covered and preserved Pompeii and Herculaneum, and eventually allowed for their resurfacing, to the liquefaction of saintly blood, changing states of matter fed the grand stage of Neapolitan natural, religious, and antiquarian wonder. By displaying blood vessels that were purportedly visualized through the

[165] De Felice, *Encyclopédie*, vol. 28, 484.

[166] Charles Marie de La Condamine, *Journal of a Tour to Italy, translated from the French* (Dublin: J. Potts at Swift's Head, 1763), 103–7 (citation p. 104).

[167] Ibid., 105. [168] Ibid., 107.

[169] In 1769, Lalande generically referred to the author of the replica of the miracle as a savant 'equally illustrious for his birth as for his knowledge ("lumières")'; see Lalande, *Voyage d'un François en Italie*, vol. 6, 283–4. On the remark in the second edition of Lalande's work, see Lalande, *Voyage en Italie*, vol. 7, 112.

[170] [Miller], *Letters from Italy*, vol. 2, 142–3. [171] Ibid.

hardening of injected materials, the anatomical machines seemingly linked material transformation with anatomical regeneration. In doing so, they added to a setting that invested much in the revelatory power of physical transformation.[172] It would be beyond the scope of this study to explore in depth the variety of meanings associated with blood as a powerful symbol related, among other things, to life, death, and rebirth.[173] But in order to further explore the historical significance of the anatomical machines, it is worth considering the import of di Sangro's engagement with the investigation of blood in light of his involvement with Freemasonry, which held the notion of regeneration among its chief philosophical tenets.

REGENERATION

After his exposure as the Grand Master of the Neapolitan lodge, di Sangro's abjuration of Freemasonry was hasty and dramatic. Reactions to di Sangro's disclosure of the names of Masonic adepts were equally fierce. His portrait was sent to the various lodges and his effigy was burnt in Berlin in a public square.[174] Yet, despite his repudiation, di Sangro's attitude towards Freemasonry remained somewhat fluid. While a German visitor, who was in Naples in 1753, reported having had the honour of being welcomed by di Sangro as a fellow Freemason, another Freemason traveller complained that he had been rebuffed by di Sangro on account that he already had too many duties as a man and a citizen and did not intend to take on more with regard to 'a particular society'.[175] Both before and after his abjuration, echoes of Freemasonic philosophy and symbology continued to permeate di Sangro's activities and natural pursuits.[176] Art historian Rosanna Cioffi has suggested

[172] For a different reading of di Sangro's inquiries into blood, his replica of the miracle of Saint Januarius, and the anatomical machines, see Rossi, 'O' principe'; Clorinda Donato, 'Esoteric Reason, Occult Science, and Radical Enlightenment: Seamless Pursuits in the Work and Networks of Raimondo di Sangro, the Prince of San Severo', *Philosophica*, 89 (2014), 179–237. Donato's article appeared shortly after the completion of this chapter and offers an alternative account of the anatomical machines in the context of views of regeneration.

[173] On blood and its histories see, for instance, Mariacarla Gadebusch Bondio (ed.), *Blood in History and Blood Histories*, in Micrologus' Library 13 (Florence: Sismel/Edizione del Galluzzo, 2005); Caroline W. Bynum, *Wonderful Blood: Theology and Practice in Late Medieval Northern Germany and Beyond* (Philadelphia: University of Pennsylvania Press, 2007).

[174] Giuseppe De Blasis, 'Le prime loggie dei liberi muratori a Napoli', in Giuseppe Giarrizzo (ed.), *I liberi muratori di Napoli nel secolo XVIII* (Naples: Società Napoletana di Storia Patria di Napoli, 1998), 465–6.

[175] Biblioteca della Società Napoletana di Storia Patria (Naples), ms. XXX, B 18, 'Lettere a Ferdinando Galiani', Letter of 3 July 1753 from Domenico Sanseverino in Rome, 188.

[176] See for instance [Tschudy, Théodore Henri de], *L'étoile flamboyante, ou la société des Francs-Maçons, considérée sous tous les aspects*, vol. 1 (Frankfurt and Paris: Antoine Boudet, 1766), 36 and 179. On di Sangro's involvement in Freemasonry, see Venturi, *Settecento riformatore*, 542ff; Cioffi, *La Cappella Sansevero*; Giarrizzo (ed.), *I liberi muratori di Napoli*; Francovich, *Storia della Massoneria in Italia*, 98ff; Vincenzo Ferrone, *I profeti dell'illuminismo: Le metamorfosi della ragione nel tardo Settecento italiano* (Bari: Laterza, 1989), 217ff; Di Castiglione, *La Massoneria nelle Due Sicilie*, esp. vols. 1 and 2; Rossi and Li Vigni (eds.), *I veli di pietra*; Donato, 'Esoteric Reason'. On Freemasonry in the Kingdom of Naples see also Anna Maria Rao, 'La Massoneria nel Regno di Napoli', in Cazzaniga (ed.), *Storia d'Italia*, 513–42.

that di Sangro's family chapel—its monuments, coloured marbles, paintings, and especially the statues which were sculpted either veiled or engaged in the act of unveiling—was enmeshed in a web of Freemasonic evocations.[177] Some of the arenas in which di Sangro couched his interests as a natural inquirer, such as his writings and cabinet of curiosities, similarly echoed Freemasonic themes like initiation, regeneration, and illumination. Some of the curiosities displayed in his palace were themselves evocative of Freemasonic philosophy. In some cases, they also provided material complements to the claims di Sangro had advanced in his writings. As we have seen, in his writings di Sangro discussed the discovery of perpetual lamps, a theme that resonated with the Masonic vocabulary of enlightenment. In the early 1770s, visitors could catch a glimpse of one of these 'inextinguishable lamps' glittering in the San Severo Chapel.[178]

The anatomical machines equally brought some of the themes associated with the display of blood vessels and injected specimens to bear on di Sangro's claims to have carried out experiments on rebirth and regeneration. As we have seen, in the eyes of early modern anatomists, anatomical knowledge could provide insights into how to create as well as cure bodies.[179] Anatomical injections promised to add to the scope of such claims. Fontenelle emphasized that whereas Ruysch's mummies protracted life, those of ancient Egypt prolonged death.[180] As late as 1824, the Italian poet and literato Giacomo Leopardi conjured up the awakening of Ruysch's anatomical specimens in his 'Dialogue between Frederick Ruysch and his mummies'.[181] When Guillaume Desnoües injected the body of a woman who had died in childbirth, he hoped that he could 'somehow revive her'.[182] Mid-eighteenth-century commentators similarly described Salerno's anatomical specimens in terms of revivification. In his letter of 1762 to the physician Agostino Giuffrida, Giuseppe di Gregorio e Russo remarked that in Salerno's skeleton the injection of 'an artificial liquid' made the veins and arteries coloured and 'turgid' so as to create the impression of 'a new man' generated out of the dead.[183] Later in the century, the Sicilian Marquis of Villabianca, author of a multi-volume chronicle of eighteenth-century Palermo, similarly referred to Salerno's anatomical specimens as 'revivified skeletons'.[184]

Appropriately displayed in the Apartment of the Phoenix, the mythical bird that was reborn out of its own ashes, and regarded as reanimated anatomies, the anatomical machines seemingly evoked one of the most salient symbols of Freemasonry: regeneration. Just like the phoenix, in Freemasonic philosophy the newly initiated adept was supposed to rise from the ashes and defy death. Although banned in 1751, Freemasonry continued to operate more or less overtly in Naples.[185] In

[177] Cioffi, *La Cappella Sansevero*.
[178] [Grosley], *New Observations*, vol. 2, 231.
[179] Bellini, *Discorsi di Anatomia*, 78.
[180] Fontenelle, 'Éloge de M. Ruysch', 103.
[181] Giacomo Leopardi, 'Dialogo di Federico Ruysch e delle sue mummie', in *Operette morali* (Milan: Ant. Fort. Stella e Figli, 1827), 163–71.
[182] Desnoües, *Lettres de G. Desnoües*, 82. On anatomical injections' capacity to restore the appearance of life, see also Medici, 'Elogio d'Ercole Lelli', 164.
[183] De Gregorio e Russo, 'Ad Augustinum Giuffrida', 247.
[184] Biblioteca Comunale di Palermo (henceforth BCP), ms. Qq D 109 , Francesco Maria Emanuele Gaetani (Marchese di Villabianca), 'Diario Palermitano', vol. 17, 532.
[185] Giarrizzo (ed.), *I liberi muratori di Napoli*.

1763, the Masonic ship *Fenix* was stationed for a period in the city's port.[186] In the same year, di Sangro acquired the second anatomical machine from Salerno. Arguably, while writings such as the *Lettera apologetica* generated controversy and plunged di Sangro into trouble, the degree of fluidity and variability that accompanied the meanings of material objects such as the anatomical machines could convey messages that might otherwise be perceived as contentious. Indeed, while the anatomical machines generated words of praise also because of their capacity to stage 'reanimated skeletons', di Sangro's claims to have carried out experiments related to the regeneration of life did not go down particularly well. In particular, his assertion to have carried out 'beautiful experiences' concerning natural and artificial palingenesis, or the regeneration of plants and animals that were reborn out of their ashes, ran the risk of upsetting the carefully interwoven network of credit that he had patiently constructed around his cabinet and his investigations.

JUGGLER OR PHILOSOPHER

Palingenesis, the alchemical resurrection of plants and animals, was discussed by Athanasius Kircher in his *Mundus subterraneus* (1665), which included an account of Kircher's exploration of Mount Vesuvius. In the early eighteenth century, Pierre Le Lorrain, abbé de Vallemont, built on Kircher's work to present a variety of experiences that concerned the 'vegetal Phoenix' and the palingenesis of plants and animals.[187] Di Sangro's claim to have replicated life dated back at least to the appearance of Origlia's *Istoria dello studio di Napoli* (1754). Here, di Sangro was said to have enacted both vegetable and animal palingenesis by replicating fennels and carbonizing crabs, and adding oxblood to their ashes.[188] The text also hinted at di Sangro's ideas on the palingenesis of humans, suggesting that 'to see the image of Cesar, Cicero, or of other ancients [...] it was enough to procure one of their bones'.[189] The final section of the *Breve nota* equally alluded to di Sangro's experiments on palingenesis.[190] Di Sangro did discuss the matter with some travellers. Lalande was among those who enjoyed this privilege but remained perplexed. He referred to di Sangro's 'most extraordinary discoveries' made with regard to 'a natural and real palingenesis of plants and animals'.[191] However, since he had not received satisfactory clarifications, he decided to mention the matter only in passing. Others did not feel any more persuaded.

In the mid-1750s, di Sangro sent a letter to the British natural philosopher Stephen Hales (1677–1761) in which he claimed that the infusion of ashes into

[186] Di Castiglione, *La Massoneria nelle Due Sicilie*, vol. 1, chapter 5.

[187] Pierre Le Lorrain de Vallemont, *Curiositez de la nature et de l'art sur la vegetation*, 2nd edn. (Paris: par la Société, 1711). In his *La Palingénésie philosophique* (1769), the Swiss naturalist Charles Bonnet (1720–1793) placed palingenesy at the centre of the debate on generation by suggesting that living beings relied on preformed germ-like seeds that survived death; see Charles Bonnet, *La Palingénésie philosophique, ou idées sur l'état passé et future des êtres vivants* (Geneva: C. Philibert and B. Chirol, 1769).

[188] Origlia Paolino, *Istoria*, vol. 2, 379.

[189] Ibid., 382.

[190] *Breve nota*, 50–1.

[191] Lalande, *Voyage d'un François en Italie*, vol. 6, 249.

some plants and animals led to their regeneration. Hales' reaction was one of shock. When the savant Pietro Paolo Celesia, a friend of di Sangro, met Hales during his tour of Britain, he diplomatically explained that di Sangro's words needed careful interpretation. However, when he reported the episode to Galiani, he expressed some qualms about di Sangro's claims:

> With his palingeneses, *archee*, and perpetual lamps, this illustrious literato dreamer will make us Italians look like many Raymond Lullys.[192]

To some, di Sangro's assertions about palingenesis felt like one claim too many. After travelling in Italy, in the 1770s Maximilian Joseph von Lamberg made no mystery of his belief that the majority of travellers with whom he had spoken had exaggerated the value of the curiosities displayed in the San Severo Palace.[193] Eager to prove them wrong, he published in his *Mémorial d'un mondain*, a letter from Paul-Joseph Vallet, lieutenant in Grenoble and author of a *Méthode pour faire promptement des progrès dans les sciences et dans les arts* (1767), who had himself expressed reservations about the cabinet. Vallet was the author of the French translation of the *Breve nota* that had appeared in *Le Journal encyclopédique* (1768). His translation helped to spread knowledge about di Sangro's pursuits and his cabinet across the Alps. However, Vallet's goal had been altogether different, as he had hoped to reveal that di Sangro's claims about palingenesis were deceitful. Likewise, he had wanted to show that among the marvels of the San Severo Palace there was 'a considerable quantity of knacks' ('*tours de main*'), which were 'lavishly employed for no other reason than to take advantage of the gullibility of the vulgar'.[194]

In fact, by the time Vallet's translation was published, di Sangro's activities and pursuits had already been plagued by adverse circumstances. In September 1762, di Sangro was arrested for having hosted gambling activities in his palace in order to pay back his growing debts.[195] Apparently, even before the sentence was commuted into house arrest, di Sangro acquired the second anatomical machine from Salerno. In that period, his health began to fail him. As his spouse Carlotta noticed, by February 1766 di Sangro's complexion had deteriorated 'to the point of generating tears': he had become so weak that just 'going to the domestic chapel, not to talk of parties, or even visiting the theatre, which he has not attended for years', had made him so ill that the doctors as well as the family feared the worst.[196] The *Breve nota* was published in the same year. As di Sangro's health continued to worsen, his encounters with visitors likely became less frequent. Meanwhile, the *Breve nota*

192 Salvatore Rotta (ed.), *L'illuminismo a Genova: Lettere di P. P. Celesia a F. Galiani*, vol. 1 (Florence: La Nuova Italia, 1973), 175. Raymond Lully (or Ramon Lull) was a medieval Catalan theologian and alchemist.

193 Lamberg, *Mémorial d'un mondain*, vol. 1, 167ff.

194 Letter of 10 April 1772 from Paul-Joseph Vallet in Grenoble, published in Lamberg, *Mémorial d'un mondain*, vol. 1, 167–8.

195 Archivio di Stato di Napoli (henceforth ASN), Segreteria di Stato di Casa Reale, Affari Diversi, busta n. 862, Letters of 19 September 1762 and 18 November 1762 from the Prince of San Severo.

196 ASN, Segreteria di Stato di Casa Reale, Affari Diversi, busta n. 870, Letter of 27 February 1766 from the Princess of San Severo in Portici.

acquired increasing importance as a means of introducing viewers to the display.[197] The Marquis de Sade, who visited the San Severo premises after di Sangro's death, found it for sale at the entrance to the Palace.[198]

The end of di Sangro's polite encounters and demonstrations marked the beginning of a season in which visitors adopted an increasingly critical attitude towards his claims and creations, though the trend did not involve the anatomical machines. In 1776, de Sade noticed 'two very curious skeletons' in one of the run-down apartments of the palace but disapproved of the chapel and its statues, which, although praised by Richard, in his view were nothing but the high point of 'unreasoning and bad taste'.[199] Upon his visit to the San Severo premises, in 1788 the British politician Charles Abbot, first Baron of Colchester, similarly noted in his diary that he had seen upstairs 'two injected skeletons' but overall regarded the San Severo Palace and Chapel as 'a collection of bad taste in all the Arts'.[200] Over time, some of di Sangro's other pursuits also encountered disapproval. Like Lamberg, who had expressed doubts about the '*merveilles*' on display at the San Severo Palace, in the 1780s the English botanist James Edward Smith (1759–1828), founder of the Linnean Society of London, remained unimpressed and concluded:

> De la Lande mentions the last prince of this family as having been very curious in the chemistry, and as having discovered several ingenious methods of encaustic painting, printing in colour, &c. all of which he kept secret, and therefore deserves to be reckoned a juggler, and not a philosopher.[201]

Smith's remark on the secrecy of di Sangro's methods may sound somewhat surprising. It is true that a halo of secrecy surrounded di Sangro's activities: he joined a secret society like Freemasonry, his replica of the miracle of liquefaction was initially treated as a matter of great secrecy, he was involved in the exchange of 'secrets' and claimed to have recovered the ancient secret of inextinguishable lamps. At the same time, much of di Sangro's pursuit of a reputation as a savant entailed engaging with audiences and publicizing his activities. The doors of the Palace of San Severo were opened wide to visitors and guests. Di Sangro delighted in introducing them to the outcomes of his undertakings, and engaged in sharing his views by corresponding with savants. Such a pairing of secrecy and openness was not unusual. As historians have remarked, well into the eighteenth century these categories were

[197] Anna Riggs Miller, for instance, was on the San Severo premises just days before di Sangro's death, and visited the curiosities of the palace and the chapel with the *Breve nota* in her hands; see [Miller], *Letters from Italy*, vol. 2, 144.

[198] Sade, *Voyage d'Italie*, vol. 16, 430–1. In the period following di Sangro's death, some travellers were taken around the San Severo Palace by di Sangro's son Vincenzo. Björnståhl described him as 'a very polite man' who showcased all his father's experiences and inventions, but did not 'carry on his pursuits'; see Björnståhl, *Lettere ne' suoi viaggj*, vol. 2, 151.

[199] Sade, *Voyage d'Italie*, vol. 16, 429–30. See also Beinecke Rare Book & Manuscript Library, Yale University (New Haven), Osborn ms. c. 332, Phillip Hardwick, 3rd Earl of Yorke, 1778–9, 'January 13, 1779'.

[200] The National Archives (London), PRO 30/9/21, 'Italy, Journal', 1788, vol. 3, fol. 21r.

[201] James Edward Smith, *A Sketch of a Tour on the Continent, in the Years 1786 and 1787*, vol. 2 (London: printed for the author by J. Davis' sold by B. and J. White, 1793), 83.

fluid and mutually related, and coexisted and intersected in complex ways.[202] Although some eighteenth-century savants stigmatized it, secrecy continued to inform practices of knowledge production, transfer, and exchange.[203] Di Sangro's own pursuits were characterized by a taste for theatricality that addressed audiences and evoked some of the features that were associated with the early modern world of secrecy such as duplicity and dissimulation.[204] As Koen Vermeir has suggested, 'cunning use of the rhetoric of secrecy was a powerful means of building a reputation, by advertising that one has a secret as widely as possible and at the same time carefully controlling access to the content of the secret'.[205] The *Breve nota* offers an intriguing example of such dynamics: the final part of the booklet advertised di Sangro's findings on palingenesis, though it refrained from presenting them in detail. Rather, it announced that in order to be introduced to them one had to have familiarity (*confidenza*) with the prince. In the case of di Sangro, this strategy of concealment and revelation also became the object of scrutiny.

In the *Encyclopédie d' Yverdon*, Fortunato Bartolomeo De Felice presented his friend di Sangro as 'the oracle of nature and the art' and described his numerous inventions. De Felice also reported that for six years he had personally witnessed di Sangro's 'admirable discoveries' and had prayed him in vain to publish his findings. However, di Sangro had always refrained from doing so out of modesty, claiming that they were not worth the attention.[206] When Smith lamented that di Sangro had kept his methods secret, he was likely pointing to the Prince of San Severo's failure to publicize his findings in writing. While some of di Sangro's writings had generated controversy, engagement in the making and display of objects may have allowed him to convey meanings that could have otherwise been regarded as contentious. Yet, failure to comply with the codes of communication that had come to characterize academic protocol, such as publishing, ran the risk of jeopardizing his aspiration to consolidate his reputation as a savant.[207]

[202] On secrets in the early modern period, see William Eamon, *Science and the Secrets of Nature: Books of Secrets in Medieval and Early Modern Culture* (Princeton: Princeton University Press, 1994); Pamela O. Long, *Openness, Secrecy, Authorship: Technical Arts and the Culture of Knowledge from Antiquity to the Renaissance* (Baltimore: Johns Hopkins University Press, 2001); Alisha Rankin and Elaine Leong (eds.), *Secrets and Knowledge in Medicine and Science, 1500–1800* (Farnham: Ashgate, 2011); Koen Vermeir and Dániel Margócsy (eds.), 'States of Secrecy', special issue, *The British Journal for the History of Science*, 45:2 (2012); Bertucci, 'Enlightened Secrets'.

[203] See, for instance, Bertucci, 'Enlightened Secrets'.

[204] On theatricality and secrecy in the early modern period, see Koen Vermeir, 'Openness versus Secrecy? Historical and Historiographical Remarks', in Vermeir and Margócsy (eds.), 'States of Secrecy', 165–88. On the role of dissimulation as a template for early modern courtly virtues of civility, manners, and conversation, see Jon R. Snyder, *Dissimulation and the Culture of Secrecy in Early Modern Europe* (Berkeley: University of California Press, 2009). For an analysis of how theatrical and marvellous effects continued to raise concerns about duplicity and dissimulation into the eighteenth century, see, for instance, Simon Schaffer, 'Enlightened Automata', in William Clark, Jan Golinski, and Simon Schaffer (eds.), *The Sciences in Enlightened Europe* (Chicago: University of Chicago Press, 1999), 126–65.

[205] Vermeir, 'Openness versus Secrecy?', 180.

[206] De Felice, *Encyclopédie*, vol. 28, 482–5 (citation p. 484).

[207] On publishing as a way of securing early modern artificers' credibility and reputation, see Long, *Openness, Secrecy, Authorship*. On the relationship between publishing, secrecy, and reputation in the eighteenth century, see Bertucci, 'Enlightened Secrets'.

On the other hand, di Sangro's pursuit of recognition as a savant and a natural inquirer did not just end in grief. As De Felice engaged in rescuing his friend's memory, he presented di Sangro to the readers of his *Encyclopédie d'Yverdon* as not only a 'member of an academy' but 'an academy in his own right'.[208] Björnståhl similarly wrote that di Sangro made so many inventions that one would need a book to describe all of them.[209] Also, perhaps thanks to his capacity to weave a transnational network of savant friends and correspondents, di Sangro seemingly had a plant named after him posthumously, though this apparently happened by mistake. As is well known, the naming of plants inscribed politics of inclusion and exclusion and involved configurations of power and patronage as well as patterns of exchange and reciprocation.[210] The story has it that in 1788 the Neapolitan botanist Vincenzo Petagna sent a new plant to the Swedish naturalist Carl Peter Thunberg with a suggestion to name it 'Sanseverina' after Pietro Antonio Sanseverino, Count di Chiaromonte, a collector of rare plants of whom Petagna was a protégé. But Thunberg, who may have heard about di Sangro from the reports of Swedish travellers like Björnståhl, may have confused Sanseverino with the Prince of San Severo, and in 1794 he named the plant as Sansevieria.[211]

THE NATURAL AND THE ARTIFICIAL

The story of the anatomical machines may be similarly situated in the context of the theatrical convergence of duplication and duplicity, veiling and unveiling that, in the eyes of some viewers, characterized di Sangro's pursuits. It raises questions about anatomical models' capacity to conceal as well as to reveal, and their complicated place in the relationship between the power of spectacle and the role of objects in in mediating notions of authenticity and creating and conveying knowledge beyond words. It is worth recalling that while injecting techniques remained somewhat secretive, by the time di Sangro acquired Salerno's pricy skeletons, anatomical preparations made by injections had come to be regarded as the ultimate source of revelation of corporeal knowledge. By displaying the anatomical machines in his cabinet, and presenting them as made by injection, di Sangro may have hoped to transfer some of that truthfulness and authenticity to the rest of his collection and his own pursuits. Yet, a degree of ambiguity marked contemporaries' accounts of the nature and making of these specimens.

While the *Breve nota* presented these objects as the result of anatomical injections, others highlighted their artificial character as manufactured artefacts. The Neapolitan

[208] De Felice, *Encyclopédie*, vol. 28, 484. On De Felice's relationship with di Sangro's, see Donato, 'Esoteric Reason'.

[209] Björnståhl, *Lettere ne' suoi viaggj*, vol. 2, 149.

[210] See, for instance, Londa Shiebinger, 'Naming and Knowing: The Global Politics of Eighteenth-Century Botanical Nomenclatures', in Smith and Schmidt (eds.), *Making Knowledge in Early Modern Europe*, 90–105.

[211] Michele Tenore, *Catalogo delle piante che si coltivano nel R. Orto botanico di Napoli* (Naples: Tipografia dell'Aquila di V. Puzziello, 1845), 95. See also Acton, *The Bourbons of Naples*, 99; De Sangro, *Raimondo de Sangro*, 93–4.

protomedico Buoncuore, for instance, compared Salerno's skeleton to the king of Denmark's artificial skeleton, which displayed veins and arteries made in white iron.[212] In 1792, a new edition of the famous guide-book of the seventeenth-century lawyer and literato Carlo Celano, *Notizie del bello, dell'antico e del curioso della città di Napoli*, referred to the anatomical machines as both 'the skeletons of a woman and a man worked by injection' and as showing all the arteries and veins of the human body 'covered by a silver net'.[213] Likewise, in his *Vicende della coltura nelle Due Sicilie*, the writer Pietro Napoli Signorelli (1731–1815) mentioned that in the anatomical machines one could see 'all the veins and arteries made by injection artificiously placed'.[214] Early and mid-nineteenth-century Sicilian historians further described Salerno's skeleton as 'artificial', or 'manufactured with all the veins and arteries, and their intricacies, or ramifications', worked with so much mastery that it looked 'true and natural'.[215] Read against the *Breve nota*'s presentation of the anatomical machines as made by injections, such accounts complicate our historical understanding of these objects. They also invite us to ponder the significance of terms such as 'natural' and 'artificial' when they refer to eighteenth-century anatomical displays.

The interplay between art and nature was, of course, a feature of early modern cabinets of curiosities, where artificers and collectors delighted in the blending of naturalia and artificialia.[216] As historians have suggested, incidental to the development of distinct notions of order and patterns of classification was the emergence of a widening gap between nature and art.[217] However, in the case of anatomy, the blurring of art and nature continued to characterize collections and displays well into the eighteenth century. In 1777, on the occasion of the grand opening celebrating the Institute of the Sciences' acquisition of the anatomical collection of Anna Morandi, Luigi Galvani paraphrased a well-known theme: he referred to anatomical modelling by wondering 'whether this art owes more to nature, or nature to this art'.[218] By then, the issue of the relationship between art and nature had informed

[212] Buoncuore, 'Lettera di Francesco Buoncuore', 127.

[213] Carlo Celano, *Delle notizie del Bello, dell'Antico, e del Curioso della città di Napoli*, 4th edn., vol. 3 (Naples: a spese di Salvatore Palermo, 1792), 90.

[214] Pietro Napoli Signorelli, *Vicende della coltura nelle Due Sicilie: Dalla venuta delle Colonie straniere sino a' nostri giorni*, 2nd edn., vol. 7 (Naples: n.p., 1811), 18. Here Napoli Signorelli presented Salerno as one of the famous Sicilian wax modellers.

[215] Andrea Barbacci, *Prospetto della storia dell'Accademia Jatro-fisica di Palermo, ora detta delle scienze mediche, col primo rapporto dei travagli da giugno 1831 a dicembre 1832* (Palermo: Salvatore Barcellona, 1833), 15; Scinà, *Prospetto della storia letteraria di Sicilia*, vol. 1, 276. On the manufacturing of the anatomical machines, see also Lucia Dacome and Renata Peters, 'Fabricating the Body: The Anatomical Machines of the Prince of Sansevero', in Virginia Greene et al., *Objects Specialty Group: Proceedings of the Objects Specialty Group Session, 35th Annual Meeting of the American Institute of Conservation* (Washington: American Institute for Conservation of Historic & Artistic Works, 2008), 161–77.

[216] See, for instance, Daston and Park, *Wonders and the Order of Nature*; Smith and Findlen (eds.), *Merchants and Marvels*; Claudia Swan, *Art, Science, and Witchcraft in Early Modern Holland: Jacques de Gheyn II (1565–1629)* (Cambridge: Cambridge University Press, 2005), 93–4; Goldgar, *Tulipmania*, 123.

[217] See, for instance, Daston and Park, *Wonders and the Order of Nature*, esp. chapter 7.

[218] Galvani, *De Manzoliniana supellectili*, 49.

well-established motifs and tropes, and redesigned views of art and nature alongside their shifting boundaries. Eighteenth-century anatomical cabinets continued to display many such instances of the blurring of art and nature. On the one hand, anatomical models included parts of the natural body that were not subject to rapid decay such as bones, teeth, and hair as well as materials such as wax and clay. On the other hand, anatomical preparations employed 'artificial' materials in order to visualize and preserve the inner body. Moreover, anatomical models could themselves be portrayals of anatomical preparations made by injection.

In the late eighteenth century, William Hunter's enthusiasm for injections as the ultimate medium of anatomical truth, and his dismissal of waxworks on account of their inaccuracy, pointed to the creation of new boundaries between artificial and natural anatomy.[219] However, the very emergence of such boundaries was affected by circumstances related to place.[220] We may wonder whether in Naples such distinctions mattered. At a time in which marvel continued to be a trademark of a colonial capital like Naples, the boundaries between the artificial and the natural may have not been as sharp there as they appeared in London. Indeed, while being presented as the result of anatomical injections, the anatomical machines participated in the grand stage of Neapolitan wonder that thrived on material transformation and continued to blend natural and artificial domains. Acting as both Grand Tour attractions and precious anatomical specimens that unveiled nature, they lured viewers and promised to act as testimonials of the reliability of di Sangro's engagements and the authenticity of the curiosities displayed in the San Severo Palace. Yet, as di Sangro receded from his role as a mediator of their meanings and his claims became the object of scrutiny, ultimately even the anatomical machines fell short of their promise to act as vehicles of credit. In the end, di Sangro's reputation as a savant remained volatile; and while some took him to be a philosopher, others regarded him as a juggler.

[219] Hunter, *Two Introductory Lectures*, 56.

[220] On eighteenth-century varying geographies of wonder, see James Delbourgo, *A Most Amazing Scene of Wonders: Electricity and Enlightenment in Early America* (Cambridge, MA: Harvard University Press, 2006). See also Bertucci, 'The Architecture of Knowledge'.

Epilogue
Becoming Obsolete

Giuseppe Salerno never made it to Bologna. Having gained a lifetime pension, he travelled back home, ready to make the most out of the fame and fortune he had found in Naples.[1] This turned out to be a wise plan. Back in Palermo, Salerno made three new anatomical skeletons, two females and a male, which were even 'more complete and perfect that the first ones'.[2] He then demonstrated them in the Grand Hall of the Palermitan Senate, and promised that two of them, a female and the male, would not leave the city.[3] Just like the anatomical machines displayed in Naples, the new anatomical specimens Salerno made in Palermo became tourist attractions and appealed to a wide audience. In 1777, when the French naturalist Charles-Nicolas-Sigisbert Sonnini de Manoncourt stopped in Palermo on his way back from Egypt, he 'noticed an anatomical injection of a man and another of a woman, remarkably well executed by a Sicilian physician, who was still alive'.[4] Some five years later, the Moroccan ambassador Mohamed Ibn Uthmân Al-Meknassî visited Palermo and was stunned by the 'absolute wonder' of 'a human being, as if weaved in a net of veins': 'a man and woman', with their flesh 'removed from their bones' and their veins 'restored as they once were'.[5]

When, on 19 December 1789, Sálerno organized a new spectacular 'angiological' demonstration of his skeletons at the Palermitan Senate, the event seemed to mark the high point of a successful career. A large crowd, including the 'Viceroy, almost all nobility, and the best literati' gathered alongside the professors of medicine to attend

[1] Buoncuore, 'Lettera di Francesco Buoncuore', 127.

[2] 'Lo stampatore a chi legge', in *Opuscoli di autori siciliani*, vol. 7, xv–xvi.

[3] Ibid. See also Giovanni Gorgone, *Notizie sulle statue angiografiche e la vita di Giuseppe Salerno* (Palermo: Presso gli eredi Graffeo, 1830), 9; BCP, ms. Qq D 109, Francesco Maria Emanuele Gaetani (Marchese di Villabianca), 'Diario Palermitano', vol. 17, 530–2.

[4] Charles Sigisbert Sonnini, *Travels in Upper and Lower Egypt undertaken by Order of the Old Government of France*, trans. Henry Hunter, vol. 1 (London: J. Debrett, 1800), 29.

[5] Al-Meknassî was sent by Sidi Mohammed Ben Abdallah, the Sultan of Morocco, on a diplomatic mission to Malta, Naples, and Sicily. He concluded his report of the anatomical skeletons with a comment based on the Quran: '"Such is the creation of God: Now show me what is there that others besides Him have created". And the Almighty said: "As also in your own selves: will you not then see?"', Mohammed Ibn Uthmân Al-Meknassî, *Al-bâdr Assâfir lî hîdayat al-mûsafir li fikak al-asâra min yadî al-adoui al-kâfir*, ed. Malika Ezzahidi (Mohammedia: Publications de la Faculté des Lettres et des Sciences Humaines, 2005), 638–9. I am grateful to Malika Ezzahidi for drawing my attention to these passages of Al-Meknassî's text and to Muna Salloum for translating them.

the event.[6] Everything was organized with the greatest care and nothing was left to chance. As the surviving chart of the seating plan shows, even the seating arrangement was thought out down to the smallest detail (Plate 54). A Senate delegation was to welcome the viceroy and accompany him to his seat, a damask-fitted chair in front of the stage where the demonstration would take place. The nobility, the ministers, the literati, and the professors of medicine would then take their places around him, according to their rank.[7] And yet, despite all of this careful planning and staging, things did not unfold in quite the way that Salerno might have wished. Critics apparently mocked the show as a déjà vu, an outdated repetition of the past, evoking the demonstrations that Graffeo and Salerno himself had done some thirty years earlier.[8]

By then, other collections had started to gain prominence. Notably, the anatomical collection of the Royal Museum of Physics and Natural History in Florence had begun to compete with the displays of Bologna, Naples, and Palermo, introducing new approaches to anatomical modelling. As we have seen, in Bologna and Naples artificers maintained control over all of the phases of the production and display of their anatomical models, namely from the dissection of cadavers and the actual modelling, to the dramatic performances in which they showcased their creations.[9] Conversely, the Florentine collection was characterized by reliance on 'the division of labour between those who dissected the cadavers, those who made the waxworks and those who showed them to the public'.[10] Moreover, the process of model production relied on the systematic use of casting, a technique that throughout the early modern period had been regarded as a privileged medium for producing authentic representations of nature.[11] Division of labour and regular use of casting techniques also allowed the Florentine workshop to engage in a conspicuous production of copies.[12] Over a few decades, copies of the Florentine models started to appear in different cities, including Cagliari, Montpellier, Pavia, and Vienna. By contrast, in Bologna and Naples trustees and collectors remained concerned with safeguarding the 'uniqueness' of their models, and accordingly limited the number of copies made.[13] 'Uniqueness' was taken to accrue the models'

[6] The event was reported in local chronicles and the Marquis of Villabianca dedicated to it an entry of his *Diario Palermitano*; see BCP, ms. Qq D 108, Francesco Maria Emanuele Gaetani (Marchese di Villabianca), 'Diario Palermitano', vol. 16, 248.

[7] Archivio Storico del Comune di Palermo, Cerimoniali (1789), vol. 38, 12 December 1789, 505–16; BCP, ms. Qq D 108, Francesco Maria Emanuele Gaetani (Marchese di Villabianca), 'Diario Palermitano', vol. 16, 248.

[8] Giuseppe Pitré, *La vita in Palermo cento e più anni fa*, vol. 2 (Palermo: Alberto Reber, 1905), 392.

[9] Dacome, 'Waxworks'.

[10] Ibid., 34. On the models' production in the Florentine workshop, see Mazzolini, 'Plastic Anatomies and Artificial Dissections'; Maerker, *Model Experts*. It seems that Morandi may have made use of casting techniques. However, I could not find evidence that such techniques were employed in Bologna in as systematic and comprehensive a fashion as in Florence. On the suggestion that Morandi may have used casting techniques, see Armaroli (ed.), *Le cere anatomiche bolognesi*, 59; Focaccia, 'Anna Morandi Manzolini', 71 and 54 n. 196.

[11] Pamela H. Smith and Tonny Beentjes, 'Nature and Art, Making and Knowing: Reconstructing Sixteenth-Century Life-Casting Techniques', *Renaissance Quarterly*, 63:1 (2010), 128–79.

[12] See for instance; Maerker, *Model Experts*.

[13] When, in 1765, Galli offered advice to the Milanese Hospital Maggiore about the possibility of creating a collection like his own, he warned his correspondents that in Bologna the *Assunti* of the

value and was closely related to specific views about artificers' special skills, craft, and expertise, and the models' own role as special tools of knowledge.[14] However, as the models of the Florentine workshop started to circulate across Europe, emphasis on 'uniqueness' ran the risk of becoming a drawback. For one thing, what made the models 'unique' also caused them to be very expensive and time consuming, making it difficult for the modellers to keep up with growing demand. For another, emphasis on uniqueness exposed the highly crafted nature of the models, and could raise doubts about their capacity to imitate nature.

In his celebratory speech on Morandi's collection, Luigi Galvani argued that her models would never become obsolete because they perfectly imitated nature. As a consequence, they could not become outdated because nature 'is always one, and remains the same and identical'.[15] Galvani reckoned that other artificers could perhaps make more elegant, beautiful, and pleasant models, but surely they could not create more truthful ones. As we have seen, in Galvani's view anatomical models were to be preferred over anatomical preparations on account of their material properties—such as solidity, malleability, and reliable colouring—which enabled them to better express crucial anatomical features such as shape, position, direction, and development.[16] In fact, according to Galvani, such features allowed the models to be even truer than the natural body itself. In the following years, however, opinions as to whether anatomical waxworks had the capacity to perfectly imitate nature, and to do so in an everlasting way, became a matter of debate.

The British anatomist and man-midwife William Hunter was willing to acknowledge the value of casting, and he reckoned that 'the wax-work art of the moderns might deserve notice in any history of Anatomy'.[17] However, he dismissed many of the waxworks made by his contemporaries on the grounds that their makers had been 'so careless in their imitation', and in fact, their wax models looked 'tawdry',

Institute of the Sciences had forbidden the use of the existing models for making copies. In 1776, when the Institute's *Assunti* heard of a new collection of midwifery models being made in the home of Dr. Mondini for the neighbouring city of Modena, they wondered whether this could be detrimental to the Institute's own midwifery collection. Moreover, as we saw in Chapter 6, when the Polish Princess Anna Sapieha Jablonowska contacted Girolamo Ranuzzi to inquire about the possibility of finalizing the copy of the senses that she had commissioned from Morandi, Ranuzzi was reluctant to oblige her on the ground that this may lessen their value 'as unique things in Europe'. In Naples, Salerno's anatomical machines were equally presented as 'unique things in Europe'; see ASM, Luoghi pii, p.a., Cartella 382, '1765. Osservazioni per le scuole di Chirurgia ed Ostetricia nell'Ospital Maggiore di Milano', 'Informazione del Dottore Galli di Bologna'; ASB, Assunteria d'Istituto, Atti 7 (1776–9), fols. 27r and 28r–v; ASB, Archivio Ranuzzi, Carte di Famiglia, Lettere di Casa, 1770, Letter of June 20, 1770; ASB, Archivio Ranuzzi, Scritture diverse spettanti alla Nobil Casa Ranuzzi, Lib. 125, 1774–8, 'Pro-memoria al Monsig. Illmo e Rmo Ranuzzi' and 'Risposta alla pro-memoria indirizzata a Mon. Ranuzzi, da Monsig. Lascaris'; *Breve nota*, 20.

[14] To be sure, some of the models displayed in Bologna and Naples ended up being copied and duplicated: Lelli made copies of his anatomical statuette, Morandi created a number of copies of some of her models such as the series of the senses, and Salerno duplicated his anatomical specimens for the city of Palermo. Yet, in these cases the making of copies apparently happened to be on a relatively small scale, and in many ways these artefacts remained 'unique' in the sense that they were carefully manufactured, they involved a high level of skill, they were limited in number, and they remained closely linked with the names of their makers.

[15] Galvani, *De Manzoliniana supellectili*, 55–6.

[16] Ibid., 48–50.

[17] Hunter, *Two Introductory Lectures*, 56.

had 'unnatural colours', and were incorrect with regard to 'the circumstances of figure, situation and the like': in short, 'though they strike a vulgar eye with admiration, they must appear ridiculous to an Anatomist'.[18] Having embarked on a Grand Tour along with the eighth Duke of Hamilton, the Scottish physician John Moore, who had attended William Hunter's lectures in London, further downplayed the anatomical value of the Bolognese wax models. In his *View of Society and Manners in Italy* (1781), Moore remarked that the Bolognese 'waxen models could not stand in comparison with the preparations of the real parts in Dr. Hunter's museum'. Rather,

> if brought to that test, the Bologna waxworks, though admirable in their kind, would appear as their best casts of the Vatican Apollo and Laocoön would, if placed beside the originals. Indeed, the real preparations to be seen here, are far inferior to those of that great anatomist; who is now possessed of the most complete, and most accurate collection of anatomical preparations, that ever was made by human skill and industry.[19]

Moore's comment may have been partly motivated by his loyalty to his teacher and fellow citizen. Still, it was a far cry from Galvani's comments on Morandi's models' capacity to perfectly imitate nature—and to do so even more truthfully than the natural body itself—and his conviction that, as a consequence, they would defy time.

In the same period, other travellers engaged in endless comparisons and rankings of anatomical collections: the Florentine versus the Bolognese; the Bolognese versus the Parisian, the Florentine, and the Neapolitan; the models of Marie Marguerite Bihéron in Paris versus the models of Anna Morandi in Bologna and those of Dr Showell in Philadelphia; the Florentine models versus all the rest; etc.[20] In doing so, they raised doubts as to the capacity of some collections to account for the truth of the body and hinted that some might have already become obsolete.[21] When, in 1793, René-Nicolas Desgenettes enjoyed the privilege of a private visit to the Florentine museum, he wholeheartedly supported the initiative of having a copy of the collection made for France, and concluded that the collection in Florence was 'infinitely superior, in every respect, to any other collection scattered around Europe'.[22] Along with copies of the models, the skills developed by Florentine

[18] Ibid.

[19] John Moore, *A View of Society and Manners in Italy*, vol. 1 (London: W. Strahan and T. Cadell, 1781), 304–5.

[20] On the travellers' comparison among the various anatomical collections, see, for instance, Ferber, *Travels through Italy*, 74; Björnståhl, *Lettere ne' suoi viaggj [...]*, vol. 3, 147; François Jean de Beauvoir, marquis de Chastellux, *Voyages de M. le marquis de Chastellux dans l'Amérique Septentrionale, dans les années 1780, 1781 et 1782*, 2nd edn., vol. 1 (Paris: Prault, 1788), 196; Adam Walker, *Ideas, Suggested on the Spot in a Late Excursion through Flanders, Germany, France, and Italy* (London: J. Robson et al., 1790), 349–50; Thomas Charles Morgan, 'Appendix: On the State of Medicine in Italy, with Brief Notices of Some of the Universities and Hospitals', in Lady Morgan [Sydney Owenson], *Italy*, vol. 1, 327.

[21] By the turn of the nineteenth century, Galli's midwifery collection had also started to be considered obsolete, and in 1801 the surgeon Tarsizio Riviera proposed to recreate the collection; see Bortolotti, 'Il maestro alla lavagna', 19.

[22] Desgenettes, 'Réflexions générales', esp. 233–52. As Maerker has suggested, Desgenettes may have written his report in consultation with the museum's director Felice Fontana; see Maerker, *Model Experts*, 128–9. The habit of making copies may also have been handy in situations in which the original collection was at risk, like during the period in which Napoleonic troops were present in

artificers also started to travel and transfer styles and techniques around the Italian peninsula and beyond.[23] Notably, the family of Giuseppe Ferrini—the first modeller of the Florentine anatomical workshop—set off to follow prestigious and lucrative commissions. Gennaro Ferrini, the son of Giuseppe, ended up making anatomical models in Paris and in Naples, and in 1788 Gaetano Ferrini, Giuseppe's brother, travelled from Milan to Palermo where local authorities entrusted him with the task of creating an 'anatomical theatre in wax'.[24] At the end of August 1792, Gaetano was again commissioned twenty-four midwifery models (*fantocci*) in Palermo.[25]

It would be hard to judge whether it was by mere coincidence that about a month later, on 25 September 1792, Giuseppe Salerno took his life by leaping from the balcony of his home in the centre of Palermo. To some, the tragedy came as no surprise, since it followed a period in which Salerno had developed a 'strong hypochondria that had turned into a perfect mania'.[26] Still, taking place about three years after Salerno's grand anatomical demonstration at the Palermitan Senate, which had apparently generated mixed responses, Salerno's suicide seemed to point to the end of an era. In the following years, the spaces and publics of anatomical displays started to change. In 1796, the Palermitan local authorities decided to restrict access to the 'anatomical theatre in wax' and to limit attendance to medical students and their instructors, forbidding the presence of both those 'teachers from other schools' who occasionally attended out of 'caprice' and lay people who participated in demonstrations just out of 'mere curiosity'.[27] This kind of rulings marked the end of an age in which artificers had occupied the centre stage of a new space of anatomical encounter, a venue of viewing and learning where anatomical specimens' beauty and capacity to embody knowledge and defy decay had been core features of their success. As a characteristic mark of this era, different audiences had been encouraged to acquire knowledge about their bodies

the Italian peninsula and sent many precious objects as booty to France. One may wonder whether this may have been the background for the note signed 'Bonaparte' reporting about the proposal to make a copy of the Florentine anatomical collection for France, which is included in a folder of documents related to the shipment of confiscated 'objects of art and science' from Italy to France during the Napoleonic period; see Archives Nationales, Paris, F/17/1279. It is worth noting that when the Florentine models were duplicated and started to circulate, they sometimes generated mixed reactions. As Anna Maerker has shown, when copies of the Florentine anatomical models were presented at the Josephinum in Vienna, they left some wondering about the value of objects that looked to them more like toys than tools of knowledge; see Maerker, *Model Experts*, chapter 5. On the circulation of copies of the famous Florentine Venus, see De Ceglia, 'The Importance of Being Florentine'.

[23] On the transformation of the adjective 'Florentine' into a brand of anatomical modelling, see De Ceglia, 'The Importance of Being Florentine'.

[24] Soprintendenza Archivistica della Sicilia-Archivio di Stato di Palermo (henceforth SAAS-SIPA), Commissione di pubblica istruzione ed educazione, vol. 3, fol. 75r (28 August 1788). See also *Effemeridi scientifiche e letterarie per la Sicilia*, 65 (1839), 80–1; *Archivio storico siciliano*, 2 (1874), 223 n. 2.

[25] SAAS-SIPA, Commissione di pubblica istruzione ed educazione, vol. 7, fols. 87v–89v (31 August 1792). On Gaetano Ferrini, *Enciclopedia metodica critico-ragionata delle belle arti* (Parma, Tipografia Ducale, 1821), part I, vol. 8, 258.

[26] BCP, ms. Qq D 109, Francesco Maria Emanuele Gaetani (Marchese di Villabianca), 'Diario Palermitano', vol. 17, 529.

[27] SAAS-SIPA, Commissione di pubblica istruzione ed educazione, filza 480 (1778–1804), fols. 57r–59v (citation fol. 58v). In Bologna, during the Napoleonic period, the Institute of the Sciences was abolished and its anatomical collections were relocated; see Focaccia, 'Anna Morandi Manzolini', 23.

by attending modellers' anatomical demonstrations and, while doing so, had ensured the modellers' celebrity and success. The Palermitan ruling sheds light on a shift in attitude towards anatomical modelling. Drawing attention to the changing relationship between models, modellers, and their audiences, it highlights the transient nature of models' meanings.

Galvani's speech on Morandi highlighted that an important aspect of the lure of anatomical models lay in their capacity to defy time in the sense that they both resisted physical decay and promised to provide lasting and timeless sources of corporeal knowledge. Galvani maintained that thanks to their capacity to express natural features with absolute precision, and to do so in an imperishable way, Morandi's anatomical models would never become outdated.[28] However, in the end his prediction turned out to be overly optimistic. Later collections would hardly match the beauty and elegance of Morandi's models. Yet, as mid-eighteenth-century anatomical displays started to withdraw from the public eye, and new ideas of accuracy and authenticity began to emerge, they fell short of the promise that they would never become obsolete.

[28] Galvani, *De Manzoliniana supellectili.*

Select Bibliography

PRIMARY SOURCES

Manuscript Sources: Archives and Libraries

Académie Nationale de Médecine, Paris
Accademia della Crusca, Florence
Archives du Palais Princier, Principality of Monaco
Archives Nationales, Paris
Archivio Arcivescovile di Bologna
Archivio dell'Accademia di Belle Arti di Bologna
Archivio di Stato di Bologna
Archivio di Stato di Firenze
Archivio di Stato di Milano
Archivio di Stato di Napoli
Archivio di Stato di Torino
Archivio Segreto Vaticano, Rome
Archivio Storico del Banco di Napoli
Archivio Storico del Comune di Palermo
Archivio Storico dell'Università di Torino
Archivio Storico del Monte del Matrimonio, Bologna
Beinecke Rare Book & Manuscript Library, Yale University, New Haven
Biblioteca Ambrosiana, Milan
Biblioteca Apostolica Vaticana, Rome
Biblioteca Civica Gambalunga, Rimini
Biblioteca Comunale 'Aurelio Saffi', Forlì
Biblioteca Comunale dell'Archiginnasio di Bologna
Biblioteca Comunale di Palermo
Biblioteca della Società Napoletana di Storia Patria, Naples
Biblioteca di Archeologia e Storia dell'Arte, Rome
Biblioteca Reale, Turin
Biblioteca Universitaria di Bologna
Bibliothèque Nationale de France, Site Richelieu-Louvois, Paris
Bodleian Library, Oxford
British Library, London
Getty Research Institute, Los Angeles
Soprintendenza Archivistica della Sicilia—Archivio di Stato di Palermo
The National Archives, London
The National Library of Malta, Valletta
The Wellcome Library, London

Printed Primary Sources

Al-Meknassî, Mohammed Ibn Uthmân, *Al-bâdr Assâfîr lî hîdayat al-mûsafîr li fîkak al-asâra min yadî al-adoui al-kâfîr*, ed. Malika Ezzahidi (Mohammedia: Publications de la Faculté des Lettres et des Sciences Humaines, 2005).

Algarotti, Francesco, *Il newtonianismo per le dame, ovvero, Dialoghi sopra la luce e i colori* (Naples [Milan]: n.p., 1737).

Algarotti, Francesco, *Saggio sopra la pittura*, 2nd edn. (Livorno: Marco Coltellini, 1763).

Algarotti, Francesco, *Opere del conte Algarotti*, vol. 10 (Venice: Carlo Palese, 1794).

Andrés, Juan, *Cartas familiares del Abate D. Juan Andrés s a su hermano D. Carlos Andrés* (Madrid: Don Antonio de Sancha, 1786).

Angelelli, Giuseppe, *Notizie dell'origine, e progressi dell'Instituto delle Scienze di Bologna e sue accademie* (Bologna: Instituto delle Scienze, Bologna, 1780).

Annonces, affiches, et avis divers, 6, 20 Janvier 1755, 42–6.

Archenholz, Johann Wilhelm von, *A Picture of Italy*, trans. J. Trapp (London: G.G.J. and J. Robinson, 1791).

Azzoguidi, Germano, *Observationes ad uteri constructionem pertinentes* (Bologna: Longhi, 1773).

[Azzoguidi, Germano], *Lettres de Madame Cunégonde écrites de B [...] à Madame Paquette à F*, in Paul Mengal (ed.), *Giacomo Casanova: Lana Caprina; Une controverse médicale sur l'utérus pensant à l'Université de Bologne en 1771–1772*, trans. Roberto Poma (Paris: Honoré Champion, 1999).

Barbacci, Andrea, *Prospetto della storia dell'Accademia Jatro-Fisica di Palermo, ora detta delle scienze mediche, col primo rapporto dei travagli da giugno 1831 a dicembre 1832* (Palermo: Salvatore Barcellona, 1833).

Baretti, Giuseppe Marco Antonio, *An Account of the Manners and Customs of Italy: With Observations on the Mistakes of Some Travellers, with Regard to That Country* (London: T. Davies, L. Davis, and C. Rymers, 1768).

Barry, James, *A Letter to the Dilettanti Society: Respecting the Obtention of Certain Matters Essentially Necessary for the Improvement of Public Taste, and for Accomplishing the Original Views of the Royal Academy of Great Britain*, 2nd edn. (London: J. Walker, 1799).

Baudeau, Nicolas, *Analyse de l'ouvrage du Pape Benoit XIV, sur les béatifications et canonisations: Approuvée par lui-même, et dédié au Roi* (Paris: Hardy, 1759).

Beauvoir, François Jean de, marquis de Chastellux, *Voyages de M. le marquis de Chastellux dans l'Amérique Septentrionale, dans les années 1780, 1781 et 1782* (Paris: Prault, 1788).

Bellini, Lorenzo, *Discorsi di Anatomia*, 2 vols. (Florence: Francesco Moüke, 1741–4).

Bernoulli, Jean, *Zusätze zu den neuesten Reisebeschreibungen von Italien*, vol. 1 (Leipzig: Caspar Fritsch, 1777).

Bianchi, Giovanni, 'Lettera del Signor Dottor Giovanni Bianchi di Rimino scritta da Bologna ad un suo amico di Firenze', *Novelle letterarie, pubblicate in Firenze*, 15 (1754), 707–11.

Bianchini, Francesco, *La istoria universale provata con monumenti, e figurata con simboli degli Antichi* (Rome: Antonio de' Rossi, 1697).

Bianconi, Giovanni Lodovico, *Lettere del consigliere Gian Lodovico Bianconi* [...] *sopra il libro del Canonico Luigi Crespi, Bolognese, intitolato Felsina pittrice* (Milan: Tipografia de' Classici italiani, 1802).

Björnståhl, Jacob Jonas, *Lettere ne' suoi viaggj stranieri di Giacomo Giona Bjoernstaehl, professore di Filosofia in Upsala, scritte al Signor Gjörwell, bibliotecario regio in Istocolma, tradotte dallo svezzese in tedesco da Giusto Ernesto Groskurd e dal tedesco in italiano recate da Baldassar Domenico Zini di Val di Non*, trans. Baldassar Domenico Zini (Poschiavo: Giuseppe Ambrosioni, 1782–7).

Blainville, [Henry] de, *Travels through Holland, Germany, Switzerland, and Other Parts of Europe, but Especially Italy*, trans. William Guthrie, vol. 2 (London: printed by W. Strahan for the Proprietor, 1743).

Bolletti, Giuseppe Gaetano, *Dell'origine e de' progressi dell'Istituto delle Scienze di Bologna* (Bologna: Lelio dalla Volpe, 1751).

Bottari, Giovanni Gaetano, *Sculture e pitture sagre estratte dai cimiteri di Roma pubblicate già dagli autori della Roma sotterranea e ora nuovamente date in luce colle spiegazioni*, vol. 3 (Rome: Niccolò e Marco Pagliarini, 1754).

Bottari, Giovanni Gaetano and Stefano Ticozzi, *Raccolta di lettere sulla pittura, scultura ed architettura scritte da' più celebri personaggi dei secoli XV, XVI, e XVII*, vol. 2 (Milan: Giovanni Silvestri, 1822).

Bouchard, Jean-Jacques, *Journal II: Voyage dans le Royaume de Naples; Voyage dans la campagne de Rome*, ed. Emanuele Kanceff (Turin: G. Giappichelli, 1976).

Boyle, John, Earl of Corke and Orrery, *Letters from Italy in the Years 1754 and 1755* (London: B. White, 1773).

Breve nota di quel che si vede in casa del Principe di Sansevero D. Raimondo di Sangro nella città di Napoli ([Naples]: n.p., 1766).

Buffon, Georges-Louis Leclerc and Louis-Jean-Marie Daubenton, *Histoire naturelle, générale et particulière, avec la description du cabinet du roi*, vol. 3 (Paris: Imprimerie Royale, 1749).

Buoncuore, Francesco, 'Lettera di Francesco Buoncuore medico del nostro re Carlo Borbone indirizzata a S. E. sig. marchese Fogliani vicerè, e capitan generale di Sicilia', in Francisco Maria Vesco, *De eloquentia apud siculos, orta, aucta, et absoluta [...]* (Palermo: Solli, 1797), 125–8.

Caraccioli, Louis-Antoine, *Éloge historique de Benoît XIV* (Liège: J. Fr. Bassompière, 1766).

Caraccioli, Louis-Antoine, *The Life of Pope Clement XIV (Ganganelli). Translated from the French* (London: J. Johnson and J.P. Coghlan, 1776).

Caraccioli, Louis-Antoine, *La vie du pape Benoît XIV, Prosper Lambertini* (Paris: Rue et Hôtel Serpente, 1783).

Catherine II, 'Lettres de l'impératrice Catherine II à Grimm (1774–1796), publiées avec les notes explicatives de Grote', in *Recueil de la Société Impériale russe d'histoire*, vol. 2 (St Petersburg: n.p., 1878).

Celano, Carlo, *Delle notizie del bello, dell'antico, e del curioso della città di Napoli*, 4th edn., vol. 3 (Naples: a spese di Salvatore Palermo, 1792).

Cocchi, Antonio, *Dell'anatomia* (Florence: Gio. Batista Zannoni, 1745).

Cochin, Charles-Nicolas, *Voyage d'Italie, ou recueil de notes sur les ouvrages de peinture et de sculpture, qu'on voit dans les principales villes d'Italie*, vol. 2 (Paris: Ch. Ant Jombert, 1758).

Cotugno, Domenico, 'Iter Italicum Patavinum', in Felice Lombardi (ed.), *Le scoperte anatomiche di Domenico Cotugno e il suo 'Iter Italicum Patavinum'* (Naples: R. Licenziato, 1964).

Crespi, Luigi, *Felsina pittrice: Vite de' pittori bolognesi*, vol. 3 (Rome: Marco Pagliarini, 1769).

Crimaldi, Bruno (ed.), *Chartulae desangriane: Il principe committente* (Naples: Alòs, 2006).

D'Audierne, Joseph, *Lettres curieuses, utiles et théologiques sur la béatification des serviteurs de Dieu et la canonisation des beatifies, ou, Abrégé du grand Ouvrage du Cardinal Prosper Lambertini, Pape, sous le nom de Benoist XIV, sur la même matière* (Rennes: J. Vatar, 1758–64).

De Brosses, Charles, *Le président de Brosses en Italie: Lettres familières écrites d'Italie en 1739 et 1740*, 12th edn., vol. 1 (Paris: Didier et Cie., 1858).

De Felice, Fortunato Bartolomeo, *Encyclopédie, ou dictionnaire universel raisonné des connoissances humaines*, 58 vols. (Yverdon: n.p., 1770–80).

De Gregorio e Russo, Giuseppe, 'Ad Augustinum Giuffrida Ex Archiatris Catanensibus, Epistola, De notatu dignis Regalis Panh. Medicorum Academiae', in *Opuscoli di autori siciliani*, vol. 7 (Palermo: Stamperia de' Ss. Apostoli in Piazza Vigliena per Pietro Bentivegna, 1762), 237–50.

De La Porte, Joseph, *Le voyageur françois, ou la connoissance de l'ancien et du nouveau monde mis au jour par l'Abbé Delaporte*, vol. 26 (Paris: L. Cellot, 1779).

De Rinaldis, Rinaldo, *Memorie del viaggio in Italia (1779–1780)*, ed. Pier Giorgio Sclippa (Pordenone: Accademia di San Marco, 2000).

De Tipaldo, Emilio (ed.), *Biografia degli italiani illustri nelle scienze, lettere ed arti del secolo XVIII, e de' contemporanei, compilata da letterati italiani di ogni provincia*, vol. 8 (Venice: Alvisopoli, 1841).

De' Vegni, Leonardo, 'Lettera preliminare in cui alquanto discorresi del celebre Ercole Lelli al Ch. Sig. Cav. Onofrio Boni', in *Memorie per le belle arti*, vol. 4 (Rome: Pagliarini, 1788), iii–xx.

Del Pozzo, Luigi, *Cronaca civile e militare delle Due Sicilie sotto la dinastia Borbonica dall'anno 1734 in poi* (Naples: Stamperia Reale, 1857).

Denon, Vivant, *Viaggio nel Regno di Napoli, 1777–1778*, trans. Teresa Leone (Naples: Paparo, 2001).

Desgenettes, René-Nicolas, 'Réflexions générales sur l'utilité de l'anatomie artificielle; et en particulier sur la collection de Florence, et la nécessité d'en former de semblables en France', *Journal de médecine, chirurgie et pharmacie*, 94 (1793), 162–76 and 233–52.

Desnoües, Guillaume, *Lettres de G. Desnoües, Professeur d'Anatomie, & de Chirurgie, de l'Académie de Bologne; et de Mr Guglielmini, Professeur de Medecine & de Mathematiques à Padoüe, de L'Académie Royale des Sciences, et d'autres Sâvans sur differentes nouvelles découvertes* (Rome: Antoine Rossi, 1706).

Di Sangro, Raimondo, *Lettere del signore D. Raimondo di Sangro Principe di Sansevero di Napoli sopra alcune scoperte chimiche indirizzate al signor cavaliere Giovanni Giraldi fiorentino e riportate ancora nelle Novelle letterarie di Firenze del 1753* (Naples: n.p., after 1753).

Di Sangro, Raimondo, *Lettres écrites par Monsieur le Prince de S. Sevère de Naples à Mons.r l'Abbé Nollet de l'Académie des Sciences à Paris, contenant la rélation d'une découverte, qu'il a faite par le moyen de quelques expériences chimiques & l'explication physique de ses circonstances* (Naples: Joseph Raimondi, 1753).

Di Sangro, Raimondo, *Dissertation sur une lampe antique trouvée à Munich en l'année 1753, écrite par M. le Prince de St-Sévère, pour servir de suite à la première partie de ses lettres à M. l'Abbé Nollet, à Paris, sur une découverte qu'il a faite dans la Chimie* (Naples: Morelli, 1756).

Di Sangro, Raimondo, *Supplica a Benedetto XIV*, ed. Leen Spruit (Naples: Alòs, 2006 [1753]).

Di Sangro, Raimondo, *Lettera apologetica dell'Esercitato accademico della Crusca contenente la difesa del libro intitolato Lettere d' una Peruana per rispetto alla supposizione de' Quipu scritta dalla duchessa di S**** e dalla medesima fatta pubblicare*, ed. Leen Spruit (Naples: Alòs, 2010 [1750]).

Diario bolognese, ecclesiastico e civile (Bologna: Lelio dalla Volpe, 1759–1800).

'Discours prononcé à la réception de plusieurs Apprentifs, à la loge du Prince de S.S. à Naples, en 1745', in [Théodore Henri de Tschudy], *L'étoile flamboyante, ou la société des Francs-Maçons, considérée sous tous les aspects*, vol. 2 (Paris: À L'orient chez Le Silence, 1780), 31–4.

Fantuzzi, Giovanni, *Notizie degli scrittori bolognesi raccolte da Giovanni Fantuzzi*, 9 vols. (Bologna: San Tommaso d'Aquino, 1781–94).

Ferber, Johan Jakob, *Travels through Italy, in the Years 1771 and 1772*, trans. R.E. Raspe (London: L. Davis, 1776).

[Fontana, Felice], *Saggio del Real Gabinetto di Fisica e di Storia naturale di Firenze* (Rome: Giovanni Zempel, 1775).

Fontenelle, Bernard Le Bovier de, 'Éloge de M. Ruysch', in *Histoire de l'Académie Royale des Sciences, Année 1731* (Paris: Imprimerie Royale, 1733), 100–9.

Galen, Claudius, 'On Mixtures, Book 1', in *Selected Works*, ed. and trans. P.N. Singer (Oxford: Oxford University Press, 1997), 202–31.

Galvani, Luigi, *De Manzoliniana supellectili, oratio, habita in Scientiarum et Artium Instituto cum ad anatomen in tabulis ab Anna Manzolina perfectis pubblice tradendam aggrederetur anno MDCCLXXVII*, in *Opere edite ed inedite del professore Luigi Galvani, raccolte e pubblicate per cura dell'Accademia delle Scienze dell'Istituto di Bologna* (Bologna: Emidio Dall'Olmo, 1841), 41–58.

Ganganelli, Giovanni Vincenzo Antonio, *Interesting Letters of Pope Clement XIV (Ganganelli): To Which Are Prefixed, Anecdotes of His Life*, trans. Lottin Le Jeune, 3rd edn., vol. 1 (London: T. Becket, 1777).

Ganganelli, Giovanni Vincenzo Antonio, *Interesting Letters of Pope Clement XIV (Ganganelli): To Which Are Prefixed, Anecdotes of his Life*, trans. Lottin Le Jeune, 5th edn., vol. 2 (London: T. Becket, 1781).

Genovesi, Antonio, *Autobiografia, lettere e altri scritti*, ed. Gennaro Savarese (Milan: Feltrinelli, 1962).

Giordani, Gaetano, Articolo di biografia *a lode dell'Anna Morandi Manzolini, celebre anatomica* (Bologna: Nobili e Comp., 1835).

Goethe, Johann Wolfgang von, *Goethe's Travels in Italy: Together with His Second Residence in Rome and Fragments on Italy*, trans. A.J.W. Morrison and Charles Nisbet (London: George Bell and Sons, 1892).

Goethe, Johann Wolfgang von, *Wilhelm Meisters Wanderjahre*, in *Sämtliche Werke, Briefe, Tagebücher und Gespräche*, ed. Gerhard Neumann und Hans-Georg Drewitz, vol. 10 (Frankfurt am Main: Deutcher Klassiker Verlag, 1989).

Gorgone, Giovanni, *Notizie sulle statue angiografiche e la vita di Giuseppe Salerno* (Palermo: Presso gli eredi Graffeo, 1830).

Gray, Thomas, *Correspondence of Thomas Gray*, ed. Paget Toynbee and Leonard Whibley, vol. 1 (Oxford: Clarendon Press, 1935).

[Grosley, Pierre Jean], *New Observations on Italy and its Inhabitants. Written in French by two Swedish Gentleman*, trans. Thomas Nugent, 2 vols. (London: L. Davis and C. Reymers, 1769 [1764]).

Hervey, Christopher, *Letters from Portugal, Spain, Italy and Germany, in the Years 1759, 1760, and 1761*, vol. 3 (London: Printed by J. Davis for R. Faulder, 1785).

Hunter, William, *Two Introductory Lectures Delivered by Dr. William Hunter, to His Last Course of Anatomical Lectures, at His Theatre in Windmill-Street: As They Were Left Corrected for the Press by Himself* (London: Printed by the Order of Trustees for J. Johnson, 1784).

'Journal de voyage d'un médecin bruxellois de Munich à Rome en 1755', ed. Charles Terlinden, *Bulletin de l'Institut historique belge de Rome*, 23 (1944–6), 123–59.

Keyssler, Johann Georg, *Travels through Germany, Bohemia, Hungary, Switzerland, Italy, and Lorrain: Giving a True and Just Description of the Present State of Those Countries; Carefully Translated from the Second Edition of the German*, 2nd edn., 4 vols. (London: A. Linde and T. Field, 1756–7).

Kraus, Franz Xaver (ed.), *Lettere di Benedetto XIV scritte al canonico Pier Francesco Peggi a Bologna, 1729–1758* (Freiburg: J.C.B. Mohr, 1884).

La Condamine, Charles-Marie de, 'Extrait d'un journal de voyage en Italie', in *Histoire de l'Académie Royale des Sciences, Année 1757* (Paris: L'Imprimerie Royale, 1762), 336–410.

La Condamine, Charles-Marie de, *Journal of a Tour to Italy, translated from the French* (Dublin: Printed by J. Potts at Swift's Head, 1763).

Laghi, Tommaso, 'De perficienda injectionum anatomicarum methodo', in *De Bononiensi Scientiarum et Artium Instituto atque Academia Commentarii*, vol. 4/I (Bologna: Lelio dalla Volpe, 1757), 120–32.

Lalande, Joseph Jérôme Lefrançois de, *Voyage d'un François en Italie, fait dans les années 1765 et 1766*, 8 vols. (Venice: Desaint, 1769).

Lalande, Joseph Jérôme Lefrançois de, *Voyage en Italie [...]. Second Edition corrigée & augmentée*, 2nd edn., 9 vols. (Paris: Desaint, 1786).

Lamberg, Maximilian Joseph von, *Mémorial d'un mondain*, 2nd edn., vol. 1 (London [i.e. Paris?]: n.p., 1776 [1774]).

Lambertini, Prospero, 'Delle Ostetrici, o Mammane, o sieno Comari da Putti [...]', in *Raccolta di alcune notificazioni, editti, ed istruzioni pubblicate dall'Eminentissimo, e Reverendissimo Signor Cardinale Prospero Lambertini, Arcivescovo di Bologna, e Principe del S.R.I. pel buon governo della sua Diocesi*, vol. 1 (Bologna: Longhi, 1733), 78–85.

Lambertini, Prospero, *De servorum Dei beatificatione et beatorum canonizatione*, 4 vols. (Bologna: Longhi, 1734–8).

Lambertini, Prospero, 'Sopra la Notomia da farsi nelle pubbliche Scuole [...]', in *Raccolta di alcune notificazioni, editti, ed istruzioni pubblicate dall'Eminentissimo, e Reverendissimo Signor Cardinale Prospero Lambertini [...] pel buon governo della sua diocesi*, vol. 3 (Bologna: Longhi, 1737), 263–8.

Lambertini, Prospero, "Sopra il portare i corpi de' defunti alla sepoltura, e Messe da celebrarsi per le anime loro [...]", in *Raccolta di alcune notificazioni, editti, ed istruzioni pubblicate pel buon governo della sua diocesi dall'Eminentissimo e Reverendissimo Signor Cardinale Prospero Lambertini, Arcivescovo di Bologna, ora Benedetto XIV, sommo Pontefice*, 10th edn., vol. 1 (Naples: a spese di Andrea Migliaccio, 1772), 175–80.

Lambertini, Prospero, 'Sopra le Immagini della Santissima Croce, e de' Santi, che nei muri delle Case si dipingono [...]', in *Raccolta di alcune notificazioni, editti, ed istruzioni pubblicate pel buon governo della sua diocese [...]*, 10th edn., vol. 2 (Naples: a spese di Andrea Migliaccio, 1772), 77–9.

Lambertini, Prospero, 'Sopra l'Esposizione del SS. Sagramento dell'Eucaristia [...]', in *Raccolta di alcune notificazioni, editti, ed istruzioni pubblicate pel buon governo della sua diocese [...]*, 10th edn., vol. 1 (Naples: a spese di Andrea Migliaccio, 1772), 138–46.

Lambertini, Prospero, 'Motuproprio, col quale Ercole Lelli Artefice delle otto Statue Anatomiche, esistenti per liberalità di Nostro Signore nell'Instituto delle Scienze, con altri lavori rappresentanti le parti del Corpo Umano, viene costituito Custode ed Ostensore di dette Statue [...]', in Annarita Angelini (ed.), *Anatomie Accademiche: L'Istituto delle Scienze e l'Accademia*, vol. 3 (Bologna: Il Mulino, 1993), 535–40.

Lambertini, Prospero, 'Motuproprio pel quale s'istituisce in Bologna una Scuola di Chirurgia, e si prescieglie per la prima volta alla carica di Dimostratore delle Operazioni Chirurgiche il Dottore Pietro Paolo Molinelli', in Annarita Angelini (ed.), *Anatomie Accademiche: L'Istituto delle Scienze e l'Accademia*, vol. 3 (Bologna: Il Mulino, 1993), 524–8.

Leopardi, Giacomo, 'Dialogo di Federico Ruysch e delle sue mummie', in *Operette morali* (Milan: Ant. Fort. Stella e Figli, 1827), 163–71.

Macchiavelli, Alessandro, *Effemeridi sacro-civili perpetue bolognesi* (Bologna: Lorenzo Martelli, 1739).

Maffei, Scipione, *Museum Veronense, hoc est, Antiquarum inscriptionum atque anaglyphorum collectio: cui taurinensis adiungitur et vindobonensis: accedunt monumenta id genus plurima nondum vulgata, et ubicumque collecta* (Verona: Typis Seminarii, 1749).

Malvasia, Carlo Cesare, *Le pitture di Bologna [...]*, 5th edn. (Bologna: Longhi, 1766).
Mandeville, Bernard, *The Virgin Unmask'd: Or, Female Dialogues Betwixt an Elderly Maiden Lady, and her Niece*, 2nd edn. (London: Printed and sold by G. Strahan, W. Mears, and F. Stagg, 1724 [1709]).
Martuscelli, Domenico, *Biografia degli uomini illustri del Regno di Napoli, ornata de loro rispettivi ritratti*, vol. 6 (Naples: Nicola Gervasi, 1813).
Martyn, Thomas, *The Gentleman's Guide in his Tour through Italy: With a Correct Map, and Directions for Travelling in that Country* (London: Printed for and sold by G. Kearsley, 1787).
Mazzetti, Serafino, *Memorie storiche sopra l'Università e l'Istituto delle Scienze di Bologna* (Bologna: San Tommaso d'Aquino, 1840).
Medici, Michele, 'Elogio d'Ercole Lelli', in *Memorie della Accademia delle Scienze dell'Istituto di Bologna*, vol. 7 (Bologna: San Tommaso d'Aquino, 1856), 157–86.
Medici, Michele, 'Elogio di Gian Antonio Galli', in *Memorie dell' Accademia delle Scienze dell'Istituto di Bologna*, vol. 8 (Bologna: San Tommaso d'Aquino, 1857), 423–50.
Medici, Michele, 'Elogio di Giovanni, e di Anna Morandi coniugi Manzolini', in *Memorie della Accademia delle Scienze dell'Istituto di Bologna*, vol. 8 (Bologna: San Tommaso d'Aquino, 1858), 3–26.
Melli, Sebastiano, *La comare levatrice istruita nel suo ufizio secondo le regole più certe, e gli ammaestramenti più moderni* (Venice: Gio. Battista Recurti, 1721).
Meloni, Antonio (ed.), *Raccolta ferrarese di opuscoli scientifici e letterari*, vol. 4 (Venice: Coleti, 1780).
Mengal, Paul (ed.), *Giacomo Casanova, Lana Caprina: Une controverse médicale sur l'utérus pensant à l'Université de Bologne en 1771–1772*, trans. Roberto Poma (Paris: Honoré Champion, 1999).
Metastasio, Pietro, *Lettere*, in *Tutte le opere di Pietro Metastasio*, ed. Bruno Brunelli, 5 vols. (Milan: Arnoldo Mondadori Editore, 1943–54).
[Miller, Anna Riggs], *Letters from Italy, Describing the Manners, Customs, Antiquities, Paintings, &c. of that Country, in the Years MDCCLXX and MDCCLXXI, to a Friend Residing in France, by an English Woman*, 2nd edn., 2 vols. (London: Edward and Charles Dilly, 1777).
Mongitore, Antonino, *Memorie dei pittori, scultori, architetti, artefici in cera siciliani*, ed. Elvira Natoli (Palermo: S.F. Flaccovio, 1977).
Monro, Alexander, 'An Essay on the Art of Injecting the Vessels of Animals', in *Medical Essays and Observations, Revised and Published by a Society in Edinburgh*, 2nd edn., vol. 1 (Edinburgh: T. and W. Ruddimans for W. Monro and W. Drummond et al., 1737), 94–111.
Moore, John, *A View of Society and Manners in Italy*, vol. 1 (London: W. Strahan and T. Cadell, 1781).
Morgagni, Giambattista and Francesco Maria Zanotti, *Carteggio tra Giambattista Morgagni e Francesco M. Zanotti* (Bologna: Zanichelli, 1875).
Morgan, John, *The Journal of Dr. John Morgan of Philadelphia, from the City of Rome to the City of London, 1764* (Philadelphia: Printed for private circulation by J.B. Lippincott, 1907).
Morgan, Lady [Sydney Owenson], *Italy*, vol. 1 (London: Henry Colburn and Co., 1821).
Morgan, Thomas Charles, 'Appendix: On the State of Medicine in Italy, with Brief Notices of Some of the Universities and Hospitals', in Lady Morgan [Sydney Owenson] *Italy*, vol. 1 (London: Henry Colburn and Co., 1821), 311–48.
Muratori, Ludovico Antonio, *Della forza della fantasia umana* (Venice: Giambatista Pasquali, 1745).

Muratori, Ludovico Antonio, *Della pubblica felicità, oggetto de' buoni principi* (Lucca: n.p., 1749).

[Muratori, Ludovico Antonio], Lamindo Pritanio, pseud., *Della regolata divozion de' cristiani* (Venice: Giambattista Albrizzi & Gir., 1747).

Napoli Signorelli, Pietro, *Vicende della coltura nelle Due Sicilie, o sia storia ragionata della loro legislazione e polizia, delle lettere, del commercio, delle arti, e degli spettacoli dalle colonie straniere insino a noi*, vol. 4 (Naples: Vincenzo Flauto, 1785).

Napoli Signorelli, Pietro, *Vicende della coltura nelle Due Sicilie: Dalla venuta delle Colonie straniere sino a' nostri giorni*, 2nd edn., vol. 7 (Naples: n.p., 1811).

Origlia Paolino, Giovanni Giuseppe, *Istoria dello Studio di Napoli; in cui si comprendono gli avvenimenti di esso più notabili da' primi suoi principi fino a' tempi presenti, con buona parte della Storia Letteraria del Regno*, vol. 2 (Naples: Giovanni di Simone, 1754).

Orlandi, Cesare, 'Anatomia', in Cesare Ripa, *Iconologia del cavaliere Cesare Ripa, perugino; notabilmente accresciuta d'immagini, di annotazioni, e di fatti dall'Abate Cesare Orlandi*, vol. 1 (Perugia: Piergiovanni Costantini, 1764), 127–30.

Orlandi, Cesare, *Delle città d'Italia e sue isole adjacenti compendiose notizie*, vol. 4 (Perugia: Stamperia Augusta, 1775).

Patoun, William, 'Advice on Travel in Italy', in John Ingamells (ed.), *A Dictionary of British and Irish Travellers in Italy, 1701–1800* (New Haven: Yale University Press, 1997), xxxix–lii.

Pentolini, Francesco Clodoveo Maria, *Donne illustri: Canti dieci*, vol. 2 (Livorno: Gio. Vincenzo Falorni, 1776–7).

Pilati, Carlo Antonio, *Voyages en différens pays de l'Europe, en 1774, 1775 et 1776; ou Lettres écrites de l'Allemagne, de la Suisse, de l'Italie, de Sicile et de Paris*, vol. 1 (The Hague: C. Plaat et Comp., 1777).

Pini, Ermenegildo, *Dell'architettura: Dialoghi* (Milan: Marelliana, 1770).

Piozzi, Hester Lynch, *Observations and Reflections Made in the Course of a Journey through France, Italy, and Germany*, vol. 1 (London: A. Strahan and T. Cadell, 1789).

Pisarri, Carlo, *Dialoghi tra Claro, e Sarpiri per istruire chi desidera d'essere un eccellente pittore figurista* (Bologna: Ferdinando Pisarri, 1778).

Pitré, Giuseppe, *La vita in Palermo cento e più anni fa* (Palermo: Alberto Reber, 1905).

Poullain de la Barre, François, *De l'égalité des deux sexes: Discours physique et moral, où l'on voit l'importance de se défaire des préjugéz* (Paris: Jean Du Puis, 1673).

Poullain de la Barre, François, *De l'éducation des dames pour la conduite de l'esprit dans les sciences et dans les moeurs: Entretiens* (Paris: Jean Du Puis, 1674).

Pritanio, Lamindo, pseud. [Muratori, Ludovico Antonio], *Della regolata divozion de' cristiani* (Venice: Giambattista Albrizzi & Gir., 1747), see Muratori, Ludovico Antonio.

Quillet, Claude, *Callipaedia: or, the Art of Getting Beautiful Children; a Poem, in Four Books, Written in Latin by Claudius Quillet*, trans. N. Rowe, 3rd edn. (London: W. Feales, 1733).

'Remarques sur quelques-unes des curiosités observées en 1766, à Naples, dans le Palais de San-Severo, seigneur Raimond de Sangro, Prince de San-Sévero', *Journal encyclopédique*, vol. 8 (1768), 108–15.

Richard, Jérôme, *Description historique et critique de l'Italie, ou Nouveaux mémoires sur l'etat actuel de son gouvernement, des sciences, des arts, du commerce, de la population & de l'histoire naturelle*, 2nd edn., 6 vols. (Paris: Saillant, Desaint, J.M. Coru de la Goibrie, 1769 [1766]).

'Riflessioni sopra i sensi umani', in *Giornale de' letterati per l'anno MDCCXLIV, pubblicato col titolo di Novelle Letterarie Oltramontane* (Rome: Fratelli Pagliarini, 1744), 263–70.

Sade, Donatien Alphonse François, Marquis de, *Voyage d'Italie*, in *Oeuvres complètes du Marquis de Sade*, ed. Gilbert Lely, vol. 16 (Paris: Cercle du livre précieux, 1967).

Saint-Non, Jean Claude Richard de, *Panopticon italiano: Un diario di viaggio ritrovato, 1759–1761* (Rome: Elefante, 1986).

[Schiavo, Domenico], *Memorie per servire alla storia letteraria di Sicilia*, vol. 2 (Palermo: Stamperia de' SS. Apostoli per Pietro Bentivenga, 1756).

Scinà, Domenico, *Prospetto della storia letteraria di Sicilia nel secolo decimottavo*, vol. 1 (Palermo: Lo Bianco, 1859).

Smith, James Edward, *A Sketch of a Tour on the Continent, in the Years 1786 and 1787*, vol. 2 (London: Printed for the author by J. Davis, 1793).

Sonnini, Charles Sigisbert, *Travels in Upper and Lower Egypt undertaken by Order of the Old Government of France*, trans. Henry Hunter, vol. 1 (London: J. Debrett, 1800).

Strange, Robert, *An Inquiry into the Rise and Establishment of the Royal Academy of Arts: To Which is Prefixed, a Letter to the Earl of Bute* (London: E. and C. Dilly; J. Robson, and J. Walter, 1775).

'Suites des remarques sur quelques unes de curiosités observes en 1766, à Naples, &c', *Journal encyclopédique*, vol. 8 (1768), 117–27.

Sydenham, Thomas, 'Anatomie, 1688', in Kenneth Dewhurst (ed.), *Dr. Thomas Sydenham (1624–1689): His Life and Original Writings* (Berkeley: University of California Press, 1966), 85–93.

Tanucci, Bernardo, *Epistolario I: 1723–1746*, ed. Romano Paolo Coppini et al. (Rome: Edizioni di Storia e Letteratura, 1980).

Tanucci, Bernardo, *Epistolario III: 1752–1756*, ed. Anna Vittoria Migliorini (Rome: Edizioni di Storia e Letteratura, 1982).

Taylor, John, 'The Life &c.', in *The History of the Travels and Adventures of the Chevalier John Taylor, Ophthalmiater*, vol. 1 (London: J. Williams, 1761).

[Tschudy, Théodore Henri de], *L'étoile flamboyante, ou la société des Francs-Maçons, considérée sous tous les aspects*, vol. 1 (Frankfurt and Paris: Antoine Boudet, 1766); vol. 2 (Paris: À L'orient chez Le Silence, 1780).

Tumiati, Giovanni, *Elementi d'anatomia*, vol. 2 (Ferrara: Francesco Pomatelli, 1800).

Vallisneri, Antonio, *Istoria della generazione dell'uomo, e degli animali; se sia da'vermicelli spermatici, o dalle uova* (Venice: Gio. Gabbriel Hertz, 1721).

Vasari, Giorgio, *Le vite de' più eccellenti pittori scultori e architettori*, 2nd edn., 3 vols. (Florence: Giunti, 1568 [1550]).

Vespa, Giuseppe, *Dell'arte ostetricia* (Florence: Andrea Bonducci, 1761).

Vigée-Lebrun, Louise-Élisabeth, *Souvenirs de Madame Vigée Le Brun*, vol. 1 (Paris: Charpentier et Cie, 1869).

Volkmann, Johann Jacob, *Historisch-kritische Nachrichten von Italien* [...], vol. 1 (Leipzig: Caspar Fritsch, 1770).

Winckelmann, Johann Joachim, *Reflections on the Imitation of Greek Works in Painting and Sculpture*, trans. Elfriede Heyer and Roger C. Norton (La Salle, IL: Open Court, 1987).

Wright, Edward, *Some Observations Made in Travelling Through France, Italy*, &c. *in the years 1720, 1721, and 1722*, vol. 2 (London: Tho. Ward and E. Wicksteed, 1730).

Zaccaria, Francesco Antonio, *Storia letteraria d'Italia*, vol. 5 (Venice: Poletti, 1753).

Zanotti, Francesco Maria, 'De iis, quae Instituto jam condito adjuncta sunt', in *De Bononiensi Scientiarum et Artium Instituto atque Academia Commentarii*, vol. 1 (Bologna: Lelio dalla Volpe, 1731), 22–32.

Zanotti, Francesco Maria, 'De anatome in Institutum introducenda', in *De Bononiensi Scientiarum et Artium Instituto atque Academia Commentarii*, vol. 2/I (Bologna: Lelio dalla Volpe, 1745), 44–50.

Zanotti, Francesco Maria, 'De Professoribus Instituti', in *De Bononiensi Scientiarum et Artium Instituto atque Academia Commentarii*, vol. 3 (Bologna: Lelio dalla Volpe, 1755), 7–11.

Zanotti, Francesco Maria, 'De re obstetricia', in *De Bononiensi Scientiarum et Artium Instituto atque Academia Commentarii*, vol. 3 (Bologna: Lelio dalla Volpe, 1755), 87–9.

Zanotti, Francesco Maria, 'De Senatoribus Instituti Praefectis', in *De Bononiensi Scientiarum et Artium Instituto atque Academia Commentarii*, vol. 3 (Bologna: Lelio dalla Volpe, 1755), 4–7.

Zanotti, Giampietro, *Storia dell'Accademia Clementina di Bologna* (Bologna: Lelio dalla Volpe, 1739).

Zanotti, Giampietro, *Avvertimenti di Giampietro Cavazzoni Zanotti, per lo incamminamento di un giovane alla pittura* (Bologna: Lelio dalla Volpe, 1756).

SECONDARY SOURCES

Acton, Harold Mario Mitchell, *The Bourbons of Naples, 1734–1825* (London: Methuen, 1974 [1956]).

Alberti, Samuel J.M.M., 'The Museum Affect: Visiting Collections of Anatomy and Natural History', in Aileen Fyfe and Bernard V. Lightman (eds.), *Science in the Marketplace: Nineteenth-Century Sites and Experiences* (Chicago: University of Chicago Press, 2007), 371–403.

Alberti, Samuel J.M.M., 'Wax Bodies: Art and Anatomy in Victorian Medical Museums', *Museum History Journal*, 2:1 (2009), 7–36.

Alberti, Samuel J.M.M., *Morbid Curiosities: Medical Museums in Nineteenth-Century Britain* (Oxford: Oxford University Press, 2011).

Algazi, Gadi, 'Scholars in Households: Refiguring the Learned Habitus, 1480–1550', *Science in Context*, 16:1/2 (2003), 9–42.

Andretta, Elisa, 'Anatomie du Vénérable dans la Rome de la Contre-réforme: Les autopsies d'Ignace de Loyola et de Philippe Neri', in Maria Pia Donato and Jill Kraye (eds.), *Conflicting Duties: Science, Medicine and Religion in Rome, 1550–1750* (London: Warburg Institute, 2009), 275–300.

Angelini, Annarita (ed.), *Anatomie Accademiche*, vol. 3, *L'Istituto delle Scienze e l'Accademia* (Bologna: Il Mulino, 1993).

Angelini, Annarita, 'L'Institut des Sciences de Bologne entre les "théâtres du monde" et les laboratoires de science expérimentale', in Daniel-Odon Hurel and Gérard Laudin (eds.), *Académies et sociétés savantes en Europe (1650–1800)* (Paris: Honoré Champion, 2000), 177–97.

Angelini, Massimo, 'Il potere plastico dell'immaginazione nelle gestanti tra XVI e XVIII secolo: La fortuna di un'idea', *Intersezioni*, 14:1 (1994), 53–69.

Appadurai, Arjun (ed.), *The Social Life of Things: Commodities in Cultural Perspective* (Cambridge: Cambridge University Press, 1986).

Armaroli, Maurizio (ed.), *Le cere anatomiche bolognesi del Settecento: Catalogo della mostra organizzata dall'Università degli Studi di Bologna nell'Accademia delle Scienze* (Bologna: CLUEB, 1981).

Azzaroli Puccetti, Maria Luisa, 'Gaetano Giulio Zumbo: La vita e le opere', in Paolo Giansiracusa (ed.), *Gaetano Giulio Zumbo* (Milan: Fabbri Editori, 1988), 17–46.

Babini, Valeria P., 'Anatomica, medica, chirurgica', in Walter Tega (ed.), *Anatomie Accademiche*, vol. 2 (Bologna: Il Mulino, 1987), 59–85.

Bambi, Anna Rosa, 'Il conte Girolamo Ranuzzi, un eclettico bolognese del 700', *Il Carrobbio*, 24 (1998), 137–56.

Barker-Benfield, G.J., *The Culture of Sensibility: Sex and Society in Eighteenth-Century Britain* (Chicago: University of Chicago Press, 1992).

Barry, Elizabeth, 'Celebrity, Cultural Production and Public Life', *International Journal of Cultural Studies*, 11:3 (2008), 251–8.

Barry, Elizabeth, 'From Epitaph to Obituary: Death and Celebrity in Eighteenth-Century British Culture', *International Journal of Cultural* Studies, 11:3 (2008), 259–75.

Baxandall, Michael, *Painting and Experience in Fifteenth Century Italy: A Primer in the Social History of Pictorial Style* (Oxford: Oxford University Press, 1988).

Beaurepaire, Pierre-Yves, '"Grand Tour", République des Lettres e reti massoniche: Una cultura della mobilità nell'Europa dei Lumi', in Gian Mario Cazzaniga (ed.), *Storia d'Italia, Annali 21: La massoneria* (Turin: Einaudi, 2006), 31–89.

Belloni, Luigi, 'Italian Medical Education after 1600', in Charles Donald O'Malley (ed.), *The History of Medical Education* (Berkeley: University of California Press, 1970), 105–19.

Benassi, Stefano, *L'Accademia Clementina: La funzione pubblica e l'ideologia estetica* (Bologna: Minerva Edizioni, 2004).

Benimeli, José Antonio Ferrer, 'Origini, motivazioni ed effetti della condanna vaticana', in Gian Mario Cazzaniga (ed.), *Storia d'Italia, Annali 21*: *La massoneria* (Turin: Einaudi, 2006), 143–65.

Bennett, James A., 'Shopping for Instruments in Paris and London', in Pamela H. Smith and Paula Findlen (eds.), *Merchants and Marvels: Commerce Science and Art in Early Modern Europe* (New York: Routledge, 2002), 370–95.

Bensaude-Vincent, Bernadette and Christine Blondel, 'Introduction: A Science Full of Shocks, Sparks and Smells', in Bernadette Bensaude-Vincent and Christine Blondel (eds.), *Science and Spectacle in the European Enlightenment* (Aldershot: Ashgate, 2008), 1–24.

Bensaude-Vincent, Bernadette and Christine Blondel (eds.), *Science and Spectacle in the European Enlightenment* (Aldershot: Ashgate, 2008).

Berg, Maxine and Helen Clifford (eds.), *Consumers and Luxury: Consumer Culture in Europe, 1650–1850* (Manchester: Manchester University Press, 1999).

Berg, Maxine and Elizabeth Eger (eds.), *Luxury in the Eighteenth Century: Debates, Desires and Delectable Goods* (Basingstoke: Palgrave Macmillan, 2003).

Berkowitz, Carin, 'The Beauty of Anatomy: Visual Displays and Surgical Education in Early Nineteenth-Century London', *Bulletin of the History of Medicine*, 85:2 (2011), 248–78.

Berkowitz, Carin, 'Systems of Display: The Making of Anatomical Knowledge in Enlightenment Britain', *The British Journal for the History of Science*, 46:3 (2013), 359–87.

Bermingham, Ann, 'The Aesthetics of Ignorance: The Accomplished Woman in the Culture of Connoisseurship', *Oxford Art Journal*, 16:2 (1993), 3–20.

Bermingham, Ann, *Learning to Draw: Studies in the Cultural History of a Polite and Useful Art* (New Haven: Yale University Press, 2000).

Bernabeo, Raffaele A. and I. Romanelli, 'Considerazioni di Giovanni Manzolini (1700–1755) sull'anatomia dell'orecchio in condizioni normali e patologiche', in *Atti del XXVII° Congresso Nazionale di Storia della Medicina: Estratto* (Capua: n.p., 1977), 1–8.

Berti Logan, Gabriella, 'The Desire to Contribute: An Eighteenth-Century Italian Woman of Science', *The American Historical Review*, 99:3 (1994), 785–812.

Berti Logan, Gabriella, 'Women and the Practice and Teaching of Medicine in Bologna in the Eighteenth and Early Nineteenth Centuries', *Bulletin of the History of Medicine*, 77:3 (2003), 506–35.

Bertoli Barsotti, Anna Maria, 'La figura di Ercole Lelli e la nascita del Museo Anatomico', in Raffaele A. Bernabeo (ed.), *Atti del XXXI Congresso internazionale di Storia della Medicina, Bologna, 30 agosto–4 settembre 1988* (Bologna: Monduzzi Editore, 1990), 57–64.

Bertoloni Meli, Domenico, 'Mechanistic Pathology and Therapy in the Medical *Assayer* of Marcello Malpighi', *Medical History*, 51:2 (2007), 165–80.

Bertoloni Meli, Domenico, *Mechanism, Experiment, Disease: Marcello Malpighi and Seventeenth-Century Anatomy* (Baltimore: Johns Hopkins University Press, 2011).

Bertucci, Paola, *Viaggio nel paese delle meraviglie: Scienza e curiosità nell'Italia del Settecento* (Turin: Bollati Boringhieri, 2007).

Bertucci, Paola, 'The Architecture of Knowledge: Science, Collecting and Display in Eighteenth-Century Naples', in Melissa Calaresu and Helen Hills (eds.), *New Approaches to Naples c.1500–c.1800: The Power of Place* (Farnham: Ashgate, 2013), 149–74.

Bertucci, Paola, 'Enlightened Secrets: Silk, Intelligent Travel, and Industrial Espionage in Eighteenth-Century France', *Technology and Culture*, 54:4 (2013), 820–52.

Bertucci, Paola, 'The In/visible Woman: Mariangela Ardinghelli and the Circulation of Knowledge between Paris and Naples in the Eighteenth Century', *Isis*, 104:2 (2013), 226–49.

Biagi Maino, Donatella, 'Arte, scienza e potere: Le risoluzioni di Benedetto XIV per le istituzioni accademiche bolognesi', in Philippe Koeppel (ed.), *Papes et papauté au XVIIIe siècle: Vie colloque franco-italien, Société française d'étude du XVIIIe siècle, Université de Savoie, Chambéry, 21–22 septembre 1995* (Paris: Honoré Champion, 1999), 27–50.

Biagi Maino, Donatella, 'La rifondazione dell'Accademia in età benedettina', in Donatella Biagi Maino (ed.), *L'immagine del Settecento da Luigi Ferdinando Marsili a Benedetto XIV* (Turin: Umberto Allemandi, 2005), 81–98.

Biagi Maino, Donatella, 'Luigi Ferdinando Marsili e le arti del disegno: La nuova visione del mondo', in Donatella Biagi Maino (ed.), *L'immagine del Settecento da Luigi Ferdinando Marsigli a Benedetto XIV* (Turin: Umberto Allemandi, 2005), 29–49.

Biagi Maino, Donatella (ed.), *Benedetto XIV e le arti del disegno: Convegno internazionale di studi di storia dell'arte, Bologna 28–30 novembre 1994* (Rome: Quasar, 1998).

Biagioli, Mario, 'Scientific Revolution, Social Bricolage, and Etiquette', in Roy Porter and Mikuláš Teich (eds.), *The Scientific Revolution in National Context* (Cambridge: Cambridge University Press, 1992), 11–54.

Biagioli, Mario, *Galileo's Instruments of Credit: Telescopes, Images, Secrecy* (Chicago: University of Chicago Press, 2006).

Bianchi, Ilaria, 'Femminea natura degli studi sopra i cadaveri: L'arte della scienza di Anna Morandi Manzolini', *Annuario della scuola di specializzazione in storia dell'arte dell'Università di Bologna*, 3 (2002), 21–41.

Biliński, Bronisław, 'Bologna nel ritrovato manoscritto "Journaux des Voyages" di Michele Mniszech (1767)', in Riccardo Casimiro Lewanski (ed.), *Laudatio Bononiae: Atti del Convegno storico italo-polacco svoltosi a Bologna dal 26 al 31 maggio 1988 in occasione del Nono Centenario dell'Alma Mater Studiorum* (Bologna: Università degli Studi di Bologna/ Warsaw: Istituto Italiano di Cultura di Varsavia, 1990), 355–73.

Bisogni, Fabio, 'Ex voto e la scultura in cera nel tardo Medioevo', in Andrew Ladis and Shelley E. Zuraw (eds.), *Visions of Holiness: Art and Devotion in Renaissance Italy* (Athens: Georgia Museum of Art, 2001), 67–91.

Black, Jeremy, *The British Abroad: The Grand Tour in the Eighteenth Century* (Stroud: The History Press, 2003).

Black, Jeremy, *Italy and the Grand Tour* (New Haven: Yale University Press, 2003).

Bleichmar, Daniela, 'Training the Naturalist's Eye in the Eighteenth Century: Perfect Global Visions and Local Blind Spot', in Cristina Grasseni (ed.), *Skilled Visions: Between Apprenticeship and Standards* (Oxford: Berghahn Books, 2007), 166–90.

Bleichmar, Daniela, 'Learning to Look: Visual Expertise across Art and Science in Eighteenth-Century France', *Eighteenth-Century Studies*, 46:1 (2012), 85–111.

Bleichmar, Daniela, *Visible Empire: Botanical Expeditions & Visual Culture in the Hispanic Enlightenment* (Chicago: University of Chicago Press, 2012).

Boespflug, François, *Dieu dans l'art: Sollicitudini Nostrae de Benoît XIV (1745) et l'affaire Crescence de Kaufbeuren* (Paris: Éditions du Cerf, 1984).

Bohn, Babette, 'Female Self-Portraiture in Early Modern Bologna', *Renaissance Studies*, 18:2 (2004), 239–86.

Bonfait, Olivier, *Les exposition de peintures a Bologne au XVIIIe siécle* (Mémoire de l'Ecole du Louvre, 1990).

Bordini, Silvia, '"Studiare in un istesso luogo la Natura, e ciò che ha saputo far l'Arte": Il museo e l'educazione degli artisti nella politica culturale di Benedetto XIV', in Donatella Biagi Maino (ed.), *Benedetto XIV e le arti del disegno: Convegno internazionale di studi di storia dell'arte, Bologna 28–30 Novembre 1994* (Rome: Quasar, 1998), 385–94.

Bortolotti, Marco, 'Insegnamento, ricerca e professione nel museo ostetrico di Giovanni Antonio Galli', in *I materiali dell'Istituto delle Scienze: Catalogo della mostra, Bologna, settembre-novembre 1979* (Bologna: CLUEB, 1979), 239–47.

Bortolotti, Marco, 'Il maestro alla lavagna. Il museo Galli dall'inventario al catalogo', in Marco Bortolotti et al., *Ars obstetricia bononiensis: Catalogo ed inventario del Museo Ostetrico Giovan Antonio Galli* (Bologna: CLUEB, 1988), 14–23.

Bortolotti, Marco et al., *Ars obstetricia bononiensis: Catalogo ed inventario del Museo Ostetrico Giovan Antonio Galli* (Bologna: CLUEB, 1988).

Boulinier, Georges, 'Une femme anatomiste au siècle des Lumières: Marie Marguerite Bihéron (1719–1795)', *Histoire des sciences médicales*, 35:4 (2001), 411–23.

Bourguet, Marie-Noëlle, Christian Licoppe and H. Otto Sibum (eds.), *Instruments, Travel and Science: Itineraries of Precision from the Seventeenth to the Twentieth Century* (London: Routledge, 2002).

Brambilla, Elena, 'La medicina del Settecento: Dal monopolio dogmatico alla professione scientifica', in Franco della Peruta (ed.), *Storia d'Italia, Annali 7: Malattia e medicina* (Turin: Einaudi, 1984), 5–147.

Brambilla, Elena, *Corpi invasi e viaggi dell'anima: Santità, possessione, esorcismo dalla teologia barocca alla medicina illuminista* (Rome: Viella, 2010).

Brighetti, Antonio, 'Ercole Lelli e le cere bolognesi in carteggi inediti del Settecento', in *La ceroplastica nella scienza e nell'arte: Atti del I Congresso Internazionale, Firenze, 3–7 giugno 1975*, vol. 1 (Florence: Leo S. Olschki, 1977), 207–13.

Brizzi, Gian Paolo, 'Lo Studio di Bologna tra *orbis academicus* e mondo cittadino', in Adriano Prosperi (ed.), *Storia di Bologna*, vol. 3: *Bologna nell' età moderna (secoli XVI–XVIII)*, part II: *Cultura, istituzioni culturali, Chiesa e vita religiosa* (Bologna: Bononia University Press, 2008), 5–113.

Brock, Claire, *The Feminization of Fame, 1750–1830* (Basingstoke: Palgrave Macmillan, 2006).

Busacchi, Vincenzo, 'Le cere anatomiche dell'Istituto delle Scienze', in *I materiali dell'Istituto delle Scienze* (Bologna: CLUEB, 1979), 230–8.

Bynum, Caroline Walker, 'Material Continuity, Personal Survival, and the Resurrection of the Body: A Scholastic Discussion in Its Medieval and Modern Contexts', *History of Religions*, 30:1 (1990), 51–85.

Bynum, Caroline Walker, *The Resurrection of the Body in Western Christianity, 200–1336* (New York: Columbia University Press, 1995).

Bynum, Caroline Walker, *Christian Materiality: An Essay on Religion in Late Medieval Europe* (New York: Zone Books, 2011).

Cabré, Montserrat, 'Women or Healers? Household Practices and the Categories of Health Care in Late Medieval Iberia', *Bulletin of the History of Medicine*, 82:1 (2008), 18–51.

Calaresu, Melissa, 'Looking for Virgil's Tomb: The End of the Grand Tour and the Cosmopolitan Ideal in Europe', in Jaś Elsner and Joan Pau Rubiés (eds.), *Voyages and Visions: Towards a Cultural History of Travel* (London: Reaktion Books, 1999), 138–61.

Calaresu, Melissa and Helen Hills (eds.), *New Approaches to Naples c.1500–c.1800: The Power of Place* (Farnham: Ashgate, 2013).

Canetti, Luigi, 'Reliquie, martirio e anatomia: Culto dei santi e pratiche dissettorie fra tarda Antichità e primo Medioevo', *Micrologus*, 7 (1999), 113–53.

Carlino, Andrea, *Books of the Body: Anatomical Ritual and Renaissance Learning*, trans. Anne Tedeschi and John A. Tedeschi (Chicago: University of Chicago Press, 1999).

Cavallo, Sandra, *Artisans of the Body in Early Modern Italy: Identities, Families and Masculinities* (Manchester: Manchester University Press, 2007).

Cavallo, Sandra and Tessa Storey, *Healthy Living in Late Renaissance Italy* (Oxford: Oxford University Press, 2013).

Cavallo, Sandra and Lyndan Warner (eds.), *Widowhood in Medieval and Early Modern Europe* (New York: Longman, 1999).

Cavazza, Marta, 'La "Casa di Salomone" realizzata?', in *I materiali dell'Istituto delle Scienze: Catalogo della mostra, Bologna, settembre–novembre 1979* (Bologna: CLUEB, 1979), 42–54.

Cavazza, Marta, *Settecento inquieto: Alle origini dell'Istituto delle Scienze di Bologna* (Bologna: Il Mulino, 1990).

Cavazza, Marta, 'Dottrici e lettrici dell'Università di Bologna nel Settecento', *Annali di Storia delle università italiane*, 1 (1997), 109–26.

Cavazza, Marta, 'La ricezione della teoria halleriana dell'irritabilità nell'Accademia delle Scienze di Bologna', *Nuncius*, 12 (1997), 359–77.

Cavazza, Marta, 'The Uselessness of Anatomy: Mini and Sbaraglia Versus Malpighi', in Domenico Bertoloni Meli (ed.), *Marcello Malpighi: Anatomist and Physician* (Florence: Leo S. Olschki, 1997), 129–45.

Cavazza, Marta, 'Women's Dialectics or the Thinking Uterus: An Eighteenth-Century Controversy on Gender and Education', in Lorraine Daston and Gianna Pomata (eds.), *The Faces of Nature in Enlightenment Europe* (Berlin: BWV-Berliner Wissenschafts-Verlag, 2003), 237–57.

Cavazza, Marta, 'Between Modesty and Spectacle: Women and Science in Eighteenth-Century Italy', in Paula Findlen, Wendy Wassyng Roworth, and Catherine M. Sama (eds.), *Italy's Eighteenth Century: Gender and Culture in the Age of the Grand Tour* (Stanford: Stanford University Press, 2009), 275–302.

Cavazza, Marta, 'Aspetti dell'insegnamento dell'anatomia a Bologna nel Seicento e Settecento', in Giuseppe Olmi and Claudia Pancino (eds.), *Anatome: Sezione, scomposizione, raffigurazione del corpo nell'età moderna* (Bologna: Bononia University Press, 2012), 59–77.

Cecchelli, Marco (ed.), *Benedetto XIV (Prospero Lambertini): Convegno internazionale di studi storici, sotto il patrocinio dell'archidiocesi di Bologna: Cento, 6–9 dicembre 1979*, 2 vols. (Cento: Centro studi 'Girolamo Baruffaldi', 1981–2).

Cellini, Antonia Nava, *La scultura del Settecento* (Turin: UTET, 1982).

Cenacchi, Giuseppe, 'Benedetto XIV e l'Illuminismo', in Marco Cecchelli (ed.), *Benedetto XIV (Prospero Lambertini): Convegno internazionale di studi storici, sotto il patrocinio dell'archidiocesi di Bologna: Cento, 6–9 dicembre 1979*, vol. 1 (Cento: Centro studi 'Girolamo Baruffaldi', 1981), 1077–102.

Ceranski, Beate, *'Und sie fürchtet sich vor niemandem': Die Physikerin Laura Bassi (1711–1778)* (Frankfurt: Campus, 1996).

Chabot, Isabelle and Massimo Fornasari, *L'economia della carità. Le doti del Monte di Pietà di Bologna (secoli XVI–XX)* (Bologna: Il Mulino, 1997).

Chaney, Edward, *The Evolution of the Grand Tour: Anglo-Italian Cultural Relations since the Renaissance* (London: Frank Cass, 1998).

Chaplin, Simon, 'Nature Dissected, or Dissection Naturalized? The Case of John Hunter's Museum', *Museum and Society*, 6:2 (2008), 135–51.

Chaplin, Simon, 'John Hunter and the "Museum Oeconomy", 1750–1800' (PhD Thesis, King's College London, 2009).

Chaplin, Simon, 'The Divine Touch, or Touching Divines: John Hunter, David Hume and the Bishop of Durham's Rectum', in Helen Deutsch and Mary Terrall (eds.), *Vital Matters: Eighteenth-Century Views of Conception, Life, and Death* (Toronto: University of Toronto Press, 2012), 222–45.

Chard, Chloe, 'Effeminacy, Pleasure and the Classical Body', in Gillian Perry and Michael Rossington (eds.), *Femininity and Masculinity in Eighteenth-Century Art and Culture* (Manchester: Manchester University Press, 1994), 142–61.

Chard, Chloe, 'Nakedness and Tourism: Classical Sculpture and the Imaginative Geography of the Grand Tour', *Oxford Art Journal*, 18:1 (1995), 14–28.

Chard, Chloe, *Pleasure and Guilt on the Grand Tour: Travel Writing and Imaginative Geography, 1600–1830* (Manchester: Manchester University Press, 1999).

Chard, Chloe, 'Women who Transmute into Tourist Attractions: Spectator and Spectacle on the Grand Tour', in Amanda Gilroy (ed.), *Romantic Geographies: Discourses of Travel, 1775–1844* (Manchester: Manchester University Press, 2000), 109–26.

Chard, Chloe and Helen Langdon (eds.), *Transports: Travel, Pleasure, and Imaginative Geography, 1600–1830* (New Haven: Yale University Press, 1996).

Chartier, Roger, *The Order of Books: Readers, Authors and Libraries in Europe between the Fourteenth and the Eighteenth Centuries*, trans. Lydia C. Cochrane (Stanford: Stanford University Press, 1994).

Chiosi, Elvira, 'Intellectuals and Academies', in Girolamo Imbruglia (ed.), *Naples in the Eighteenth Century: The Birth and Death of a Nation State* (Cambridge: Cambridge University Press, 2000), 118–34.

Chiosi, Elvira, 'Academicians and Academies in Eighteenth-Century Naples', trans. Mark Weir, *Journal of the History of Collections*, 19:2 (2007), 177–90.

Christopoulos, John, 'Abortion and the Confessional in Counter-Reformation Italy', *Renaissance Quarterly*, 65:2 (2012), 443–84.

Christopoulos, John, *Abortion in Counter-Reformation Italy* (PhD thesis, University of Toronto, December 2012).

Ciardi, Roberto, 'L'anatomista e il pittore', in *Morgagni e l'iconografia anatomica tra '600 e '800* (Forlì: Comune di Forlì, 1982), 23–33.

Cioffi, Rosanna, *La Cappella Sansevero: Arte barocca e ideologia massonica* (Salerno: Edizioni 10/17, 1987).

Clark, Stuart, *Thinking with Demons: The Idea of Witchcraft in Early Modern Europe* (Oxford: Oxford University Press, 1997).

Clark, Stuart, *Vanities of the Eye: Vision in Early Modern European Culture* (Oxford: Oxford University Press, 2007).

Cocco, Sean, *Watching Vesuvius: A History of Science and Culture in Early Modern Italy* (Chicago: University of Chicago Press, 2013).

Cohen, Elizabeth S., 'Miscarriages of Apothecary Justice: Un-separate Spaces for Work and Family in Early Modern Rome', *Renaissance Studies*, 21:4 (2007), 480–504.

Cohen, Estelle, '"What Women At All Times Would Laugh At": Redefining Equality and Difference, circa 1660–1760', *Osiris*, 12 (1996), 121–42.

Cole, Francis J., 'The History of Anatomical Injections', in Charles Joseph Singer (ed.), *Studies in the History and Method of Science*, vol. 2 (Oxford: Clarendon Press, 1921), 285–343.

Colonna di Stigliano, Fabio, 'La Cappella Sansevero e don Raimondo di Sangro', *Napoli nobilissima*, 4 (1894), 33–6, 52–8, 72–5, 90–4, 116–21, 138–42, 152–3.

Conforti, Maria, '"Affirmare quid intus sit divinare est": mole, mostri e vermi in un caso di falsa gravidanza di fine Seicento', *Quaderni storici*, 130:1 (2009), 125–51.

Conforti, Maria, 'The Biblioteca Lancisiana and the 1714 Edition of Eustachi's Plates, or, Ancients and Moderns Reconciled', in Maria Pia Donato and Jill Kraye (eds.), *Conflicting Duties: Science, Medicine and Religion in Rome, 1550–1750* (London: Warburg Institute, 2009), 303–17.

Cook, Harold J., 'Time's Bodies: Crafting the Preparation and Preservation of Naturalia', in Pamela H. Smith and Paula Findlen (eds.), *Merchants and Marvels: Commerce, Science, and Art in Early Modern Europe* (New York: Routledge, 2002), 223–47.

Cook, Harold J., *Matters of Exchange: Commerce, Medicine, and Science in the Dutch Golden Age* (New Haven: Yale University Press, 2007).

Cook, Harold J., 'The Preservation of Specimens and the Takeoff in Anatomical Knowledge in the Early Modern Period', in Pamela H. Smith, Amy Meyers, and Harold Cook (eds.), *Ways of Making and Knowing: The Material Culture of Empirical Knowledge* (Ann Arbor: University of Michigan Press, 2014), 302–29.

Corradi, Alfonso, *Dell'ostetricia in Italia dalla metà dello scorso secolo fino al presente* (Bologna: Gamberini e Parmeggiani, 1874).

Crisciani, Chiara, 'History, Novelty, and Progress in Scholastic Medicine', *Osiris*, 6 (1990), 118–39.

Cunningham, Andrew, 'The End of the Sacred Ritual of Anatomy', *Canadian Bulletin of Medical History/Bulletin canadien d'histoire de la médecine*, 18:2 (2001), 187–204.

Cunningham, Andrew, *The Anatomist Anatomis'd: An Experimental Discipline in Enlightenment Europe* (Farnham: Ashgate, 2010).

Czennia, Bärbel (ed.), *Celebrity: The Idiom of a Modern Era* (New York: AMS Press, 2013).

Dacome, Lucia, '"Un certo e quasi incredibile piacere": cera e anatomia nel Settecento', *Intersezioni*, 25:3 (2005), 415–36.

Dacome, Lucia, 'Resurrecting by Numbers in Eighteenth-Century England', *Past & Present*, 193 (2006), 73–110.

Dacome, Lucia, 'Waxworks and the Performance of Anatomy in Mid-18th-Century Italy', *Endeavour*, 30:1 (2006), 29–35.

Dacome, Lucia, 'Women, Wax and Anatomy in the "Century of Things"', *Renaissance Studies*, 21:4 (2007), 522–50.

Dacome, Lucia, 'The Anatomy of the Pope', in Maria Pia Donato and Jill Kraye (eds.), *Conflicting Duties: Science, Medicine and Religion in Rome, 1550–1750* (London: Warburg Institute, 2009), 353–74.

Dacome, Lucia, 'Ai confini del mondo naturale: anatomia e santità nell'opera di Prospero Lambertini', in Maria Teresa Fattori (ed.), *Storia, medicina e diritto nei trattati di Prospero Lambertini—Benedetto XIV* (Rome: Edizioni di Storia e Letteratura, 2013), 319–38.

Dacome, Lucia, '"Une dentelle très bien agencée et très precise": les femmes et l'anatomie dans l'Europe du dix-huitième siècle', in Adeline Gargam (ed.), *Femmes de science de l'Antiquité au XIXe siècle. Réalités et représentations* (Dijon: Editions Universitaires de Dijon, 2014), 157–75.

Dacome, Lucia and Renata Peters, 'Fabricating the Body: The Anatomical Machines of the Prince of Sansevero', in Virginia Greene et al. (eds.), *Objects Specialty Group: Proceedings of the Objects Specialty Group Session, 35th Annual Meeting of the American Institute of Conservation* (Washington: American Institute for Conservation of Historic & Artistic Works, 2008).

Dalla Torre, Giuseppe, 'Santità ed economia processuale: L'esperienza giuridica da Urbano VIII a Benedetto XIV', in Gabriella Zarri (ed.), *Finzione e santità tra medioevo ed età moderna* (Turin: Rosenberg & Sellier, 1991), 231–63.

Daninos, Andrea (ed.), *Waxing Eloquent: Italian Portraits in Wax* (Milan: Officina Libraria, 2011).

Daston, Lorraine, 'The Nature of Nature in Early Modern Europe', *Configurations*, 6:2 (1998), 149–72.

Daston, Lorraine and Peter Galison, 'The Image of Objectivity', *Representations*, in 'Seeing Science', special issue, 40 (1992), 81–128.

Daston, Lorraine and Peter Galison, *Objectivity* (New York: Zone Books, 2007).

Daston, Lorraine and Elizabeth Lunbeck (eds.), *Histories of Scientific Observation* (Chicago: University of Chicago Press, 2011).

Daston, Lorraine and Katharine Park, *Wonders and the Order of Nature, 1150–1750* (New York: Zone Books, 1998).

Daston, Lorraine and Gianna Pomata (eds.), *The Faces of Nature in Enlightenment Europe* (Berlin: BWV-Berliner Wissenschafts-Verlag, 2003).

De Bolla, Peter, *The Education of the Eye: Painting, Landscape, and Architecture in Eighteenth-Century Britain* (Stanford: Stanford University Press, 2003).

De Ceglia, Francesco, 'Rotten Corpses, a Disembowelled Woman, a Flayed Man: Images of the Body from the End of the 17th to the Beginning of the 19th Century; Florentine Wax Models in the First-Hand Accounts of Visitors', *Perspectives on Science*, 14:4 (2007), 417–56.

De Ceglia, Francesco, 'The Importance of Being Florentine: A Journey around the World for Wax Anatomical Venuses', *Nuncius*, 26:1 (2011), 83–108.

De Ceglia, Francesco, 'Thinking with the Saint: The Miracle of Saint Januarius of Naples and Science in Early Modern Europe', *Early Science and Medicine*, 19:2 (2014), 133–73.

De Chadarevian, Soraya, 'Microstudies Versus Big Picture Accounts?', *Studies in History and Philosophy of Science, Part C: Studies in History and Philosophy of Biological and Biomedical Sciences*, 40:1 (2009), 13–19.

De Chadarevian, Soraya and Nick Hopwood (eds.), *Models: The Third Dimension of Science* (Stanford: Stanford University Press, 2004).

De Munck, Bert, 'Artisans, Products and Gifts: Rethinking the History of Material Culture in Early Modern Europe', *Past & Present*, 224:1 (2014), 39–74.

De Renzi, Silvia, 'Witnesses of the Body: Medico-Legal Cases in Seventeenth-Century Rome'. *Studies in History and Philosophy of Science, Part A*, 33:2 (2002), 219–42.

De Renzi, Silvia, 'Medical Competence, Anatomy and the Polity in Seventeenth-Century Rome', *Renaissance Studies*, 21:4 (2007), 551–67.

De Renzi, Silvia, 'Medical Expertise, Bodies, and the Law in Early Modern Courts', *Isis*, 98:2 (2007), 315–22.

De Renzi, Silvia, 'Resemblance, Paternity and Imagination in Early Modern Courts', in Staffan Müller-Wille and Hans-Jörg Rheinberger (eds.), *Heredity Produced: At the Crossroads of Biology, Politics, and Culture, 1500–1870* (Cambridge, MA: MIT Press, 2007), 61–83.

De Renzi, Silvia, 'The Risks of Childbirth: Physicians, Finance, and Women's Deaths in the Law Courts of Seventeenth-Century Rome', *Bulletin of the History of Medicine*, 84:4 (2010), 549–77.

De Sangro, Oderisio, *Raimondo de Sangro e la Cappella Sansevero* (Rome: Bulzoni, 1991).

De Vos, Paula, 'Natural History and the Pursuit of Empire in Eighteenth-Century Spain', *Eighteenth-Century Studies*, 40:2 (2007), 209–39.

Delbourgo, James, *A Most Amazing Scene of Wonders: Electricity and Enlightenment in Early America* (Cambridge, MA: Harvard University Press, 2006).

Di Castiglione, Ruggiero, *La Massoneria nelle Due Sicilie e i 'fratelli' meridionali del '700*, 6 vols. (Rome: Gangemi Editore, 2014).

Di Macco, Michela, 'Il "Museo Accademico" delle Scienze nel Palazzo dell'Università di Torino. Progetti e istituzioni nell'età dei Lumi', in Giacomo Giacobini (ed.), *La Memoria della scienza: Musei e collezioni dell' Università di Torino* (Turin: Fondazione CRT, 2003), 29–52.

Didi-Huberman, Georges, 'Viscosities and Survivals: Art History Put to the Test by the Material', in Roberta Panzanelli (ed.), *Ephemeral Bodies: Wax Sculpture and the Human Figure* (Los Angeles: Getty Publications, 2008), 154–69.

Ditchfield, Simon, 'Sanctity in Early Modern Italy', *Journal of Ecclesiastical History*, 47:1 (1996), 98–112.

Ditchfield, Simon, 'Il mondo della Riforma e della Controriforma', in Anna Benvenuti et al. (eds.), *Storia della santità nel cristianesimo occidentale* (Rome: Viella, 2005), 261–330.

Ditchfield, Simon, 'Tridentine Worship and the Cult of the Saints', in Ronnie Po-Chia Hsia (ed.), *The Cambridge History of Christianity*, vol. 6: *Reform and Expansion, 1500–1600* (Cambridge: Cambridge University Press, 2007), 201–24.

Ditchfield, Simon, 'Thinking with the Saints: Sanctity and Society in the Early Modern World', *Critical Inquiry*, 35:3 (2009), 552–84.

Donato, Clorinda, 'Esoteric Reason, Occult Science, and Radical Enlightenment: Seamless Pursuits in the Work and Networks of Raimondo di Sangro, the Prince of San Severo', *Philosophica*, 89 (2014), 179–237.

Donato, Maria Pia, 'Gli "strumenti" della politica di Benedetto XIV (1742–1759)', in Marina Caffiero and Giuseppe Monsagrati (eds.), 'Dall'erudizione alla politica: Giornali, giornalisti ed editori a Roma tra XVII e XX secolo', special issue, *Dimensioni e problemi della ricerca storica*, 1 (1997), 39–61.

Donato, Maria Pia, *Accademie romane: Una storia sociale, 1671–1824* (Naples: Edizioni Scientifiche Italiane, 2000).

Donato, Maria Pia, 'The Mechanical Medicine of a Pious Man of Science: Pathological Anatomy, Religion and Papal Patronage in Lancisi's *De subitaneis mortibus* (1707)', in Maria Pia Donato and Jill Kraye (eds.), *Conflicting Duties: Science, Medicine and Religion in Rome, 1550–1750* (London: Warburg Institute, 2009), 319–52.

Donato, Maria Pia, *Sudden Death: Medicine and Religion in Eighteenth-Century Rome* (Farnham: Ashgate, 2014).

Duden, Barbara, *The Woman Beneath the Skin: A Doctor's Patients in Eighteenth-Century Germany*, trans. Thomas Dunlap (Cambridge, MA: Harvard University Press, 1991).

Duffin, Jacalyn, 'The Doctor Was Surprised; or, How to Diagnose a Miracle', *Bulletin of the History of Medicine*, 81: 4 (2007), 699–729.

Duffin, Jacalyn, *Medical Miracles: Doctors, Saints, and Healing in the Modern World* (Oxford: Oxford University Press, 2009).

Dupré, Sven and Christoph Herbert Lüthy (eds.), *Silent Messengers: The Circulation of Material Objects of Knowledge in the Early Modern Low Countries* (Berlin: LIT Verlag, 2011).

Ebenstein, Joanna, 'Ode to an Anatomical Venus', *Women's Studies Quarterly*, 40:3/4 (2012), 346–52.

Emiliani, Andrea, 'Ritratti in cera del 700 bolognese', *Arte Figurativa*, 44 (1960), 28–35.

Engel, Laura, *Fashioning Celebrity: Eighteenth-Century British Actresses and Strategies for Image Making* (Columbus: Ohio State University Press, 2011).

Falabella, Susanna 'Ercole Lelli', *Dizionario Biografico degli Italiani*, vol. 64 (2005), 332–5.

Fanti, Mario, 'Sulla figura e l'opera di Marcello Oretti: Spigolature d'archivio per la storia dell'arte di Bologna', *Il Carrobbio*, 8 (1982), 125–43.

Fattori, Maria Teresa, 'Cronologia della vita e delle opera di Prospero Lambertini', in Maria Teresa Fattori (ed.), *Le fatiche di Benedetto XIV: Origine ed evoluzione dei trattati di Prospero Lambertini (1675–1758)* (Rome: Edizioni di Storia e Letteratura, 2011), lv–lxvi.

Fattori, Maria Teresa, 'Introduzione', in Maria Teresa Fattori (ed.), *Le fatiche di Benedetto XIV: Origine ed evoluzione dei trattati di Prospero Lambertini (1675–1758)* (Rome: Edizioni di Storia e Letteratura, 2011), xiii–liv.

Fattori, Maria Teresa (ed.), *Storia, medicina e diritto nei trattati di Prospero Lambertini-Benedetto XIV* (Rome: Edizioni di Storia e Letteratura, 2013).

Ferrari, Giovanna, 'Public Anatomy Lessons and the Carnival: The Anatomy Theatre of Bologna', trans. Chris Woodall, *Past & Present*, 117 (1987), 50–106.

Ferrer Benimeli, José Antonio, 'Origini, motivazioni ed effetti della condanna vaticana', in Gian Mario Cazzaniga (ed.), *Storia d'Italia, Annali 21: La massoneria* (Turin: Einaudi, 2006), 143–65.

Ferretti, Massimo, 'Il notomista e il canonico', in *I materiali dell'Istituto delle Scienze: Catalogo della mostra, Bologna, settembre-novembre 1979* (Bologna: CLUEB, 1979), 100–14.

Filippini, Nadia Maria, 'Levatrici e ostetricanti a Venezia tra Sette e Ottocento', *Quaderni storici*, 58 (1985), 149–80.

Filippini, Nadia Maria, 'The Church, the State and Childbirth: The Midwife in Italy During the Eighteenth Century', in Hilary Marland (ed.), *The Art of Midwifery: Early Modern Midwives in Europe* (London: Routledge, 1993), 152–75.

Filippini, Nadia Maria, *La nascita straordinaria: Tra madre e figlio la rivoluzione del taglio cesareo, sec. XVII–XIX* (Milan: Franco Angeli, 1995).

Filippini, Nadia Maria, 'Sanctuaire de la nature ou prison du fœtus': nature et corps féminin sous le combat sur la césarienne en France au XVIIIe siècle', in Lorraine Daston and Gianna Pomata (eds.), *The Faces of Nature in Enlightenment Europe* (Berlin: Berliner Wissenschafts-Verlag, 2003), 259–82.

Findlen, Paula, 'Science as a Career in Enlightenment Italy: The Strategies of Laura Bassi', *Isis*, 84:3 (1993), 441–69.

Findlen, Paula, *Possessing Nature: Museums, Collecting, and Scientific Culture in Early Modern Italy* (Berkeley: University of California Press, 1994).

Findlen, Paula, 'Translating the New Science: Women and the Circulation of Knowledge in Enlightenment Italy', *Configurations*, 3 (1995), 167–206.

Findlen, Paula, 'The Scientist's Body: The Nature of a Woman Philosopher in Enlightenment Italy', in Lorraine Daston and Gianna Pomata (eds.), *The Faces of Nature in Enlightenment Europe* (Berlin: BWV-Berliner Wissenschafts-Verlag, 2003), 211–36.

Findlen, Paula, 'Listening to the Archives: Searching for the Eighteenth-Century Women of Science', in Paola Govoni and Zelda Alice Franceschi (eds.), *Writing about Lives in Science: (Auto)biography, Gender, and Genre* (Göttingen: V&R Unipress, 2014), 87–116.

Findlen, Paula, Wendy Wassyng Roworth and Catherine M. Sama (eds.), *Italy's Eighteenth Century: Gender and Culture in the Age of the Grand Tour* (Stanford: Stanford University Press, 2009).

Finucci, Valeria, 'Maternal Imagination and Monstrous Birth: Tasso's *Gerusalemme Liberata*', in Valeria Finucci and Kevin Brownlee (eds.), *Generation and Degeneration: Tropes of Reproduction in Literature and History from Antiquity to Early Modern Europe* (Durham: Duke University Press, 2001), 41–77.

Fioni, Alessandra, 'L'Inquisizione a Bologna: Sortilegi e superstizioni popolari nei secoli XVII–XVIII', *Il Carrobbio*, 18 (1992), 141–50.

Fiorentini, Erna (ed.), *Observing Nature—Representing Experience: The Osmotic Dynamics of Romanticism, 1800–1850* (Berlin: Reimer Verlag, 2007).

Fischer, Jean-Louis, *L'art de faire de beaux enfants: Histoire de la callipèdie* (Paris: Albin Michel, 2009).

Fissell, Mary E., 'Hairy Women and Naked Truths: Gender and the Politics of Knowledge in Aristotle's *Masterpiece*', *The William and Mary Quarterly*, 60:1 (2003), 43–74.

Fissell, Mary E., *Vernacular Bodies: The Politics of Reproduction in Early Modern England* (Oxford: Oxford University Press, 2004).

Focaccia, Miriam, 'Anna Morandi Manzolini: Una donna fra arte e scienza', in Miriam Focaccia (ed.), *Anna Morandi Manzolini: Una donna fra arte e scienza; immagini, documenti, repertorio anatomico* (Florence: Leo S. Olschki, 2008), 1–73.

Focaccia, Miriam (ed.), *Anna Morandi Manzolini: Una donna fra arte e scienza; immagini, documenti, repertorio anatomico* (Florence: Leo S. Olschki, 2008).

Francovich, Carlo, *Storia della Massoneria in Italia: Dalle origini alla Rivoluzione francese* (Florence: La Nuova Italia, 1974).

French, Roger, *Dissection and Vivisection in the European Renaissance* (Aldershot: Ashgate, 1999).

Frutaz, Pietro Amato, 'Le principali edizioni e sinossi del *De servorum Dei beatificatione et beatorum canonizatione* di Benedetto XIV: Saggio per una bio-bibliografia critica', in Marco Cecchelli (ed.), *Benedetto XIV (Prospero Lambertini)*, vol. 1 (Cento: Centro Studi 'Girolamo Baruffaldi, 1981–2), 27–90.

Garms-Cornides, Elisabeth, 'Storia, politica e apologia in Benedetto XIV: Alle radici della reazione cattolica', in Philippe Koeppel (ed.), *Papes et papauté au XVIIIe siècle: VIe colloque franco-italien; Société française d'étude du XVIIIe siècle, Université de Savoie, Chambéry, 21–22 septembre 1995* (Paris: Champion, 1999), 145–61.

Gavrus, Delia, *Men of Strong Opinions: Identity, Self-Representation, and the Performance of Neurosurgery, 1919–1950* (PhD thesis, University of Toronto, 2011).

Geary, Patrick, 'Sacred Commodities: The Circulation of Medieval Relics', in Arjun Appadurai (ed.), *The Social Life of Things: Commodities in Cultural Perspective* (Cambridge: Cambridge University Press, 1988), 169–94.

Gelbart, Nina Rattner, *The King's Midwife: A History and Mystery of Madame Du Coudray* (Berkeley: University of California Press, 1998).

Gentilcore, David, *From Bishop to Witch: The System of the Sacred in Early Modern Terra d'Otranto* (Manchester: Manchester University Press, 1992).

Gentilcore, David, 'Contesting Illness in Early Modern Naples: Miracolati, Physicians and the Congregation of Rites', *Past & Present*, 148 (1995), 117–48.

Gentilcore, David, *Healers and Healing in Early Modern Italy* (Manchester: Manchester University Press, 1998).

Gentilcore, David, *Medical Charlatanism in Early Modern Italy* (Oxford: Oxford University Press, 2006).

Giacobini, Giacomo (ed.), *La memoria della scienza: Musei e collezioni dell' Università di Torino* (Turin: Fondazione CRT, 2003).

Giansiracusa, Paolo (ed.), *Vanitas vanitatum: Studi sulla ceroplastica di Gaetano Giulio Zumbo* (Syracuse: Lombardi, 1991).

Giarrizzo, Giuseppe (ed.), *I liberi muratori di Napoli nel secolo XVIII* (Naples: Società Napoletana di Storia Patria di Napoli, 1998).

Ginzburg, Carlo, 'Microhistory: Two or Three Things That I Know About It', trans. John Tedeschi and Anne C. Tedeschi, *Critical Inquiry*, 20:1 (1993), 10–35.

Giovannucci, Pierluigi, 'Dimostrare la santità per via giudiziaria', in Maria Teresa Fattori (ed.), *Storia, medicina e diritto nei trattati di Prospero Lambertini-Benedetto XIV* (Rome: Edizioni di Storia e Letteratura, 2013), 277–95.

Golinski, Jan, 'A Noble Spectacle: Phosphorus and the Public Cultures of Science in the Early Royal Society', *Isis*, 80:1 (1989), 11–39.

Golinski, Jan, *Science as Public Culture: Chemistry and Enlightenment in Britain, 1760–1820* (Cambridge: Cambridge University Press, 1992).

Gorce, Jean-Denys, *L'oeuvre médicale de Prospero Lambertini (Pape Benoît XIV)* (Bordeaux: Destout, 1915).

Gosden, Chris and Yvonne Marshall (eds.), 'The Cultural Biography of Objects', *World Archaeology*, 31:2 (1999), 169–78.

Gotor, Miguel, *I beati del papa: Santità, Inquisizione e obbedienza in età moderna* (Florence: Leo S. Olschki, 2002).

Grandi, Renzo et al. (eds.), *Presepi e terrecotte nei Musei Civici di Bologna* (Bologna: Nuova Alfa Editoriale, 1991).

Green, Monica, *Making Women's Medicine Masculine: The Rise of Male Authority in Pre-Modern Gynaecology* (Oxford: Oxford University Press, 2008).

Guerrini, Anita, 'Anatomists and Entrepreneurs in Early Eighteenth-Century London', *Journal of the History of Medicine and Allied Sciences*, 59:2 (2004), 219–39.

Guerrini, Anita, 'Alexander Monro Primus and the Moral Theatre of Anatomy', *The Eighteenth Century*, 47:1 (2007), 1–18.

Guerrini, Anita, 'Inside the Charnel House: The Display of Skeletons in Europe, 1500–1800', in Rina Knoeff and Robert Zwijnenberg (eds.), *The Fate of Anatomical Collections* (Farnham: Ashgate, 2015), 93–109.

Guerzoni, Guido Antonio, 'Uses and Abuses of Beeswax in the Early Modern Age: Two Apologues and a Taste', in Andrea Daninos (ed.), *Waxing Eloquent: Italian Portraits in Wax* (Milan: Officina Libraria, 2012), 43–59.

Hanson, Craig Ashley, *The English Virtuoso: Art, Medicine, and Antiquarianism in the Age of Empiricism* (Chicago: University of Chicago Press, 2009).

Harcourt, Glenn, 'Andreas Vesalius and the Anatomy of Antique Sculpture', in 'The Cultural Display of the Body,' special issue, *Representations*, 17 (1987), 28–61.

Harkness, Deborah E., 'Managing an Experimental Household: The Dees of Mortlake and the Practice of Natural Philosophy', *Isis*, 88:2 (1997), 247–62.

Haskell, Francis. *Patrons and Painters: Art and Society in Baroque Italy* (New Haven: Yale University Press, 1980).

Haskell, Francis and Nicholas Penny, *The Most Beautiful Statues: The Taste for Antique Sculpture, 1500–1900: An Exhibition Held at the Ashmolean Museum from 26 March to 10 May 1981* (Oxford: Ashmolean Museum, 1981).

Haskell, Francis and Nicholas Penny, *Taste and the Antique: The Lure of Classical Sculpture, 1500–1900*, 5th edn. (New Haven: Yale University Press, 1998 [1981]).

Haviland, Thomas N. and Lawrence Charles Parish, 'A Brief Account of the Use of Wax Models in the Study of Medicine', *Journal of the History of Medicine and Allied Sciences*, 25:1 (1970), 52–75.

Hendriksen, Marieke M.A., 'The Fabric of the Body: Textile in Anatomical Models and Preparations, ca. 1700–1900', *Histoire, médecine et santé*, 5 (2014), 21–31.

Hilaire-Pérez, Liliane, 'Technology as a Public Culture in the Eighteenth Century: The Artisans' Legacy', *History of Science*, 45:2 (2007), 135–53.

Hilaire-Pérez, Liliane, 'Technology, Curiosity and Utility in France and England in the Eighteenth Century', in Bernadette Bensaude-Vincent and Christine Blondel (eds.), *Science and Spectacle in the European Enlightenment* (Aldershot: Ashgate, 2008), 25–42.

Hills, Helen, 'Through a Glass Darkly: Material Holiness and the Treasury Chapel of San Gennaro in Naples', in Melissa Calaresu and Helen Hills (eds.), *New Approaches to Naples c.1500–c.1800: The Power of Place* (Farnham: Ashgate, 2013), 31–62.

Holmes, Megan, 'Ex-votos: Materiality, Memory and Cult', in Michael W. Cole and Rebecca E. Zorach (eds.), *The Idol in the Age of Art: Objects, Devotions and the Early Modern World* (Farnham: Ashgate, 2009), 159–82.

Hopwood, Nick, *Embryos in Wax: Models from the Ziegler Studio* (Cambridge: Whipple Museum of the History of Science/Bern: Institute of the History of Medicine, University of Bern, 2002).

Hopwood, Nick, 'Artist Versus Anatomist, Models against Dissection: Paul Zeiller of Munich and the Revolution of 1848', *Medical History*, 51:3 (2007), 279–308.

Huet, Marie-Hélène, *Monstrous Imagination* (Cambridge, MA: Harvard University Press, 1993).

Iliffe, Robert, 'Material Doubts: Hooke, Artisan Culture and the Exchange of Information in 1670s London', *The British Journal for the History of Science*, 28:3 (1995), 285–318.

Iliffe, Robert and Frances Willmoth, 'Astronomy and the Domestic Sphere: Margaret Flamsteed and Caroline Herschel as Assistant-Astronomers', in Lynette Hunter and Sarah Hutton (eds.), *Women, Science and Medicine, 1500–1700* (Stroud: Sutton Publishing, 1997), 235–65.

I materiali dell'Istituto delle Scienze: Catalogo della mostra, Bologna, settembre–novembre 1979 (Bologna: CLUEB, 1979).

Imbruglia, Girolamo (ed.), *Naples in the Eighteenth Century: The Birth and Death of a Nation State* (Cambridge: Cambridge University Press, 2000).

Inglis, Fred, *A Short History of Celebrity* (Princeton: Princeton University Press, 2010).

Jacobs, Fredrika H., 'Woman's Capacity to Create: The Unusual Case of Sofonisba Anguissola', *Renaissance Quarterly*, 47:1 (1994), 74–101.

Johns, Christopher M.S., *Papal Art and Cultural Politics: Rome in the Age of Clement XI* (Cambridge: Cambridge University Press, 1993).

Jones, Colin, 'The Great Chain of Buying: Medical Advertisement, the Bourgeois Public Sphere and the Origins of the French Revolution', *American Historical Review*, 101:1 (1996), 13–40.

Jordanova, Ludmilla, 'Gender, Generation and Science: William Hunter's Obstetrical Atlas', in William F. Bynum and Roy Porter (eds.), *William Hunter and the Eighteenth-Century Medical World* (Cambridge: Cambridge University Press, 1985), 385–412.

Jordanova, Ludmilla, *Sexual Visions: Images of Gender in Science and Medicine between the Eighteenth and Twentieth Centuries* (Madison: University of Wisconsin Press, 1989).

Jordanova, Ludmilla, 'Museums: Representing the Real?' in George Lewis Levine (ed.), *Realism and Representation: Essays on the Problem of Realism in Relation to Science, Literature, and Culture* (Madison: University of Wisconsin Press, 1993), 255–78.

Jordanova, Ludmilla, 'Medicine and Genres of Display', in Lynne Cooke and Peter Wollen (eds.), *Visual Display: Culture Beyond Appearances* (New York, The New Press, 1995), 202–17.

Jordanova, Ludmilla, *The Look of the Past: Visual and Material Evidence in Historical Practice* (Cambridge: Cambridge University Press, 2012).

Joy, Jody, 'Reinvigorating Object Biography: Reproducing the Drama of Object Lives', *World Archaeology*, 41:4 (2009), 540–56.

Keller, Eve, 'The Subject of Touch: Medical Authority in Early Modern Midwifery', in Elizabeth D. Harvey (ed.), *Sensible Flesh: On Touch in Early Modern Culture*. (Philadelphia: University of Pennsylvania Press, 2003), 62–80.

Kelly, Jason M., *The Society of Dilettanti: Archaeology and Identity in the British Enlightenment* (New Haven: Yale University Press, 2009).

Kemp, Martin, 'A Drawing for the Fabrica; and Some Thoughts Upon the Vesalius Muscle-Men', *Medical History*, 14:3 (1970), 277–88.

Kemp, Martin, '"The Mark of Truth": Looking and Learning in Some Anatomical Illustrations from the Renaissance and the Eighteenth Century', in William F. Bynum and Roy S. Porter (eds.), *Medicine and the Five Senses* (Cambridge: Cambridge University Press, 1993), 85–121.

Kemp, Martin, 'Style and Non-Style in Anatomical Illustration: From Renaissance Humanism to Henry Gray', *Journal of Anatomy*, 216:2 (2010), 192–208.

Kemp, Martin and Marina Wallace, *Spectacular Bodies: The Art and Science of the Human Body from Leonardo to Now* (Berkeley: University of California Press, 2000).

King, Helen, *Midwifery, Obstetrics and the Rise of Gynaecology: The Uses of a Sixteenth-Century Compendium* (Aldershot: Ashgate, 2007).

Klapisch-Zuber, Christiane, *Women, Family, and Ritual in Renaissance Italy*, trans. Lydia Cochrane (Chicago: University of Chicago Press, 1985).

Klein, Ursula and Emma C. Spary (eds.), *Materials and Expertise in Early Modern Europe: Between Market and Laboratory* (Chicago: University of Chicago Press, 2010).

Klestinec, Cynthia, 'A History of Anatomy Theatres in Sixteenth-Century Padua', *Journal of the History of Medicine and Allied Sciences*, 59:3 (2004), 375–412.

Klestinec, Cynthia, *Theaters of Anatomy: Students, Teachers, and Traditions of Dissection in Renaissance Venice* (Baltimore: Johns Hopkins University Press, 2011).

Knappett, Carl, 'Photographs, Skeuomorphs and Marionettes: Some Thoughts on Mind, Agency and Object', *Journal of Material Culture*, 7:1 (2002), 97–117.

Knoeff, Rina, 'The Visitor's View: Early Modern Tourism and the Polyvalence of Anatomical Exhibits', in Lissa Roberts (ed.), *Centres and Cycles of Accumulation in and around the Netherlands during the Early Modern Period* (Berlin: LIT Verlag, 2011), 155–76.

Knoeff, Rina, 'Touching Anatomy: On the Handling of Preparations in the Anatomical Cabinets of Frederik Ruysch (1638–1731)', *Studies in History and Philosophy of Science, Part C: Studies in History and Philosophy of Biological and Biomedical Sciences*, 49 (2015), 32–44.

Knoeff, Rina and Robert Zwijnenberg (eds.), *The Fate of Anatomical Collections* (Farnham: Ashgate, 2015).

Kopytoff, Igor, 'The Cultural Biography of Things: Commoditization as Process', in Arjun Appadurai (ed.), *The Social Life of Things: Commodities in Cultural Perspective* (Cambridge: Cambridge University Press, 1986), 64–91.

Kornmeier, Uta, 'Almost Alive: The Spectacle of Verisimilitude in Madame Tussaud's Waxworks', in Roberta Panzanelli (ed.), *Ephemeral Bodies: Wax Sculpture and the Human Figure* (Los Angeles: Getty Research Institute, 2008), 67–81.

Kornmeier, Uta, 'The Famous and the Infamous: Waxworks as Retailers of Renown', *International Journal of Cultural Studies*, 11:3 (2008), 276–88.

Kümin, Beat and Cornelie Usborne, 'At Home and in the Workplace: A Historical Introduction to the "Spatial Turn"', *History and Theory*, 52:3 (2013), 305–18.

Kusukawa, Sachiko, *Picturing the Book of Nature: Image, Text and Argument in Sixteenth-Century Human Anatomy and Medical Botany* (Chicago: University of Chicago Press, 2012).

La ceroplastica nella scienza e nell'arte: Atti del I Congresso Internazionale, Firenze, 3–7 giugno 1975, 2 vols. (Florence: Leo S. Olschki, 1977).

Lafuente, Antonio, 'Enlightenment in an Imperial Context: Local Science in the Late-Eighteenth-Century Hispanic World', *Osiris*, 15 (2000), 155–73.

Landes, Joan B., 'Wax Fibers, Wax Bodies and Moving Figures: Artifice and Nature in Eighteenth-Century Anatomy', in Roberta Panzanelli (ed.), *Ephemeral Bodies: Wax Sculpture and the Human Figure* (Los Angeles: Getty Research Institute, 2008), 41–65.

Lanzarini, Viviana, 'Un museo per la didattica e la sanità ostetrica', in Bortolotti et al., *Ars obstetricia bononiensis: Catalogo ed inventario del Museo Ostetrico Giovan Antonio Galli* (Bologna: CLUEB, 1988), 32–47.

Latour, Bruno, *Reassembling the Social: An Introduction to Actor-Network-Theory* (Oxford: Oxford University Press, 2005).

Lemire, Michel, *Artistes et mortels* (Paris: Chabaud, 1990).

Leong Elaine, 'Making Medicines in the Early Modern Household', *Bulletin of the History of Medicine*, 82:1 (2008), 145–68.

Leong Elaine and Alisha Rankin (eds.), *Secrets and Knowledge in Medicine and Science, 1500–1800* (Farnham: Ashgate, 2011).

Levi, Giovanni, 'On Microhistory', in Peter Burke (ed.), *New Perspectives on Historical Writing* (Cambridge: Polity Press, 2001 [1991]), 97–119.

Lieske, Pam, '"Made in Imitation of Real Women and Children": Obstetrical Machines in Eighteenth-Century Britain', in Andrew Mangham and Greta Depledge (eds.), *The Female Body in Medicine and Literature* (Liverpool: Liverpool University Press, 2011), 69–88.

Lightbown, R.W., 'Gaetano Giulio Zumbo—I: The Florentine Period', *The Burlington Magazine*, 106:740 (1964), 486–96.

Lightbown, R.W., 'Gaetano Giulio Zumbo—II: Genoa and France', *The Burlington Magazine*, 106:741 (1964), 563–9.

Lilti, Antoine, *Figures publiques: l'invention de la célébrité, 1750–1850* (Paris: Fayard, 2014).

Lincoln, Evelyn, 'Invention and Authorship in Early Modern Italian Visual Culture', *DePaul Law Review*, 52:4 (2003), 1093–119.

Long, Pamela O., *Openness, Secrecy, Authorship: Technical Arts and the Culture of Knowledge from Antiquity to the Renaissance* (Baltimore: Johns Hopkins University Press, 2001).

Loriga, Sabina, 'A Secret to Kill the King: Magic and Protection in Piedmont in the Eighteenth Century', in Edward Muir and Guido Ruggiero (eds.), *History from Crime*, trans. Corrada Biazzo Curry et al. (Baltimore: Johns Hopkins University Press, 1994), 88–109.

McClive, Cathy, 'The Hidden Truths of the Belly: The Uncertainties of Pregnancy in Early Modern Europe', *Social History of Medicine*, 15:2 (2002), 209–27.

McClive, Cathy, 'Blood and Expertise: The Trials of the Female Medical Expert in the Ancien-Regime Courtroom', *Bulletin of the History of Medicine*, 82:1 (2008), 86–108.

McTavish, Lianne, *Childbirth and the Display of Authority in Early Modern France* (Aldershot: Ashgate, 2005).

Maerker, Anna, 'The Anatomical Models of la Specola: Production, Uses and Reception', *Nuncius*, 21:2 (2006), 295–321.

Maerker, Anna, '"Turpentine Hides Everything": Autonomy and Organization in Anatomical Model Production for the State in Late Eighteenth-Century Florence', *History of Science*, 45:3 (2007), 257–86.

Maerker, Anna, *Model Experts: Wax Anatomies and Enlightenment in Florence and Vienna, 1775–1815* (Manchester: Manchester University Press, 2010).

Maerker, Anna, 'Florentine Anatomical Models and the Challenge of Medical Authority in Late Eighteenth-Century Vienna', *Studies in History and Philosophy of Science, Part C: Studies in History and Philosophy of Biological and Biomedical Sciences*, 43:3 (2012), 730–40.

Maerker, Anna, 'Anatomizing the Trade: Designing and Marketing Anatomical Models as Medical Technologies, c.1700–1900', *Technology and Culture*, 54:3 (2013), 531–62.

Mandressi, Rafael, *Le regard de l'anatomiste: Dissections et invention du corps en Occident* (Paris: Éditions du Seuil, 2003).

Margócsy, Dániel, 'Advertising Cadavers in the Republic of Letters: Anatomical Publications in the Early Modern Netherlands', *The British Journal for the History of Science*, 42:2 (2009), 187–210.

Margócsy, Dániel, 'A Museum of Wonders or a Cemetery of Corpses? The Commercial Exchange of Anatomical Collections in Early Modern Netherlands', in Sven Dupré and Christoph H. Lüthy (eds.), *Silent Messengers: The Circulation of Material Objects of Knowledge in the Early Modern Low Countries* (Berlin: LIT Verlag, 2011), 185–215.

Margócsy, Dániel, *Commercial Visions: Science, Trade, and Visual Culture in the Dutch Golden Age* (Chicago: University of Chicago Press, 2014).

Marland, Hilary (ed.), *The Art of Midwifery: Early Modern Midwives in Europe* (London: Routledge, 1993).

Martinotti, Giovanni, *L'insegnamento dell'anatomia in Bologna prima del secolo XIX* (Bologna: Cooperativa Tipografica Azzoguidi, 1911).

Martinotti, Giovanni, *Prospero Lambertini (Benedetto XIV) e lo studio dell'anatomia in Bologna* (Bologna: Cooperativa Tipografica Azzoguidi, 1911).

Massey, Lyle, 'On Waxes and Wombs: Eighteenth-Century Representations of the Gravid Uterus', in Roberta Panzanelli (ed.), *Ephemeral Bodies: Wax Sculpture and the Human Figure* (Los Angeles: Getty Research Institute, 2008), 83–105.

Mazzolini, Renato G., 'Plastic Anatomies and Artificial Dissections', in Soraya de Chadarevian and Nick Hopwood (eds.), *Models: The Third Dimension of Science* (Stanford: Stanford University Press, 2004), 43–70.

Mazzotti, Massimo, 'Maria Gaetana Agnesi: Mathematics and the Making of the Catholic Enlightenment', *Isis*, 92:4 (2001), 657–83.

Mazzotti, Massimo, *The World of Maria Gaetana Agnesi, Mathematician of God* (Baltimore: Johns Hopkins University Press, 2007).

Meli, Domenico Bertoloni, 'Mechanistic Pathology and Therapy in the Medical *Assayer* of Marcello Malpighi', *Medical History*, 51:2 (2007), 165–80.

Meli, Domenico Bertoloni, *Mechanism, Experiment, Disease: Marcello Malpighi and Seventeenth-Century Anatomy* (Baltimore: Johns Hopkins University Press, 2011).

Messbarger, Rebecca, 'Waxing Poetic: Anna Morandi Manzolini's Anatomical Sculptures', *Configurations*, 9:1 (2000), 65–97.

Messbarger, Rebecca, 'Re-Membering a Body of Work: Anatomist and Anatomical Designer Anna Morandi Manzolini', *Studies in Eighteenth Century Culture*, 32:1 (2003), 123–54.

Messbarger, Rebecca, *The Lady Anatomist: The Life and Work of Anna Morandi Manzolini* (Chicago: University of Chicago Press, 2010).

Messbarger, Rebecca, 'The Re-Birth of Venus in Florence's Royal Museum of Physics and Natural History', *Journal of the History of Collections*, 25:2 (2013), 195–215.

Messbarger, Rebecca and Paula Findlen (eds.), *The Contest for Knowledge: Debates over Women's Learning in Eighteenth-Century Italy* (Chicago: University of Chicago Press, 2005).

Mole, Tom, 'Lord Byron and the End of Fame', *International Journal of Cultural Studies*, 11:3 (2008), 343–61.

Momigliano, Arnaldo, 'Ancient History and the Antiquarian', *Journal of the Warburg and Courtauld Institutes*, 13:3/4 (1950), 285–315.

Mommertz, Monika, 'The Invisible Economy of Science: A New Approach to the History of Gender and Astronomy at the Eighteenth-Century Berlin Academy of Sciences', trans. Julia Baker, in Judith P. Zins'ser (ed.), *Men, Women, and the Birthing of Modern Science* (DeKalb: Northern Illinois University Press, 2005), 159–78.

Montroni, Giovanni, 'The Court: Power Relations and Forms of Social Life', in Girolamo Imbruglia (ed.), *Naples in the Eighteenth Century: The Birth and Death of a Nation State* (Cambridge: Cambridge University Press, 2000), 22–43.

Morello, Giovanni, 'Il "Museo Cristiano" di Benedetto XIV nella Biblioteca Vaticana', in Marco Cecchelli (ed.), *Benedetto XIV (Prospero Lambertini): Convegno internazionale di studi storici, sotto il patrocinio dell'archidiocesi di Bologna: Cento, 6–9 Dicembre 1979*, vol. 2 (Cento: Centro studi 'Girolamo Baruffaldi', 1981–2), 1119–51.

Morello, Giovanni, 'La creazione del Museo Cristiano', in Donatella Biagi Maino (ed.), *Benedetto XIV e le arti del disegno: Convegno internazionale di studi di storia dell'arte, Bologna 28–30 novembre 1994* (Rome: Quasar, 1998), 263–75.

Moser, Stephanie, 'Making Expert Knowledge through the Image: Connections Between Antiquarian and Early Modern Scientific Illustration', *Isis*, 105:1 (2008), 58–99.

Mostra del Settecento bolognese (Bologna: Mareggiani, 1935).

Muir, Edward and Guido Ruggiero (eds.), *Microhistory and the Lost Peoples of Europe: Selections from Quaderni Storici* (Baltimore: Johns Hopkins University Press, 1991).

Murard, Ambre, *La collection du médicin-chirurgien Giovan Antonio Galli à Bologne* (Paris: Mémoire de maîtrise en Langue et Civilisation italiennes, Université de Paris III, 1997).

Murard, Ambre, 'La rappresentazione del corpo femminile nell'ostetricia settecentesca', in Claudia Pancino (ed.), *Corpi: Storia, metafore, rappresentazioni fra Medioevo ed età contemporanea* (Venice: Marsilio, 2000), 41–54.

Musacchio, Jacqueline Marie, *The Art and Ritual of Childbirth in Renaissance Italy* (New Haven: Yale University Press, 1999).

Naddeo, Barbara Ann, 'Cultural Capitals and Cosmopolitanism in Eighteenth-Century Italy: The Historiography and Italy on the Grand Tour', *Journal of Modern Italian Studies*, 10:2 (2005), 183–99.

Nappi, Eduardo, 'La famiglia, il palazzo e la cappella dei principi di Sansevero', *Revue Internationale d'Histoire de la Banque*, 11 (1975), 100–61.

Neveu, Bruno, *Érudition et religion aux XVIIe et XVIIIe siècles* (Paris: Albin Michel, 1994).

Niccoli, Ottavia, *La vita religiosa nell'Italia moderna: Secoli XV–XVIII* (Rome: Carocci, 1998).

Nussbaum, Felicity, *Rival Queens: Actresses, Performance, and the Eighteenth-Century British Theater* (Philadelphia: University of Pennsylvania Press, 2010).

O'Malley, Michelle and Evelyn S. Welch (eds.), *The Material Renaissance* (Manchester: Manchester University Press, 2007).

Olmi, Giuseppe, *L'inventario del mondo: Catalogazione della natura e luoghi del sapere nella prima età moderna* (Bologna: Il Mulino, 1992).

Ottani, Vittoria and Gabriella Giuliani-Piccari, 'L'opera di Anna Morandi Manzolini nella ceroplastica anatomica bolognese', in *Alma Mater Studiorum: La presenza femminile dal XVIII al XX secolo; Ricerche sul rapporto Donna/Cultura universitaria nell'Ateneo Bolognese* (Bologna: CLUEB 1988), 81–103.

Pagden, Anthony, *Spanish Imperialism and the Political Imagination: Studies in European and Spanish-American Social and Political Theory, 1513–1830*, 2nd edn. (New Haven: Yale University Press, 1998).

Palazzi, Maura, 'Solitudini femminili e patrilignaggio: Nubili e vedove fra Sette e Ottocento', in Marzio Barbagli and David I. Kertzer (eds.), *Storia della famiglia italiana, 1750–1950* (Bologna: Il Mulino, 1992), 129–58.

Palmer, Richard, 'Medicine at the Papal Court in the Sixteenth Century', in Vivian Nutton (ed.), *Medicine at the Courts of Europe, 1500–1837* (London: Routledge, 1990), 49–78.

Pancino, Claudia, *Il bambino e l'acqua sporca: Storia dell'assistenza al parto dalle mammane alle ostetriche (secoli XVI–XIX)* (Milan: Franco Angeli, 1984).

Pancino, Claudia, *Voglie materne: Storia di una credenza* (Bologna: CLUEB, 1996).

Pancino, Claudia, 'Questioni di genere nell'anatomia plastica del Settecento bolognese', *Studi tanatologici*, 2 (2007), 317–32.

Pancino, Claudia, 'Malati, medici, mammane, saltimbanchi: Malattia e cura nella Bologna d'età moderna', in Adriano Prosperi (ed.), *Storia di Bologna*, vol. 3: *Bologna nell'età moderna (secoli XVI–XVIII)*, part II: *Cultura, istituzioni culturali, Chiesa e vita religiosa* (Bologna: Bononia University Press, 2008), 719–24.

Pancino, Claudia and Jean d' Yvoire, *Formato nel segreto: Nascituri e feti fra immagini e immaginario dal XVI al XXI secolo* (Rome: Carocci, 2006).

Panzanelli, Roberta, 'Compelling Presence: Wax Effigies in Renaissance Florence', in Roberta Panzanelli (ed.), *Ephemeral Bodies: Wax Sculpture and the Human Figure*. Los Angeles: Getty Research Institute, 2008, 13–39.

Panzanelli, Roberta (ed.), *Ephemeral Bodies: Wax Sculpture and the Human Figure* (Los Angeles: Getty Research Institute, 2008).

Panzanelli, Roberta, 'Introduction: The Body in Wax, the Body of Wax', in Roberta Panzanelli (ed.), *Ephemeral Bodies: Wax Sculpture and the Human Figure* (Los Angeles: Getty Research Institute, 2008), 1–12.

Park, Katharine, 'The Criminal and the Saintly Body: Autopsy and Dissection in Renaissance Italy', *Renaissance Quarterly*, 47:1 (1994), 1–33.

Park, Katharine, 'The Life of the Corpse: Division and Dissection in Late Medieval Europe', *Journal of the History of Medicine and Allied Sciences*, 50:1 (1995), 111–32.

Park, Katharine, 'Impressed Images: Reproducing Wonders', in Peter Galison and Caroline A. Jones (eds.), *Picturing Science, Producing Art* (New York: Routledge, 1998), 254–71.

Park, Katharine, 'Relics of a Fertile Heart: The "Autopsy" of Clare of Montefalco', in Anne L. McClanan and Karen Rosoff Encarnación (eds.), *The Material Culture of Sex, Procreation, and Marriage in Premodern Europe* (New York: Palgrave, 2002), 115–33.

Park, Katharine, *Secrets of Women: Gender, Generation and the Origins of Human Dissection* (New York: Zone Books, 2006).

Pastor, Ludwig Freiherr von, *The History of the Popes: From the Close of the Middle Ages; Drawn from the Secret Archives of the Vatican and Other Original Sources*, trans. E.F. Peeler, vol. 35 (London: Routledge and Kegan Paul, 1949).

Pastore, Alessandro, *Il medico in tribunale: La perizia medica nella procedura penale d'antico regime (secoli XVI–XVIII)* (Bellinzona: Edizioni Casagrande, 2004 [1998]).

Peiffer, Jeanne, 'L'âme, le cerveau et les mains: l'autoportrait d'Anna Morandi', in Thérèse Chotteau et al., *Rencontres entre artistes et mathématiciennes: Toutes un peu les autres* (Paris: L'Harmattan, 2001), 72–7.

Peiffer, Jeanne, 'La recherche dans et hors ses murs', *Cahiers art et science*, 7 (2002), 47–63.

Peiffer, Jeanne and Véronique Roca, 'Corps moulés, corps façonnés: Autoportraits de femmes', in Thérèse Chotteau et al., *Rencontres entre artistes et mathématiciennes: Toutes un peu les autres* (Paris: L'Harmattan, 2001), 56–91.

Pilbeam, Pamela, *Madame Tussaud and the History of Waxworks* (London: Hambledon & London, 2003).

Pimentel, Juan, 'The Iberian Vision: Science and Empire in the Framework of a Universal Monarchy, 1500–1800', in Roy MacLeod (ed.), *Nature and Empire: Science and the Colonial Enterprise, Osiris*, 15 (2000), 17–30.

Pinto-Correia, Clara, *The Ovary of Eve: Egg and Sperm and Preformation* (Chicago: University of Chicago Press, 1997).

Plongeron, Bernard, 'Recherches sur l' "Aufklärung" catholique en Europe occidentale (1770–1830)', *Revue d'histoire moderne et contemporaine*, 16:4 (1969), 555–605.

Plongeron, Bernard, 'Questions pour l'Aufklärung catholique en Italie', *Il Pensiero Politico: Rivista di Storia delle Idee Politiche e Sociali*, 3:1 (1970), 30–58.

Pointon, Marcia, 'Casts, Imprints and the Deathliness of Things: Artefacts at the Edge', *Art Bulletin*, 96 (2014), 170–95.

Pomata, Gianna, 'Barbieri e comari', in *Cultura popolare nell'Emilia Romagna: Medicina, erbe e magia* (Milan: Silvana Editoriale, 1981), 161–83.

Pomata, Gianna, *Contracting a Cure: Patients, Healers, and the Law in Early Modern Bologna*, trans. Gianna Pomata with the assistance of Rosmarie Foy and Anna Taraboletti-Segre (Baltimore: Johns Hopkins University Press, 1998).

Pomata, Gianna, 'Family and Gender', in John A. Marino (ed.), *Early Modern Italy: 1550–1796* (Oxford: Oxford University Press, 2002), 69–86.

Pomata, Gianna, 'Malpighi and the Holy Body: Medical Experts and Miraculous Evidence in Seventeenth-Century Italy', *Renaissance Studies*, 21:4 (2007), 568–86.

Pomata, Gianna, 'Observation Rising: Birth of an Epistemic Genre, 1500–1650', in Lorraine Daston and Elizabeth Lunbeck (eds.), *Histories of Scientific Observation* (Chicago: University of Chicago Press, 2011), 45–80.

Pomata, Gianna, 'A Word of the Empirics: The Ancient Concept of Observation and Its Recovery in Early Modern Medicine', *Annals of Science*, 68:1 (2011), 1–25.

Pomata, Gianna and Nancy G. Siraisi (eds.), *Historia: Empiricism and Erudition in Early Modern Europe* (Cambridge, MA: MIT Press, 2005).

Pratt, Mary Louise, *Imperial Eyes: Travel Writing and Transculturation*, 2nd edn. (London: Routledge, 2008).

Prodi, Paolo, 'Carità e galateo: La figura di papa Lambertini nelle lettere al marchese Paolo Magnani (1743–1748)', in Marco Cecchelli (ed.), *Benedetto XIV (Prospero Lambertini): Convegno internazionale di studi storici, sotto il patrocinio dell'archidiocesi di Bologna, Cento, 6–9 Dicembre 1979*, vol. 1 (Cento: Centro studi 'Girolamo Baruffaldi', 1981–2), 445–71.

Prodi, Paolo, *The Papal Prince: One Body and Two Souls. The Papal Monarchy in Early Modern Europe*, trans. Susan Haskins (Cambridge: Cambridge University Press, 1987).

Prodi, Paolo and Maria Teresa Fattori (eds.), *Le lettere di Benedetto XIV al marchese Paolo Magnani* (Rome: Herder, 2011).

Prosperi, Adriano, *Tribunali della coscienza: Inquisitori, confessori, missionari* (Turin: Einaudi, 1996).

Prosperi, Adriano, 'Battesimo e identità tra Medio evo e prima età moderna', in Peter von Moos (ed.) *Unverwechselbarkeit: Persönliche Identität und Identifikation in der vormodernen Gesellschaft* (Cologne: Böhlau, 2004), 325–54.

Prosperi, Adriano (ed.), *Storia di Bologna*, vol. 3, *Bologna nell'età moderna (secoli XVI–XVIII*, part II: *Cultura, Istituzioni culturali, Chiesa e vita religiosa* (Bologna: Bononia University Press, 2008).

Raj, Kapil, 'Introduction: Circulation and Locality in Early Modern Science', in Kapil Raj and Mary Terrall (eds.), 'Circulation and Locality in Early Modern Science', special issue, *The British Journal for the History of Science*, 43:4 (2010), 513–17.

Rankin, Alisha, *Panaceia's Daughters: Noblewomen as Healers in Early Modern Germany* (Chicago: University of Chicago Press, 2013).

Rao, Anna Maria, *Il Regno di Napoli nel Settecento* (Naples: Guida, 1984).

Rao, Anna Maria, 'La Massoneria nel Regno di Napoli', in Gian Mario Cazzaniga (ed.), *Storia d'Italia, Annali 21*: *La massoneria* (Turin: Einaudi, 2006), 513–42.

Ray, Meredith K., *Daughters of Alchemy*: *Women and Scientific Culture in Early Modern Italy* (Cambridge, MA: Harvard University Press, 2015).

Redford, Bruce, *Dilettanti: The Antic and the Antique in Eighteenth-Century England* (Los Angeles: Getty Research Institute, 2008).

Riccomini, Eugenio, *Mostra della scultura bolognese del Settecento*: *Catalogo* (Bologna: Tamari, 1966).

Roberts, Lissa, Simon Schaffer, and Peter Robert Dear (eds.), *The Mindful Hand: Inquiry and Invention from the Late Renaissance to Early Industrialization* (Amsterdam: Koninkliijke Nederlandse Akademie van Wetenschappen, 2007).

Röhrl, Boris, *History and Bibliography of Artistic Anatomy: Didactics for Depicting the Human Figure* (Hildesheim: G. Olms, 2000).

Roodenburg, Herman W., 'The Maternal Imagination: The Fears of Pregnant Women in Seventeenth-Cenatury Holland', *Journal of Social History*, 21:4 (1988), 701–16.

Rosa, Mario, 'Benedetto XIV', in *Dizionario biografico degli italiani* (*DBI*), vol. 8 (Rome: Istituto della Enciclopedia Italiana, 1966), 393–408.

Rosa, Mario, *Riformatori e ribelli nel '700 religioso italiano* (Bari: Edizioni Dedalo, 1969).

Rosa, Mario, 'Introduzione all'Aufklärung cattolica in Italia', in Mario Rosa (ed.), *Cattolicesimo e lumi nel Settecento italiano* (Rome: Herder, 1981), 1–47.

Rosa, Mario, *Settecento religioso: Politica della ragione e religione del cuore* (Venice: Marsilio, 1999).

Rosa, Mario, 'The Catholic *Aufklärung* in Italy', in Ulrich L. Lehner and Michael Printy (eds.), *A Companion to the Catholic Enlightenment in Europe* (Leiden: Brill, 2010), 215–50.

Rossi, Paolo A., 'O' principe "haravec": le machine anatomiche e il sangue di San Gennaro', in Rossi and Ida Li Vigni (eds.), *I veli di pietra: Raimondo di Sangro* (Genoa: Nova Scripta Edizioni, 2011), 20–61.

Saccenti, Riccardo, 'La lunga genesi dell'opera sulle canonizzazioni', in Maria Teresa Fattori (ed.), *Le fatiche di Benedetto XIV* (Rome: Edizioni di Storia e Letteratura, 2011), 3–47.

Saccenti, Riccardo, 'Le fonti del *De Servorum Dei* e il loro uso nel trattato lambertiniano', in Maria Teresa Fattori (ed.), *Storia, medicina e diritto nei trattati di Prospero Lambertini-Benedetto XIV* (Rome: Edizioni di Storia e Letteratura, 2013), 247–75.

Sallmann, Jean-Michel, *Naples et ses saints à l'âge baroque (1540–1750)* (Paris: Presses Universitaires de France, 1994).

Sampolo, Luigi, *La R. Accademia degli Studi di Palermo* (Palermo: Tipografia dello Statuto, 1888).

San Juan, Rose Marie, 'The Horror of Touch: Anna Morandi's Wax Models of Hands', *Oxford Art Journal*, 34:3 (2011), 433–47.

San Juan, Rose Marie, 'Dying Not to See: Anna Morandi's Wax Model of the Sense of Sight', *Oxford Art Journal*, 36:1 (2013), 39–54.

Sanlorenzo, Olimpia, *L'insegnamento di ostetricia nell'Università di Bologna* (Bologna: Alma Mater Studiorum Saecularia Nona, 1988).

Santing, Catrien, '*Tirami sù*: Pope Benedict XIV and the Beatification of the Flying Saint Giuseppe Da Copertini', in Andrew Cunningham and Ole Peter Grell (eds.), *Medicine and Religion in Enlightenment Europe* (Aldershot: Ashgate, 2007), 79–100.

Sarti, Raffaella, *Europe at Home: Family and Material Culture, 1500–1800*, trans. Allan Cameron (New Haven: Yale University Press, 2002).

Sawday, Jonathan, *The Body Emblazoned: Dissection and the Human Body in Renaissance Culture* (London: Routledge, 1995).

Schaffer, Simon, 'Natural Philosophy and Public Spectacle in the Eighteenth Century', *History of Science*, 21:1 (1983), 1–43.

Schaffer, Simon, 'Experimenters' Techniques, Dyers' Hands, and the Electric Planetarium', *Isis*, 88:3 (1997), 456–83.

Schaffer, Simon, 'Regeneration: The Body of Natural Philosophers in Restoration England', in Christopher Lawrence and Steven Shapin (eds.), *Science Incarnate: Historical Embodiments of Natural Knowledge* (Chicago: University of Chicago Press, 1998), 83–120.

Schaffer, Simon, 'Enlightened Automata', in William Clark, Jan Golinski, and Simon Schaffer (eds.), *The Sciences in Enlightened Europe* (Chicago: University of Chicago Press, 1999), 126–65.

Schaffer, Simon, 'Easily Cracked: Scientific Instruments in States of Disrepair', *Isis*, 102:4 (2011), 706–17.

Schaffer, Simon, Lissa Roberts, Kapil Raj, and James Delbourgo (eds.), *The Brokered World: Go-Betweens and Global Intelligence, 1770–1820* (Sagamore Beach, MA: Science History Publications, 2009).

Schlosser, Julius von, 'History of Portraiture in Wax', in Roberta Panzanelli (ed.), *Ephemeral Bodies: Wax Sculpture and the Human Figure* (Los Angeles: Getty Publications, 2008), 171–314.

Schnalke, Thomas, *Diseases in Wax: The History of the Medical Moulage*, trans. Kathy Spatschek (Carol Stream, IL: Quintessence Publishing, 1995).

Schnalke, Thomas, 'Casting Skin: Meanings for Doctors, Artists, and Patients', in Soraya de Chadarevian and Nick Hopwood (eds.), *Models: The Third Dimension of Science* (Stanford: Stanford University Press, 2004), 207–41.

Schnapp, Alain, 'Introduction: Neapolitan Effervescence', trans. Mark Weir, *Journal of the History of Collections*, 19:2 (2007), 161–4.

Schutte, Anne Jacobson, *Aspiring Saints: Pretense of Holiness, Inquisition, and Gender in the Republic of Venice, 1618–1750* (Baltimore: Johns Hopkins University Press, 2001).

Secord, Anne, 'Botany on a Plate: Pleasure and the Power of Pictures in Promoting Early Ninenteenth-Century Scientific Knowledge', *Isis*, 93:1 (2002), 28–57.

Shapin, Steven, 'The House of Experiment in Seventeenth-Century England', *Isis*, 79:3 (1988), 373–404.

Shaw, James and Evelyn S. Welch, *Making and Marketing Medicine in Renaissance Florence* (Amsterdam: Rodopi, 2011).

Sibum, Heinz Otto, 'Reworking the Mechanical Value of Heat: Instruments of Precision and Gestures of Accuracy in Early Victorian England', *Studies in History and Philosophy of Science*, 26:1 (1995), 73–106.

Simon, Jonathan, 'The Theatre of Anatomy: The Anatomical Preparations of Honoré Fragonard', *Eighteenth-Century Studies*, 36:1 (2002), 63–79.

Siraisi, Nancy G., 'History, Antiquarianism, and Medicine: The Case of Girolamo Mercuriale', *Journal of the History of Ideas*, 64:2 (2003), 231–51.

Siraisi, Nancy G., *History, Medicine, and the Traditions of Renaissance Learning* (Ann Arbor: University of Michigan Press, 2007).

Smith, Pamela H., *The Body of the Artisan: Art and Experience in the Scientific Revolution* (Chicago: University of Chicago Press, 2004).

Smith, Pamela H. and Tonny Beentjes, 'Nature and Art, Making and Knowing: Reconstructing Sixteenth-Century Life-Casting Techniques', *Renaissance Quarterly*, 63:1 (2010), 128–79.

Smith, Pamela H. and Paula Findlen (eds.), *Merchants and Marvels: Commerce, Science, and Art in Early Modern Europe* (New York: Routledge, 2002).

Smith, Pamela H. and Benjamin Schmidt (eds.), *Making Knowledge in Early Modern Europe: Practices, Objects, and Texts, 1400–1800* (Chicago: University of Chicago Press, 2007).

Spary, Emma C., 'Scientific Symmetries', *History of Science*, 42 (2004), 1–46.

Stephens, Elizabeth, *Anatomy as Spectacle: Public Exhibitions of the Body from 1700 to the Present* (Liverpool: Liverpool University Press, 2011).

Stevens, Scott Manning, 'Sacred Heart and Secular Brain', in David Hillman and Carla Mazzio (eds.), *The Body in Parts: Fantasies of Corporeality in Early Modern Europe* (New York: Routledge, 1997), 263–82.

Stewart, Larry, *The Rise of Public Science: Rhetoric, Technology, and Natural Philosophy in Newtonian Britain* (Cambridge: Cambridge University Press, 1992).

Stewart, Larry, 'The Laboratory, the Workshop and the Theatre of Experiment', in Bernadette Bensaude-Vincent and Christine Blondel (eds.), *Science and Spectacle in the European Enlightenment* (Aldershot: Ashgate, 2008), 11–24.

Stewart, Larry and Paul Weindling, 'Philosophical Threads: Natural Philosophy and Public Experiment among the Weavers of Spitalfields', *The British Journal for the History of Science*, 28:1 (1995), 37–62.

Stolberg, Michael, 'A Woman Down to Her Bones: The Anatomy of Sexual Difference in the Sixteenth and Early Seventeenth Centuries', *Isis*, 94:2 (2003), 274–99.

Strocchia, Sharon T., *Death and Ritual in Renaissance Florence* (Baltimore: Johns Hopkins University Press, 1992).

Strocchia, Sharon T. (ed.), 'Women and Healthcare in Early Modern Europe', special issue, *Renaissance Studies*, 28:4 (2014), 579–96.

Sutton, Geoffrey V., *Science for a Polite Society: Gender, Culture, and the Demonstration of Enlightenment* (Boulder: Westview Press, 1995).

Sweet, Rosemary, *Cities and the Grand Tour: The British in Italy, c.1690–1820* (Cambridge: Cambridge University Press, 2012).

Taddia, Elena, 'Corpi, cadaveri, chirurghi stranieri e ceroplastiche: L'Ospedale di Pammatone a Genova tra Sei e Settecento', *Mediterranea*, 6:15 (2009), 157–94.

Terpstra, Nicholas, *Lay Confraternities and Civic Religion in Renaissance Bologna* (Cambridge: Cambridge University Press, 1995).

Terpstra, Nicholas, *Abandoned Children of the Italian Renaissance: Orphan Care in Florence and Bologna* (Baltimore: Johns Hopkins University Press, 2005).

Terpstra, Nicholas (ed.), *The Art of Executing Well: Rituals of Execution in Renaissance Italy* (Kirksville, MO: Truman State University Press, 2008).

Terrall, Mary, 'Gendered Spaces, Gendered Audiences: Inside and Outside the Paris Academy of Sciences', *Configurations*, 3:2 (1995), 207–32.

Terrall, Mary, *The Man Who Flattened the Earth: Maupertuis and the Sciences in the Enlightenment* (Chicago: University of Chicago Press, 2002).

Terrall, Mary, 'The Uses of Anonymity in the Age of Reason', in Mario Biagioli and Peter Galison (eds.), *Scientific Authorship: Credit and Intellectual Property in Science* (London: Routledge, 2003), 91–112.

Terrall, Mary, 'Public Science in the Enlightenment', *Modern Intellectual History*, 2:2 (2005), 265–76.

Terrall, Mary, 'Material Impressions: Conception, Sensibility, and Inheritance', in Helen Deutsch and Mary Terrall (eds.), *Vital Matters: Eighteenth-Century Ideas about Conception, Life and Death* (Toronto: University of Toronto Press, 2012), 109–29.

Mary Terrall, *Catching Nature in the Act: Réaumur and the Practice of Natural History in the Eighteenth Century* (Chicago: University of Chicago Press, 2014).

Thomas, Nicholas, *Entangled Objects: Exchange, Material Culture, and Colonialism in the Pacific* (Cambridge, MA: Harvard University Press, 1991).

Tillyard, Stella, 'Celebrity in 18th-Century London', *History Today*, 55:6 (2005), 20–7.

Toscano, Maria, 'The Figure of the Naturalist-Antiquary in the Kingdom of Naples: Giuseppe Giovene (1753–1837) and His Contemporaries', trans. Mark Weir, *Journal of the History of Collections*, 19:2 (2007), 225–37.

Traub, Valerie, 'The Nature of Norms in Early Modern England: Anatomy, Cartography, *King Lear*', *South Central Review*, 26:1/2 (2009), 42–81.

Trentmann, Frank, 'Materiality in the Future of History: Things, Practices, and Politics', special issue on Material Culture, *Journal of British Studies*, 48:2 (2009), 283–307.

Tripaldi, Agostino, *Le cere anatomiche bolognesi del Settecento tra arte e scienza* (Tesi di Laurea, Storia della Scienza, Università di Bologna, 1997–8).

Trivellato, Francesca, 'Is There a Future for Italian Microhistory in the Age of Global History?', *California Italian Studies*, 2:1 (2011), 1–26.

Tumidei, Stefano, 'Terrecotte bolognesi di Sei e Settecento: Collezionismo, produzione artistica, consumo devozionale', in Renzo Grandi (ed.), *Presepi e terrecotte nei Musei Civici di Bologna* (Bologna: Nuova Alfa Editoriale, 1991), 21–51.

Valverde, Nuria, 'Small Parts: Crisóstomo Martínez (1638–1694), Bone Histology, and the Visual Making of Body Wholeness', *Isis*, 100:3 (2009), 45–80.

Vassena, Elio, *La fortuna dei ceroplasti bolognesi del Settecento* (Tesi di Laurea, Storia della Critica d'Arte, Università di Bologna, 1996–7).

Venturi, Franco, *Settecento riformatore: Da Muratori a Beccaria*, 2nd edn., vol. 1 (Turin: Einaudi, 1998 [1969]).

Venturi, Giampaolo, 'Benedetto XIV e le collezioni universitarie di Bologna', in Marco Cecchelli (ed.), *Benedetto XIV (Prospero Lambertini): Convegno internazionale di studi storici, sotto il patrocinio dell'Archidiocesi di Bologna, Cento, 6–9 Dicembre 1979*, vol. 1 (Cento: Centro studi 'Girolamo Baruffaldi', 1981–2), 1197–208.

Vermeir, Koen, 'Openness versus Secrecy? Historical and Historiographical Remarks', in Koen Vermeir and Dániel Margócsy (eds.), 'States of Secrecy', special issue, *The British Journal for the History of Science*, 45:2 (2012), 165–88.

Vermeir, Koen and Dániel Margócsy (eds.), 'States of Secrecy', special issue, *The British Journal for the History of Science*, 45:2 (2012).

Vidal, Fernando, 'Brains, Bodies, Selves, and Science: Anthropologies of Identity and the Resurrection of the Body', *Critical Inquiry*, 28:4 (2002), 930–74.

Vidal, Fernando, 'Miracles, Science, and Testimony in Post-Tridentine Saint-Making', *Science in Context*, 20:3 (2007), 481–508.

Vidal, Fernando, 'Prospero Lambertini's "On the Imagination and Its Powers"', in Maria Teresa Fattori (ed.), *Storia, medicina e diritto nei trattati di Prospero Lambertini-Benedetto XIV* (Rome: Edizioni di Storia e Letteratura, 2013), 297–318.

Vila, Anne C. (ed.), *A Cultural History of the Senses in the Age of Enlightenment, 1650–1800* (New York: Bloomsbury Academic, 2014).

Von Düring, Monika, Georges Didi-Huberman, and Marta Poggesi, *Encyclopaedia Anatomica: A Complete Collection of Anatomical Waxes* (Cologne: Taschen, 1999).

Werrett, Simon, 'Healing the Nation's Wounds: Royal Ritual and Experimental Philosophy in Restoration England', *History of Science*, 38 (2000), 377–99.

Werrett, Simon, *Fireworks: Pyrotechnic Arts and Sciences in European History* (Chicago: University of Chicago Press, 2010).

Werrett, Simon, 'Recycling in Early Modern Science', *The British Journal for the History of Science*, 46:4 (2013), 627–46.

Wilson, Adrian, *The Making of Man-Midwifery: Childbirth in England, 1660–1770* (London: UCL Press, 1995).

Wilson, Philip K., '"Out of Sight, out of Mind?": The Daniel Turner-James Blondel Dispute over the Power of the Maternal Imagination', *Annals of Science*, 49:1 (1992), 63–85.

Wilton, Andrew and Ilaria Bignamini (eds.), *Grand Tour: The Lure of Italy in the Eighteenth Century* (London: Tate Gallery Publishing, 1996).

Zanotti, Andrea, 'Tra terra e cielo: Prospero Lambertini e i processi di beatificazione', in Andrea Zanotti (ed.), *Prospero Lambertini: Pastore della sua città, pontefice della cristianità* (Bologna: Minerva, 2004), 233–53.

Zarri, Gabriella, *Le sante vive: Profezie di corte e devozione femminile tra '400 e '500* (Turin: Rosenberg & Sellier, 1990).

Zarri, Gabriella (ed.), *Finzione e santità tra medioevo ed età moderna* (Turin: Rosenberg & Sellier, 1991).

Zemon Davis, Natalie, *The Gift in Sixteenth-Century France* (Oxford: Oxford University Press, 2000).

Ziegler, Joseph, 'Practitioners and Saints: Medical Men in Canonization Processes in the Thirteenth to Fifteenth Centuries', *Social History of Medicine*, 12:2 (1999), 191–225.

Ziegler, Joseph, 'Medicine and Immortality in Terrestriak Paradise', in Peter Biller and Joseph Ziegler (eds.), *Religion and Medicine in the Middle Ages* (York: York Medieval Press, 2001), 201–42.

Index

Page numbers in italics refer to images
References to plates are in bold typeface

Abbot, Charles (first Baron of Colchester) 249
Accademia Capitolina del Nudo (Rome) 51
Accademia Clementina (Bologna) 60–1, 69, 84, 90, 152, 194 (*see also* Institute of the Sciences)
Accademia dei Gelati (Bologna) 213
Accademia dei Ricoverati (Padua) 137
Accademia del Disegno (Florence) 84, 195
Accademia della Crusca (Florence) 224, 225
Accademia di San Luca (Milan) 149
Accademia di San Luca (Rome) 51, 88
Academy of Liberal Arts (Augsburg) 84
Academy of the Sciences (Bologna) 31, 116, 167–8, 178, 187 (*see also* Institute of the Sciences)
Academy of the Sciences (Paris) 57, 59, 217, *219*, 231–2, 239
Addison, Joseph 242, 244
advertising 12, 250
  medical 124
  self-advertising 124
affects 3, 10, 20, 85, 112, 122, 126, 132, 139, 153, 155, 166–7
agency 20, 96, 130, 142, 212
Agnesi, Maria Gaetana 93–4, 103, 159, 182, 195
  and Lambertini 132, 136, 212
Agnus Dei 143
Alacoque, Marguerite Marie 139, 162
Albani, Alessandro 39
Alberti, Vincenzo Camillo 205, 206
Aldrovandi, Niccolò 31–2, 62, 76
Algarotti, Francesco 8, 80, 84, 86, 87
Al-Meknassî, Mohamed Ibn Uthmân ix, 254
anatomical books 18, 51, 117–18, 145, 171, 199
anatomical collections, *passim*
anatomical demonstrations 38, 101, 123, 125, 134, 155, 190, 195, 199, 204, 215, 220, 223, 258–9, **Plate 54**
anatomical dissections 3, 18, 32, 33–4, 76, 87, 104, 106, 110, 121, 124, 125–7, 161–2
  cadavers used in 34–5
  and claims of expertise 134, 145
  familiarity with 113, 117, 120, 123, 132
  as spectacle 73
  versus anatomical models 47–8, 64, 112
anatomical injections
  and bodily visualization 216–17, 234–5, 236–8, 246, 251–3, **Plates 50–3**
  and chemistry 239–40
  and microscopes 216, 237–8
  and the 'querelle des Anciens et des Modernes' 237
anatomical machines ix, 64, 234–5, 241, 244–54 *passim*
anatomical modellers 15, 17–19, 22, 38, 58, 65, 69, 84, 90, 100, 112, 118–20, 124, 126 151–2, 217, 256, 258–9 (*see also* Ferrini, Gaetano; Lelli, Ercole; Manzolini, Giovanni; Morandi, Anna; Salerno, Giuseppe)
  authority of 119
  celebrity of. *See* celebrity
  division of labour 127
  and the Grand Tour 14, 19, 58, 71, 128, 208, 215
  manual skills of 58, 211 (*see also* Lelli, Ercole)
anatomical models, *passim* (*see also* anatomical injections; anatomical machines; midwifery models; skeletons; wax models)
  beauty of 8, 86, 111–12, 153, 258–9
  as bodily spectacles 18, 180, 251
  and devotional objects 17, 132, 153–4
  and the Fall 57, 85–6
  and the Grand Tour 5, 11–16, 19, 23, 48, 57, 91, 94, 121, 253, 257
  as home decorations 5, 111
  and human nature 10, 14, 22, 30, 52, 57, 112, 155, 180
  lighting of 76–7
  as luxury goods 5, 12, 124, 193, 201
  and malleability 5–9, 132, 216, 256
  as markers of the natural world 6, 11, 30, 48, 55, 132–3, 142, 153–4
  and polite sociability 90, 112, 121, 124, 126–7
  and saint-making 30, 47–8 (*see also* anatomy)
  of the senses 65, 106, 111, 116, 122, 146–7, 154, 218
  as sources of knowledge 11, 154, 171, 251, 259
  and symmetry 65, 87–8, 111–12
  as teaching tools 5, 40, 56, 78, 100–1, 183–4, 193, 195, 211
anatomical theatres 50–1, 76, 105, 116, 121
  Bologna 33, 34, 57, 62, 73, 75, 92, 105, **Plate 7**, **Plate 16**
  Mantua 76
anatomy, *passim*
  allegory of 107, 114, *115*
  and art 5, 7–8, 11, 15–19, 22–3, 30, 110–11

anatomy (*cont.*)
  and childbearing 103, 106, 164, 166
  and the Church 30, 32–4, 41, 47, 134
  and classical sculpture 14, 39, 83, 85–7, 235
  and domestic spaces 19, 22, 93–124
  and embroidery 104–11, 154
  and the Fall 57, 85–6
  language of 3, 23, 79, 121–2, 165n14, 191
  and medical expertise 113
  and needlework 97, 106, 108, 110
  and pre-lapsarian bodily perfection 86
  and saint-making 29–30, 43–6, 131–2 (*see also* Benedict XIV, beatification and canonization; *De servorum Dei beatificatione et beatorum canonizatione;* miracles; sacred anatomy; sanctity)
anatomy room (Institute of the Sciences) 22, 30–2, 38, 40, 47–8, 56–8, 63–71, *72*, 72–3, 76, 77–9, 80–2, 90–2, 101, 145, 149, 163, 172, 181, 223, 235, 236, **Plate 4**, **Plates 8–15**
  and artistic training 83–6, 89
  and the Grand Tour 57
anatomy room in hospital of Santa Maria della Morte, (*see* hospital of Santa Maria della Morte)
Angelelli, Giuseppe 213
Annonces, affiches, et avis divers 103, 124
Antichità di Ercolano 221
antiquarian culture 5, 10, 11, 53, 86, 87, 115n119, 150
antiquities 14, 30, 39, 51, 55, 58, 82, 91, 221–2
Apocynum 228
Appadurai, Arjun 20
Archenholz, Johann Wilhelm von 53
artisanal culture
  aspects of 5, 10–11, 17–18, 22, 58–9, 70, 96, 101
  and natural knowledge 18, 57–9, 191
artisans 16–18, 22, 57–8, 96, 133
Assunteria dei Magistrati 211
Assunti di Studio 74–5, 133–4, 169, 186
Assunti of the hospital of Santa Maria della Morte 15, 134–5
Assunti of the Institute of the Sciences 38, 49, 63–4, 67, 183, 210, 255n13
Assunti of the orphanage of San Bartolomeo di Reno 130
Astruc, Jean 119, 176
audiences, *passim*
authenticity 54, 156, 259
  anatomical models as sites of 9
  of divine inspiration, concerns for 131, 136–42 *passim*, 144–6
  of holy images and objects 150
  ideas of 259
  objects as media of 251, 253
  of objects on display 150
  of relics 149
automata 234
Azzoguidi, Germano 119, 123, 158, 185, 195, 196, 200
Azzoguidi, Giuseppe 158

Baker, Malcolm 88
Balbi, Paolo Battista 35
Bambi, Anna Rosa 201
baptism 99, 114, 187–8, 209, 235
  emergency. *See* midwives
  in utero. *See* midwives
Baretti, Giuseppe 79
Barry, James 56, 91
Bartholin, Thomas 236
basilica of San Petronio (Bologna) 85, 149
Bassi, Ferdinando 101, 120, 202
Bassi, Laura 93–4, 102, 103, 123, 158–161, 189, 195, 199, 212–13
  and anatomy 104–5
  and *Insignia* 33, 73, 75, 104–5, 145, **Plate 5**
  and the Institute of the Sciences 160–161, 182
  and papal patronage 33, 93, 132, 135, 159, 182
  public demonstrations by 33, 73, 75, 104, 123, 160, 200, 212–13
  wax portrait of 158–9
Bath 202, 203, 207
Baxandall, Michael 87
beatification and canonization 24, 29, 31, 41, 42, 43, 44, 45, 49, 54, 55, 131, 152, 156 (*see also* Benedict XIV; *De servorum Dei beatificatione et beatorum canonizatione*; miracles; saint-making; saints; sanctity)
  celebration of 54–5, *54*
  and medical expertise 30, 46
Beccari, Jacopo Bartolomeo 120
  and Agnesi, Maria Gaetana 94
  and Galli's collection 163, 164, 169, 172–3, 176, 180, 185
  and Institute of the Sciences 40
  and Morandi, Anna 120, 134, 207
  and Ranuzzi, Girolamo 202
Bellini, Lorenzo 103
  and bodily embroidery 107, 154
Belvedere Torso (statue) 82, 87
Benedict XIV, pope (Prospero Lambertini) 1, 3, 24–55 *passim*
  assessor of sanctity 10, 22, 29, 131, 139
  and Catholic Enlightenment 28–9
  and display of holy objects and images 140–3, 148–50
  election to pontificate 25, 28
  and Galli's midwifery collection 176, 181, 189
  images of 24, *25–7*, **Plate 3**
  and midwifery licensing 186–9
  notification on anatomy 32–5, 37, 46–7, 134
  patronage; of academies of Christian erudition in Rome 51–2; of anatomical collections 10, 22, 29, 38, 40, 47, 49, 52, 55; of anatomy 10, 22, 50; of antiquarian

displays 22, 52, 54; of the Institute of the Sciences 30–2, 38, 40, 47, 56, 63, 68, 82, 149–50, 181–2, 189, 194; of learned women, *see* Agnesi, Maria Gaetana; Bassi, Laura; Morandi, Anna; of natural knowledge 38, 50, 55, 148, 150
as promoter of faith 31, 41–3, 45, 131–2, 137–9
on saint-making 29–30, 41–8, 55, 131 (*see also* anatomy; beatification and canonization; *De servorum Dei beatificatione et beatorum canonizatione*; saints; sanctity)
and school of surgery 38, 134
Berengario da Carpi, Jacopo 236
Bermingham, Ann 91
Berti Logan, Gabriella 97, 199
Bianchi, Giovanni (Janus Plancus) 80, 101–4, 119–21, 123–4, 126, 133, 154, 159, 194, 195, 202, 211, 222
Bianconi, Giovanni Lodovico 129
Bihéron, Marie Marguerite 105, 106, 107, 123, 209, 213, 223, 257
Björnstâhl, Jacob Jonas 223, 231, 251
blindness 46, 174
blood 44, 52, 216, 240
bloodletting 106, 185
circulation of 216, 240
di Sangro's experiments with 241
miraculous liquefaction of 241–3 (*see* Naples; Saint Januarius)
replica of blood miracle, (*see* di Sangro, Raimondo; Saint Januarius)
blood vessels 216
demonstration of 235
as displayed by anatomical machines 234–5, 241, 244, 246
visualization of 216–18, 234–5, 237, 240, 241, 246 (*see also* anatomical injections)
Boccalaro, Antonio 143
Bolletti, Giuseppe Gaetano 66, 70, 71, 213
Bologna (Italy), *passim*
Bologna (gazette) 192
Bolognese Senate 38, 189
bombasari 60nn.17&18, 90
Bonazzoli, Lorenzo 31, 61, 67, 77, 185
Boniface VIII (pope)
bull of. See *Detestandae feritatis abusum*
and dissecting practices 32–3
Bonnet, Charles 237
Borghese Gladiator (statue) 82, 87, *89*, 89–90
Borsieri di Kanifeld, Giovanni Battista 196
Boswell, James 160
Bottari, Giovanni Gaetano 52
Bouchard, Jean-Jacques 241
Boyle, John, Earl of Corke and Orrery 39, 40, 78
Brambilla, Elena 136, 137
Breve nota di quel che si vede in casa del Principe di Sansevero 233–5, 241, 247–9, 250, 251–2
Broschi, Carlo (Farinelli) 197
Brugnoli, Domenico 58–9, 60, 92
Buffon, Georges Louis Leclerc de 218, *219*
Buoncuore, Francesco 218, 252
burial 32, 36–7
Lambertini's notification on 36
and rites for dissected bodies 34
Burney, Charles 170, 181

cabinets 11, 13, 40, 68, 96, 152, 206, 218, 233
anatomical 13, 15, 63–4, 94, 101–2, 118, 121, 123–4, 152, 154, 170, 194, 197–8, 218, *219*, 223, 236, 240, 253 (*see also* di Sangro, Raimondo; Morandi, Anna)
of curiosities 7, 15, 96, 201, 216, 224, 233–5, 241, 246, 248, 252 (*see also* di Sangro, Raimondo)
cadavers 9, 15, 18, 32–3, 36–7, 44, 73–4, 105, 112, 123, 127, 236
access to 33–5
burial of 36–7
decay of 104, 114, 127, 238
dissection of 61–2, 64, 102, 118–20, 168, 255
supply of 123, 134–5, 158
Caldani, Leopoldo Marco Antonio 126, 203
Calegari Zucchini, Anna Maria 156
callipaedia 167
Callipaedia (Quillet) 179
Campani, Giuseppe 39, 68
Campani, Maria Vittoria 68
candlelight viewing 83, 88–9, *89*
Cangiamila, Francesco Emanuele 187, 235
canonization. *See* beatification and canonization; Benedict XIV; *De servorum Dei beatificatione et beatorum canonizatione*; saint-making; sanctity
Canova, Antonio 83
Caraccioli, Louis-Antoine 24, *27*, 42, 136, 137, 140, 212
carnival 73, 75–6
Cartolari, Antonio 170
midwifery machine by 174, **Plate 39**
Casanova, Giacomo 140, 200
Cassini, Giovanni Domenico 68, 136
casting 31, 67, 82, 100, 170, 255, 256
Catherine II, Russian Empress, 12, 209
Catholic Enlightenment 28–9
Cavallazzi, Petronio 192
Cavazza, Marta 125, 212
Cavazzoni, Angelo Michele 18, 61, 116–17
Celano, Carlo 252
celebrity 10, 16, 91, 93, 128, 159, 200, 212, 259 (*see also* Morandi, Anna)
culture of 10, 16, 19, 159
versus fame 17n55
Celesia, Pietro Paolo 248
Chard, Chloe 123
charities 97–8, 130, 135, 157–8, 159, 196

Charles de Bourbon, king of Naples and Sicily 12, 124, 194, 218, 220, 222, 224, 226n58, 227–9, 242
Charles Emmanuel III of Savoy, king of Sardinia 12, 64, 124, 194, 208, 209, 230
Chiarini, Laura 91
  healing power of 144
  invisible hand of 144–5
  odour of sanctity 144–5, 156
  visionary inspiration of 145
  as wax-modeller 91, 145, 167
  wax-portrait of 145, 156
childbirth 100, 106, 163–8, 170–1, 173, 176, 180, 188, 190, 235, 246 (*see also* midwifery machines; midwifery models; Morandi, Anna)
  natural 166
  preternatural 166, 168, 180, **Plate 38**, **Plate 40**, **Plate 45**, **Plate 46**
children, malleable bodies of 178–80
chocolate 74
Christian Museum 51–2
church of San Gabriele (Bologna) 37, 99
church of San Nicolò degli Albari (Bologna) 98
church of San Procolo (Bologna) 192
church of Santo Stefano (Bologna) 149
Cioffi, Rosanna 245
Clark, Stuart 43, 137
classical sculpture 14, 86–7, 235
classical statues 14, 39, 56, 81–3, 85–8, 235 (*see also* anatomy; candlelight viewing; Polykleitos)
  and proportions 14, 83, 87–8
  and symmetry 87
clay 5, 100, 163, 164, 166, 167, 170, 173–4, 180, 253 (*see also* midwifery models)
Cocchi, Antonio 35, 113, 202
Cochin, Charles-Nicolas 71
Cohen, Elizabeth 96
Coigny, Countess de 105–6
College of Physicians (Bologna) 114, 184–6, 189
College of Physicians (Rome) 46
Colombo, Realdo 45
commerce 12, 124, 151
Congregation of Rites 31, 41–4, 48, 131, 138–9
Congregazione di Gabella Grossa 133, 134, 197
connoisseur 22, 56–9, 79, 81, 83–4, 88–91, 221
connoisseurship 56, 91
consumption 6, 12, 59, 95, 124
Controni, Domenico 203–4
corpses. *See*, cadavers
Corradini, Antonio 234
Cotugno, Domenico 66, 78, 81, 116, 117, 119, 223
Count of Falkenstein. *See* Joseph II, Holy Roman Emperor
Crescentia (Maria Crescentia Höss) 139, 141
Crespi, Giuseppe Maria 24
Crespi, Luigi 71, 79, 98–9, 104, 108, 122, 129, 154
curiosities 5, 7, 11, 14, 58, 124, 226, 232–3, 246, 248, 253 (*see also* cabinets of curiosities)

d'Agreda, Maria 139, 140
Dal Sole, Giovan Gioseffo 60, 99
Dardani, Luigi 69
Daubenton, Louis-Jean-Marie 218, *219*
De aure humana tractatus (Valsalva) 46, 63, 116
De Bononiensi Scientiarum et Artium Instituto atque Academia Commentarii 2, 61, 78, 86, 101, 111, 167, 170, 181, 236
de Brosses, Charles 50, 62, 242
De Felice, Fortunato Bartolomeo 195, 250–1
de Graaf, Reinier 237
de Graffigny, Françoise 228
de Julianis, Caterina 105, 222
de la Faye, Georges 117, 217
de La Porte, Joseph 49, 73
De l'éducation des dames (Poullain de la Barre) 106
De l'egalité des deux sexes (Poullain de la Barre) 106
de' Liuzzi, Mondino 32, 94
Della forza della fantasia umana (Muratori) 141
Della pubblica felicità (Muratori) 169
della Quercia, Jacopo 85
Della regolata devozione de' cristiani (Muratori) 141–2
della Torre, Giovanni Maria 221
Dell'origine e progressi dell'Istituto delle Scienze di Bologna (Bolletti) 66, 71
de Mandeville, Bernard 106
De Rinaldis, Rinaldo 152
de' Rossi, Properzia 98
Description historique et critique de l'Italie (Richard) 174, 196
De servorum Dei beatificatione et beatorum canonizatione (Lambertini) 24, 29, 42, 44, 46–9, 54, 137–9, 146
  responses to 48–9
Desgenettes, René-Nicolas 6n13, 128, 257
Desnoües, Guillaume 70, 238–9, 246
Detestandae feritatis abusum (*see also* Boniface VIII) 32–3
de' Vegni, Leonardo 110
devotional objects 7, 17, 132, 140–4, 148–50, 153–4, 162, 167, 222 (*see also* holy objects)
Diario bolognese 151, 194, 195
Dì geniali. Della Dialettica delle Donne ridotta al suo vero principio (Zecchini) 199–200
Di Gregorio e Russo, Giuseppe 238, 246
di Sangro, Raimondo, seventh Prince of San Severo 13, 23, 195, 201, 215–53 *passim*, **Plate 48**
  and Accademia della Crusca 224–45
  acquisition of Salerno's skeletons 215–16, 218, 220, 223, 226, 231, 240, 247–8, 251

cabinet of curiosities of 201, 216, 224, 233–5, 241, 246–8, 251, 253
and Charles de Bourbon 227, 229
failing health of 248
and freemasonry 229, 243, 245–6, 249
and the Grand Tour 216, 231–3, 253
and palingenesis 247–8, 250
and Ranuzzi, Girolamo 195, 201, 216, 232
and regeneration 245–7
and replica of the miracle of Saint Januarius 243–5
and secrecy 225, 249–50
disputatio 73, 76
Dissertation sur une lampe antique 230, 231
Ditchfield, Simon 140
domesticity 19, 124, 196, 212
domestic setting 93–7, 99, 101, *109*, 110, 112
Doria, Paolo Mattia 227, 242
Dotti, Carlo Francesco 158
dry preparations 46, 63, 101, 116n121, 154, 236 (*see also* Valsalva, Antonio Maria)
du Coudray, Angélique-Marguerite Le Boursier (Madame du Coudray) 107, 164, **Plate 20**

écorchés 7, 62, 65–6, 76, 88, 235, **Plate 7**, **Plates 10–13**
Egyptian mummy 39
Embriologia sacra (Cangiamila) 235
embroidery 104, 106–8, 110
and anatomical skill 108
and anatomy 106–7
the human body as divine 107, 154
Encyclopédie d' Yverdon (De Felice) 195, 250–1
Engel, Laura 212
entangled lives 19–22
Essay on Painting (Algarotti) 84
Eucharist 162
display of 151
Eustachi, Bartolomeo 50, 65
Eve and Adam 65, 85, 88, **Plates 8 and 9**, **Plate 17**

fabric 66, 153, 228, 233
in anatomical models 153, 164, 167, **Plate 20**
of the body 103, 107–8, 111, 116, 127, 177, 218
fame 16, 201, 215, 254 (*see also* celebrity)
and Bassi, Laura 160
and Galli, Giovanni, Antonio 183
and the Institute of the Sciences 38, 40, 63, 79, 182
and Lambertini, Prospero 40
and Lelli, Ercole 56, 79, 81, 84
and Morandi, Anna 18, 93, 106, 119, 124, 127–8, 197, 210, 214
versus celebrity 17n55
Fantuzzi, Giovanni 71, 114, 171
Farinelli. *See* Broschi, Carlo
Farnese Hercules (statue) 82, 87
Farsetti, Filippo Vincenzo 82
Felsina pittrice (Crespi; Malvasia) 71, 98, 129
Fenix (Masonic ship) 247
Ferrari, Giovanna 35, 74, 75
Ferrini, Gaetano 258
Ferrini, Gennaro 258
Ferrini, Giuseppe 258
Florence (Italy) 3, 4, 28, 63, 81, 84, 118, 128, 151, 156, 195, 203, 205, 217, 223, 225, 255, 257
Focaccia, Miriam 126
Fogliano, Giovanni 218
Fontana, Felice 223
Fontana, Lavinia 98
Fontenelle, Bernard le Bovier de 237, 246
Fortino, Anna 105
Frederick Christian, prince-elector of Saxony
Insignia degli Anziani 62, **Plate 6**
Frederick the Great 80, 227, 243
Freemasonry. *See*, di Sangro, Raimondo
French Academy in Rome 50, 79, 82

Gaetani dell'Aquila d'Aragona, Carlotta, Princess of San Severo 201, 232, 248
Galeati, Domenico Maria 35
Galeazzi, Domenico Maria Gusmano 73, 116, 120, 144
Galiani, Ferdinando 225, 228, 248
Galli, Giovanni Antonio 23, 38, 40, 77–8, 81, 100, 120, 128, 163–92 *passim*, 205, **Plate 43**
as *accoucher* of Princess Maria Caterina (Monaco) 183
and blindfolding 174–7
and caesarean section 187
and crystal womb. *See* midwifery machines
and forceps 176
and Institute of the Sciences 38, 182, 189
and midwifery books 171
midwifery collection of 100–1, 128, 163–91 *passim*, 194–5, 234, 236, **Plate 38**, **Plate 44**
Galvani, Luigi 9, 76, 77
as demonstrator of anatomy 78, 184
on Morandi, Anna 108, 111, 205, 252, 256–7, 259
Ganganelli, Giovanni Vincenzo Antonio 221, 224, 228, 233
Garofali, Alessandro 158
Garzoni, Tommaso 142
Gazette van Gendt 103
gender 8, 19, 96, 108, 212
generation 102–3, 106, 168, 177–9, 188, 190 (*see also* childbirth; pregnancy)
models of 64–5, 155, 163–4, 166–7, 172–3, 180–1
parts of 77, 169, 172
uncertainties of 164–7, 180, 190

Genlis, Madame de (Stéphanie Félicité Ducrest de St-Aubin) 105, 106
Genovesi, Antonio 224, 229, 242
gestural knowledge. *See* knowledge, gestural
Giannotti, Silvestro 62, **Plate 7**
Gibbon, Edward 238
gift exchange 90, 203, 207–10
Giliani, Alessandra 94, 236
Giornale de' Letterati 44, 49, 195
Giornale Enciclopedico 192
Giovannini, Rosa 97
Giuffrida, Agostino 246
Goethe, Johann Wolfgang von 88, 111, 121
Goldoni, Carlo 49, 94–5
Graffeo, Paolo 218, 255
Grand Tour 11, 13–15, 161 (*see also* anatomical modellers; anatomical models; di Sangro, Raimondo; Lelli, Ercole; Morandi, Anna)
  and anatomical collections 5, 12, 23, 58, 128, 180, 183, 215–16, 223
  and antiquarianism 220
  and connoisseurship 91
  and di Sangro 231–3, 253
  and the Institute of the Sciences 40, 48–9, 57
  travellers 28, 71, 79, 88, 231, 257; map for 5, **Plate 2**
  and women 91, 123
Gray, Thomas 28
Grifoni, Lucia 199
Grimm, Friedrich Melchior, Baron von 210
Grosholtz, Marie (Madame Tussaud) 159
Guarnacci, Mario 207, 208
Guglielmini, Domenico 236, 238
Guidotti Luigi 92

Habermas, Jürgen 95
Hales, Stephen 247, 248
Haller, Albrecht von 126
Hamilton, William 221, 226, **Plate 49**
Harvey, William 240
health 14, 95, 201, 234
  and the Grand Tour 5, 14, 201
  and the Porretta spa 204
  of progeny 167, 179
Herculaneum 220–2
Hervey, Christopher 78
Histoire naturelle, générale et particulière (Buffon and Daubenton) 218, *219*
holy objects 11, 132, 141, 148, 153 (*see also* devotional objects; relics)
  attitude toward 142
  control of 149–50
  power of 141–2
  public display of 149
Homberg, Wilhelm 239
Hopwood, Nick 20
hospital Maggiore (Milan) 173, 186
hospital of San Giacomo Apostolo (Naples) 223
hospital of Santa Maria della Morte (Bologna) 74, 78, 135, *157*, 158, 168, 184, 236
  and anatomical dissections 38, 48
  anatomy room of 15; improper use of 134
  and cadavers, supply of 123, 134–5
  Scuola della Confortaria 158
hospital of Santa Maria della Vita (Bologna) 38, 113
  surgical instruments 38, 47; public display of 50
hospital of Santo Spirito (Rome)
  and Biblioteca Lancisiana 51
  and écorché 88
  enlargement of 51
  and salt of the lion 203
hospital of the Esposti (Bologna) 188
hospital of the Incurabili (Naples) 223
hospital of the Incurabili (Rome) 120
human nature
  and anatomical models 30, 52, 112, 155, 180
  investigation of 57
  knowledge of 10, 14, 22
Hunter, William 122, 176, 240, 253, 256, 257
Hussey, Giles 56

Iconologia (Ripa; Orlandi) 107, 114, *115*
Il Pasquino 24
imagination 53, 95, 117, 132, 136–7, 141, 145–6, 239, 243
  as agent of illusion 137
  control of 132
  disturbance of 142
  excesses of 137, 224
  and experience 53
  Lambertini on 42, 137–8, 141, 146
  Muratori on 141–2
  power of 140, 224
  unruly 132, 136, 138
  and visionary claims 132, 145
  and women 139, 141–2 (*see also* maternal imagination)
Insignia degli Anziani (*see also* Bassi Laura, Frederick Christian)
  portraying women at work in a silk factory 108, **Plate 21**
Institute of the Sciences (Bologna) *passim, 2,* **Plate 6** (*see also* Accademia Clementina; Academy of the Sciences (Bologna); anatomy room; *Assunti* of the Institute of the Sciences; Bassi, Laura; Benedict XIV; Galli, Giovanni Antonio; Grand Tour; Marsigli, Luigi Ferdinando)
  anatomy room 30–2, 38–40, 47–8, 56, 58, 64–92 *passim*, 99, 100–1, 145, 149, 163, 172, 181, 184, 235–6, **Plate 4**
  astronomical observatory 39
  as a 'Cyclopaedia of the senses' 53
  drawing school 60
  Egyptian mummy 39
  gallery of the statues 82–4

library 39, 60, 82
midwifery room 71, 78, 128, 182, 184
optical instruments 39, 68, 77, 82
rooms of physics 77
as 'Solomon's house' 1
instruments
anatomical 114, 125, 199, 217
for anatomical injections 81, 235, 237–9
of Christian martyrdom 52
experimental 40, 60
optical 39, 68, 77, 82
surgical 38, 47, 50, 209 (*see also* hospital of Santa Maria della Vita)
Isolani, Ercole 156, 199
Istoria dello Studio di Napoli (Origlia Paolino) 225, 247
Istoria universale provata con monumenti (Bianchini) 53

Jablonowska, Anna (née Sapieha) 206, 208
James, Robert 238
Johnson, Samuel 12, 160
Jones, Colin 124
Jordanova, Ludmilla 150
Jörg, Carl 105
Joseph II, Holy Roman Emperor 12, 152, 160, 204–6, 220
Josephinum 205, 258n22

Kantorowicz, Ernst 158, 158n150
Keill, James 107
Keyssler, Johann Georg 75, 231
kidneys 1, 236–7
horseshoe kidney 31, 61, 67, **Plate 1**
Kircher, Athanasius 224, 247
Klapisch-Zuber, Christiane 166
knowledge, *passim*
anatomical, *passim*
gestural 167, 174, 189–91 (*see also* midwives)
natural, *passim*
tacit 23, 167, 191
Kopytoff, Igor 20
Kusukawa, Sachiko 117

La comare levatrice (Melli) 143, 169
La Condamine, Charles-Marie de 14, 104, 228, 232, 243, 244
La donna di garbo (Goldoni) 94
Laghi, Tommaso 81, 119, 120, 236, 240
Lalande, Joseph Jérôme Lefrançois de 71
and Bologna's learned women 160
and *Diario Bolognese* 151
and di Sangro 233, 244, 247
and Galli's midwifery collections 181
midwifery models, misattribution of 128
and Morandi, Anna 128, 170
and Southern Italian aristocracy, depiction of 227
Lamberg, Maximilian Joseph von 160, 248–9
Lambertini, Prospero, *see* Benedict XIV, pope
Lami, Giovanni 102, 229
Lancisi, Giovanni Maria 50–1
Laocoön (statue) 82, 87, 257
La piazza universale di tutte le professioni del mondo (Garzoni) 142
La Santa. See Vigri, Caterina
La Specola. *See* Royal Museum of Physics and Natural History
Laurenti, Marco Antonio 69, 72, 114, 181, 185
leisure 202
Le Journal encyclopédique 234, 248
Lelli, Ercole 18, 22, 56–92 *passim*
anatomical models of 31–2, 34, **Plate 1**, **Plate 7**, **Plates 8 and 9**, **Plates 10–13**, **Plates 14 and 15**
anatomical statuette of 83, 90
and anatomy room 56–8, 63–8, *72*, 93, 99, 181
and celebrity 91
as coiner 64
and Grand Tour travellers 79
as harquebus maker 56, 58–60
journey to Rome 68, 80
manual skills of 59, 90 (*see also* anatomical modellers)
and optical theatre 81, 91–2
rivalry with Manzolini and Morandi 69–71
school of drawing 56, 60, 69, 83–4
self-portrait of 90, **Plate 18**
Le Lorrain, Pierre (abbé de Vallemont) 247
Leopardi, Giacomo 246
Le pitture di Bologna (Malvasia) 71
Lettera apologetica (di Sangro) 228–9, 247
Letter to the Society of Dilettanti (Barry) 56
Letters from Italy (Riggs Miller) 204
Lettres écrites par Monsieur le Prince de S. Sevère (di Sangro) 231
Le voyageur françois (de la Porte) 49, 73
Levret, André 176
lifelikeness 5–6, 6n13, 144, 145n92, 152
Lini, Elena 63
Linnaeus, Carl 223
Locke, John 45, 103, 147, 175
Loriga, Sabina 143
Lusitanus, Amatus 236
luxury
debates about 12
luxury goods 124, 201 (*see also* anatomical models)

Macchiavelli, Alessandro
and anatomical injections 236
and forgery 94
and story of Alessandra Giliani 94, 236
McClive, Cathy 165
McKeon, Michael 96
McTavish, Lianne 175, 180
Madonna di San Luca
icon of 149
sanctuary of 158

Maerker, Anna 4, 151
Maffei, Scipione 51–2
Magnani, Paolo 67, 69
malleability 5–6, 8–9, 132, 139, 145n92, 177, 179–80, 216, 256
Malpighi, Marcello 45, 46, 115, 117, 237
Malvasia, Carlo Cesare 71, 98
Malvasia family 98
Malvezzi, Laura Pepoli 157
Malvezzi, Sigismondo 181–2
Manfredi, Eraclito 194
Manfredi, Eustachio 212
Manget, Jean-Jacques 117–18
Manningham, Richard 164
Mantua (Italy), theatre 76
Manzolini, Anna Morandi. *See* Morandi, Anna
Manzolini, Carlo 102, 199, 214
Manzolini, Giovanni 18, 22, 37, 67, 93–130 *passim*, 153, 159, 163, 170, 194 (*see also* Morandi, Anna)
  anatomical expertise of 113–16, 211
  authorship, misattribution of 128
  and carious bone, drawing of 120
  clay womb of 170
  death of 124, 128, 130
  and dissection 103, 112
  and domestic space 93–6, 100–1, 111
  and Lelli, Ercole, rivaly with 69–71, 181
  library of 117–18
  and marriage to Morandi 93, 97–100
  as melancholic 104
  as member of congregation 37
  wax portrait of 125–6, 127, 155, 208, **Plate 30**, **Plate 31**
  waxworks of 153, **Plate 32**
maritime carriage 230, *230*
Marquis Dauvet 221
Marsigli, Luigi Ferdinando
  and Bolognese authorities, conflict with 39
  and the Institute of the Sciences, founder of 1, 38, 59
  and the mechanical arts 60
  military career of 59
Martyn, Thomas 128
marvels 42, 52, 117, 123, 153–4, 205, 220, 226, 239, 253 (*see also* wonder)
  and midwifery models 163–4, 180
  and the San Severo Palace 231, 248
masonic lodge 224, 229
Mastiani, Giuseppe
  models at the Cabinet du Roi 218
  model of the ear 217–18, *219*
maternal imagination 138, 177–80
maternity 19, 97, 102–3, 144, 166, 212
Mayer, Anthonius (or Majer) 15, 223
Mazzotti, Massimo 132
Mehus, Lorenzo 225
Melli, Sebastiano 143, 169
Mellini, Maria Flaminia 186
Mémorial d'un mondain (Lamberg) 248
Menghini, Vincenzo Antonio 68
Messbarger, Rebecca 19, 126
Metastasio, Pietro 205–6
metropolitan cathedral of San Pietro 101
microhistory 8
midwifery machines 164, 170, 172, 174, 177, 234
  crystal womb 164, 174, 191
midwifery manuals 169, 171
midwifery models 23, 38, 78, 100, 107, 163–4, 166–7, 169, 176, 181, 191, 258
  in clay 163, 166, 170, 172, 173, **Plate 38**, **Plate 40, Plate 41, Plate 42, Plate 45, Plate 46**
  of pelvis 163, 172, **Plate 36**
  translating gestural knowledge 189–91
  in wax 163, 170, 173, **Plate 37**, **Plate 44**
midwifery schools 165n14, 170–1, 176, 190–1
midwives 23, 163–91 *passim*
  baptism in utero 187
  blindfolding of 174
  emergency baptism 187–8, 235
  and gestural knowledge 189–91
  and instruments 176
  and manual dexterity 173–4, 176–7, 190
  and medical licensing 184–6
  and the *portella* 182–3, 191
  and religious licensing 186–9
  and skill 173–4
  and tacit knowledge 23, 167, 191
  training of 143, 164, 167, 169, 171–3, 182, 184
Millo, Giovanni Giacomo 181–2
mineral waters 202 (*see also* salt of the lion)
miracles 41, 43–6, 144, 154, 241–4, 249 (*see also* beatification and canonization; Benedict XIV; *De servorum Dei beatificatione et beatorum canonizatione*; Saint Januarius; supernatural)
miraculous healing 46, 144
Mitelli, Giuseppe Maria 147
  'Vedere' ('Seeing') *148*
Mniszech, Michal 79, 154
Mocenigo, Alvise Giovanni 106, 194
Mocenigo, Pisana (Corner) 106
modesty 75, 210–14, 250
Molinari, Innocenzo 228
Molinelli, Pier (or Pietro) Paolo 38, 61, 77, 100, 120, 170, 181, 183
Momigliano, Arnaldo 53
Mondini, Carlo 76, 157, 255–6n13
Monro, Alexander, *primus* 122, 237, 240
Monti, Francesco 69, 98
Montroni, Giovanni 242
Moore, John 257
Morand, Sauveur-François 209, 217
Morandi, Anna
  anatomical collection of 93–129 *passim*, 154, 194, 197–8, 223, 236, **Plate 25**, **Plate 26**,

Plate 27, **Plate 28**, **Plate 29** (*see also* Manzolini, Giovanni)
anatomical collection, sale of 198–201, 204, 207
anatomical demonstrations of 96, 101, 121–6, 134, 148, 154–5, 195, 197, 199, 204
and anatomical sociability 112
and celebrity 16, 19, 93, 95, 121–2, 124, 127–9, 159, 192, 194, 197–8, 204, 206, 208–13
and childbearing 103, 144
and children 100, 102, 104, 130, 196–7, 198, 214
death of 192
and devotional waxworks 91, 132, 144, 153–4
and domestic setting 100–4
dowry of 98, 135
and the Grand Tour 40, 94, 121, 123, 128, 196, 204, 208
and marriage with Giovanni Manzolini 97–100
and the microscope 114
and needlework 104–11 *passim*
papal patronage of 22, 38, 40, 130–6, 144, 159 (*see also* Benedict XIV)
portraits of *110*, 208–10
and Ranuzzi, Girolamo 199, 205–6, 207–8, 209–10
self-portrait (wax) of 108, 110, 124–9, 145, 154–5, 157–9, 161, 208–9, **Plate 22**, **Plate 23**, **Plate 24**
self-portrait, hand gesture 108, 154
wax portrait of Giovanni Manzolini. *See* Manzolini, Giovanni
Morandi, Antonio 113
Morgagni, Giambattista 18, 46, 61, 106, 117, 118, 120, 126, 178, 195–6
Morgan, John 71, 128
motherhood 102–3
Mount Vesuvius 220–2, 242, 244, 247, **Plate 47**, **Plate 49**
Muratori, Ludovico Antonio (pseud. Lamindo Pritanio) 139, 141–142, 171
on displays of sacred images 143, 149–50
on Giuseppe da Copertino 44
and imagination 141–2, 178
on midwifery practice 169
and the senses 53
Musacchio, Jacqueline Marie 166
mystical women 131–2, 136, 139–41, 145

Naples (Italy)
and blood miracles 241–2
as the 'city of bloods' 241
as colonial capital 220, 253
court of 217, 221–2, 225–9, 232
as Grand Tour destination 220, 223, 233
as a site of wonder 220, 226, 231, 241, 244, 253
Napoli Signorelli, Pietro 252
needlework 97, 106–10, *109*, 110, *110*
Nelle, Florian 151
Nollekens, Joseph 208
Nollet, Jean-Antoine 231
Notizie del bello, dell'antico e del curioso della città di Napoli (Celano) 252
Novelle letterarie 102, 113, 124, 133, 194, 222, 225, 229
Nussbaum, Felicity 212

observation
anatomical 61, 78, 83, 89, 118, 119–20, 124, 132, 145, 196
of Mount Vesuvius 222
practices of 13, 57, 78, 83, 85, 88–9, 118, 120
Observationes ad uteri constructionem pertinentes (Azzoguidi) 119, 195–6
obsolescence 8, 22, 75–6, 254, 256–7, 259
oil of turpentine 66, 74, 157, 216, 235, 237, 239
Oretti, Marcello 104, 144, 153, 197–8, 206
Origlia Paolino, Giovanni Giuseppe 225, 247
Orlandi, Cesare 107, 114, *115*, 126–7
orphanage of San Bartolomeo di Reno 130, 133, 196

Palermitan Senate 217, 254, 258
Palermo (Italy) 5, 11, 14, 22, 105, 215, 217–18, 246, 254–5, 258
palingenesis. *See* di Sangro
Panzacchi, Anna 60
Panzacchi, Maria Elena 60–1
papal patronage. *See* Benedict XIV
Paré, Ambroise 179
Parenti, Paolo Andrea 113–14
Park, Katharine 32
Pastore, Alessandro 172
Patoun, William 122, 213
Pazienza, Giuseppe 213
Pedretti, Giuseppe 69, 98
Peggi, Pier Francesco 149
Pentolini, Francesco Clodoveo Maria 213
Perpignani, Galgano 99, 110
Peter the Great, Russian Emperor 12, 209, 238
Pether, William 89, *89*
phoenix 246–7 (*see also* San Severo Palace)
Piaggio, Antonio 220
Pietro Leopoldo, Grand Duke of Tuscany 151, 205
Pilati, Carlo Antonio 49
Piò, Angelo 153
Sacra Famiglia 153–4, **Plate 34**, **Plate 35**
Piò, Domenico 65
Piozzi, Hester Lynch 160–1
Pisarri, Carlo 67, 71, 80
Plongeron, Bernard 28
Polykleitos (or Polycleitus) 14, 14n43, 87
Pomata, Gianna 114, 152, 185
Pompeii 220–2, 244
Porretta spa 201–4, 207, 216

portella. *See* midwives
Poullain de la Barre, François 106
preformationism 177–8
pregnancy 163–190 *passim* (*see also* generation; maternal imagination; midwifery machines; midwifery models)
 and anatomical knowledge 106
 and anatomical models 163, 167, 172–4
 uncertainties of 164–7, 180, 190
Prestini, Elisabetta 172
preternatural 43, 132, 142, 166, 168
Prince of San Severo. *See* di Sangro, Raimondo
Princess of San Severo. *See* Gaetani dell'Aquila d'Aragona, Carlotta
private anatomy sessions 77–8
problem of Molyneux 175
promoter of faith 41–2, 45 (*see also* Benedict XIV)
Protomedicato 184–6, 188
protomedico 46, 106, 169, 185, 218, 252
public anatomy lesson 3, 33–4, 73, 121, **Plate 5** (*see also* Bassi, Laura)
 argumentation in 74–5
 and carnival 73, 75–6
 as complement to models 116
 decline of 74–6
 decorum of 74–5
 moral tone of 57

Quaestiones medico-legales (Zacchia) 46
Queirolo, Francesco 223, 234
Quesnay, François 240

Ranuzzi, Girolamo 23, 193, 195
 and contract with Morandi 199, 205–6, 207–8
 and Morandi's collection 193, 198–201, 209–10
 and Poretta spa 201–4
 and salt of the lion 201–4, 206–7
Ranuzzi Palace 193, 199, 201, 203–4, 206–7, 209
Ranuzzi, Vincenzo 209, 210
Reale Accademia Ercolanese 221
relics 52, 55, 140, 241 (*see also* holy objects)
 authenticity of 150
 contained in wax portraits 156–7
 and the cult of saints 30, 156
 devotion of 140–3, 148
 display of 150, 152–3
 incorrupt body of Caterina Vigri 152 (*see also* Vigri, Caterina)
 skull of St Anna 148, 152
resemblance 137, 146, 178
Respublica Literaria Umbrorum 195
resurrection 36–7, 247
Reynier, Albertino 62
Richard, Jérôme 71
 on di Sangro 232–3
 on Galli's collection 186
 on midwives 174
 on Morandi 115, 122–3, 158, 196, 208
Riggs Miller, Anna 204, 244
Rinuccini, Alessandro 228, 232
Ripa, Cesare 107, 114, *115*
Roman College 48, 224
Rome (Italy) 24, 28, 45, 49, 67–70, 81–2, 87–8, 111, 139–140, 149, 160, 203–5, 208–210, 220, 223–4, 238
 and antiquarian displays 22, 30, 52, 54, 55
 and Christian museum 52
 Lambertini and 49–52, 54–55
Rouhault, Pierre Simon 239
Rousseau, Jean-Jacques 212
Royal Academy of Arts (London) 56
Royal Academy of Painting, Sculpture, and Architecture (Parma) 84
Royal Academy of Physicians (Palermo) 218
Royal Museum (Portici) 221
Royal Museum of Physics and Natural History (La Specola) (Florence) 3–4, 118, 151, 205, 215, 255
Royal Palace of Caserta 230
Royal Society (London) 57, 59, 75
Royal Theatre of San Carlo (Naples) 226
Ruysch, Frederik 209, 237–8, 246

sacred anatomy 33, 44
Sacred Heart of Jesus 139, 162
Sade, Donatien Alphonse François, Marquis de 127, 233, 249
Saggio sopra la pittura (Algarotti) 86–7
saint-making 29–30, 43, 45–6, 55, 131, 156 (*see also* anatomy; beatification and canonization; Benedict XIV; *De servorum Dei beatificatione et beatorum canonizatione*; miracles; saints; sanctity; supernatural)
saints 41, 52, 131, 241 (*see also* sanctity)
 anatomies of 36, 44
 aspiring 44, 131, 137
 canonization of 54 (*see also* beatification and canonization)
 cult of 30, 33, 41, 132, 140, 142, 162, 187
 images of 143–4, 149
 incorrupt bodies of 36
 lives of 52, 156, 159, 241
 relics of 140, 149, 152, 156
Saint Januarius 242
 blood miracle of 241–3
 order of 228, 242–3
 replica of blood miracle of 243–5
Saint-Non, Jean Claude Richard de 79, 243
Salerno, Giuseppe
 anatomical demonstrations 218, 226
 anatomical injections 216, 240, 246
 anatomical skeletons 23, 215, 217–20, 234–5, 247–8, 252, 254, **Plates 50–3**
 anatomical skeletons, sale of 220, 223, 251
 death of 258

Sallmann, Jean-Michel 241
salt of the lion 201–4, 206–7 (*see also* mineral waters)
Sammartino, Giuseppe 234
Sandri, Giovanni Battista 170
Sandri, Margherita 190
San Juan, Rose Marie 147
San Severo Chapel 231, 246
San Severo Palace
  and anatomical specimens 234, 240–1, 249
  apartment of the phoenix 234, 246
  curiosities displayed in 232–3, 248, 253
  as Grand Tour destination 231–3
sanctity (*see also* beatification and canonization; Benedict XIV; *De servorum Dei beatificatione et beatorum canonizatione*; saint-making; saints)
  assessment of 10, 22, 29, 41–5, 47–8, 52, 131, 137, 139
  claims to 41, 42, 145, 152, 156
  odour of 33, 44, 140, 153, 156–7 (*see also* Chiarini, Laura)
  simulated 138, 141
Sansevieria 251
Santa Maria Maddalena 70, 99–100
Sarti, Raffaella 108
Savorini, Domenico 157
Sbaraglia, Giovanni Girolamo 45
Scagliarini, Veronica 35–6
Scandellari, Filippo 65, 90, 145, 156
Scarselli, Flaminio 40, 163, 181
senses, the 3, 53, 118, 121–2, 137, 140–1, 147, *148*, 151, 155, 167, 173, 175, 178
  Anna Morandi's models of 106, 111, 125, 146–8, 161, 194, 206, 208
  correct use of 132, 145, 147, 155
  hearing 47, 56, 116–117, *219*
  and the imagination 132, 137, 141, 145–6, 178
  as moral mementos 147
  sight 56, 126, 137, 173, 175–6, 190
  smell 3, 39, 127
  touch 125–6, 146–7, 161, 173, 175–6, 190
  training of 145 (*see also* observation; training of the eye)
  vision, uncertainty of 137
Serao, Francesco 221
Serra, Carlo 119–20
Severino, Marco Aurelio 223
sewing 97, 106, 108, *109*, 110
skeletons 15, 56, 88, 154 (*see also* Salerno, Giuseppe)
  at the Institute of the Sciences 65–6, 67, 85, **Plates 14 and 15**
  owned by the king of Denmark 218, 252
Sirani, Elisabetta 98, 158
Smellie, William 164
Smith, James Edward 249–50
Society of Dilettanti 56, 91
softness (tenderness) 6, 6n13, 8, 66, 107, 139, 146–7, 152, 162, 164, 167, 177–80, 235–6, 239
solidification 142, 235–7, 239, 241, 244, 256
solidity 8–9, 107, 234, 238, 256
Solimei, Flaminio 196
Solimei, Giuseppe (Manzolini) 196, 214
Somis, Ignazio 194
Sonnini, Charles-Nicolas-Sigisbert 254
Spanish empire 220–2, 228
Spanish monarchy 220, 222, 226, 242
St Peter's Basilica 24, *26*, 54, *54*
Storia dell'Accademia Clementina (Zanotti) 60–1
Strange, Robert 79
supernatural 43–4, 132, 142, 144, 242 (*see also* miracles)
surgery 45, 50, 209, 218
  and anatomical knowledge 65
  professorship in 114
  school of 38, 134
  teaching of 168, 211
Swammerdam, Jan 237
symmetry. *See* anatomical models; classical statues
Sydenham, Thomas 45, 103
Sylvius, Franciscus 236

Tacconi, Gaetano 104
tacit knowledge. *See* knowledge, tacit
Taylor, John 13
tenderness. *See* softness
Theatrum Anatomicum (Manget) 118
The King's Two Bodies (Kantorowicz) 158
Thunberg, Carl Peter 251
Torri, Bartolomeo 112
Toselli, Nicola 170
Toselli, Ottavio 170
training of the eye 22, 91–2
Trattato di medicamenti spettanti alla chirurgia (Parenti) 114
Traub, Valerie 14
Turin (Italy) 143, 194, 203, 206, 230
  anatomy room 63–4
  Morandi's models 194, 206, 208–9
  Museum for the Royal University 62

Unione di Sant'Anna 135, *157*, 157–8 (*see also* hospital of Santa Maria della Morte)
University of Bologna 34, 114, 133–4, 136, 168, 199–200 (*see also* Bassi, Laura; Morandi, Anna; public anatomy lessons)
Urban VIII, pope 42, 140

Vallet, Paul-Joseph 248
Vallisneri, Antonio
  as defender of ovism 178
  and support for women 137
Valsalva, Antonio Maria 46, 61, 119
  and anatomical representation 116–17
  and cure of deafness 47
  dry preparations of 63, 81, 116, 236

variatio 111–12
Vasari, Giorgio 112
Vassena, Elio 198
Venice (Italy) 83, 94, 106, 140, 142, 203
Veratti, Giuseppe 160
Verri, Pietro 212
Vesalius, Andreas 65, 87, 117
Vespa, Giuseppe 176
Vicende della coltura nelle Due Sicilie (Napoli Signorelli) 252
Vico, Giambattista 232
View of Society and Manners in Italy (Moore) 257
Vigri, Caterina (*La Santa*) 98, 152, 161
Villabianca, Marquis of (Francesco Maria Emanuele Gaetani) 246
visionary inspiration 140, 145–6
  claims of 132, 144–5
visions 131, 136, 138–9, 141, 145, 162
Volkmann, Johann Jacob 170
von Zweibrücken, Friedrich Michael (Count Palatine) 105
Voyage d'un François en Italie (Lalande) 128, 151, 227, 233, 244
Voyer d'Argenson, Madame de (Marie-Jeanne-Constance) 106

Walpole, Horace 28
wax, *passim*
  cultures of 132, 152–5
  of the Levant 6, 66
  lost wax technique 7n22
  properties of 142, 256
  use in devotional practices 5–6, 22, 90, 132, 142–3, 153–4
wax dolls 142–3, 167, 179
wax portraits 155–62 (*see also* Bassi, Laura; Chiarini, Laura; Manzolini, Giovanni; Morandi, Anna)
  of Bolognese citizens 158
  and celebrity culture 124, 127–8, 159–60, 208–10
  as funerary effigies 158
  of individuals who died in 'odour of sanctity' 145, 153, 156–7
  role in royal rituals 158
wax-votives 7, 143–4
Wilhelm Meisters Wanderjahre (Goethe) 121
Willis, Thomas 125
Winckelmann, Johann Joachim 86
Winslow, Jacques-Bénigne 117, 217–18
women. *See* Agnesi, Maria; Bassi, Laura; Benedict XIV; childbirth; embroidery; generation; maternity; needlework; midwives; Morandi, Anna; motherhood; mystical women; pregnancy
wonder 102, 154, 164, 173, 220, 224, 226, 231, 241, 244, 253–4 (*see also* marvels; Naples)
Wright of Derby, Joseph 89, *89*

Zaccaria, Francesco Antonio 171, 180–1
Zacchia, Paolo 46
Zanotti, Francesco Maria 61, 78, 81, 86, 88, 101, 104, 111, 122, 167, 170, 181
Zanotti, Giampietro 61, 71, 122–3, 148
Zecchini, Petronio Ignazio 123, 199–200
Zumbo, Gaetano Giulio (or Zummo) 70, 127, 217, 222, 239